Human Spermatozoa in Assisted Reproduction

Human Spermatozoa in Assisted Reproduction

2nd edition

Anibal A. Acosta
Department of Obstetrics and Gynecology
The Jones Institute for Reproductive Medicine
Eastern Virginia Medical School
Virginia, USA

and

Thinus F. Kruger
Reproductive Biology Unit
Department of Obstetrics and Gynecology
Tygerberg Hospital/University of Stellenbosch
Tygerberg, South Africa

The Parthenon Publishing Group
International Publishers in Medicine, Science & Technology

NEW YORK LONDON

Library of Congress Cataloging-in-Publication Data

Human spermatozoa in assisted reproduction /
[edited by] Anibal A. Acosta and Thinus F. Kruger.
– 2nd ed.
p. cm.
Includes bibliographical references and index.
ISBN 1-85070-590-9
1. Human reproductive technology. 2. Spermatozoa.
I. Acosta, Anibal A. II. Kruger, Thinus.
[DNLM: 1. Spermatozoa. 2. Fertilization in Vitro.
WJ 834 H918 1996]
RG133.5.H88 1996
612.6′1–dc20
DNLM/DLC
for Library of Congress 95-39885
CIP

British Library Cataloguing in Publication Data

Human Spermatozoa in Assisted
Reproduction. – 2Rev.ed
I. Acosta, Anibal A. II. Kruger, Thinus F.
616.692

ISBN 1-85070-590-9

Published in North America by
The Parthenon Publishing Group Inc.
One Blue Hill Plaza
PO Box 1564 Pearl River
New York 10965, USA

Published in the UK and Europe by
The Parthenon Publishing Group Limited
Casterton Hall, Carnforth
Lancs. LA6 2LA, UK

First edition published 1990
Second edition published 1996

Composed by Servis Filmsetting Ltd, Longsight, Manchester
Printed and bound by The Bath Press, Bath, UK

Contents

List of contributors

A. A. Acosta
Department of Obstetrics and Gynecology
The Jones Institute for Reproductive Medicine
Eastern Virginia Medical School
601 Colley Avenue
Norfolk, Virginia 23507
USA

R. J. Aitken
MRC Reproductive Biology Unit
Centre for Reproductive Biology
37 Chalmers Street
Edinburgh EH3 9EW
UK

R. H. Asch
Department of Obstetrics and Gynecology
Division of Reproductive Endocrinology and Infertility
UCI Center for Reproductive Health
College of Medicine
University of California, Irvine
101 The City Drive
Orange, California 92668
USA

H. W. G. Baker
Reproductive Biology Unit
The Royal Women's Hospital
132 Grattan Street
Carlton, Victoria 3053
Australia

E. Bosmans
Eurogenetics
Transportstraat 4
3980 Tessenderlo
Belgium

J. C. Calamera
Laboratorio de Estudios en Reproduccion
Avenue Cordoba 2077 1 P 'E'
1120 Buenos Aires
Argentina

O. E. Claassens
Reproductive Biology Unit
Department of Obstetrics and Gynecology
Tygerberg Hospital / University of Stellenbosch
Tygerberg 7505
South Africa

K. Coetzee
Reproductive Biology Unit
Department of Obstetrics and Gynecology
Tygerberg Hospital/University of Stellenbosch
Tygerberg 7505
South Africa

F. H. Comhaire
Universiteit Gent
Dienst Voor Inwendige Ziekten
Endocrinologies-Stofwisselingszietken
De Pintelaan 185
9000 Gent
Belgium

A. Cox
Gent Institute for Fertility Technology (GIFT)
Department of Obstetrics and Gynecology
St Jans Hospital
Schlepse Bos 2
3600 Gent
Belgium

M. del Carmen Quiros
Laboratorio de Estudios en Reproduccion
Avenue Cordoba 2077 1 P 'E'
1120 Buenos Aires
Argentina

P. Devroey
Centre for Reproductive Medicine
Medical School and University Hospital
Dutch-speaking Brussels Free University (VUB)
Laarbeeklaan 101
B-1090 Brussels
Belgium

G. F. Doncel
Sperm Biology and Contraceptive Research Laboratory
Contraceptive Research and Development (CONRAD) Program
and Department of Obstetrics and Gynecology
Eastern Virginia Medical School
601 Colley Avenue
Norfolk, Virginia 23507
USA

T. C. du Toit
Reproductive Biology Unit
Department of Obstetrics and Gynecology
Tygerberg Hospital / University of Stellenbosch
Tygerberg 7505
South Africa

M. E. Enginsu
Department of Cell Biology and Genetics
3X Building
University of Limburg
6200 MD Maastricht
The Netherlands

J. L. H. Evers
Professor of Obstetrics and Gynaecology
Academisch Ziekenhuis Maastricht
and The University of Limburg
PO Box 5800
NL 6202 AZ
Maastricht
The Netherlands

D. R. Franken
Reproductive Biology Unit
Department of Obstetrics and Gynecology
Tygerberg Hospital / University of Stellenbosch
Tygerberg 7505
South Africa
and The Jones Institute for Reproductive Medicine
Eastern Virginia Medical School
601 Colley Avenue
Norfolk, Virginia 23507
USA

L. K. Gabriel
Reproductive Biology Unit
Department of Obstetrics and Gynecology
Tygerberg Hospital / University of Stellenbosch
Tygerberg 7505
South Africa

R. R. Henkel
Department of Dermatology and Andrology
Justus Liebig University
Giessen, 35392
Gaffkystrasse 14
Germany

G. D. Hodgen
The Jones Institute for Reproductive Medicine
Department of Obstetrics and Gynecology
Eastern Virginia Medical School
601 Colley Avenue
Norfolk, Virginia 23507
USA

D. S. Irvine
MRC Reproductive Biology Unit
Centre for Reproductive Biology
37 Chalmers Street
Edinburgh EH3 9EW
UK

M. Janssen
Gent Institute for Fertility Technology (GIFT)
Department of Obstetrics and Gynecology
St Jans Hospital
Schlepse Bos 2
3600 Gent
Belgium

R. S. Jeyendran
Department of Obstetrics and Gynecology
Northwestern University Medical Center
333 East Superior Street
Chicago, Illinois 60611
USA

H. Joris
Department of Reproductive Biology
Centre for Reproductive Medicine
Medical School and University Hospital
Dutch-speaking Brussels Free University (VUB)
Laarbeeklaan 101
B-1090 Brussels
Belgium

K. Kaskar
Reproductive Biology Unit
Department of Obstetrics and Gynecology
Tygerberg Hospital / University of Stellenbosch
Tygerberg 7505
South Africa

W. G. Kearns
Assistant Professor
Center for Pediatric Research
Department of Pediatrics
Eastern Virginia Medical School
855 West Brambleton Avenue
Norfolk, Virginia 23510
USA
and Center for Medical Genetics
Johns Hopkins University School of Medicine
Baltimore, Maryland
USA

T. F. Kruger
Reproductive Biology Unit
Department of Obstetrics and Gynecology
Tygerberg Hospital / University of Stellenbosch
Tygerberg 7505
South Africa

J. W. Lens
Free University Hospital
PO Box 7057
Amsterdam
The Netherlands

I. Liebaers
Department of Medical Genetics
Medical School and University Hospital
Dutch-speaking Brussels Free University (VUB)
Laarbeeklaan 101
B-1090 Brussels
Belgium

D. Y. Liu
University of Melbourne
Department of Obstetrics and Gynecology
Royal Women's Hospital
132 Grattan Street
Melbourne, Victoria 3053
Australia

J. Liu
Department of Reproductive Biology
Centre for Reproductive Medicine
Medical School and University Hospital
Dutch-speaking Brussels Free University (VUB)
Laarbeeklaan 101
B-1090 Brussels
Belgium

R. Menkveld
Reproductive Biology Unit
Department of Obstetrics and Gynecology
Tygerberg Hospital / University of Stellenbosch
Tygerberg 7505
South Africa

J. F. Moreau
Eurogenetics
Transportstraat 4
3980 Tessenderlo
Belgium

M. Morshedi
Cry Laboratory
Department of Obstetrics and Gynecology
Eastern Virginia Medical School
601 Colley Avenue
Norfolk, Virginia 23507
USA

P. Nagy
Department of Reproductive Biology
Centre for Reproductive Medicine
Medical School and University Hospital
Dutch-speaking Brussels Free University (VUB)
Laarbeeklaan 101
B-1090 Brussels
Belgium

S. Oehninger
Department of Obstetrics and Gynecology
The Jones Institute for Reproductive Medicine
Eastern Virginia Medical School
601 Colley Avenue
Norfolk, Virginia 23507
USA

D. A. Ohl
Section of Urology
and Electroejaculation Program
University of Michigan Medical School
2918 G Taubman Center
Box 0330
Ann Arbor, Michigan 48109
USA

W. Ombelet
Genk Institute for Fertility Technology (GIFT)
Department of Obstetrics and Gynecology
St Janshospital
Schiepse Bos 2
3600 Genk
Belgium

T. Ord
IVF Laboratory
Centers for Reproductive Health
University of California, Irvine
and Saddelback Memorial Medical Center
101 The City Drive
Orange, California 92668
USA

J. W. Overstreet
Department of Obstetrics and Gynecology
Division of Reproductive Biology and Medicine
University of California, Davis
School of Medicine
Davis, California 95616
USA

P. Patrizio
Male Infertility Service
Department of Obstetrics and Gynecology
University of California, Irvine
101 The City Drive
Orange, California 92668
USA

J. Sønksen
Department of Urology
Righospitalet
National University Hospital
University of Copenhagen
Denmark

E. Van Assche
Cytogenetics Laboratory
Department of Medical Genetics
Medical School and University Hospital
Dutch-speaking Brussels Free University (VUB)
Laarbeeklaan 101
B-1090 Brussels
Belgium

H. Vandeput
Gent Institute for Fertility Technology (GIFT)
Department of Obstetrics and Gynecology
St Jans Hospital
Schlepse Bos 2
3600 Gent
Belgium

J. P. Van der Merwe
Reproductive Biology Unit
Department of Obstetrics and Gynecology
Tygerberg Hospital / University of Stellenbosch
Tygerberg 7505
South Africa

A. Van Steirteghem
Department of Radioimmunology and Reproductive Biology
Centre for Reproductive Medicine
Medical School and University Hospital
Dutch-speaking Brussels Free University (VUB)
Laarbeeklaan 101
B-1090 Brussels
Belgium

J. P. W. Vermeiden
IVF Laboratory
Free University Hospital
PO Box 7057
1007 MB Amsterdam
The Netherlands

M.-L. Windt
Reproductive Biology Unit
Department of Obstetrics and Gynecology
Tygerberg Hospital / University of Stellenbosch
Tygerberg 7505
South Africa

A. Wisanto
Fertility Clinic
Centre for Reproductive Medicine
Medical School and University Hospital
Dutch-speaking Brussels Free University (VUB)
Laarbeeklaan 101
B-1090 Brussels
Belgium

W.-R. Yeh
Department of Obstetrics and Gynecology
Taipei City Ho-Ping Hospital
Taipei
Taiwan

J. L. Zackowski
Cytogenetics
Division of Genetics
Department of Pediatrics
Eastern Virginia Medical School
601 Colley Avenue
Norfolk, Virginia 23507
USA

L. J. D. Zaneveld
Obstetrics and Gynecology Research
Rush-Presbyterian/St Luke's Medical Center
Rush-University
1653 West Congress Parkway
Chicago, Illinois 60612
USA

Acknowledgements

The authors wish to thank the following members of The Jones Institute for Reproductive Medicine: William E. Gibbons, MD, Chairman of the Department of Obstetrics and Gynecology, for his support and encouragement; Mrs Nell Reece for her secretarial assistance; Ms Debi Jones for data processing; Mrs Rosita Acosta, Mrs Carmen Fallahy, and Ms Carol Montgomery for their outstanding work in the Andrology Laboratory; Mrs Beverly Cox and Mrs Ruth Shaw from the Endocrine Laboratory for their excellent cooperation; and all medical, nursing and secretarial personnel who contributed to this effort.

On behalf of the Tygerberg Research Team and the University of Stellenbosch, we wish to thank Ms Helena Krüger for her assistance to Ms Pauline M. Clynes in the preparation of the manuscripts. We also wish to thank all participants for their enthusiasm in making this project a success.

Editorial Advisors: Ms Pauline M. Clynes and Mrs Helena Krüger.

Preface to first edition

The field of andrology as a discipline has moved and developed slowly and laboriously since its inception in 1891, in spite of tremendous efforts made by many excellent basic and clinical investigators. During all these years, the final judgment on sperm quality and the determination of normality in sperm parameters in the various tests depended on the ability of the patient to establish a pregnancy in his partner. That was the only available yardstick. There are significant drawbacks to this approach. On one hand, female fertility is not always easy to determine. On the other hand, unless artificial insemination is used the quality of the sperm which established a pregnancy is, for the most part, unknown. Therefore, this endpoint by which sperm is judged – the ability to produce a gestation – is quite unreliable, particularly when conception is not achieved.

The situation changed dramatically in the late 1970s when *in vitro* fertilization (IVF) and embryo transfer came into being, followed by other methods of assisted reproduction. For the first time, investigators interested in male infertility were able to judge human oocyte–sperm interaction. Regardless of whether or not pregnancy was established, the capability of normal or abnormal sperm to fertilize the female gamete could be readily determined. A new and more reliable endpoint was now at our disposal. New approaches to diagnosis and treatment of male factors, and also new procedures for sperm evaluation, manipulation and preparation were designed. Interest began to drift away from pregnancy as a yardstick by which to measure sperm quality, and the evaluation of the many sperm tests was done by comparing their results with the results of IVF in the human system. The era of using animals for that purpose was ending. Clinicians began to look for new criteria to predict results in IVF and to develop guidelines for the acceptability of male factors into the rapidly moving field of assisted reproduction.

In spite of all efforts, a group of patients were still unable to achieve fertilization *in vitro*. The interest of scientists shifted once again to developing methods to allow abnormal sperm to fertilize, and a new field – assisted fertilization – emerged.

With these new developments in the area of andrology, because of assisted reproduction and assisted fertilization, it seems timely to compile, summarize, review critically and set forth this knowledge for gynecologists, urologists, andrologists, reproductive endocrinologists, basic scientists and laboratory technologists. Such a book may be crucial for consolidating information and establishing a platform for future explorations in the field.

The collective experience of the Andrology Laboratories of Eastern Virginia Medical School and Old Dominion University, the program of assisted reproduction at The Jones Institute for Reproductive Medicine, the Tygerberg Clinic at the University of Stellenbosch and many outstanding clinicians and researchers from other institutions who generously contributed to this book has been compiled to update the knowledge in the field and to describe the diagnostic and therapeutic tests now in use. This collaborative effort stresses the need for a multidisciplinary–multicenter approach to solve the intricacies of the male infertility problem.

We have come a long way since sperm was discovered as one of the main elements of human reproduction, but we still have a long way to go to unveil all the scientific facts of sperm function. Past and future, ignorance and knowledge, despair and hope, faith and skepticism, empiricism and science have been the extremes through which we have moved in this very delicate area of reproduction and perhaps represent the extremes through which we will continue to move, at least in the near future. To make these efforts worthwhile, this work was conceived and published.

A. A. Acosta T. F. Kruger
R. J. Swanson J. A. van Zyl
S. B. Ackerman R. Menkveld

Preface to second edition

Four years have passed since the original edition of this book was published. The goals and ideas that triggered that effort are still alive and valid. The reception has been excellent and, for the most part, the objectives were fulfilled. Complacency, none the less, should not interfere with renewed challenges and needs; a careful new look at the field of andrology gives clear evidence of areas where knowledge should be updated critically, as the approach to male factor diagnosis and treatment enters the era of assisted reproduction and assisted fertilization.

Many important centers and distinguished researchers have made substantial contributions to our understanding of this problem, but the majority of those contributions have been in seminology. Knowledge of physiology and pathophysiology of the testis contains enormous gaps in understanding; we have not made substantial progress in those fields. The fact that we are finding pure technical solutions to complex male reproductive function problems has given technology an edge over basic sciences. Nevertheless, although we continue to look at the sperm in assisted reproduction in this edition of the book, it does not mean that we fail to recognize the need to upgrade our knowledge of testicular physiology and pathophysiology to understand the roots of these deficiencies. Technology, although extremely useful, should never be allowed to replace scientific knowledge; same-way empiricism should never be allowed to replace sound scientifically based diagnosis and treatment.

Molecular genetics has now invaded medical science and the possibilities of true preventive medicine seem to be around the corner. A whole new field in andrology is now widely open and should be looked upon in a careful and hopeful manner; scrutiny is certainly warranted.

Once again, the andrology programs of the Eastern Virginia Medical School and the Tygerberg Clinic at the University of Stellenbosch join this effort. A long history of collaborative work has made this endeavor easier.

We timidly asked the best centers of the world to cooperate with us in updating this long list of subjects; the response was unanimous, generous and unrestricted: we could not have put together a better group of invited scientists and clinicians. The discipline still requires a multidisciplinary approach; otherwise, this book would have been incomplete and, in some areas, not at the level of excellence required. We are very grateful to all our contributors.

The extremes through which the field is moving, mentioned in the preface to the first edition, are still present. As the past is used for launching new ideas, the future looks brighter. As ignorance decreases, knowledge opens new doors for research therapies, despair is yielding to hope, faith is overcoming skepticism and science is fortunately replacing empiricism in our discipline.

Let us review again what we have learned in the last four years. Put it into the hands of an avid younger generation of physicians and scientists, and let them carry the torch and make its light brighter. This is a challenge that will prevent complacency. The second edition of this book is aimed to accomplish all this; the editors were mere instruments.

A kind invitation from the Chairman of the Department of Obstetrics and Gynecology at the University of Stellenbosch, Professor Hein Odendaal, to one of us (AAA) to become a Visiting Professor at his department for one month allowed us to get together to complete the task. It was an excellent and rewarding opportunity for which we are most grateful.

T. F. Kruger
A. A. Acosta

Introduction

When the second edition of *Human Spermatozoa in Assisted Reproduction* was considered we recognized that the scope of the field has widened, that the experience in many areas has increased substantially, and that attention has been refocussed according to that experience in either old or newer aspects of the male factor in assisted reproduction. Therefore, it was mandatory to reconsider carefully and replan the book's contents.

The book is still intended to target the same group of clinicians working in Reproductive Medicine, Andrology, Urology, General Gynecology, Reproductive Endocrinology and General Endocrinology, as well as scientists and technical personnel working in related areas.

Three fundamental parts were considered: (1) basic concepts of spermatology and gamete interaction; (2) diagnostic aspects of the male factor; and (3) therapeutic considerations applicable to the correction of sperm abnormalities impairing reproductive function.

Concepts of spermatogenesis and intratesticular, as well as extratesticular, sperm maturation in the human have changed dramatically, and although they cannot be applied in diagnosis and treatment for the time being, it is important to the interested reader to be aware of them. That has been done in Chapter 1.

The understanding of the anatomy of the sperm as viewed by light, transmission and scanning electron microscopy is germane to understanding physiology, testing and therapeutic approaches of sperm defects and, therefore, Chapter 2 was maintained.

The changes that sperm experience during transport in the human female genital tract have been reconsidered and reinvestigated recently and, as a result, our understanding of the process has changed substantially, new tests have been designed, and re-evaluation of the interpretation of old tests has been proposed. This is updated in Chapter 3.

Similarly, if we are going to understand the concept of failed fertilization in assisted reproduction as well as in assisted fertilization, and if we are going to attempt to predict it and treat the problem, it is mandatory to update the knowledge of that complicated process in the human. That has been attempted in Chapter 4.

After many years of experience with the male factor in natural and assisted reproduction we are still struggling with the definition of normality, the prediction of fertilizing capacity and the minimal thresholds required for fertilization and pregnancy; and more importantly, as far as this book is concerned, with the definition of male factor in assisted reproduction. If we do not reach a consensus in a relatively short period of time the past efforts, the formulation of indications for using these procedures in the treatment of the male factor and the evaluation of results will be extremely difficult. It is time to tackle this problem, and that has been attempted in Chapter 5.

The approach to basic semen analysis is certainly one of the main aspects of the book but, in the main, new developments have been considered. For instance, new ways to define sperm motility, the description of sperm abnormalities under light microscopy by technician reading and by computer analysis, as well as an update of its predictive value for the outcome of fertilization are the subjects of Chapters 6, 7, 8, 9 and 10.

The importance of detecting, evaluating and treating male genital tract infections is emphasized in Chapter 11.

New findings, tests and interpretations of results in the field of antisperm antibodies in assisted reproduction have been developed in the evaluation of immunological factors, both from a laboratory and a clinical point of view. Chapters 12 and 13 try to address and update those issues.

The sperm enzymes and substrate systems involved in locomotion, transport and fertilization, as well as the physiological role and evaluation of sperm membrane integrity, is reviewed in Chapters 14 and 15.

The concept of sperm nuclear maturation and DNA packaging is quite pertinent to the physiological changes of the sperm head after ooplasmic penetration, and this is reviewed in Chapter 16.

The study of cervical mucus penetration and the testing of sperm capacity is relevant to the process of normal fertilization, but it has also become important as a way to measure the toxic effect on sperm of different agents, and to evaluate the efficiency of some contraceptives in blocking sperm transport. This is reviewed in Chapter 17.

The evaluation of acrosomal status, although not widely used as a sperm test in most laboratories, is an indicator of the sperm's ability to react normally to physiological and pharmacological agents; its relevance to assisted reproduction and assisted fertilization is considered in Chapter 18.

The utilization of the old hamster-egg penetration assay and the new sperm-zona pellucida binding and penetration assays, and their predictive value for human *in vitro* fertilization have been addressed in Chapters 19 and 20.

An important and relatively new concept in terms of the physiological significance and the pathological implications of the presence of reactive oxygen species in the sperm and the different ways to decrease their impact when produced in abnormally high quantities is the subject of Chapter 21.

Sperm separation techniques for capacitation and selection of the motile sperm fraction, as well as for attempts to separate the X and Y chromosome-bearing sperm populations are updated in Chapter 22.

An attempt to establish the present concept of evaluation of the sperm fertilizing potential and the test to predict that is reviewed in Chapter 23.

It is important to understand the new physiological concepts, as well as the new testing capabilities that are being pursued in the field of spermatology, and Chapters 24 and 25 are devoted to that aspect.

The role of cytokines in the physiology and pathology of the sperm seems to be emerging and therefore we have devoted Chapter 26 to that subject.

The use of abnormal sperm in assisted reproduction, the problems involved and the evaluation of results are described in Chapters 27 and 28.

The use of artificial insemination (husband and donor), the oldest method of assisted reproduction used in the clinical arena, is reviewed in Chapters 29 and 30.

One of the few breakthroughs that we have witnessed recently in the field of assisted reproduction is the improvement in the technical aspects and results of assisted fertilization; Chapter 31 reviews those accomplishments.

Another interesting source of evaluation of sperm extratesticular maturation and fertilizing ability, as well as study of the implications of the genetic aspects of male genital tract malformations triggered by the use of assisted fertilization, is updated in Chapter 32.

New concepts in the physiology and pathophysiology of idiopathic oligo-astheno-teratozoospermia, its diagnosis and treatment by systemic therapy of the patient are reviewed in Chapter 33.

The use of assisted reproduction in conjunction with new techniques of sperm collection in patients with ejaculatory dysfunctions is updated in Chapter 34.

An attempt to look into the immediate and longer-term future of these therapies is the objective of Chapter 35.

Laboratory techniques that have not been described in detail in their respective chapters are listed in the Appendix.

We hope that we have covered all the pertinent fields regarding the use of normal and abnormal sperm in assisted reproduction and assisted fertilization. We feel that, with our experience of the first edition, we have improved in determining and fulfilling the objectives of this work, but even if this has not been fully accomplished the attempt to meet the challenge and to review the field has been both rewarding and worthwhile.

T. F. Kruger
A. A. Acosta

Section 1

Basic concepts of spermatology and fertilization

Spermatogenesis and intratesticular sperm maturation

1

A. A. Acosta

INTRODUCTION

The process of spermatogenesis in humans is still poorly understood and the causes for the formation of a morphological heterogeneous population that is so characteristic of the human species are, for the most part, unknown. The normal spermatogenic process requires an intact hypothalamic–pituitary–testicular axis with all its feedback, regulatory and modulating interactions intact.

THE HYPOTHALAMIC PULSE GENERATOR

The hypothalamic pulse generator in normal human males shows a mean interpulse interval of 61 min±2.9 min (SEM), mean peak 50 min±2.5 (SEM), the pulse amplitude calculated as percentage increase from baseline 163%±4.9 (SEM) and incremental amplitude measure in mIU/mL 2.8±0.22 (SEM); furthermore, the luteinizing hormone (LH) pulses are non-uniform and have a non-Gaussian distribution in each individual[1]. Talbot *et al.*[2] investigated the hypothalamic pituitary axis in normal males by measuring the pulsatile secretion of LH by bio- and radioimmunoassay of FSH and testosterone by immunoassay, and the results found in terms of pulse frequency, duration, amplitude, fractional amplitude, maximum peak and interpulse interval duration are shown in Table 1.

The pulse generator is modulated by suprahypothalamic (adrenergic, cholinergic, dopaminergic, opioidergic and gabaergic influences) and through the pulsatile secretion of gonadotropin releasing hormone (GnRH) gonadotropin synthesis, storage and release is controlled. The action of those gonadotropins, both of which are fundamental for normal spermatogenesis, on the gonads, as well as the intracellular, ultra-short, short and long feedback mechanisms of follicle stimulating hormone (FSH) and LH regulations, and the receptor-mediated effect on the hormonogenic and gametogenic functions of the testicles have been extensively studied, are well understood, and are not within the scope of this chapter. We will focus the discussion on the gonadal aspects of spermatogenesis in the human, assuming that the axis is normal.

SPERMATOGENESIS

Spermatogenesis takes place inside the seminiferous tubules, in a very close relationship and interaction with the interstitial cell compartment in which Leydig cells, blood vessels and lymphatics are the most prominent components. The seminiferous tubules are surrounded by a basement membrane with collagen-I, fibronectin, proteoglycans and protease inhibitor components (Figure 1). The basement membrane is surrounded by myofibrils which are under oxytocin (from Leydig cells) control and constitute an important part of the system for propulsion of the tubular content. Within the basement membrane the two basic components of the tubular structure are present, namely the supporting Sertoli cells and the spermatogenic cell line. The Sertoli cells are interconnected by tight junctions (Figure 1), and this intercellular sealing system divides the tubule into an adluminal inner compartment and a basal external one. The basal compartment, in contact with the basement membrane, has extensive communications with the systemic environment and certainly with the immunological system; meanwhile, the tight junction network prevents such communication with the adluminal compartment, and therefore this creates a microenvironment within the seminiferous tubule that is completely different in its physiological composition

Table 1 Hormones bio-LH, I-LH, I-FSH and I-T pulsatile secretion in normal males[2]

	Bio-LH	*I-LH*	*I-FSH*	*I-T*
Frequency (pulses/6 h)	2(1–3)	2(1–2)	2(0–3)	3(2–3)
Duration (min)	110(40–200)	110(60–180)	80(40–200)	105(40–210)
Amplitude (IU/L)	7.9(2.0–18.5)	3.1(1.5–7.0)	0.5(0.2–2.7)	6.1(3.1–9.3)
Fractional amplitude (%)	67(20–197)	90(35–177)	26(17–79)	51(23–125)
Peak maxima (IU/L)	16.2(8.7–35.9)	6.8(4.1–13.8)	2.5(1.0–6.3)	16.8(11.9–20.5)
Interpulse time (min)	125(40–200)	155(70–200)	80(40–230)	120(100–260)

to what can be measured in the systemic peripheral compartment. In some fashion, it mimics the intrafollicular compartment in the ovary, created by the presence of the basement membrane within the follicle.

The whole germ cell line proliferation and intratesticular intratubular maturation takes place in relationship with the supporting Sertoli cell. Only spermatogonia and the very early stages of spermatocytes are present in the basal compartment. As the process of spermatogenesis proceeds, the cells are able to cross the barrier and enter the adluminal compartment and, from then on, they are selectively and partially isolated from systemic communication.

The Sertoli cell is mainly under FSH control, and the different functions it stimulates are adenosine 3′, 5′-cyclic monophosphate (cAMP)-dependent or directly FSH-dependent (Figure 1). FSH stimulates cAMP, the aromatase system through which estrogen levels are increased inside of the adluminal compartment, the calcium reserve, the piruvate–lactate system and the synthesis of androgen-binding protein, ceruloplasmin, inhibin, plasminogen activator and transferrin. FSH receptors have also been described at the level of spermatogonia.

At the interstitial level the two main cellular components present are the Leydig cells and macrophages. The Leydig cells (Figure 1) have LH plus human chorionic gonadotropin (hCG) receptors through which these gonadotropins stimulate testosterone synthesis, cAMP, the aromatase system which is also present in the Leydig cells, as well as corticotropin-releasing factor (CRF) and endorphins. Lactogen, epidermal growth factor (EGF) and β-adrenergic receptors are also present. Stimulation of the EGF receptor is a powerful contributor to testosterone synthesis and, in turn, down-regulates the LH/hCG receptor.

NON-STEROIDAL GONADAL PEPTIDES AND GROWTH FACTORS

A large number of non-steroidal gonadal peptides and growth factors have been described as present in the testicular compartments. Some of them seem to have a well defined function and favor intercompartmental and intercellular communication (Table 2)[3]; for an extensive list of others, the physiological significance has not been established (Table 3)[3].

Pro-opiomelanocortin (POMC) messenger ribonucleic acids (mRNAs) have been found in both the Leydig cells and in the initial phases of spermatogenesis (spermatogonia and spermatocytes)[3]. β-Endorphin, adrenocorticotropic hormone (ACTH) and melanocyte-stimulating hormone (MSH) are produced in the Leydig cells, and their receptors are on the Sertoli cells; therefore, this may be one of the intercompartmental communication systems. β-Endorphin inhibits FSH-stimulated Sertoli cell division and other cAMP-dependent FSH functions; ACTH and α-MSH stimulate Sertoli cell division, androgen-binding protein synthesis and inhibin production[3]. Endorphins may stimulate GnRH production; gonadotropins and steroids can similarly regulate β-endorphin production.

Pro-enkephalin mRNA is expressed in round spermatids and pachytene spermatocytes, and may

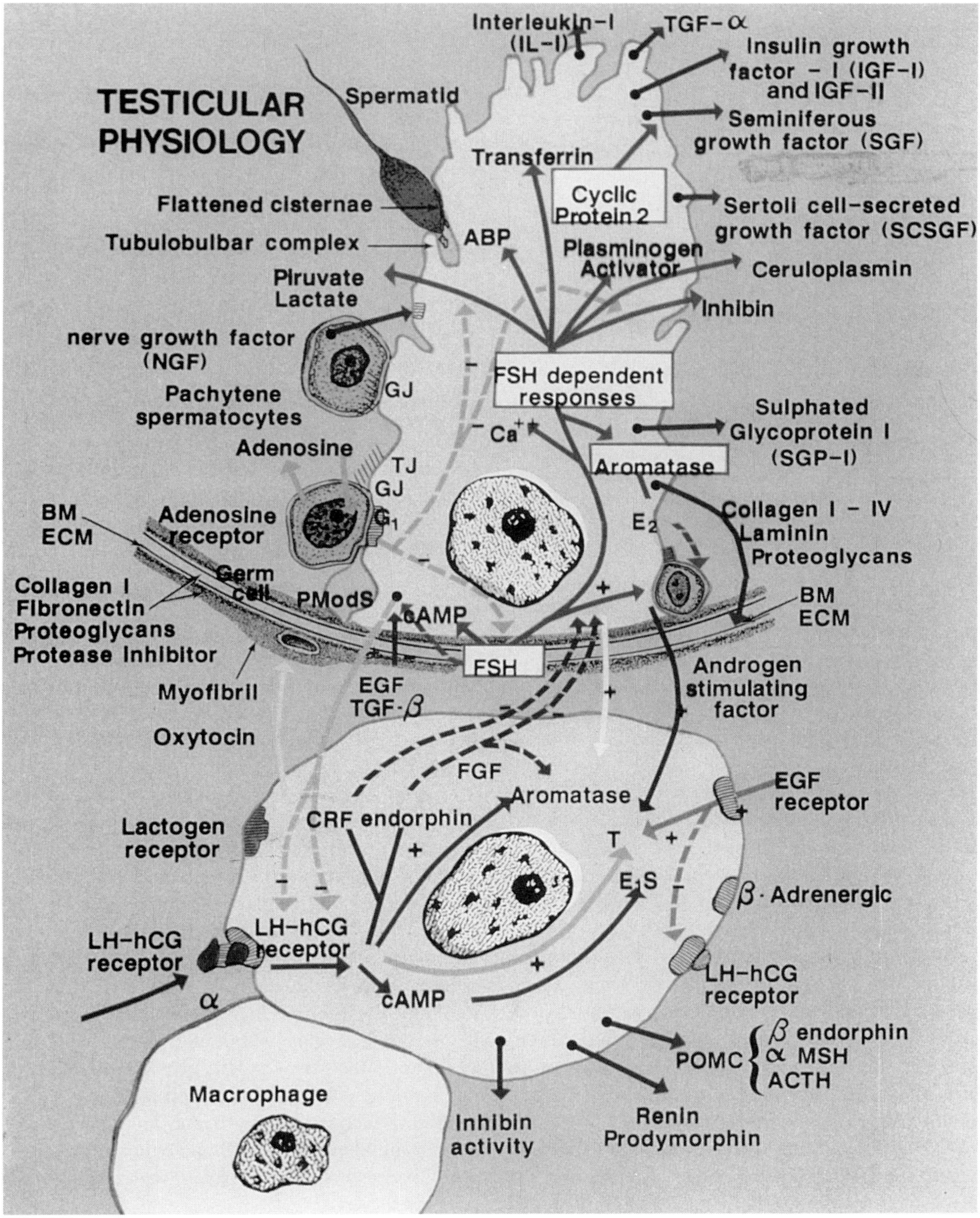

Figure 1 Testicular physiology

Table 2 Paracrine factors involved in spermatogenesis[3]

- Pro-opiomelanocortin (POMC)
- POMC derived peptides
  - β-endorphin
  - ACTH
  - MSH
- Pro-enkephalins and enkephalins
- Oxytocin and vasopressin
- Inhibins and activins
- Growth factors
  - TGF-α
  - TGF-β
  - EGF
  - IGF-I
  - IGF-II

Table 3 Factors and enzymes present in testis with no function identified[3]

• Renin-angiotensin	• Gonadotropin-binding inhibitors
• Caeruloplasmin	• Sulfated glycoproteins -1 and -2
• Calmodulin	• Plasminogen activator
• Actins	• Transferrin
• Tubulins	• Prodynorphins A and B
• X_2-macroglobulin	• Thyrotropin releasing hormone
• Cyclic protein-2	• Corticotropin releasing hormone

therefore be involved in germ cell development. The pro-enkephalin produced by the germ cells may be an intercellular communication mechanism between them and the Sertoli cells or between different stages of the germ cell lines[3]. Enkephalins stimulate the production and secretion of testicular LHRH-like factor by Sertoli cells, which in turn binds to specific receptors on the Leydig cell modulating steroid production and inhibiting β-endorphin production by the Leydig cells[3].

The germ cells seem to modulate the production of inhibin by the Sertoli cells. Transforming growth factor (TGF)-α is present in Sertoli cells and peritubular cells, and induces proliferation in peritubular cells. TGF β-1 has been demonstrated in peritubular and Sertoli cells. It stimulates the secretion of proteins by peritubular cells.

EGF binding sites are present on Sertoli[4], Leydig[5] and germ cells; there are few data on the effect of EGF in humans. Other functions assigned to EGF, at least in laboratory animals, refer to the stabilization of the Wolffian duct system and testicular descent[6]. In humans, EGF stimulates testosterone production by the Leydig cells[7].

IGF-1 is secreted by Leydig and Sertoli cells and is also present in primary spermatocytes; a receptor has been found in Sertoli cells, Leydig cells, secondary spermatocytes and early spermatids. It may exert a priming effect on the Sertoli cell to respond to FSH. It may also stimulate mitogenesis in both immature Leydig and Sertoli cells and stimulate transferrin secretion.

In terms of intratesticular control of steroidogenesis, as stated above, the list of other regulatory peptides described as present in the testes for which no known function has been described is given in Table 3[3].

SECRETORY PRODUCTS OF SERTOLI CELLS

In terms of the different secretory products of the Sertoli cells, the androgen-binding protein (ABP), very similar to the steroid hormone binding protein (SHBP) in peripheral blood, places a very important role in the transport and localization of androgens within the tubule.

The characteristics of its secretion by human Sertoli cells *in vitro* have already been described[8]. In rats, it has been shown that this protein is internalized by spermatogenic cells; in the adluminal component, they are found in the endocytic and nuclear compartment. In the latest stages of spermiogenesis (elongated spermatids) it is located mainly in the cytoplasm[9]. Transferrin transports iron molecules from the Sertoli cell to the spermatogenic cell line; receptors for transferrin have been found in adluminal germ cells[10]. Ceruloplasmin, which participates in the transfer of copper, is secreted into the lumen of the seminiferous tubules where it binds to spermatozoa, detaching from that surface in the lumen of the efferent duct. Sulfated glycoprotein-1 plays a role in single lipid binding; plasminogen activator activates plasminogen; glycoprotein-2 has a cathepsin activity; β-2 microglobulin is a protease inhibitor; lactate and pyruvate are part of the energy metabolism system; and sulfated glycoprotein-2 is a sperm coating protein with immunosuppressant activity.

The seminiferous tubules end through the transitional distal seminiferous segment into the septal rete (tubuli recti) that carry the sperm into the dip and then the superficial mediastinal rete. The last one communicates with the extratesticular rete, which is drained by the ductuli efferentes into the epididymis.

GERM CELL LINE

Sex determination in humans is not fully understood. The testicular determining factor has not been identified and different theories have been advanced. A sex-determining gene called SRY (sex-determining region for the Y chromosome) has been identified[11–14]. It is located within a 35-kilobase interval on the short arm of the Y chromosome, very close to the boundary of the pseudo-autosomal region (Figure 2). Nevertheless, experience with intersexual patients suggests that this is not the only gene involved in testicular determination, and that there might be other factors in this cascade that have not yet been identified clearly. Genes controlling the morphology and motility of the sperm may also be located in the SRY. Furthermore, an azoospermia gene has been described in the long arm of the Y chromosome[15].

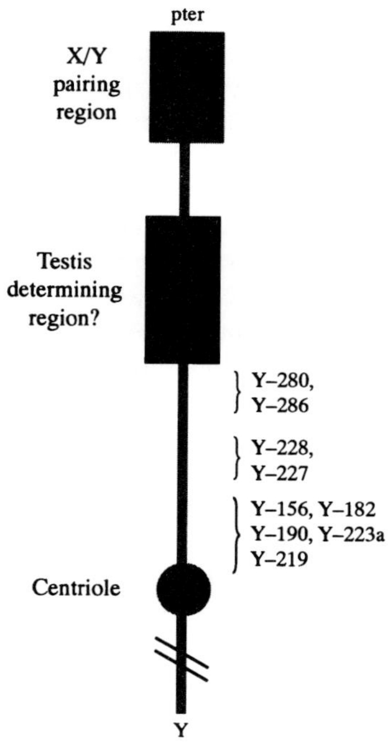

Figure 2 Schematic diagram of the relative arrangement of Y-chromosomal DNA sequencing

In mice it has been suggested that at least two autosomal genes control testis size by regulating the number of Sertoli cells[16].

Gametogenesis in humans shows clear sexual dimorphism. Gonocytes in the female enter meiosis at around 12 weeks. In the male they remain at rest until puberty, except when they are in a high steroidogenic milieu; for instance, when transferred into the adrenal gland where they do enter meiosis.

In the female during meiosis, the two sex chromosomes are transcriptionally active since the inactive X is reactivated in the prophase of meiosis I; the two sex chromosomes are fully paired and, therefore, recombination occurs along the whole length of the chromosomes. In the male, on the other hand, the sex chromosomes are transcriptionally inactive at meiosis, since they are sequestered in the sex vesicle within the nucleus and the chromosome pairing, as well as recombination, are limited since only the pseudo-autosomal region of the Y is paired with the homologous segment of the X.

The process of spermatogenesis in the human starts at puberty and proceeds through the whole life span of the individual. Very early in embryonic development, once the gonocytes have differentiated into fetal spermatogonia, there is an active process of mitotic replication which seems to be under FSH control and will establish the baseline number of precursor cells (reserve cells) of the testicle. This mitotic component will proceed, once the baseline number of spermatogonia is established after puberty, in order to continue to provide precursor cells and to start the process of differentiation and maturation. This mitotic phase involves spermatogonia types A and B and primary spermatocytes (spermatocyte I).

This is followed by a meiotic phase involving primary spermatocytes until spermatids are formed and, during this process, chromosome pairing, crossing over and genetic exchange is accomplished until a new genome is determined. In turn, a post-meiotic phase involving spermatids all the way up to spermatozoa develops, ending in the formation of a specialized cell.

Figure 3 summarizes the male germ cell line proliferation, genomic determination and intratesticular maturation until a fully formed spermatozoon is available.

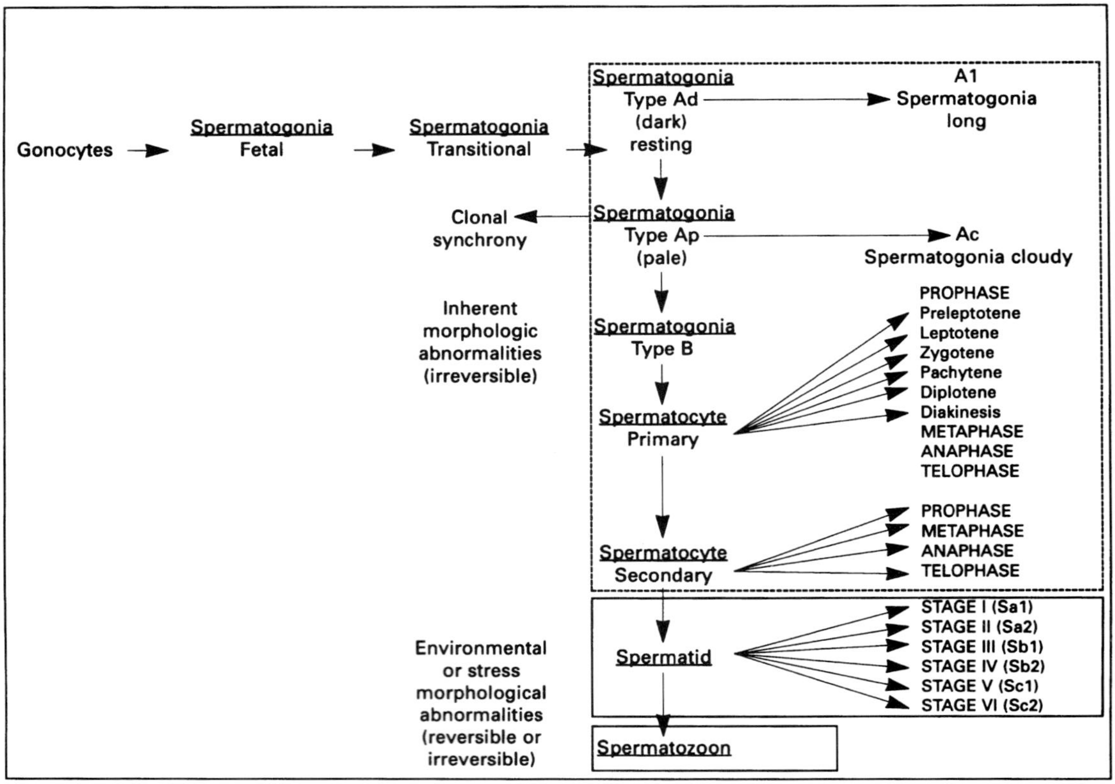

Figure 3 Germ cell line

EMBRYOGENESIS

During embryogenesis the gonocytes are converted into fetal spermatogonia and then into transitional spermatogonia and finally into spermatogonia type Ad (dark), which represent the resting germ cell in the adult gonad. By mitotic division, they give rise to one spermatogonia that will be another resting one, and one type Ap (pale) that will initiate the active process of spermatogenesis; in other species, they will keep connections and will maintain clone synchrony. They will be converted into spermatogonia type B that in turn will differentiate into primary spermatocytes. At this point the mitotic phase ends. Several factors are involved in this process: a maturation-promoting factor (MPF) that has mitotic-promoting activity and is most probably represented by a protein kinase[17]; a CV-2 protein, also a protein kinase, and cyclins. The spermatogonia show the presence of nuclear histones and also human menopausal gonadotropin (hMG), a group of non-histone proteins maintaining a higher-order chromatin structure. Several transcriptional regulatory factors have been mentioned, most of them being proto-oncogenes: namely *c-myc* mRNA and protein[18], *c-raf* proto-oncogene[19], *c-fos*, *c-jun*[18,19] and β-actin mRNA.

Entering meiosis the primary spermatocyte, with a DNA content equivalent to 2-N (diploid content) and having a diploid number of chromosomes, replicates DNA to 4-N, initiating the meiotic prophase that will go through the well known stages of preleptotene, zygotene, pachytene, diplotene and diakinesis. Chromosome pairing and crossing over occurs during these phases. The process of crossing over, perhaps the most critical in gametogenesis, is completed during pachytene with the formation of a recombination module having a lateral and central component that will facilitate the exchange of DNA during that phase. At diplotene the process is completed, the cell proceeds to metaphase, anaphase and telophase and completes the first meiotic division. Two secondary spermatocytes are formed in which the number of chromosomes is reduced to the haploid complement, but the DNA content is still diploid. The second meiotic division starts, giving origin to four spermatids with a haploid number of chromosomes, a haploid DNA content and a new genome different from the maternal and paternal contribution due to crossing-over.

Meiosis-inducing substances and meiosis-preventing substances have been described, although their final characterization and identification have not been performed in the human. Another proto-oncogene, *c-mos*[19], has been mentioned as one of the possible meiosis-triggering factors. During the process of crossing over and recombination, other factors have been mentioned. An endonuclease is involved in the initial phases of the process; a U protein seems to help in the unwinding of DNA; an R protein helps in the recombination of the single-stranded DNA; a REC-A protein (M-meiotic-recombinant) catalyzes recombination between homologous chromosomes; and DNA polymerase-B assists in DNA repair. During this process, the somatic type of nuclear histones are converted into the germ cell type of histones. Several genes are expressed at different stages of the process. PKG-2 mRNA, a phosphoglycerate kinase, is expressed in spermatocytes; PKG protein is expressed in spermatids; LDG-C gene mRNA and LDH C-4 isozyme appear in preleptotene spermatocytes up to the stage of elongated spermatids; RSA-1 (rabbit sperm autoantigen) and sulfogalactosyl-glyceril-phospholipid and binding protein are also expressed during these stages.

SPERMIOGENESIS

Once the process of meiosis is completed spermiogenesis begins. Six different stages have been described in the human in the process of spermatid maturation, also known as Sa-1 and 2, Sb-1 and 2 and Sc-1 and 2 (Figure 3). Each of these stages can be identified by morphological characteristics. During the Sa stage the Golgi complex and the mitochondria are well developed and differentiated, the acrosomal vesicle appears, the chromatoid body develops in one pole of the cell opposite from the acrosomal vesicle, and the proximal centriole and the axial filament appears. During Sb-1 and Sb-2 stages formation of the acrosome is completed, the intermediate piece is formed and the tail develops. The process is completed during the Sc stages, and some authors also recognize Sd-1 and Sd-2 phases. Once the spermatozoon completes maturation, it detaches from the Sertoli cell and floats freely in the seminiferous tubule lumen.

During the process (post-meiotic phase) there is a progressive condensation of the nucleus with inactivation of the genome, the histones are converted into transitional proteins and, finally, into protamines with well developed disulfide bonds. The spermatids originating from the same spermatogonia remain connected by bridges which allow cytoplasmic products to be transported from one to the others, until final spermatozoa formation and separation from the Sertoli cell occurs (spermiation).

During this extensive process of spermatogenesis three peaks of RNA synthesis occur:

(1) During the spermatogonia phase, due mainly to proliferation and growth;

(2) At the mid-pachytene spermatocyte stage due to cell enlargement and expression of germ cell-specific genes; and

(3) At spermiogenesis.

In the mouse some sperm cell differentiation genes have been described. While this has not been done in humans, it is important to understand that at different stages of spermatogenesis some genes are present, although their function is not completely understood. A list of these genes is given in Table 4.

The duration of the process of spermatogenesis in the human has been estimated for different stages. The duration of spermatogonia development phase is not known in the human, but seems to take around 16.5 days in the monkey. Spermatocyte maturation in the human takes 25.3 days, spermiogenesis 21.6 days. Total estimated time is approximately 74 days.

Table 4 The process of spermatogenesis: sperm cell differentiation genes (mouse)

	c-fos nuclear proto-oncogene	Type A spermatogonia Type B spermatogonia $\uparrow$ Pachytene spermatocyte
Nuclear transcription regulatory factors???	*c-raf* *c-ras*	Spermatogonia Later in spermatogenesis
Type β spermatogonia	*c-myc* nuclear proto-oncogene *c-gun* nuclear proto-oncogene	Type B spermatogonia Early preleptotene spermatocytes
	c-mos proto-oncogene	Regulation of meiosis Round spermatids $\uparrow$ Primary spermatocyte
	HOX-1.4 homeobox containing gene	Round spermatid Elongating spermatid
	int-1 proto-oncogene	Round spermatid Residual bodies
	c-abl (tyrosine kinase)	Round spermatid Elongating spermatid Residual bodies

References

1. Veldhuis, J. D., Evans, W. S., Urban, R. J., Rogol, A. D. and Johnson, M. L. (1988). Physiologic attributes of the luteinizing hormone pulse signal in the human. *J. Androl.*, **9**, 69–77
2. Talbot, J. A., Rodger, R. S., Shalet, S. M., Littley, M. D. and Robertson, W. R. (1990). The pulsatile secretion of bioactive luteinizing hormone in normal adult men. *Acta Endocrinol. Copenh.*, **22**, 643–50
3. Spiteri-Grech, J. and Nieschlag, E. (1993). Paracrine factors relevant to the regulation of spermatogenesis – a review. *J. Reprod. Fertil.*, **98**, 1–14
4. Foresta, C., Caretto, A., Varoto, A., Rossato, M. and Scandellari, C. (1991). Epidermal growth factor receptors (EGFR) localization in human testis. *Arch. Androl.*, **27**, 17–24
5. Stubbs, S. C., Hargreave, T. B. and Habib, F. K. (1990). Localization and characteristics of epidermal growth factor receptors on human testicular tissue by biochemical and immunohistochemical techniques. *J. Endocrinol.*, **125**, 485–92
6. Cain, M. P., Kramer, S. A., Tindall, D. J. and Husmann, D. A. (1994). Alterations in maternal epidermal growth factor (EGF) affect testicular descent and epididymal development. *Urology*, **43**, 375–8
7. Syed, V., Khan, S. A. and Nieschlag, E. (1991). Epidermal growth factor stimulates testosterone production of human Leydig cells in vitro. *J. Endocrinol. Invest.*, **14**, 93–7
8. Santiemma, V., Rosati, P., Guerzoni, C., Mariani, S., Beligotti, F., Magnanti, M., Garufi, G., Galoni, T. and Fabbrini, A. (1992). Human Sertoli cells *in vitro*: morphological features and androgen binding protein secretion. *J. Steroid Biochem. Mol. Biol.*, **43**, 423–9
9. Gerard, H., Gerard, A., En-Nya, A., Felden, F. and Gueant, J. L. (1994). Spermatogenic cells do internalize Sertoli androgen-binding protein: a transmission electron-microscopy autoradiographic study in the rat. *Endocrinology*, **134**, 1515–27
10. Forti, G., Vanelli, G. B., Barni, T., Balboni, G. C., Orlando, C. and Serio, M. (1992). Sertoli-germ cells interactions in the human testis. *J. Steroid. Biochem. Mol. Biol.*, **43**, 419–22
11. Sinclair, A. H., Berta, P., Palmer, M. S., Hawkins, J. R., Griffiths, B. L., Smith, M. J., Foster, J. W., Frischauf, A. M., Lovell-Badge, R. and Goodfellow, P. N. (1990). A gene from the human sex-determining region encodes a protein with homology to a conserved DNA-binding motif. *Nature*, **346**, 216–17
12. Berta, P., Hawkins, J. R., Sinclair, A. H., Taylor, A., Griffiths, B. L., Goodfellow, P. N. and Fellous, M. (1990). Genetic evidence equating SRY and the testis-determining factor. *Nature*, **348**, 448–50
13. Palmer, M. S., Berta, P., Sinclair, A. H., Pym, B. and Goodfellow, P. N. (1990). Comparison of human ZFY and ZFX transcripts. *Proc. Natl Acad. Sci. USA*, **87**, 1681–5

14. Goodfellow, P. N. and Lovell-Badge, R. (1993). SRY and sex determination in mammals. *Ann. Rev. Genet.*, **27**, 71–92
15. Nakagome, Y. and Nakahori, Y. (1993). Human Y chromosome in reproduction and development. *Nippon-Rinsho*, **51**, 3301–7
16. Chubb, C. (1992). Genes regulating testis size. *Biol. Reprod.*, **47**, 29–36
17. Nishimoto, T., Uzawa, S. and Schlegel, R. (1992). Mitotic checkpoints. *Curr. Opin. Cell Biol.*, **4**, 174–9
18. Kumar, G., Patel, D. and Naz, R. K. (1993). c-Myc mRNA is present in human sperm cells. *Cell Mol. Biol. Res.*, **39**, 111–17
19. Bellve, A. R. (1993). Purification, culture and fractionation of spermatogenic cells. *Methods Enzymol.*, **225**, 84–113

Anatomy of the mature spermatozoon 2

T. F. Kruger, R. Menkveld and S. Oehninger

INTRODUCTION

A summary of light microscopic and electron microscopic features is given in this chapter outlining the basic characteristics of the anatomy of the human spermatozoon.

LIGHT AND ELECTRON MICROSCOPIC MORPHOLOGICAL CHARACTERISTICS OF SPERMATOZOA

Spermatozoa are highly specialized and condensed cells which do not grow or divide. A spermatozoon consists of a head, containing the paternal heredity material (DNA), and a tail, which provides motility (Figures 1 and 2). The spermatozoon is endowed with a large nucleus but lacks the large cytoplasm which is characteristic of most body cells. Men are unique among mammals in the degree of morphological heterogeneity of the ejaculate[1–3].

SPERM HEAD

Light microscopy

Human spermatozoa are classified using bright field microscope optics on fixed, stained specimens[2,3].

The heads of stained human spermatozoa are slightly smaller than the heads of living spermatozoa in the original semen, although the shapes are not appreciably different[5]. The normal head should be oval in shape. Allowing for the slight shrinkage that fixation and staining induce, the length of the head is about 4.0–5.5 μm, and the width 2.5–3.5 μm. The normal length-to-width ratio is about 1.50–1.75. These values span the 95% confidence limits of comparative data for both Papanicolaou stained and living sperm heads[5]. Two slightly different types of normal spermatozoal head forms have been described based on spermatozoa found in endocervical canal mucus post-coitally[3]. The first and most common form, as identified under the microscope with bright field illumination, is the perfectly smooth oval head; the second form is oval, still having a smooth or regular contour but slightly tapered at the postacrosomal end[3]. Since diversity is a fact of all biological systems, trivial variations must be regarded as normal[3].

The following head aberrations can be observed: head shape/size defects, including large, small, tapering, pyriform, amorphous, vacuolated (>20% of the head surface occupied by unstained vacuolar areas), and double heads, or any combination of these[4].

Human spermatozoa have a well-defined acrosomal region comprising about two-thirds of the anterior head area[2–4]. It does not exhibit an apical thickening like many other species, but shows a uniform thickness/thinning towards the end forming the equatorial segment. Because of this

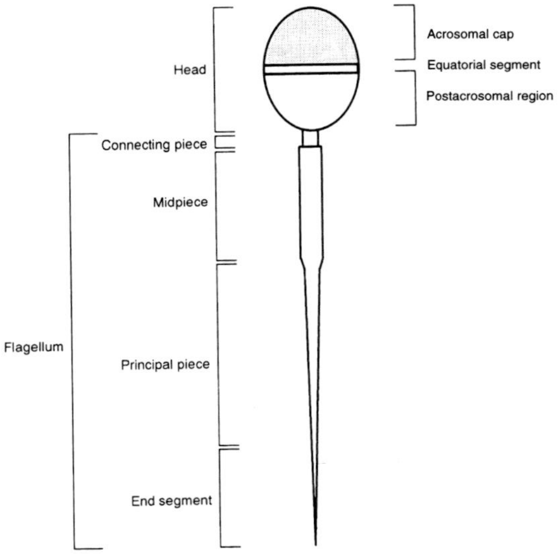

Figure 1 Schematic drawing of light microscopic human spermatozoon

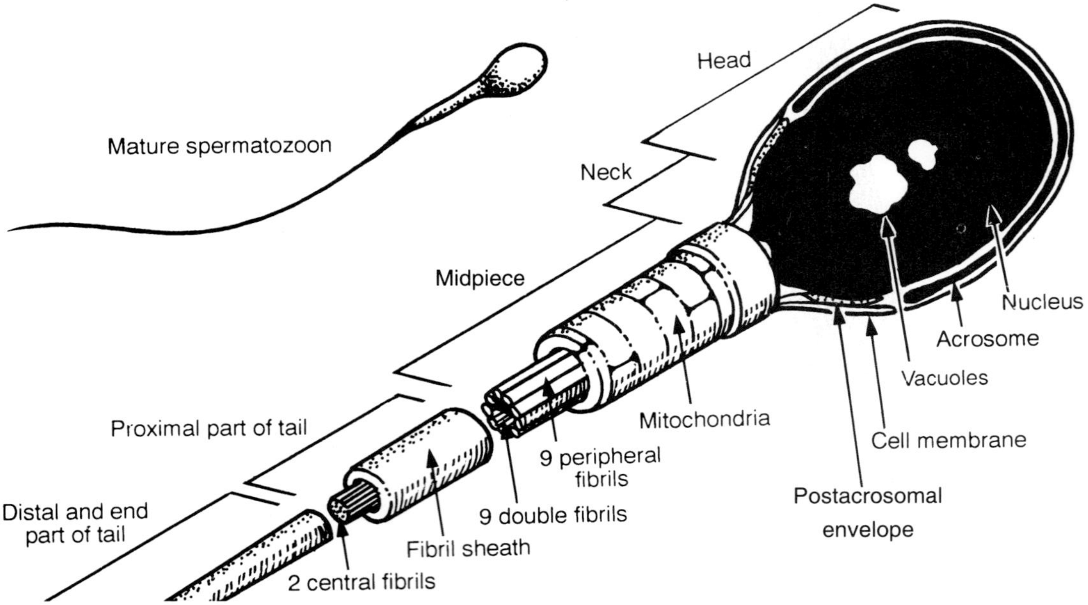

Figure 2 Light and electron microscopic diagram of human spermatozoon

thinning, the area will appear more intensely stained when examined with the light microscope. Depending on this staining intensity, the acrosome will appear to cover 40–70% of the sperm head.

Scanning electron microscopy

Scanning electron microscopy (SEM) is useful for the demonstration of surface structures of spermatozoa in great detail. Due to its three-dimensional picture, furthermore, it is possible to observe and interpret the complex structure of a human spermatozoon more easily and completely than with either light or transmission electron microscopy.

The sperm head is divided into two unequal parts by a furrow that completely encircles the head, i.e. the acrosomal and postacrosomal regions. The acrosomal region can represent up to two-thirds of the head length and in some cases a depression is noted in this area which is regarded as morphologicaly normal. The equatorial segment is not always clearly visible with SEM. Just after the equatorial segment is the beginning of the postacrosomal region, which is marked by maximal thickness and width of the spermatozoon. The postacrosomal region is divided into two parts by the posterior ring forming two equal bands. The band closest to the acrosome often stands out[1].

The surface of human spermatozoa, washed free of seminal plasma, appears smooth without coarse particles. The only exception is the acrosome and especially the anterior part that may frequently appear rough[1].

Electron transmission microscopy

The electron microscopic morphological characteristics of human spermatozoa are presented in Figures 2–6. The sperm head is a flattened ovoid structure consisting primarily of the nucleus. The acrosome is a caplike structure covering the anterior two-thirds of the sperm head (Figures 2 and 3), which arises from the Golgi apparatus of the spermatid as it differentiates into a spermatozoon. Unlike that in many other mammalian species, the acrosome of human spermatozoa does not exhibit an apical thickening, but has an anterior segment of uniform thickness. The acrosome contains several hydrolytic enzymes, including hyaluronidase and proacrosin, which are necessary for fertilization[1].

During fertilization of the egg, the enzyme-rich contents of the acrosomes are released at the time of acrosome reaction. During fusion of the outer

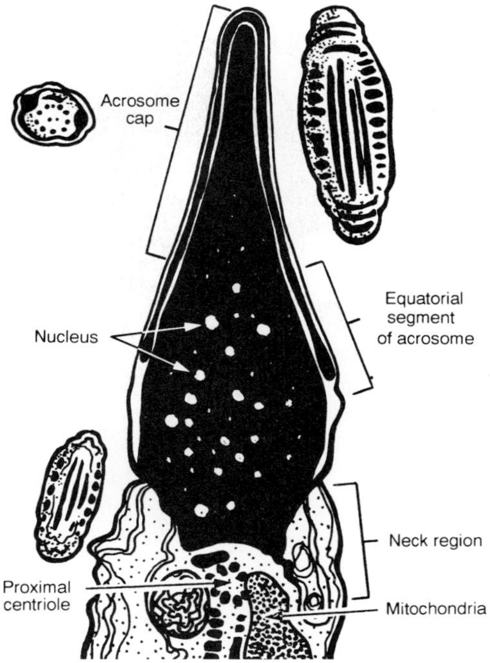

Figure 3 Schematic drawing of longitudinal section of sperm head

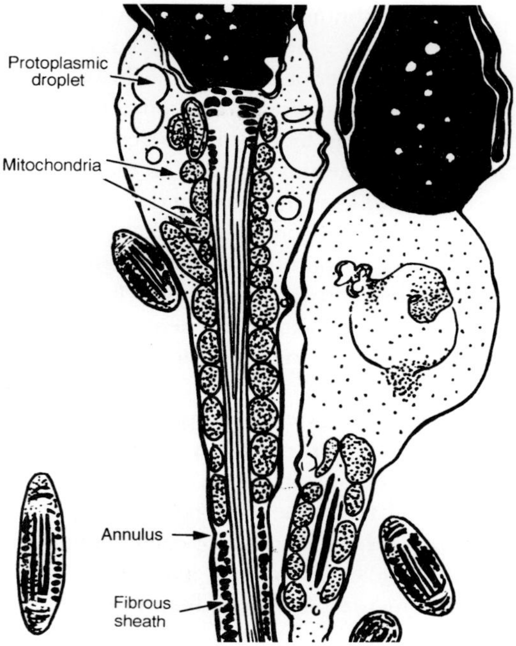

Figure 5 Longitudinal section through midpiece

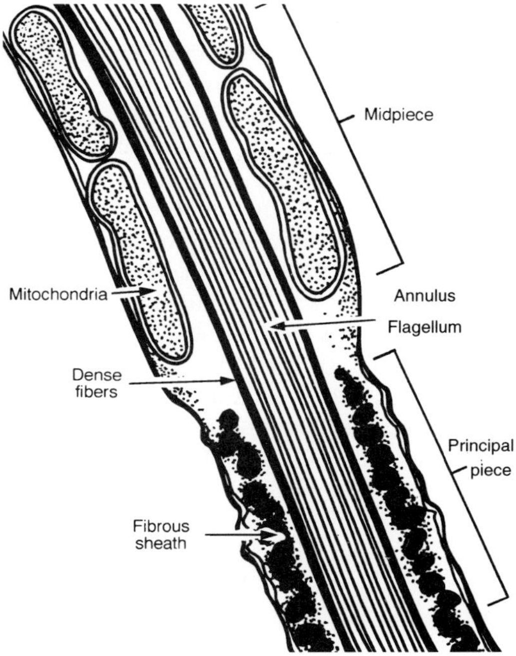

Figure 4 Longitudinal section of the region between midpiece and principal piece of human spermatozoon

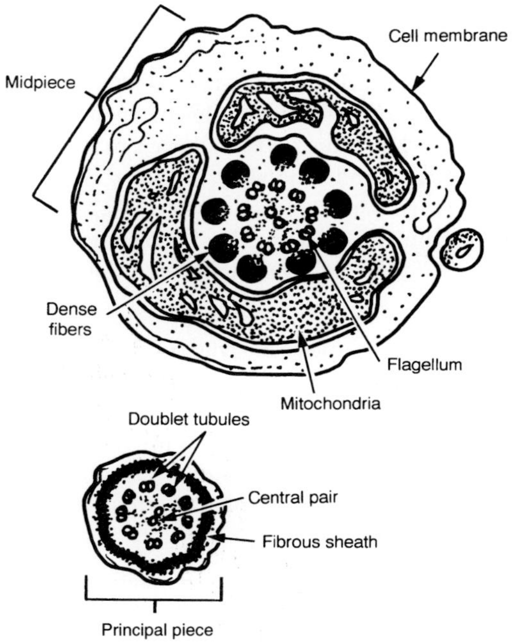

Figure 6 Cross-section of human sperm tail

acrosomal membrane with the plasma membrane at multiple sites, the acrosomal enzymes are released. The anterior half of the head is then devoid of plasma and outer acrosomal membrane and is covered only by the inner acrosomal membrane[6]. The equatorial segment of the acrosome persists more or less intact since it does not participate in acrosome reaction (Figure 3).

The posterior portion of the sperm head is covered by the postnuclear cap, which is a single membrane. The equatorial segment consists of an overlap of the acrosome and the postnuclear cap (Figure 3).

The nucleus (Figure 3), comprising 65% of the head, is composed of DNA conjugated with protein. The chromatin within the nucleus is very compact, and no distinct chromosomes are visible. Several nuclei have incomplete condensation with apparent vacuoles. The genetic information carried by the spermatozoon is 'coded' and stored in the DNA molecule, which is made up of many nucleotides. The hereditary characteristics transmitted by the sperm nucleus include sex determination[1].

SPERM TAIL

Light microscopy

The sperm tail formation arises at the spermatid stage. The centriole during spermatogenesis is differentiated into three parts: midpiece, main or principal piece, and endpiece (Figures 1,2). The midpiece has a similar length to the head, and is separated from the tailpiece by a ring, the annulus (Figure 5). The following tail aberrations can be observed:

(1) Neck and midpiece aberrations, including their absent (seen as 'free' or 'loose' heads), non-inserted or 'bent' tail (the tail forms an angle of about 90° with the long axis of the head), distended/irregular/bent midpiece, abnormally thin midpiece (i.e. no mitochondrial sheath), or any combination of these[4];

(2) Tail aberrations include short, multiple, hairpin, broken (angulation >90°) tails, irregular width, coiling tails with terminal droplets, or any combination of these[4];

(3) Cytoplasmic droplets greater than one-third the area of a normal sperm head are considered abnormal. They are usually located in the neck/midpiece region of the tail, although some immature spermatozoa may have a cytoplasmic droplet at other locations along the tail[3,4]. The endpiece is not distinctly visualized by light microscopy.

Scanning electron microscopy

With SEM the tail can be subdivided into three distinct parts, i.e. midpiece, principle piece and endpiece. In the midpiece the mitochondrial spirals can be clearly visualized. This ends abruptly at the beginning of the midpiece. The midpiece narrows towards the posterior end. A longitudinal column and transverse ribs are visible. The short endpiece has a small diameter due to the absence of outer fibers[1].

Transmission electron microscopy

The midpiece possesses a cytoplasmic portion and a lipid-rich mitochondrial sheath that consists of several spiral mitochondria, surrounding the axial filament in a helical fashion (Figures 2,5,6). The midpiece provides the sperm with the energy necessary for motility. The central axial core of 11 fibrils is surrounded by an additional outer ring of nine coarser fibrils (Figures 2,6). Individual mitochondria are wrapped around these outer fibrils in a spiral manner to form the mitochondrial sheath, which contains the enzymes involved in the oxidative metabolism of the sperm (Figures 2,4–6). The mitochondrial sheath of the midpiece is relatively short, slightly longer than the combined length of the head and neck[1].

The principal piece (mainpiece), the longest part of the tail, provides most of the propellant machinery. The coarse nine fibrils of the outer ring diminish in thickness and finally disappear, leaving only the inner fibrils in the axial core for much of the length of the principal piece (Figure 2)[8]. The fibrils of the principal piece are surrounded by a fibrous tail sheath, which consists of branching and anastomosing semicircular strands or 'ribs' held together by their attachment to two bands that run lengthwise along opposite sides of the tail[1]. The tail terminates in the endpiece with a length of 4–10 μm and a diameter of <1 μm. The small diameter is due to the absence of the outer fibers and sheath and a distal fading of the microtubules.

CONCLUSION

Although many of the structures described here, especially the ultrastructure characteristics based on electron microscopy studies, are not visible by light microscopy a basic knowledge of these structures is very important for the correct evaluation and interpretation of sperm morphology under light microscopy; in turn this will help in the determination of male fertility potential, as will be discussed in chapters to follow. These fundamental anatomic characteristics are also useful in understanding certain functional aspects of the male gamete during the fertilization process.

Original light and electron microscopy photographs, as well as schematic morphology/ anatomy drawings (light- and electron microscopy), are depicted in Figures 1–6. If followed carefully, a clear picture of the basic sperm anatomy will be obtained.

References

1. Hafez, E. S. E. (1976). *Human Semen and Fertility Regulation in Men*. (St. Louis: C. V. Mosby)
2. Kruger, T. F., Menkveld, R., Stander, F. S. H., Lombard, C. J., Van der Merwe, J. P., Van Zyl, J. A. and Smith, K. (1986). Sperm morphologic features as a prognostic factor in *in vitro* fertilization. *Fertil. Steril.*, **46**, 1118–23
3. Menkveld, R., Stander, F. S. H., Kotze, T. J. vW., Kruger, T. F. and Van Zyl, J. A. (1990). The evaluation of morphological characteristics of human spermatozoa according to stricter criteria. *Hum. Reprod.*, **5**, 586–92
4. World Health Organisation (1992). *WHO Manual for the Examination of Human Semen and Sperm–Cervical Mucus Interaction*, 2nd edn. (London: Cambridge University Press)
5. Katz, D. F., Overstreet, J. W., Samuels, S. J., Niswander, P. W., Bloom, T. D. and Lewis, E. L. (1986). Morphometric analysis of spermatozoa in the assessment of human male fertility. *J. Androl.*, **7**, 203–10
6. Barros, C. and Franklin, L. E. (1968). Behaviour of the gamete membranes during sperm entry into the mammalian egg. *J. Cell Biol.*, **37**, 13
7. Menkveld, R., Oettle, E. E., Kruger, T. F., Swanson, R. J., Acosta, A. A. and Oehninger, S. (1991). *Atlas of Human Sperm Morphology*, p. 1. (Baltimore: Williams and Wilkins)
8. White, I. G. (1974). Mammalian sperm. In Hafez, E. S. E. (ed). *Reproduction of Farm Animals*, 3rd edn. (Philadelphia: Lea & Febiger)

Physiological changes in sperm during transport through the female reproductive tract

3

J. W. Overstreet

INTRODUCTION

For ethical reasons, most studies of normal human sperm physiology in the female reproductive tract have been limited to sperm recovered from the cervix. Interpretation of data obtained in both basic and clinical studies of human sperm physiology *in vivo* is based on evidence that spermatozoa which have colonized the cervix can migrate subsequently to the upper reproductive tract and participate in fertilization. There is substantial evidence that cervical mucus can serve as a source of sperm supply for the upper reproductive tract of many mammals, including humans. This concept has important implications for understanding and treating human infertility, because the cervix is the only site of sperm accumulation in women that can be sampled non-invasively. In this chapter, these concepts will be reviewed and the observations which support them will be discussed.

Far less information is available on the functions of the uterus and uterine tubes during sperm transport in women. Although intrauterine insemination (IUI) is employed routinely to achieve pregnancy in humans and in other species, it is unknown what role sperm from the uterus may play in fertilization. Sperm physiology in the oviducts has been studied in a number of laboratory animal models, but recent observations of oviductal sperm in women suggest that concepts developed from laboratory studies may not apply to human sperm biology. Significant progress has been made in understanding the cell biology of mammalian fertilization. Almost all of this work has been carried out *in vitro* and most experiments have been performed with model species. Although many fertilization mechanisms are thought to be common to all mammals, their relevance to human sperm physiology *in vivo* remains to be established. The body of existing knowledge, although incomplete, clearly demonstrates the complexity and species variability of sperm transport and physiology in the female tract. This complexity and its implications for understanding the causes of human infertility will be emphasized in this chapter.

SPERM TRANSPORT IN THE FEMALE REPRODUCTIVE TRACT

Our understanding of the biology of sperm transport derives from a number of classical descriptive and experimental studies[1–4]. The events of sperm transport have been described as occurring in two phases. There is a brief, initial, rapid transit phase of sperm transport in which sperm reach the upper reproductive tract and/or peritoneal cavity at rates which cannot be achieved by flagellar activity alone. The succeeding phase of sustained sperm migration requires motility of the sperm cells, whose physiology may be modulated by the female environment. During this period, sperm accumulate in 'reservoirs' within the female tract including the vagina, the cervix, the uterus and the lower oviduct, depending on the species.

Rapid transit phase

Spermatozoa gain access to the reproductive tract at the moment of ejaculation, and within seconds sperm can be found throughout the female tract[3,5]. The uptake of spermatozoa into the cervix and their propulsion to the upper reproductive tract has been studied most extensively in the rabbit model and has been termed the rapid transit phase of sperm transport[6]. The studies of Settlage *et al.*[7] demonstrate that rapid sperm transport also takes place in women. In this study, volunteers were artificially inseminated intravaginally with normal donor semen prior to bilateral salpingectomy. Sperm were present in the Fallopian tubes within 5 min following insemination. This rate of sperm passage cannot be accomplished by the swimming speed of the spermatozoa, and it is assumed that contractions of the uterus and tubes are responsible[3]. Reflex-mediated pressure changes in the uterus of sufficient magnitude for passive sperm transport have been recorded during human coitus[8]. In the rabbit, experimental studies have shown that both chemical and physical stimuli may be responsible for initiating rapid sperm transport[9]. The former mechanism may involve molecules in seminal plasma; the latter mechanism may involve coital activation of vaginal stretch receptors. The reflex smooth muscular contractions appear to be mediated through the autonomic nervous system[9]. This process may be analogous in some respects to the autonomic reflexes which control emission and ejaculation in the male[10]. However, unlike the situation in males, the process in females is not closely linked to the subjective experience of orgasm, since rapid transport is the same following either artificial insemination or coitus[6].

One important sequel of rapid sperm transport is the immediate colonization of the cervical mucus by spermatozoa. This biological prediction has been confirmed clinically in reports of 'immediate post coital tests' in which sperm were observed in cervical mucus within 90 s of coitus[11]. There is an obvious relationship of these events to normal fertility because the cervical mucus offers protection from the vaginal environment, which is acidic and therefore hostile to prolonged sperm survival[12,13].

The biological importance of rapid sperm transport to the uterus and oviducts is less certain. In the few species which have been carefully studied, the evidence suggests that sperm which reach the oviducts as a consequence of rapid transport play no direct role in fertilization. In rabbits, which are reflex ovulators and do not ovulate until approximately 10 h following coitus, the rapidly transported sperm are not viable and are lost from the oviduct prior to fertilization[6]. Experimental studies in farm animals in which oviducts were transected or ligated at various intervals after mating also suggest that the functional sperm population does not reach the oviducts for several hours after coitus[14]. It has been speculated that the process of rapid sperm transport is important for reproduction because it delivers molecules to the reproductive tract from the sperm and/or seminal plasma which act as local messengers for control of sperm transport[3]. Because immunosuppressive factors have been found in seminal plasma[15] and sperm cells[16], it is possible that rapid transport is involved in suppression of the immune response of the female tract to spermatozoa[17]. If rapid sperm transport has one or more required functions for normal reproduction, abnormalities of these peri-coital events would result in infertility. Whether such abnormalities would be evident in standard clinical tests, such as the post-coital test, is not known.

Sustained migration phase

The rapid transit phase of sperm transport is confined to the peri-coital period, and thereafter sperm migration through the female tract is accomplished primarily by the flagellar activity of the sperm cells. Sperm distribution is not uniform in the female tract, but rather sperm accumulate in particular regions of the tract, which are often referred to as sperm reservoirs. Because these sperm accumulation sites result from anatomical barriers to sperm migration, there is considerable variability between species in the location of the reservoirs. The cervix is the primary block to sperm entry in primates and ruminants, and in these species the cervix is also regarded as an important sperm reservoir[4]. In other species, such as pigs, dogs, horses and rodents, semen is ejaculated either directly into the uterus or is transported across the cervix in bulk by vaginal and uterine contractions. In these species, the primary block to sperm passage is at the utero–tubal junction, and the cervix has no apparent function in sperm transport except for its valve-like action in controlling fluid passage into and out of the uterus[4].

In most species with a cervical sperm reservoir, the cervical lumen is filled with mucus. Cervical mucus is a site of sperm accumulation in non-human primates[18,19], in ruminants[20,14], and in women[21]. Cervical mucus is virtually absent in rabbits, but the survival of rabbit sperm in the vagina is as good as or better than in the cervix[22]. Therefore, the cervix may not be an important site for sperm storage in rabbits, but may act more as a valve for regulation of sperm access to the uterus.

A number of observations of human sperm in cervical mucus support the concept that this fluid is a medium in which sperm may be stored over time. Sperm swimming speeds in cervical mucus were not different when sperm were recovered at 1 h and 48 h after insemination[23]. Sperm retained fertilizing capacity in the cervix for up to 80 h, as shown by penetration of the human zona pellucida following sperm recovery from cervical mucus[24]. The sperm which are found in cervical mucus of fertile women are almost 100% viable and more than 95% have intact acrosomes[25]. The number of motile sperm observed in cervical mucus is correlated with sperm concentration in the ejaculate[26], and in artificial insemination patients there is a significant association between sperm survival for 48 h in cervical mucus and conception[27]. A similar relationship between the results of post-coital testing and fertility has been more difficult to demonstrate with infertility patients[28], perhaps because of the lack of standardization of methods and the confounding effects of other unrecognized infertility factors in these patient populations.

In species with a cervical reservoir, the uterus may function during sperm transport primarily as a conduit between the cervix and the oviduct[4]. In species such as rodents and pigs, which have bulk passage of semen into the uterus, the sperm migrate to sites of storage in the oviduct and the uterine contents are subsequently evacuated[17]. The uterus may store sperm in dogs, because motile sperm are found in uterine glands for up to 10 days after mating[20].

The isthmus of the oviduct has been identified as the likely storage site for the fertilizing sperm population in many mammals, including rodents, rabbits, pigs and ruminants[4]. Experimental evidence obtained in ruminants strongly suggests that oviductal sperm storage is a feature of reproductive biology in those species which also have a cervical sperm reservoir[14]. Nevertheless, the situation in primates is not clear. Studies of human oviducts have failed to demonstrate a site of sperm accumulation in the tubal isthmus[30]. Although sperm have been observed in the oviducts of non-human primates[31], there is also no conclusive evidence for an oviductal sperm reservoir in other primate species.

SPERM PHYSIOLOGY *IN VIVO*

Sperm capacitation

Physiological changes in sperm cells that are required for fertilization are collectively termed capacitation[32,33]. There is no agreement on the biological importance of the capacitation process *in vivo*. Bedford[34] believes that capacitation in the female is required for reversal of a stabilized state that was necessary for prolonged sperm storage in the male reproductive tract. Yanagimachi[33] has speculated that capacitation may enable the female tract to control the speed with which sperm gain fertilizing capacity and thereby enable the delivery of freshly capacitated sperm to all of the ovulated eggs, regardless of the time of mating. Sperm transport events may influence the progress of capacitation and, similarly, capacitation may be required for some of the sperm functions involved in their migration through the reproductive tract[3,33]. The acrosome reaction of the fertilizing sperm is probably induced during sperm interaction with the oocyte[33]. Premature acrosome reactions may lead to loss of sperm viability; therefore, one important interaction of capacitation and sperm transport may involve the sequestration of acrosome intact spermatozoa and their delivery to the site of fertilization in concert with ovulation.

Capacitation has often been described in terms of physiological changes that must take place in sperm as prerequisites for the acrosome reaction, although in most species there is little or no structural change in the acrosome during capacitation[33]. The control of intracellular ion concentrations is almost certainly one aspect of capacitation. There is evidence that an increase in intracellular free calcium is required for induction of the acrosome reaction[35], although calcium concentrations appear to be maintained at low levels prior to the acrosome reaction[36]. Changes in sperm metabolism, increases in adenosine 3′, 5′-cyclic monophosphate (cAMP) and activation of acrosomal enzymes all have been investigated as components of capacitation, but the importance of these individual processes is controversial and there is no widely accepted model which integrates these concepts into a functional entity[33].

There is convincing evidence that sperm membrane changes are an important part of the capacitation process. During capacitation coating substances, including seminal plasma components, are altered or removed from the sperm surface[33]. The decapacitation factors from seminal plasma[37] are well-known examples of these molecules. In the laboratory sperm washing procedures are designed to remove these surface coats and, in the female tract, sperm interaction with the cervical mucus microstructure may have a similar effect in removing sperm coating substances[21]. Phospholipids are an important component of the sperm membrane, and there is evidence that these molecules may be altered during capacitation[38]. Cholesterol may have a function in the regulation of capacitation[39]. One model proposes that albumin and high density lipoproteins in culture medium or in the female tract are involved in removal of cholesterol from the sperm membrane and that this process is a component of capacitation[40]. There is evidence that D-mannose binding lectins are involved in the binding of human sperm to the zona pellucida[41], and that the expression of these lectins on the sperm surface depends on a loss of sperm membrane cholesterol during capacitation[42].

There are no specific markers on sperm which can be used to identify an individual cell as 'capacitated'. One commonly used approach to demonstrate the presence of capacitated sperm is to expose the sperm to an agent which can induce the acrosome reaction, provided that the sperm are capacitated. These agents include human follicular fluid[43], disaggregated zona pellucida[44] and progesterone[35]. This approach has been used to evaluate the capacitation status of human sperm in cervical mucus[25]. After sperm were allowed to migrate from cervical mucus into culture media *in vitro*, the sperm suspensions were tested by dilution with follicular fluid and acrosome reactions were evaluated. The cervical mucus was recovered from women between 1 h and 72 h after insemination and the response of the sperm was identified at each time point. In all experiments, the sperm did not acrosome react in response to follicular fluid immediately after sperm migration into culture media; however, following 6 h incubation *in vitro*, 15–20% acrosome reactions were observed in response to the same follicular fluid challenge. These results were interpreted to support the concept of conservation of sperm function in the cervix, because the capacitation kinetics were the same for sperm whether they were 1 h or 72 h old[25]. Because there was no washing or other preparation of the sperm *in vitro*, the results also suggest that sperm capacitation may be initiated *in vivo* during migration through cervical mucus[21].

Although sperm capacitation *in vivo* has been studied extensively in model species[45,46], very little is known of either sperm transport or capacitation in the human uterus. There are clinical observations which suggest that sperm can re-enter the cervix after reaching the uterus. In as many as 40% of cycles there is evidence of sperm in cervical mucus 48 h following intra-uterine insemination[47]. It is possible that an equilibrium is established between the cervix and the uterus, with sperm continuously passing back and forth between the two regions. On the other hand, it is unlikely that sperm have free access to the oviducts from the uterine cavity, because the utero–tubal junction is an efficient block in most species to sperm entering the oviduct[3,4]. Observations in non-human primates suggest that the uterine sperm population may maintain longer viability than the cervical population and could serve as a source of sperm supply to the oviduct after the cervical mucus becomes non-receptive to sperm[19,48].

Sperm physiology in the oviduct

Our knowledge of sperm–oviductal interaction is based entirely on experiments in laboratory animals, and these data provide the strongest support for the sperm reservoir hypothesis in mammals. As previously discussed, sperm accumulate in the lower isthmus of the oviduct in many species and this region appears to serve as a sperm reservoir. Accumulation of sperm in the oviductal isthmus is aided by mechanical factors, such as the narrow lumen which may be filled with a mucus-like secretion[49]. The ciliary beat and muscular contractions of this region are directed primarily toward the uterus[3]. Sperm accumulation in the lower isthmus of the rabbit oviduct is associated with reversible cessation of the sperm flagellar activity[50] and sperm adherence to epithelial surfaces[51].

Although similar phenomena may occur in the mouse[52], in the hamster many isthmic sperm are irreversibly immobilized[53]. These observations strongly suggest that as a result of sperm–epithelial interaction, the female tract can immobilize swimming sperm cells and then reactivate their flagellar activity, but little is known of the cellular mechanisms which may be involved.

Sperm ascent to the site of fertilization is synchronized with ovulation in model species[3]. The physiology of these prefertilization events is not well understood, but ovulation-associated changes in the contractility of the oviductal musculature[54] and capacitation-related intracellular changes in the spermatozoa[51] appear to be involved. The time required for sperm capacitation in the female can vary, and the process may be accelerated when mating occurs after ovulation[53]. The signal for transport of the fertilizing sperm may involve the endocrine changes associated with ovulation and may be mediated by the autonomic nervous system[4]. Sperm release from isthmic binding sites may involve small changes in the oviductal temperature[4] and hyperactivated motility may enable sperm separation from the isthmic epithelium[55]. Subsequently, hyperactivated motility is also important for rapid progression of spermatozoa along the epithelial surfaces of the oviduct and for initial sperm contact with the cumulus[56].

Sperm interaction with the cumulus oophorus

Sperm ascending from the lower oviduct encounter an oocyte which is surrounded by at least two protective investments. Innermost is the acellular zona pellucida and beyond the zona is the cumulus oophorus. The cumulus is formed of granulosa cells and their extracellular matrix (ECM). The granulosa cell layer which is closest to the zona has different biochemical and structural features than the remaining cumulus[57,58], and it is termed the corona radiata.

The oviductal isthmus and utero–tubal junction strictly limit the number of spermatozoa reaching the site of fertilization and this appears to be an important function for preventing polyspermic fertilization[33]. In concert with this sperm limitation, the expanded cumulus in the tubal ampulla is thought to enhance the probability that one of the few ascending spermatozoa will encounter the oocyte within the relatively large ampullar space[34]. This function is well illustrated in the mated rat, in which the cumuli are frequently recovered with no extra sperm present, even though all oocytes are fertilized[59]. The efficiency of this fertilization process may be enhanced by gradients within the cumulus which induce both chemotaxis (attraction) and chemokinesis (motility stimulation) of the fertilizing sperm cells[60,61].

The cumulus ECM is produced by granulosa cells[62]; it is formed primarily of hyaluronic acid, but also contains some protein[58,63]. The structure of the cumulus matrix is a network with openings that are smaller than the sperm head[58,64]. Spermatozoa penetrating the cumulus display hyperactivated motility[65], and these flagellar movements may physically tear the structure of the cumulus[64] and thus facilitate sperm entry. Sperm motility may be modulated by interaction with the cumulus and may respond to chemical stimuli, as well as physical stimuli during cumulus penetration. The chemical signals which are involved may be related to the chemotactic/chemokinetic factors demonstrated in human follicular fluid[60]. The speed of sperm penetration through cumulus *in vivo* is not known, but penetration through the cumulus to the zona surface requires 3–20 min *in vitro*[66–68]. The characteristics of the sperm surface are important for penetration of the cumulus ECM. For example, non-capacitated sperm[66,69] and acrosome-reacted sperm[67,69,70] cannot enter the cumulus ECM. Some vigorously motile sperm adhere irreversibly to granulosa cells and cumulus penetration is prevented[67,68,70]. Other spermatozoa, including sperm with intact acrosomes, are phagocytosed by granulosa cells[71]. The cellular mechanisms and biological significance of these sperm–granulosa cell interactions are unknown.

Although it is controversial, the view of most reproductive biologists is that the acrosome reaction of the fertilizing sperm is induced by contact with the zona pellucida, and that the fertilizing sperm has an intact acrosome during penetration of the cumulus[33,72]. Experiments with the mouse have demonstrated that only sperm having intact acrosomes can bind to the zona[73–75]. Experiments with human gametes suggest that the sequence of events prior to fertilization in our species also includes sperm–zona binding followed by the acrosome reaction[44]. Nevertheless, there is evidence that biochemical changes in sperm enzymes may take place during interaction with the cumulus[63], and one result of such interactions may be a sensitization of the fertilizing sperm to ensure that it will acrosome react upon binding to the zona[33].

Recently, the PH-20 protein has been shown to have hyaluronidase activity[76] and this protein has been localized on the plasma membrane of acrosome intact sperm of mice and humans[76], as well as non-human primates[77]. In this location, membrane bound hyaluronidase could depolymerize the cumulus ECM in the immediate vicinity of the acrosome intact, fertilizing sperm. It has also been proposed that acrosomal enzymes, including hyaluronidase, may escape from the acrosome before completion of the morphological acrosome reaction[33]. In addition to the sperm surface enzymes which may depolymerize the cumulus ECM, vigorous sperm flagellar activity is probably required for cumulus penetration, as discussed previously.

Sperm interaction with the zona pellucida

The membranes of mammalian sperm include a number of molecules with strong affinity for the zona pellucida of the oocyte[33]. The most widely accepted model for sperm–zona binding in mammals is based on studies of fertilization in mice. In this model the specific recognition between gametes is mediated by carbohydrate binding proteins on the sperm surface and glycoconjugates on the zona pellucida[78]. Two zona components that bind to sperm have been identified. The ZP-3 glycoprotein is involved in primary binding to the plasma membrane of the acrosome intact mouse sperm[79] and ZP-3 also has the capability of inducing the acrosome reaction of bound spermatozoa[80]. Acrosome reacted mouse sperm appear to bind by the inner acrosomal membrane to the ZP-2 glycoprotein[81–83]. This phase of sperm–zona pellucida interaction is termed secondary binding and also may have a function during sperm penetration of the zona (see below).

A variety of molecules in several species have been identified as potential sperm receptors for the zona pellucida and it is possible that sperm binding may involve multiple ligands[84]. Many zona binding molecules are enzymes, although their zona binding function may not be enzymatic. These sperm enzymes include galactosyl transferase[85,86], a tyrosine kinase[87], -D-mannosidase[88] and proacrosin/acrosin[89,90], as well as the PH-20 protein[91] which has hyaluronidase activity[76].

The acrosome reaction of the fertilizing sperm is believed to result as a consequence of primary sperm–zona binding and may be controlled by signal transduction pathways which are common to other cell systems[33]. Capacitation may result in the loss of coating substances from the sperm surface and the exposure of zona receptors such as the mannose binding ligand[42]. As a result of binding to ZP-3 the sperm receptors aggregate[92]. A signal transduction cascade follows receptor aggregation and may involve a guanosyl nucleotide regulating (G) protein and phospholipase C (PLC)[93,94]. In this model, PLC acts on membrane phosphatidyl inositol diphosphate (PIP_2) to produce inositol triphosphate (IP_3) and thereby release intracellular calcium. Phospholipase C also may produce diacyl glycerol which promotes protein phosphorylation. Methylation of a part of IP_3 produces IP_4, which may open voltage-dependent membrane calcium channels[95]. Increased intracellular calcium is thought to facilitate membrane fusion by promotion of phase transition and separation of membrane phospholipids. The activated G protein may act on membrane phospholipids to produce fusogenic lipids such as lysophosphatidyl choline, arachidonic acid and phosphatidic acid. It may also act through the adenylate cyclase pathway to elevate cAMP, which is required for protein phosphorylation and the $Na+/H+$ flux that raises intra-acrosomal pH. Other models envision that receptor–ligand interactions open sperm membrane ion channels for calcium[96] or that progesterone binds and aggregates membrane steroid receptors to allow calcium influx[35].

After the acrosome reaction the sperm appears to be more firmly attached to the zona[65,67,70], and the acrosomal remnant or shroud may tether the sperm to the zona prior to penetration[65]. At the ultrastructural level this remnant can be found associated with sperm penetrating the zona[97], or on the zona surface of fertilized oocytes[98,99].

Penetration of the zona pellucida is very rapid even *in vitro*, requiring 4–11 min in hamsters[100] and 15–26 min in mice[101]. Vigorous flagellar activity is characteristic of sperm movement during zona penetration[100,101]. The highly condensed nucleus, extremely flattened head and hardened perforatorium of the mammalian sperm may facilitate shearing of the zona material[102]. The sperm flagellar movements during zona penetration have been compared to those of a lever, and they have been suggested to produce forces capable of breaking molecular bonds[103]. In some species, acrosin activity has been localized to the surface of the sperm head after the acrosome reaction[104], and this enzyme may facilitate penetration by disrupting the zona matrix surrounding the sperm head. Acrosin or proacrosin also may play a role in secondary sperm–zona binding[89,90], which could involve sequential building and release of the sperm head as it traverses the zona pellucida. Because of the location of PH-20 on the inner acrosomal membrane, this protein could also have a function in secondary sperm–zona binding[77].

Sperm fusion and incorporation into the oocyte

Following penetration of the zona pellucida, the sperm enters the perivitelline space (PVS). The composition of the fluid in the PVS is unknown, but it appears to be rich in hyaluronic acid[105]. The inner acrosomal membrane is the first region of the sperm to contact the oolemma[33], but this is not the region in which sperm–oocyte membrane fusion takes place. Although the inner acrosomal membrane is the site of sperm–oocyte fusion in all other mammalian species as well as other vertebrates and invertebrates, eutherian mammals initiate fusion beginning with the plasma membrane over the equatorial segment and continuing with the posterior region of the sperm head, midpiece and tail[33].

Only acrosome-reacted spermatozoa are capable of fusing with oocytes, but the mechanism by which the equatorial region becomes fusogenic is not known. One possibility is that acrosomal contents such as acrosin, which are released during the acrosome reaction, alter this region[106]. Another possibility is that fusogenic membrane components migrate to this region as a result of the acrosome reaction[107]. Sperm fusion is initiated immediately following sperm entry into the PVS, and within seconds of membrane fusion sperm tail movement ceases, perhaps because of a calcium influx or depolarization of the sperm tail membrane[33].

A number of molecules have been suggested to mediate sperm–oocyte fusion including galactosyl transferase in mice[108], 40-kDa protein in mice[109], 37-kDa protein in rats[110], 43-kDa protein in humans[111], fertilin (PH-30) in guinea pigs[112] and fibronectin and vitronectin in humans[113].

The oolemma of mammalian oocytes expresses integrin-like molecules[114]. Integrins are a family of cell adhesion receptors composed of two glycopeptides termed the α and β subunits[115]. Integrins bind extracellular matrix ligands such as collagen, laminin and fibronectin; their specificity is determined by their subunit composition. Integrins mediate cell–cell adhesion by binding to cellular membrane proteins, and they may also regulate cell behavior by signal transduction in response to binding of a ligand[115]. One of the amino acid recognition sequences of the integrin ligands is Arg-Gly-Asp (RGD)[116] and this sequence is present on extracellular matrix proteins including fibronectin, vitronectin, collagen type I and laminin[117]. Fibronectin and vitronectin are both expressed on human sperm[113,118]. One subunit of the fertilin protein in guinea pigs has high homology with another family of integrin ligands, the disintegrins[112,119]. The second subunit of fertilin resembles a viral fusion protein[119]. Recent experiments have demonstrated inhibition of sperm–egg fusion by small peptides with the RGD sequence[118,120] and with peptide analogs of the putative integrin binding sequence of fertilin[121].

The inner acrosomal membrane of eutherian sperm is incorporated into the oocyte by a process which is entirely different from membrane fusion and which involves engulfment by the oocyte[71]. Bedford[122] has hypothesized that unusual stability of the inner acrosomal membrane is required to produce the shearing forces needed for penetration of the resilient zona pellucida, which also is characteristic of placental mammals. This structural stability, in turn, may necessitate unique sperm incorporation mechanisms by the oocyte. The stability of the inner acrosomal membrane is clearly evident from its persistence as a recognizable structure in the ooplasm after sperm nucleus decondensation[71]. Although the sperm is frequently described as being incorporated into the oocyte in a 'phagocytic manner'[33], virtually nothing is known about the signals which initiate the process or the cellular mechanisms by which it is accomplished.

SPERM DYSFUNCTION *IN VIVO* AND INFERTILITY

The results of treatment with assisted reproductive technologies (ART) in couples with unexplained infertility and male-factor infertility suggest that sperm dysfunction *in vivo* may be a significant factor in the etiology of reproductive failure. Some investigators have reported fertilization rates for couples with unexplained infertility which are comparable to those of patients with tubal infertility[123]. In diagnosed male-factor infertility, where there are identifiable abnormalities of sperm function, spermatozoa often are capable of fertilization *in vitro*[124–126]. These outcomes are consistent with the interpretation that abnormal sperm interaction with the female is a major contributor to the infertility of these couples. In a number of studies, gamete intrafallopian transfer (GIFT) has been as successful or more successful than *in vitro* fertilization (IVF) in producing pregnancies[127–129]. These reports also support the hypothesis that disorders of sperm physiology *in vivo* as well as fertilization dysfunction play a significant role in the etiology of infertility.

There are very few therapeutic options other than ART which are currently available for management of couples with male-factor or unexplained infertility. This situation is due largely to our lack of understanding of the causes of these types of infertility. In the absence of effective medical and surgical therapy, improvements in reproductive technology which target the sperm cells rather than the patient have had the greatest impact on clinical practice. The recent advances in sperm micromanipulation suggest that patients with sperm dysfunctions of diverse etiologies can be treated successfully with ART[130,131]. It is important that research on normal sperm physiology in the female tract, as well as the abnormal cell biology of male infertility, proceeds in parallel with the development and improvement of ART. There are well recognized medical complications associated with ART and the pregnancies obtained using this technology[132] and the cost of these procedures is high. Therefore, less invasive and more economical approaches for treatment of infertility are needed, as well as reliable diagnostic tests which identify those patients for whom the benefits of assisted reproductive technologies clearly outweigh its costs. These new tests and therapeutic approaches will be developed as our basic knowledge of sperm physiology in the female increases.

References

1. Blandau, R. J. (1969). Gamete transport – comparative aspects. In Hafez, E. S. E. and Blandau, R. J. (eds.) *The Mammalian Oviduct*, pp. 129–62. (Chicago: University of Chicago Press)
2. Mortimer, D. (1978). Selectivity of sperm transport in the female genital tract. In Cohen, J. and Hendry, W. F. (eds.) *Spermatozoa, Antibodies and Infertility*, pp. 37–53. (Blackwell: Oxford)
3. Overstreet, J. W. (1983). Transport of gametes in the reproductive tract of the female mammal. In Hartmann, J. F. (ed.) *Mechanism and Control of Animal Fertilization*, pp. 499–543. (Academic Press: New York)
4. Drobnis, E. Z. and Overstreet, J. W. (1992). The natural history of mammalian spermatozoa in the female reproductive tract. In Milligan, S. (ed.) *Oxford Reviews of Reproductive Biology*, Vol. 14, pp. 1–45. (Oxford: Oxford University Press)
5. Overstreet, J. W. and Katz, D. F. (1990). Interaction between the female reproductive tract and spermatozoa. In Gagnon, C. (ed.) *Controls of Sperm Motility*, pp. 63–75. (Boca Raton: CRC Press Inc.)
6. Overstreet, J. W. and Cooper, G. W. (1978). Sperm transport in the reproductive tract of the female rabbit: I. The rapid transit phase of transport. *Biol. Reprod.*, **19**, 101–14
7. Settlage, D. S. F., Motoshima, M. and Tredway, D. R. (1973). Sperm transport from the external cervical os to the fallopian tubes in women: A time and quantitation study. *Fertil. Steril.*, **24**, 655–61
8. Fox, C. A., Wolff, H. S. and Baker, J. A. (1970). Measurement of intravaginal and intrauterine pressure during human coitus by radiotelemetry. *J. Reprod. Fertil.*, **22**, 243–51
9. Overstreet, J. W. and Tom, R. A. (1982).

Experimental studies of rapid sperm transport in rabbits. *J. Reprod. Fertil.*, **66**, 601–6
10. Oates, R. D. and Lipshultz, L. I. (1993). Emission and ejaculation. In Krane, R.J., Siroky, M. B. and Goldstein, I. (eds.) *Male Sexual Dysfunction*, 2nd edn., (Boston: Little Brown & Co.)
11. Sobrero, A. J. and MacLeod, J. (1962). The immediate post-coital test. *Fertil. Steril.*, **13**, 184–9
12. Masters, W. H. and Johnson, V. E. (1966). *Human Sexual Response*. (Boston, Little, Brown & Co.)
13. Fox, C. A., Meldrum, S. J. and Watson, B. W. (1973). Continuous measurement by radiotelemetry of vaginal pH during human coitus. *J. Reprod. Fertil.*, **33**, 69–75
14. Hunter, R. H. F. (1987). Human fertilization *in vivo*, with special reference to progression, storage and release of competent spermatozoa. *Hum. Reprod.*, **2**, 329–32
15. James, K. and Hargreave, T. B. (1984). Immunosuppression by seminal plasma and its possible clinical significance. *Immunol. Today*, **5**, 357–63
16. Witkin, S. S. (1990). Sensitization to sperm as a risk factor for the heterosexual transmission of HIV. In Alexander, N. J., Gabelnick, H. L. and Spieler, J. M. (eds.) *Heterosexual Transmission of AIDS*, pp. 205–11. (New York: Wiley-Liss)
17. Overstreet, J. W. and Mahi-Brown, C. A. (1993). Sperm processing in the female reproductive tract. In Griffin, P. D. and Johnson, P. M. (eds.) *Local Immunity in Reproduction Tract Tissues*, pp. 321–34. (Oxford: Oxford University Press)
18. Jaszczak, S. and Hafez, E. S. E. (1973). Sperm migration through the uterine cervix in the macaque during the menstrual cycle. *Am. J. Obstet. Gynecol.*, **115**, 1070–82
19. Behboodi, E., Katz, D. F., Overstreet, J. W. and Hendrickx, A. G. (1989). Movement of cynomolgus and rhesus monkey spermatozoa collected from the lower female reproductive tract. *Gamete Res.*, **24**, 333–42
20. Hawk, H. W. (1987). Transport and fate of spermatozoa after insemination of cattle. *J. Dairy Sci.*, **70**, 1487–503
21. Overstreet, J. W., Katz, D. F. and Yudin, A. I. (1991). Cervical mucus and sperm transport in reproduction. *Semin. Perinatol.*, **15**, 149–55
22. Overstreet, J. W., Cooper, G. W. and Katz, D. F. (1978). Sperm transport in the reproductive tract of the female rabbit: II. The sustained phase of transport. *Biol. Reprod.*, **19**, 115-32
23. Hanson, F. W. and Overstreet, J. W. (1981). The interaction of human spermatozoa with cervical mucus *in vivo*. *Am. J. Obstet. Gynecol.*, **140**, 173–8
24. Gould, J. E., Overstreet, J. W. and Hanson, F. W. (1984). Assessment of human sperm function after recovery from the female reproductive tract. *Biol. Reprod.*, **31**, 888–94
25. Zinaman, M., Drobnis, E. Z., Morales, P., Brazil, C., Kiel, M., Cross, N. L., Hanson, F. W. and Overstreet, J. W. (1989). The physiology of sperm recovered from the human cervix: acrosomal status and response to inducers of the acrosome reaction. *Biol. Reprod.*, **41**, 790–7
26. Tredway, D. R., Buchanan, G. C. and Drake, T. S. (1978). Comparison of the fractional postcoital test and semen analysis. *Am. J. Obstet. Gynecol.*, **130**, 647–52
27. Hanson, F. W., Overstreet, J. W. and Katz, D. F. (1982). A study of the relationship of motile sperm numbers in cervical mucus 48 hours after artificial insemination with subsequent fertility. *Am. J. Obstet. Gynecol.*, **143**, 85–90
28. Boyers, S. P. (1994). Evaluation and treatment of disorders of the cervix. In Keye, W. R., Chang, R. J., Rebar, R. W. and Soules M. (eds.) *Infertility: Evaluation and Treatment* (New York: WB Saunders)
29. Doak, R. L., Hall, A. and Dale, H. E. (1967). Longevity of spermatozoa in the reproductive tract of the bitch. *J. Reprod. Fertil.*, **13**, 51–8
30. Williams, M., Hill, C. J., Scudamore, I., Dunphy, B., Cooke, I. D. and Barratt, C. L. R. (1993). Sperm numbers and distribution within the human Fallopian tube around ovulation. *Hum. Reprod.*, **8**, 2019–26
31. Overstreet, J. W. and VandeVoort, C. A. (1993). Sperm–zona pellucida interaction in macaque. In Wolf, D. P., Brenner, R. M. and Stouffer, R. L. (eds.) *In Vitro Fertilization and Embryo Transfer in Primates*, pp. 103–9. (New York: Springer-Verlag)
32. Eddy, E. M. and O'Brien, D. A. (1994). The spermatozoon. In Knobil, E. and O'Neill, J. D. (eds.) *The Physiology of Reproduction*, 2nd edn, pp. 29–78. (New York: Raven Press)
33. Yanagimachi, R. (1994). Mammalian fertilization. In Knobil, E. and O'Neill, J. D. (eds.) *The Physiology of Reproduction*, 2nd edn, pp. 189–317. (New York: Raven Press)
34. Bedford, J. M. (1994). The contraceptive potential of fertilization: a physiological perspective. *Hum. Reprod.*, **9**, 842–58
35. Thomas, P. and Meizel, S. (1989). Phosphatidylinositol 4,5-biphosphate hydrolysis in human sperm stimulated with follicular fluid or progesterone is dependent upon Ca^{2+} influx. *Biochem. J.*, **264**, 539–46
36. Mahanes, M. S., Ochs, D. L. and Eng, L. A. (1986). Cell calcium of ejaculated rabbit spermatozoa before and following *in vitro* capacitation. *Biochem. Biophys. Res. Commun.*, **134**, 664–70
37. Kanwar, K. C., Yanagimachi, R. and Lopata, A. (1979). Effects of human seminal plasma on fertilizing capacity of human spermatozoa. *Fertil. Steril.*, **31**, 321–7
38. Bearer, E. L. and Friend, D. S. (1982). Modifications of anionic–lipid domains preceding membrane fusion in guinea pig sperm. *J. Cell Biol.*, **92**, 604–15

39. Parks, J. E. and Ehrenwalt, E. (1990). Cholesterol efflux from mammalian sperm and its potential role in capacitation. In Bavister, B. D., Cummins, J. and Raldan, E. (eds.) *Fertilization in Mammals*, pp. 155. (Norwell, MA: Serono Symposia USA)
40. Ravnik, S. E., Zarutskie, P. W. and Muller, C. H. (1992). Purification and characterization of a human follicular fluid lipid transfer protein that stimulates human sperm capacitation. *Biol. Reprod.*, **47**, 1126–33
41. Benoff, S., Cooper, G. W., Hurley, I., Napolitano, B., Rosenfeld, D. L., Scholl, G. M. and Hershlag, A. (1993). Human sperm fertilizing potential *in vitro* is correlated with differential expression of a head specific mannose–ligand receptor. *Fertil. Steril.*, **59**, 854–62
42. Benoff, S., Hurley, I., Cooper, G. W., Mandel, F. S., Hershlag, A., Scholl, G. M. and Rosenfeld, D. L. (1993). Fertilization potential *in vitro* is correlated with head-specific mannose ligand receptor expression, acrosome status, and membrane cholesterol content. *Hum. Reprod.*, **8**, 2155–66
43. Suarez, S. S., Wolf, D. P. and Meizel, S. (1986). Induction of the acrosome reaction in human spermatozoa by a fraction of human follicular fluid. *Gamete Res.*, **14**, 107–21
44. Cross, N. L., Morales, P., Overstreet, J. W. and Hanson, F. W. (1988). Induction of acrosome reactions by the human zona pellucida. *Biol. Reprod.*, **38**, 235–44
45. Bedford, J. M. (1970). Sperm capacitation and fertilization in mammals. *Biol. Reprod.*, **2** (Suppl. 2), 128–58
46. Bedford, J. M. (1983). Significance of the need for sperm capacitation before fertilization in eutherian mammals. *Biol. Reprod.*, **28**, 108–20
47. Overstreet, J. W. and Drobnis, E. Z. (1992). Sperm transport in the female tract. In Barratt, C. L. R. and Cooke, I. D. (eds.) *Advances in Donor Insemination*, pp. 33–49. (Cambridge: Cambridge University Press)
48. VandeVoort, C. A., Tollner, T. L., Tarantal, A. F. and Overstreet, J. W. (1989). Ultrasound-guided transfundal uterine sperm recovery from *Macaca fascicularis*. *Gamete Res.*, **24**, 327–31
49. Jansen, R. P. S. (1978). Fallopian tube isthmic mucus and ovum transport. *Science*, **201**, 349–51
50. Burkman, L. J., Overstreet, J. W. and Katz, D. F. (1984). A possible role for potassium and pyruvate in the modulation of sperm motility in the rabbit oviductal isthmus. *J. Reprod. Fertil.*, **71**, 367–76
51. Cooper, G. W., Overstreet, J. W. and Katz, D. F. (1979). The motility of rabbit spermatozoa recovered from the female reproductive tract. *Gamete Res.*, **2**, 35–42
52. Suarez, S. S. (1987). Sperm transport and motility in the mouse oviduct: observations *in situ*. *Biol. Reprod.*, **36**, 203–10
53. Smith, T. T. and Yanagimachi, R. (1989). Capacitation status of hamster spermatozoa in the oviduct at various times after mating. *J. Reprod. Fertil.*, **86**, 255–61
54. Battalia, D. E. and Yanagimachi, R. (1979). Enhanced and coordinated movement of the hamster oviduct during the periovulatory period. *J. Reprod. Fertil.*, **56**, 515–20
55. Suarez, S. S., Katz, D. F., Owen, D. H., Andrew, J. B. and Powell, R. L. (1991). Evidence for the function of hyperactivated motility in sperm. *Biol. Reprod.*, **44**, 375–81
56. Katz, D. F., Drobnis, E. Z. and Overstreet, J. W. (1989). Factors regulating mammalian sperm migration through the female reproductive tract and oocyte vestments. *Gamete Res.*, **22**, 443–69
57. Talbot, P. (1985). Sperm penetration through oocyte investments in mammals. *Am. J. Anat.*, **174**, 331–46
58. Cherr, G. N., Yudin, A. I. and Katz, D. F. (1990). Organization of the hamster cumulus extracellular matrix: a hyaluronate–glycoprotein gel which modulates sperm access to the oocyte. *Dev. Growth Diff.*, **32**, 353–65
59. Bedford, J. M. and Kim, H. H. (1993). Cumulus oophorus as a sperm sequestering device, *in vivo*. *J. Exp. Zool.*, **265**, 321–8
60. Ralt, D., Manor, M., Cohen-Dayag, A., Tur-Kaspa, I., Ben-Shlomo, I., Makler, A., Yuli, I., Dor, J., Blumberg, S., Mashiach, S. and Eisenbach, M. (1994). Chemotaxis and chemokinesis of human spermatozoa to follicular factors. *Biol. Reprod.*, **50**, 774–85
61. Cohen-Dayag, A., Ralt, D., Tur-Kaspa, I., Manor, M., Makler, A., Dor, J., Mashiach, S. and Eisenbach, M. (1994). Sequential acquisition of chemotactic responsiveness by human spermatozoa. *Biol. Reprod.*, **50**, 786–90
62. Eppig, J. J. (1982). The relationship between cumulus cell–oocyte coupling, oocyte meiotic maturation, and cumulus expansion. *Dev. Biol.*, **89**, 268–72
63. Drahorad, J., Tesarik, J., Cechova, D. and Vilim, V. (1991). Proteins and glycosaminoglycans in the intercellular matrix of the human cumulus oophorus and their effect on conversion of proacrosin to acrosin. *J. Reprod. Fertil.*, **93**, 253–62
64. Yudin, A. I., Cherr, G. N. and Katz, D. F. (1988). Structure of the cumulus matrix and zona pellucida in the golden hamster: A new view of sperm interaction with oocyte-associated extracellular matrices. *Cell Tissue Res.*, **251**, 555–64
65. Drobnis, E. Z., Yudin, A. I., Cherr, G. N. and Katz, D. F. (1988). Kinematics of hamster sperm during penetration of the cumulus cell matrix. *Gamete Res.*, **21**, 367–83
66. Cummins, J. M. and Yanagimachi, R. (1982). Sperm–egg ratios and the site of the acrosome reaction during *in vivo* fertilization in the hamster. *Gamete Res.*, **5**, 239–56
67. Cherr, G. N., Lambert, H., Meizel, S. and Katz, D. F. (1986). *In vitro* studies on the golden hamster sperm acrosome reaction: completion on the zona pellucida and induction by homologous soluble zonae pellucidae. *Dev. Biol.*, **114**, 119–31

68. Corselli, J. and Talbot, P. (1987). *In vitro* penetration of hamster oocyte–cumulus complexes using physiological numbers of sperm. *Dev. Biol.*, **122**, 227–42
69. Cummins, J. M. and Yanagimachi, R. (1986). Development of ability to penetrate the cumulus oophorus by hamster spermatozoa capacitated *in vitro* in relation to the timing of the acrosome reaction. *Gamete Res.*, **15**, 187–212
70. Suarez, S. S., Katz, D. F. and Meizel, S. (1984). Changes in motility that accompany the acrosome reaction in hyperactivated hamster spermatozoa. *Gamete Res.*, **10**, 253–65
71. Bedford, J. M. (1972). An electron microscopic study of sperm penetration into the rabbit egg after natural mating. *Am. J. Anat.*, **133**, 213–54
72. Saling, P. M., Bunch, D. O., Le Guen, P. and Leyton, L. (1990). ZP3-induced acrosomal exocytosis: a new model for triggering. In Bavister, B. D., Cummins, J. and Roldan, E. R. S. (eds.) *Fertilization in Mammals*, pp. 239–52. (Norwell, MA: Serono Symposia)
73. Saling, P. M., Sowinski, J. and Storey, B. T. (1979). An ultrastructural study of epididymal mouse spermatozoa binding to zonae pellucidae *in vitro*: sequential relationship to the acrosome reaction. *J. Exp. Zool.*, **209**, 229–38
74. Saling, P. M. and Storey, B. T. (1979). Mouse gamete interactions during fertilization *in vitro*. Chlortetracycline as a fluorescent probe for the mouse acrosome reaction. *J. Cell Biol.*, **83**, 544–55
75. Florman, H. M. and Storey, B. T. (1982). Mouse gamete interactions: the zona pellucida is the site of the acrosome reaction leading to fertilization *in vitro*. *Dev. Biol.*, **91**, 121–30
76. Lin, Y., Mahan, K., Lathrop, W. F., Myles, D. G. and Primakoff, P. (1994). A hyaluronidase activity of the sperm plasma membrane protein PH-20 enables sperm to penetrate the cumulus cell layer surrounding the egg. *J. Cell Biol.*, **111**, 1839–47
77. Overstreet, J. W., Lin, Y., Yudin, A. I., Meyers, S. A., Primakoff, P., Myles, D. G., Katz, D. F. and VandeVoort, C. A. (1995). Location of the PH-20 protein on acrosome intact and acrosome reacted spermatozoa of cynomolgus macaques. *Biol. Reprod.*, **52**, 105–14
78. Wassarman, P. M. (1992). Mouse gamete adhesion molecules. *Biol. Reprod.*, **46**, 86–91
79. Bleil, J. D. and Wassarman, P. M. (1980). Mammalian sperm-egg interaction: identification of a glycoprotein in mouse egg zonae pellucidae possessing receptor activity for sperm. *Cell*, **20**, 873–82
80. Bleil, J. D. and Wassarman, P. M. (1983). Sperm–egg interactions in the mouse: Sequence of events and induction of the acrosome reaction by a zona pellucida glycoprotein. *Dev. Biol.*, **95**, 317–24
81. Bleil, J. D. and Wassarman, P. M. (1986). Autoradiographic visualization of the mouse egg's sperm receptor bound to sperm. *J. Cell Biol.*, **102**, 1363–71
82. Bleil, J. D., Greve, J. M. and Wassarman, P. M. (1988). Identification of a secondary sperm receptor in the mouse egg zona pellucida: role in maintenance of binding of acrosome reacted sperm to eggs. *Dev. Biol.*, **128**, 376–85
83. Mortillo, S. and Wassarman, P. M. (1991). Differential binding of gold-labeled zona pellucida glycoproteins mZP2 and mZP3 to mouse sperm membrane compartments. *Development*, **113**, 141–9
84. O'Rand, M. G. (1989). Sperm–egg recognition and barriers to interspecies fertilization. *Gamete Res.*, **19**, 315–26
85. Shur, B. D. and Hall, N. G. (1982). A role for mouse sperm surface galactosyltransferase in sperm binding to the egg zona pellucida. *J. Cell Biol.*, **95**, 574–9
86. Lopez, L. C.,. Bayna, E. M., Litoff, D., Shaper, N. L., Shaper, J. H. and Shur, B. D. (1985). Receptor function of mouse sperm surface galactosyltransferase during fertilization. *J. Cell Biol.*, **101**, 1501–10
87. Leyton, L. and Saling, P. (1989). 95kd sperm proteins bind ZP3 and serve as tyrosine kinase substrates in response to zona binding. *Cell*, **57**, 1123–30
88. Tulsiani, D. R. P., Skudlarek, M. D. and Orgebin-Crist, M. C. (1990). Human sperm plasma membranes possess D-mannosidase activity but no galactosyltransferase activity. *Biol. Reprod.*, **42**, 843–58
89. Jones, R. (1991). Interaction of zona pellucida glycoproteins, sulphated carbohydrates and synthetic polymers with proacrosin, the putative egg-binding protein from mammalian spermatozoa. *Development*, **111**, 1155–63
90. Urch, U. A. and Patel, H. (1991). The interaction of boar sperm proacrosin with its natural substrate, the zona pellucida, and with polysulfated polysaccharides. *Development*, **111**, 1165–72.
91. Primakoff, P., Hyatt, H. and Myles, D. G. (1985). A role for the migrating sperm surface antigen PH-20 in guinea pig sperm binding to the egg zona pellucida. *J. Cell Biol.*, **101**, 2239–44
92. Leyton, L. and Saling, P. (1989). Evidence that aggregation of mouse sperm receptors by ZP3 triggers the acrosome reaction. *J. Cell Biol.*, **108**, 2163–8
93. Kopf, G. S. (1990). Zona pellucida-mediated signal transduction in mammalian spermatozoa. *J. Reprod. Fert. Suppl.*, **42**, 33–49
94. Saling, P. M. (1991). How the egg regulates sperm function during gamete interaction: facts and fantasies. *Biol. Reprod.*, **44**, 246–51
95. Florman, H. M., Corron, M. E., Kim, T. D. H. and Babcock, D. F. (1992). Activation of voltage-dependent calcium channels of mammalian sperm is required for zona pellucida-induced acrosomal exocytosis. *Dev. Biol.*, **152**, 304–14
96. Harrison, R. A. P. and Roldan, E. R. S. (1990). Phosphoinositudes and their products in the mammalian sperm acrosome reaction. *J. Reprod. Fert. Suppl.*, **42**, 51–67

97. Yanagimachi, R. and Phillips, D. M. (1984). The status of acrosomal caps of hamster spermatozoa immediately before fertilization *in vivo*. *Gamete Res.*, **9**, 1–19
98. Crozet, N. (1984). Ultrastructural aspects of *in vivo* fertilization in the cow. *Gamete Res.*, **10**, 241–51
99. Crozet, N. and Dumont, M. (1984). The site of the acrosome reaction during *in vivo* penetration of the sheep oocyte. *Gamete Res.*, **10**, 97–105
100. Yang, W. H., Lin, L. L., Wang, J. R. and Chang, M. C. (1972). Sperm penetration through zona pellucida and perivitelline space in the hamster. *J. Exp. Zool.*, **179**, 191–206
101. Sato, K. and Blandau, R. J. (1979). Time and process of sperm penetration into cumulus-free mouse eggs fertilized *in vitro*. *Gamete Res.*, **2**, 295–304
102. Moore, H. D. M. and Bedford, J. M. (1983). The interaction of mammalian gametes in the female. In Hartman, J. R. (ed.) *Mechanism and Control of Animal Fertilization*, pp. 453–92. (New York: Academic Press)
103. Drobnis, E. Z., Yudin, A. I., Cherr, G. N. and Katz, D. F. (1988). Hamster sperm penetration of the zona pellucida: kinematic analysis and mechanical implications. *Dev. Biol.*, **130**, 311–23
104. Barros, C., Capote, C., Perez, C., Crosby, J. A., Becker, M. I. and DeIoannes, A. (1992). Immunodetection of acrosin during the acrosome reaction of the hamster, guinea-pig and human spermatozoa. *Biol. Res.*, **25**, 31–40
105. Kan, F. W. K. (1990). High resolution localization of hyaluronic acid in the golden hamster oocyte–cumulus complex by use of a hyaluronidase-gold complex. *Anat. Rec.*, **228**, 370–82
106. Dravland, J. W. and Meizel, S. (1981). Stimulation of sperm capacitation and acrosome reaction *in vitro* by glucose and lactate and the inhibition by glycolytic inhibitor alpha-chlorohydrin. *Gamete Res.*, **4**, 515–23
107. Villarroya, S. and Scholler, R. (1987). Lateral diffusion of a human sperm-head antigen during incubation in a capacitation medium and induction of the acrosome reaction *in vivo*. *J. Reprod. Fertil.*, **80**, 545–62
108. Lopez, L. C. and Shur, B. D. (1987). Redistribution of mouse sperm surface galactosyltransferase after the acrosome reaction. *J. Cell Biol.*, **105**, 1663–70
109. Saling, P. M., Raines, L. M. and O'Rand, M. G. (1983). Monoclonal antibody against mouse sperm blocks a specific event in the fertilization process. *J. Exp. Zool.*, **227**, 481–6
110. Rochwerger, L., Cohen, D. J. and Cuasnicu, P. S. (1992). Mammalian sperm–egg fusion: the rat egg has complementary sites for a sperm protein that mediates gamete fusion. *Dev. Biol.*, **153**, 83–90
111. Okabe, M., Matzno, S., Nagira, M., Kohama, Y. and Mimura, T. (1990). A human sperm antigen possible involved in binding and/or fusion with zona-free hamster eggs. *Fertil. Steril.*, **54**, 1121–6
112. Primakoff, P., Hyatt, H. and Tredick-Kline, J. (1987). Identification and purification of a sperm surface protein with a potential role in sperm–egg membrane fusion. *J. Cell Biol.*, **104**, 141–9
113. Fusi, F. and Bronson, R. A. (1992). Sperm surface fibronectin: expression following capacitation. *J. Androl.*, **13**, 28–35
114. Fusi, F. M., Vignalli, M., Gailit, J. and Bronson, R. A. (1993). Mammalian oocytes exhibit specific recognition of the RGD (Arg-Gly-Asp) tripeptide and express oolemmal integrins. *Mol. Reprod. Dev.*, **36**, 212–19
115. Hynes, R. O. (1992). Integrins: Versatility, modulation, and signaling in cell adhesion. *Cell*, **69**, 11–25
116. Ruoslahti, E. and Pierschbacher, M. D. (1987). New perspectives in cell adhesion: RGD and integrins. *Science*, **238**, 491–7
117. Yamada, K. M. (1991). Adhesive recognition sequences. *J. Biol. Chem.*, **266**, 12809–12
118. Fusi, F. M., Vignalli, M., Busacca, M. and Bronson, R. A. (1992). Evidence for the presence of an integrin cell adhesion receptor on the oolemma of unfertilized human oocytes. *Mol. Reprod. Dev.*, **31**, 215–22
119. Blobel, C. P., Wolfsberg, T. G., Turck, C. W., Myles, D. G., Primakoff, P. and White, J. M. (1992). A potential fusion peptide in an integrin ligand domain in a protein active in sperm-egg fusion. *Nature (Lond.)*, **356**, 248–52
120. Bronson, R. A. and Fusi, F. (1990). Evidence that an Arg-Gly-Asp (RGD) adhesion sequence plays a role in mammalian fertilization. *Biol. Reprod.*, **43**, 1019–25
121. Myles, D. G., Kimmel, L. H., Blobel, C. P., White, J. M. and Primakoff, P. (1994). Identification of a binding site in the disintegrin domain of fertilin required for sperm–egg fusion. *Proc. Natl Acad. Sci. USA*, **91**, 4195–8
122. Bedford, J. M. (1991). The co-evolution of mammalian gametes. In Dunbar, B. S. and O'Rand, M. G. (eds.) *A Comparative Overview of Mammalian Fertilization*, pp. 3–35. (New York: Plenum Press)
123. Fishel, S. B. and Edwards, R. G. (1982). Essentials of fertilization. In Edwards, G. D. and Purdy, J. (eds.) *Human Conception* In Vitro, pp. 157–79. (London: Academic Press)
124. Mahadevan, M. M. and Trounson, A. O. (1984). The influence of seminal characteristics on the success rate of human *in vitro* fertilization. *Fertil. Steril.*, **42**, 400–5
125. Kruger, T. F., Menkveld, R., Stander, F. S., Lombard, C. J., Van der Merwe, J. P., van Zyl, J. A. and Smith, K. (1986). Sperm morphologic features as a prognostic factor in *in vitro* fertilization. *Fertil. Steril.*, **46**, 1118–23
126. Oehninger, S., Acosta, A. A., Morshedi, M., Veeck, L., Swanson, R. J., Simmons, K. and Rosenwaks, Z. (1988). Corrective measures and pregnancy

outcome in *in vitro* fertilization in patients with severe sperm morphology abnormalities. *Fertil. Steril.*, **50**, 283–7

127. Leeton, J., Rogers, P., Caro, C., Healy, D. and Yates, C. (1987). A controlled study between the use of gamete intrafallopian transfer (GIFT) and *in vitro* fertilization and embryo transfer in the management of idiopathic and male infertility. *Fertil. Steril.*, **48**, 605–7
128. Matson, P. L., Blackledge, D. G., Richardson, P. A., Turner, S. R., Yovich, J. M. and Yovich, J. L. (1987). The role of gamete intrafallopian transfer (GIFT) in the treatment of oligospermic infertility. *Fertil. Steril.*, **48**, 608–16
129. Guastella, G., Comparetto, G., Palermo, R., Cefalu, E., Ciriminna, R. and Cittadini, E. (1986). Gamete intrafallopian transfer in the treatment of infertility: the first series at the University of Palermo. *Fertil. Steril.*, **46**, 417–23
130. Van Steirteghem, A. C., Liu, J., Joris, H., Nagy, Z., Janssenswillen, C., Tournaye, H., Derde, M. P., Van Assache, E. and Devroey, P. (1993). Higher success rate by intracytoplasmic sperm injection than by subzonal insemination. Report of a second series of 300 consecutive treatment cycles. *Hum. Reprod.*, **8**, 1055–60
131. Van Steirteghem, A. C., Nagy, Z., Joris, H., Liu, J., Staessen, C., Smitz, J., Wisanto, A. and Devroey, P. (1993). High fertilization and implantation rates after intracytoplasmic sperm injection. *Hum. Reprod.*, **8**, 1061–6
132. Schenker, J. G. and Ezra, Y. (1994). Complications of assisted reproductive techniques. *Fertil. Steril.*, **61**, 411–22

The fertilization process in the human 4

A. A. Acosta

INTRODUCTION

Fertilization, chronologically a relatively short process, is a complex sequence of co-ordinated molecular events in gamete interaction starting at gamete recognition and terminating at first cleavage division. Understanding this process is relevant to clinicians, since evaluation of its steps may define the levels at which fertilization can fail and allow corrective measures, can help to design tests demonstrating different modalities of fertilization arrest, and can allow interference with the process with contraception methods at the gamete interaction level.

The natural human process is almost unknown, and events in the *in vitro* setting have to be used to understand the *in vivo* process.

Fertilization involves the fusion of the gametes with activation of the oocyte and establishes the genotype of a new individual[1]. For a normal process to occur, the gametes should normally have undergone a complex process of proliferation, chromosomal exchange and reduction at meiosis, differentiation, maturation and transport. It ends with, first, the different membrane fusion steps that occur between the sperm and the oocyte and, second, the different levels of gamete interaction, until division (cleavage) begins.

Fusion processes may happen between not fully mature sperm and oocytes; *penetration* alone is accomplished without the normal subsequent steps occurring[2].

The process of fertilization can now be redefined as the chronologically short and normal sequence of co-ordinated molecular events involving normally matured haploid male and female gametes, determining fusion and penetration of a sperm into the oocyte with its subsequent activation; the process ends with a normal first cleavage division.

THE NORMAL HAPLOID MATURE SPERMATOZOON

The physiology of intratesticular Sertoli cell-dependent male germ cell division, differentiation and maturation is better understood than fertilization, but far from clear. In physiological conditions, spermatozoa that have completed intratesticular maturation need a process of extratesticular maturation to acquire full motility and fertilization capacities. Clinically, testicular biopsies and chromosome analysis are the only methods available to evaluate intratesticular male gamete preparations.

Extratesticular maturation occurs mainly at the epididymis and during transit through the male genital tract as interaction with seminal vesicles and prostate secretions occur.

Sperm epididymal maturation is associated with loss of total or individual phospholipids, loss of total protein, increase in adenosine 3′, 5′-cyclic monophosphate (cAMP), extensive modifications of energy metabolism, changes in lipoprotein content, differentiation and changes in size, shape, and internal structure of the acrosome, variations in cohesiveness between plasma and outer acrosomal membranes, migration of cytoplasmic droplets, increased disulfide bonds in the sperm tail with motility changes, alterations in the antigenic properties of the sperm surface, and a net increase in negative surface charge, possibly due to addition of sialic acid groups. Epididymal and male genital tract interaction with sperm forms a protein-coating layer of unknown physiological significance. The multiple modalities of semen evaluation (basic semen analysis, separation of motile fraction, test of sperm function) allow the clinician to evaluate semen and sperm quality after normal ejaculation.

Capacitation

To acquire fertilizing ability, the sperm needs activation in the female genital tract during natural fertilization; in *in vitro* fertilization, it is triggered by laboratory manipulation (incubation, washing, and separation procedures) performed as preliminary steps for assisted reproduction and assisted fertilization. First in sperm activation is capacitation, a reversible phenomenon allowing capacitation and decapacitation according to the experimental set-up. This step is calcium-dependent, takes between 2 and 22 h *in vitro*[3], with a mean of 5–6 h in men, involves activation of adenosine triphosphatase (ATPase), of free surface SH and NH2, and redistribution of glycoproteins and glycolipids on the surface with subsequent permeability changes of the membranes. Other steps involved are removal of seminal plasma-coating proteins and cell surface components, alteration of membrane cholesterol/phospholipid ratios and alterations of membrane potential[3]. Angiotensin converting enzyme (ACE) present in ejaculated human sperm is released during capacitation. ACE may participate in inducing acrosome reaction and in fertilization, since its inhibition reduces the percentage of acrosome reacted to sperm and the oocyte penetration rate in the hamster assay[4]. Capacitation can be defined as the biochemical changes increasing the permeability of the membranes to calcium ions[3]. No clinical marker is available to indicate initiation, presence or completion of capacitation, making it a pure molecular change with no morphological expression. Cumulus and follicular fluid glycosidases can enhance the process. Chang[5] demonstrated that the process is reversible and decapacitation factors have been found in bovine semen[3].

Hyperactivated motility

The second step in sperm activation after capacitation is the acquisition of hyperactivated motility[6]. Different patterns of hyperactivation are described, but definition and specificities of those patterns are not generally accepted; in the human, the exact parameters are not yet established. Patterns described are: circling, high curvature, flashing, helical and star spin. Hyperactivation is one indicator of sperm capacitation and can be evaluated by high-speed videomicrography with slow motion analysis, or standard videomicrography and time exposure analysis with computer assistance.

Acrosome reaction

The third component of sperm activation is acrosome reaction. This process starts normally at the time of sperm recognition and binding to the zona pellucida surface and can be artificially triggered by laboratory methods, and *in vivo* by cumulus oophorus cells and their secretions and follicular fluid content[7]. It seems to be necessary for some sperm at least to cross the outer layers of oocyte vestments intact to reach the zona pellucida (see below). Acrosome-intact and acrosome-reacted human sperm can initiate binding to the zona pellucida[8]. Most researchers believe that acrosome-intact sperm mainly initiate it, and acrosome reaction is rapidly triggered by zona pellucida–receptor interaction. Acrosome reaction is calcium-dependent, involving massive uptake of calcium and sodium with an efflux of hydrogen generating high pH and osmotic pressure, producing negative surface charge, and partial or total release of the acrosomal enzymes. Calcium influx may activate phospholipase A_2, resulting in accumulation of unsaturated fatty acids and fusiogenic lysophospholipids contributing to acrosome reaction[3]. Calmodulin may regulate phospholipase A_2 activity in the acrosomal region. Metallo-endoprotease release during acrosome reaction may act directly or indirectly to increase the fusibility of the sperm plasma region required for subsequent sperm–egg fusion[9]. Since acrosome reaction involves fusion of the plasma and outer acrosomal membranes, rapid conversion of proacrosine to acrosine which spread acrosome reaction, it seems that complete acrosome reaction will determine the disappearance of plasma membrane in which sperm receptors for binding to the zona pellucida are present. If acrosome-reacted sperm bind to the zona pellucida, it may imply that the acrosome reaction is only partial at the time of binding, with at least areas of intact plasma membrane having functional receptors still present to make possible recognition and binding. Acrosome reaction is not reversible, and the sperm viability afterwards is short. It can be demonstrated clinically by several

Table 1 Acrosome reaction tests

• Electron microscopy
• Triple staining (trypan blue–rose bengal–bismarck brown)
• Fluorescein isocyanate (FITC) conjugated lectins
soybean agglutinin
concanavalin A
Pisum sativum agglutinin (PSA)
Ricinus communis agglutinin (RCA)
Hoechst 33258 (supravital stain)
wheat sperm agglutinin
• Indirect immunofluorescence assay
monoclonal antibodies
HS-19; HS-21
T-15
T-6
TG (keratin-like protein)
• Chlortetracycline fluorescence assay

laboratory techniques, listed in Table 1, and transmission electromicroscopy.

It has been postulated that there is activated acrosine on the sperm surface before acrosome reaction occurs, suggesting the possibility of acrosine being involved in sperm responsiveness to egg signals, in the trigger of full acrosome reaction, and in the recognition and binding of zona pellucida[10].

Species-specific receptors on the plasma membrane of the sperm have been defined in terms of molecular structure. These receptors are glycoproteins that have been identified, isolated and characterized, for the most part, in the mouse but not in humans. Proteins considered as possible sperm receptor candidates participating in recognition and binding of the zona pellucida are listed in Table 2. In humans, αD-mannosidase has been mentioned as the protein/enzyme able to recognize and bind to the zona pellucida surface as a receptor[12]. More recently, Bennof[13] has proposed mannose as a component of the glycoprotein involved in binding (Annual Meeting of The American Fertility Society, Montreal, Canada 9–14 October, 1993). Whether a two-step process recognition or attachment and binding aided by two different receptor molecules (lectin/glycoprotein receptor) is necessary for the initial fertilization process to occur is still uncertain in the human. It is possible that recognition and binding will be part of a single step in which the protein/enzyme attaches to the substrate, forming an enzyme–substrate complex to initiate the process. It is the oligosaccharide moiety that gives the sperm the species-specificity characteristic of fertilization.

Table 2 Sperm receptor candidates

PH-20
P95
FA-1
RSA
GalTase
D-mannosidase
Fucosyltransferase
Acrosin
GBP (RHL)
Fucose/fucose sulfate
Trypsin inhibitor-sensitive site

Complete acrosome reaction exposes the inner acrosomal membrane and its contents; the equatorial and post-equatorial parts of the plasma membrane remain intact with their receptors for the sperm oocyte–oolemma fusion process to be valid. Clinically, the process of acrosome reaction can be determined by the different laboratory procedures previously mentioned, by electron microscopy, and the sperm's tight binding ability to the zona pellucida can be measured by the hemizona assay described by Burkman *et al.*[14].

OOCYTE AT THE TIME OF FERTILIZATION

The oocyte–cumulus complex (OCC) in the mature, ovulated or retrieved oocyte shows the corona cells loosely attached to each other surrounding the zona pellucida and the radially expanded cumulus cells with an abundant extracellular matrix. Glycosaminoglycans constitute the most important part of it. Their production under follicle stimulating hormone (FSH) control represents one of the most important anatomical and physiological characteristics of oocyte–cumulus complex maturation[15]. The extracellular matrix is composed of granules that are trypsin-sensitive and filaments of mostly hyaluronic acid.

The oocyte–corona–cumulus complex at the time of interaction *in vitro* shows a fully expanded cumulus and corona and the oocyte itself in the metaphase stage of the second meiotic division (MII) with the first polar body extruded. In the natural process of ovulation after the oocyte is picked up from the ovarian surface or from the cul-de-sac and has been in the tube for a while, the status of the corona–cumulus complex may be quite different from the one after oocyte retrieval before actual ovulation occurs. Very scanty information is available, indicating that, at that stage, most of the cumulus and a good part of the corona have already disappeared; therefore, the conditions that the sperm encounter could be quite different from the situation *in vitro*.

Nottala *et al.*[16] have studied the ultrastructure of the human cumulus corona (CC) cells at the time of fertilization and early embryogenesis by scanning and transmission electronmicroscopy after oocyte retrieval and fertilization from patients stimulated with clomiphene citrate, human menopausal gonadotropins and human chorionic gonadotropin. Numerous expanded and highly metabolic CC cells are found around both human unfertilized and *in vitro* fertilized preovulatory oocytes. They may create a more favorable environment for gametes and early cleaving preembryos by secreting steroids, nutrients and growth factors.

In the human zona pellucida three acidic proteins have been identified: ZP3, ZP2 and ZP1. Their molecular weights seem to be 57,000–73,000, 64,000–78,000 and 90,000–110,000, respectively. This non-cellular extracellular matrix plays a fundamental role in the initial steps of fertilization, and although the pure protein structure seems to be homogeneous in composition, foreign proteins are trapped in the external mesh of the zona pellucida incorporating heterogeneous components. Each of the zona pellucida proteins shows considerable heterogeneity by isoelectric focusing due to secondary modifications (glycosylation) of the polypeptide chain; they are all probably sulfated on the oligosaccharide side-chains. After fertilization, most likely due to the discharge of the cortical granules, there is clear loss of ZP1 (the main structural component), and a new component appears in a position similar to reduced ZP2[17]. ZP3, responsible for sperm oocyte binding, belongs to a family of functionally related highly species-conserved peptides; it shows around 1 billion copies in the zona pellucida and the *O*-linked carbohydrates seem to be responsible for binding[18]. The polypeptide component seems responsible for acrosome reaction. Several epitopes may be present in each particular receptor molecule: epitope I may be responsible for T-cell response of the immune system, and perhaps for auto-immune oophoritis when present; epitope II, responsible for B-cell response and the generation of anti-zona pellucida antibodies, which may induce reversible infertility; and epitope III, responsible for fertilization, the triggering of acrosome reaction by the polypeptide component, and for the binding by the O-linked carbohydrate. Organization and expression of the gene encoding ZP3 is much better understood; it is expressed at high levels by growing oocytes and no other cell type, at least in the mouse[19].

Underneath the zona pellucida, the perivitelline space (PVS) shows an accumulation of granules and filaments of hyaluronic acid; the latter can inhibit cell fusion.

During the process of oocyte maturation, bundles of microfilaments cover the inner surface of the oolemma, preventing cortical granule release. Activation of the cortical granules approaching the surface and their release is another expression of membrane fusion that must occur when meiosis is resumed after fertilization. Marked increase in mitochondria occurs at the same time.

During the process of maturation, the oocyte acquires competence progressively for the following functions: (1) germinal vesicle breakdown; (2) completion of meiosis I; (3) completion of meiosis II; and (4) pronuclear formation. Competence in these areas may be critical for early embryo development and normal implantation.

Evaluation of oocyte maturation and competency can be measured at present only by its morphological characteristics under high-resolution magnification. Although widely used in all clinical and research laboratories, its value in terms of prediction of oocyte performance (fertilization and establishment of term pregnancy) is far from accurate.

SPERM–OOCYTE INTERACTION

When the sperm is close to the mature oocyte, *in vivo* or *in vitro*, a question arises: is the collision course simply a matter of chance, or is there some chemical messenger that signals to the sperm the presence of the oocyte, allowing a directional movement? The answers vary when different species are considered. In humans, pre-contact sperm–egg communication (chemotaxis, chemokinesis) has not been proven to occur as in species with external fertilization. Eisenbach and Ralt[11] have hypothesized that only the fertilizing spermatozoa are attracted to the egg, while the rest are either repelled or inhibited.

As already stated, the type of mature oocyte that the sperm finds *in vivo* may be different from the one it finds *in vitro*, mainly in terms of perizonal layers. Partial or total dispersion of the corona–cumulus complex may occur in the natural process before the sperm can reach the zona pellucida, and it is probable that during the process of traversing these layers most of them will undergo an acrosome reaction, releasing enzymes that will help to disperse the complex. Radial disposition and distribution of the expanded corona and cumulus and the intercellular glycosaminoglycan matrix may direct the sperm toward the center of the mass where the oocyte lies. The human sperm seems to negotiate the cumulus mainly by physical force, since White *et al.*[20] have reported that human sperm capacitation is not needed and the cumulus does not induce rapid acrosome reaction in penetrating sperm; perhaps hyaluronidase, one of the main enzyme systems present in the acrosome, is used for this purpose. During natural fertilization, hyaluronidase is also provided by the oviduct and the cumulus, as well as the follicular fluid, present in the tube may enhance acrosome reaction. Glycoproteins manufactured by human cumulus cells can bind to a small percentage of human sperm when incubated in capacitated medium and may play a role in completing sperm capacitation[21]. In spite of these barriers, some sperm are able to go through the cumulus with an intact acrosome to bind to the zona pellucida. In two normally fertilized eggs recovered from the tube, Pereda and Coppo[22] found most of the sperm present shaped normally, acrosome-free and devoid of vesicles.

Going through the corona radiata, sperm may use esterases for passage during natural fertilization, they can also be contributed by tubal fluid. Zaneveld and Williams[23] described a specific enzyme system that the sperm uses to negotiate the corona. Their finding has not been confirmed by other investigators.

The most important step in initiation of fertilization is the sperm–zona interaction. Using electron microscopy, Sathananthan *et al.*[24] described sperm tightly bound to the zona by the plasma membrane, both acrosome-reacted and unreacted. Baltz *et al.*[25] have studied and calculated the sperm-generated forces at the time of contact, comparing them with the calculated tensile strength of sperm–zona bonds. The conclusion was that the motile sperm can be tethered by a single bond; thus, the sperm may be captured by the first bond and tethered permanently by a few. The bonds should be eliminated for the sperm to penetrate the zona, but if this elimination occurs prematurely the sperm could escape. According to Baltz *et al.*[25], the chronology of these events is critical. The maximum pulling force range of motile sperm is between 11 to 28 microdyn with a mean of 20±1.5 microdyn. The bonds between the sperm and the zona are affinity bonds, non-covalent bonds of the antibody–antigen type, septal ligands and enzyme – substrate bonds.

Biochemical and molecular analysis of binding properties shows that the zona pellucida binding ability changes as maturation proceeds[26,27]. In *in vitro* fertilization programs, oocytes inseminated before meiotic maturation is completed will not fertilize afterwards. Tesarik[27] has provided evidence that this failure is mainly due to inability of the sperm to penetrate the zona pellucida and can be overcome when increasing concentration of sperm is utilized. This maturation process may be due to active secretion of proteoglycans from metaphase II oocytes and the surrounding corona cells into the zona pellucida, as demonstrated by Tesarik and Kopecny[28]. The authors propose that a softening factor is produced by the corona cells and secreted toward the zona pellucida. In the *in vitro* system, Chen and Sathananthan[29] have demonstrated that, after insemination, sperm can reach the surface of the mature oocyte within 1 h, that most were acrosome-intact (70–90%) and were either firmly bound to the zona by their plasma membranes, were lying passively outside it, or had begun entry into the zona. Between 2 and 3 h after insemination, 30–60% of the sperm had acrosome reaction, both within the cumulus and in the outer part of the zona. Acrosome-intact, partially or fully reacted sperm may enter the zona 1–3 h after insemination; only fully reacted sperm were seen penetrating the inner zona and PVS. Passage of the sperm through the zona takes less than 1 h. Sperm–oocyte membrane fusion was seen approximately 2 h after insemination, and sperm decondensation and pronuclear formation at 3 h. These findings also indicate that the sperm goes through the cumulus and corona cells using propulsion forces without the need for enzymatic action, as has also been demonstrated by White[19].

It has been postulated that mainly acrosome intact sperm bind to the zona, although occasional reports indicate that both reacted and non-reacted sperm can bind to ZP3[8], which also triggers acrosome reaction, most likely by inducing sperm – ZP3 receptor aggregation on the surface of the plasma membrane. Only acrosome-reacted sperm can bind to ZP2[30], a secondary ligand which maintains binding. Release of oocyte cortical granules after fertilization causes limited proteolysis of ZP3, converting it to ZP2.

Clinically, the hemizona assay can evaluate binding and the zona penetration assay can test the sperm's ability to cross the zona; neither can be applied routinely in clinical work.

Vitelline membrane

As soon as the sperm goes through the zona and enters the PVS, it is exposed to the vitelline membrane. In the unfertilized human egg Dandekar and Talbot[31] have described an extracellular matrix in the PVS composed of granules and filaments very similar to that found between cumulus and corona radiata cells.

After fertilization, there is evidence of cortical granules exudate in the PVS forming a new coat around the oocyte (cortical granule envelope) which persists all the way to the blastocyst stage, and disappears following hatching[31]. The extracellular matrix of the unfertilized oocyte may be secreted by the corona radiata cells or may be synthesized and secreted by the oocyte. The granules are made of proteinaceous material and the filaments may be hyaluronic acid. After crossing the PVS, the sperm faces and interacts with the oolemma.

Both the sperm acrosomal inner membrane and the vitelline membrane are far more complex than phospholipid membranes. The process of fusion begins in the post-acrosomal region of the sperm and/or the equatorial segment where the plasma membrane is still intact. The fusion process that follows is not species specific. The sperm attaches to microvilli on the surface of the egg, and the oocyte responds with the production of pseudopodal-like processes which engulf the sperm head. The two membranes need to be brought into contact for the actual process of destabilization and fusion to occur; localized dehydration at the site of contact starts hydrophobic interactions that will promote fusion. Before contact, two forces oppose fusion: electrostatic repulsion which depends on the amount of surface electric charges at the membrane level, and the hydration barrier which may disappear if dehydration takes place. The repulsion effect of these forces acting on a curved surface decreases with the degree of the radius of curvature. There is preliminary evidence that the Asp-Gly-Arg (RGD) amino acid sequence which plays a role in cell–cell and cell–matrix adhesion and is present in fibronectin may be involed in this stage[32]. Fibronectin on the sperm surface after capacitation may interact with an oolemmal receptor[32]. Fibronectin-derived RGD-containing peptides competitively inhibit sperm–oolemmal adhesion and penetration in the heterologous (human–hamster) and homologous (hamster–hamster) gamete system[32]. After capacitation, live sperm have fibronectin on the surface of the head in different patterns[31]. This may be due to unmasking of a cellular form of fibronectin. The authors suggest that fibronectin may play a role in sperm–oolemmal binding and its defects may originate sperm dysfunction, explaining some forms of human infertility[32]. Furthermore, the presence of an IgG Fc receptor in the oolemma of the hamster oocyte and the diminishing of sperm binding after this receptor is neutralized may indicate that this system is also operational in sperm–oolemma binding[33]. Bronson *et al.*[34] demonstrated the presence of FcγRI, FcγRII and FcγRIII for the Fc domain of IgG on the surface of human oocytes using monoclonal antibodies against the three human Fc receptors. Indirect immunofluorescence and indirect immunobead binding failed to show their presence on human spermatozoa, either recently ejaculated, capacitated or acrosome-reacted.

These receptors in the oolemma may play a role in fertilization using integrins and C1q receptors on the sperm, or may be responsible for oocyte phagocytic activity. Nevertheless, the presence of integrin

B_2 subunits in the sperm membrane of healthy donors has not been demonstrated[35]. C3bi, a complement protein that contains the RGD sequence and is spatially and functionally related to an IgG Fc receptor, may be linked to the sperm plasma membrane and interact with complement receptors (CR) CR1 and CR3 that are present in the oolemma of human eggs[36]. CR1 is a first membrane protein and its receptor is CRB. Human oocytes show complement receptors type 1 in the plasma membrane besides CR2, CR3, C3 and dimetrics C3β. The C3β/B1 molecule may be the intermediate ligand to the MCB present on the acrosome-reacted sperm, and the CR present on the oocyte vitelline membrane.

Sperm surface protein (PH30)

Recently, a sperm surface protein (PH30), presumably involved in sperm fusion to the vitelline membrane, was identified. Complementary DNA and reduced amino-acid sequences of the mature α- and β-subunits were reported[37]. The α-subunit contains a fusion peptide and the β-subunit has a domain related to integrin ligands. Sperm plasmalemma–oolemma fusion is stimulated by calcium, which may induce high osmotic pressure within the acrosome and shield the surface electrical charges of the post-acrosomal region. Differences in surface tension may be the main driving force of the sperm–egg fusion. Spermatozoal translocation of membrane proteins, not necessarily involving clearance, may be a preliminary step for destabilization of the membranes in preparation for fusion. Lysophosphatidyl choline and phospholipase C enzyme systems seem to be involved in this process. Fusion occurs in any area of the vitelline membrane except where the second metaphase spindle is, because it has very few microvilli present.

Immediately after contact, the sperm is enveloped by bushes of microvilli from the egg surface, establishing very close connections mainly at the level of the post-acrosomal cap. The microvilli around the sperm start to retract and it is passively engulfed into the ooplasm. The cortex of the oocyte contains actin and myosin, and the actin filaments extending into the microvilli from the cortex can contract, bringing both the microvilli and the sperm into the cytoplasm[38].

Clinically, sperm–perivitelline membrane interaction can be evaluated by the human sperm/zona-free hamster penetration test, or by using the human sperm/human zona-free oocyte test, which is not yet in use in standard clinical laboratories.

Whether a fast or rapid block to polyspermia occurs immediately after the process of fusion in humans, as happens in the sea urchin, is still debatable. Electrical changes have been detected in the human, but they are not of the same magnitude as in the sea urchin.

Cortical reaction

The cortical reaction clearly takes place in the human as a continuation or exaggeration of the secretion process from the oocyte that occurs continuously during oocyte maturation. The lysosome-like Golgi-derived organelles are distributed in the oocyte cortex and another membrane fusion process takes place as they approach the inner aspect of the oocyte vitelline membrane. Part of the cortical reaction is the release of calcium, which involves cortical granule migration toward the surface, membrane fusion with oolemma until discharge is achieved and the elongation of thousands of microvilli on the surface of the membrane. Release of cortical granules takes approximately 15 min, slow or delayed block to polyspermia after gamete fusion. The granules are rich in proteolytic enzymes, are extruded in the PVS, produce limited proteolysis of the inner third of the zona pellucida, and perhaps cause extensive reorganization of the oocyte surface. Modifications of sperm receptors in the zona pellucida (mainly ZP1 and ZP2) are also induced. The slow block to polyspermia is a reversible phenomenon that fades as time passes. New concepts, in terms of organization of the PVS and the possible formation of a cortical granule envelope as a third mechanism to block polyspermia, have been already described[31].

Changes induced by the discharge of cortical granules into PVS and the zona pellucida are referred to as zona reaction, and produce biochemical modifications of the extracellular matrix, ZP1 and ZP2. Wassarman[39,40] demonstrated in the mouse that ZP3 from fertilized oocytes loses its function as a sperm receptor and as an acrosome reaction trigger mechanism, and he suggested that specific removal of sugar residues from ZP3 derived *O*-linked oligosaccharides can prevent the binding[38]. Hardening of the zona pellucida is due to structural changes that are not well understood. ZP2 also undergoes proteolysis after cortical granule discharge, which may be responsible for hardening of the zona.

SPERM INSIDE THE OOCYTE

At the time that the sperm–oocyte fusion occurs, the oocyte MII is completed and the second polar body is extruded. The process of decondensation of maternal chromosomes to form the female pronucleus starts. Male pronucleus formation occurs almost simultaneously with disappearance of the nuclear membrane, decondensation of the chromosomes and reformation of the pronuclear membrane from oocyte endoplasmic reticulum. The fate of the sperm inner acrosomal membrane is still unknown. Entrance of the sperm head with its highly condensed nucleus into the ooplasma triggers (1) nuclear swelling, and (2) chromatin decondensation before the formation of the male pronucleus is accomplished. Male pronuclear formation seems to be controlled by ooplasmic factors[41]. Tesarik and Kopecny[42] have shown that full development of pronuclei within oocyte cytoplasm occurs only in fully matured (metaphase II) oocytes. They also demonstrated that, when clear polyspermia occurred in their experimental conditions, pronuclear development was also impaired, and if reinsemination is performed and a second wave of sperm is allowed to penetrate into the already fertilized zona-free oocytes, the development of the pronuclei in the second wave of sperm incorporated was definitely abnormal[42]. DNA synthesis, which starts in fully developed pronuclei, did not occur when high numbers of sperm were incorporated into the ooplasm. The chromatin of the sperm incorporated is organized in tightly packed fibrillae surrounded by chromatin-associated protamines. When the nuclear membrane disappears, the ooplasmic factors can reach the sperm chromatin and the process of decondensation begins, with disruption of the disulfide bonds and replacement of protamines on the sperm chromatin by histones provided by the egg. Disulfide reducing agent may be reduced glutathione, which breaks the cross-linkage of nuclear histones in the sperm chromatin. Acrosin remaining in the sperm may also play a role in chromatin decondensation by digesting sperm histones. Nucleic acid synthesis in the human male pronucleus is dependent upon the development of a pronuclear structure; DNA synthesis begins 12 h after fertilization[43].

In 1973 Thibault and Girard[44] described a male pronucleus growth factor (MPGF), and Yanagimachi[45], in 1981, reported on a sperm pronucleus development factor (SPDF). The amount of these factors available at the time of fertilization may be a rate-limiting step in the formation of pronuclei, even when the sperm have already penetrated into the ooplasm. Schmiady *et al.*[46], in 1986, described prematurely condensed human sperm chromosomes after *in vitro* fertilization as a possible cause of lack of sperm decondensation, which may be due to an oocyte not properly activated and arrested at metaphase II after sperm penetration[46]. Chromosome condensing factors are still present and the sperm cells in G0 phase of the cell cycle have their chromosomes condensed into single chromatids.

Oocytes also contain high free thiol concentration that could cleave S–S bridges; zinc blocks free thiol groups and stabilizes the membranes. Sperm are zinc depleted during transit through the human female genital tract and during penetration of the zona pellucida, perhaps as part of capacitation. Zinc depletion may unmask free thiol groups, which will destablize S–S bridges. In natural fertilization, albumin and follicular fluid can also chelate zinc. All these processes may be either facilitators or modulators of sperm decondensation.

Zenzes *et al.*, studying abnormal zygotes, showed a marked asynchrony in paternal and maternal pronuclear development, triploidy and aneuploidy. In a second study, they demonstrated that zygotes derived from immature oocytes remain inactivated after sperm penetration and, in some, individual chromosomes or chromosome regions were prematurely condensed[48]. The process of oocyte maturation is accompanied by the appearance of maturing promoting factors (MPF), which trigger chromosome condensation and nuclear membrane disintegration. The paternal and maternal DNA replication has to be synchronous after pronucleus formation.

Tesarik and Kopecny[49] divided pronucleus development into stages 1 and 2, characterized by partial and total sperm chromatin decondensation, nuclear membrane disappearance and new nuclear envelope formation at stage 2. Stage 3 shows continuous reformation of nuclear envelope, which is still immature, and chromatin is reorganized in clusters of various sizes with initiation of development of nuclear precursors. Stage 4 has a fully developed nuclear envelope with completed nuclear precursors and detection of tritiated thymidine incorporation into DNA precursors. On the other hand, tritiated adenosine was incorporated somewhat earlier at stage 3. Early incorporation of adenosine before DNA replication may indicate early pronuclear RNA synthesis. DNA synthesis began 12 h after gamete fusion. Stages 1 and 2 developed as early as 2 h after insemination, and stage 3 may persist for a long time and may progress to stage 4 or stay arrested. Stages 1 and 2 represent the period of sperm chromatin decondensation; and stages 3 and 4 the development of the male pronucleus[48]. Lasalle and Testart[50] used zona-free human oocytes that failed to fertilize *in vitro* and showed the process of decondensation starting at the interior portion of the head and progressing posteriorly in approximately 60 min to reach maximal decondensation; recondensation starts and also takes 60 min. Re-expansion after recondensation starts with the appearance of a dense outline around the condensed sperm nucleus 120 min after the original decondensation. Tail elements and mitochondria are incorporated and eventually disintegrate. Functional mitochondria are not retained, and are therefore strictly maternal.

Clinically, the process of sperm decondensation can be investigated in the laboratory by the human sperm–hamster zona-free oocyte penetration assay, or by a non-species-specific sperm decondensation assay (xenopus maturation promoting factor).

At the time of male pronucleus formation, the oocyte second polar body is extruded and the remaining chromatin organizes in the form of the female pronucleus, which move together. Male and female chromosomes condense and associate with the microtubules, giving rise to MI; syngamy occurs and a new genome is initiated.

Availability of *in situ* hybridization techniques allowed investigation of spatial distribution of DNA in human sperm-derived pronuclei using the hamster system. Fate of individual chromosomes or of the whole human genomic DNA can be followed during decondensation, recondensation during first cleavage, and redispersion during the early two-cell stage. Brandiff *et al.*[51] followed distribution of sequences of chromosome I and observed the DNA to extend dramatically into long fibers, remaining in this conformation which may allow replication and active transcription until the first cell cycle. If extended to the whole genome, this may confer totipotency to the cell at the one and early two-cell stages. Paternal and maternal chromosomes remain sequestered initially by the different positions on the spindle.

The process of fertilization as understood today should be an essential part of clinicians' knowledge in the field of infertility. Literature is dispersed and published mainly in basic sciences journals; diagnostic and clinical applications have not been clearly defined. The purpose of this review is to contribute to bringing this subject into the clinical arena.

References

1. Edwards, R. G. (1980). *Conception in the Human Female*, p. 573. (London: Academic Press)
2. Lopata, A. and Leung, P. C. (1988). The fertilization of human oocytes at different stages of meiotic maturation. *Ann. N.Y. Acad. Sci.*, **541**, 324–36
3. Bird, J. M. and Houghton, J. A. (1991). The activation of mammalian sperm. *Sci. Prog. (Oxf.)*, **75**, 107–20
4. Foresta, C., Mioni, R., Rossato, M., Varotto, A. and Zorzi, M. (1991). Evidence for the involvement of sperm angiotensin converting enzyme in fertilization. *Int. J. Androl.*, **14**, 333–9
5. Chang, M. C. (1957). A detrimental effect of seminal plasma on the fertilizing capacity of spermatozoa. *Nature*, **179**, 258–60
6. Burkman, L. J. (1984). Characterization of hyper-

activated motility by human spermatozoa during capacitation: comparison of fertile and oligozoospermic sperm population. *Arch. Androl.*, **13**, 153–65
7. Tesarik, J. (1985). Comparison of acrosome reaction-inducing activities of human cumulus oophorus, follicular fluid and ionophore A 23187 in human sperm populations of proven fertilizing ability *in vitro*. *J. Reprod. Fert.*, **74**, 383–8
8. Morales, P., Cross, N. L., Overstreet, J. W. and Hanson, F. W. (1989). Acrosome intact and acrosome-reacted human sperm can initiate binding to the zona pellucida. *Dev. Biol.*, **133**, 385–92
9. Diaz-Perez, E. and Miezel, S. (1992). Importance of mammalian sperm metalloendoprotease activity during the acrosome reaction to subsequent sperm–egg fusion: Inhibitor studies with human sperm and zona-free hamster eggs. *Mol. Reprod. Dev.*, **31**, 122–30
10. Tesarik, J., Drahorad, J., Testart, J. and Mendoza, C. (1990). Acrosin activation follows its surface exposure and precedes membrane fusion in human sperm acrosome reaction. *Development*, **110**, 391–400
11. Eisenbach, M. and Ralt, D. (1992). Precontact mammalian sperm–egg communication and role in fertilization. *Am. J. Physiol.*, C1095–101
12. Tulsiani, D. R. S., Skudlarek, M. D. and Orgebin-Crist, M. C. (1990). Human sperm plasma membranes possess α-D-mannosidase activity but no galactosyltransferase activity. *Biol. Reprod.*, **42**, 843–58
13. Benoff, S., Cooper, G. W., Hurley, I., Napolitano, B., Rosenfeld, D. L., Scholl, G. M. and Hershlag, A. (1993). Human sperm fertilizing potential *in vitro* is correlated with differential expression of a head-specific mannose-ligand receptor. *Fertil. Steril.*, **59**, 854–62
14. Burkman, L. J., Coddington, C. C., Franken, D. R., Kruger, T. F., Rosenwaks, Z. and Hodgen, G. D. (1988). The hemizona assay (HZA): Development of a diagnostic test for the binding of human spermatozoa to human hemizona pellucida to predict fertilization potential. *Fertil. Steril.*, **49**, 688–97
15. Fowler, R. E. and Grainge, C. (1985). A histochemical study of the changes occurring in the protein-carbohydrate composition of the cumulus-oocyte complex and zona pellucida in immature mice in response to gonadotropin stimulation. *Histochem. J.*, **17**, 1735–49
16. Nottola, S. A., Familiari, G., Micara, G., Aragona, C. and Motta, P. M. (1991). The ultrastructure of human cumulus-corona cells at the time of fertilization and early embryogenesis. A scanning and transmission electron microscopic study in an *in vitro* fertilization program. *Arch. Histol. Cytol.*, **54**, 145–61
17. Shabanowitz, R. B. and O'Rand, M. G. (1988). Characterization of the human zona pellucida from fertilized and unfertilized eggs. *J. Reprod. Fert.*, **82**, 151–61
18. Sacco, A. G. (1987). The zona pellucida: current status as candidate antigen for contraceptive vaccine development. *Am. J. Reprod. Immunol. Microbiol.*, **15**, 172–80
19. Konloch, R. A., Ruiz-Seiler, B. and Wassarman, P. M. (1990). Genomic organization and polypeptide primary structure of zona pellucida glycoprotein hZP3, the hamster sperm receptor. *Dev. Biol.*, **142**, 414–21
20. White, D. R., Phillips, D. M. and Bedford, J. M. (1990). Factors affecting the acrosome reaction in human spermatozoa. *J. Reprod. Fertil.*, **90**, 71–80
21. Tesarik, J., Kopecny, V. and Dvorak, M. (1984). Selective binding of human cumulus cell-secreted glycoproteins to human spermatozoa during capacitation *in vitro*. *Fertil. Steril.*, **41**, 919–25
22. Pereda, J. and Coppo, M. (1985). An electron microscopic study of sperm penetration into the human egg investments. *Anat. Embryol.* **173**, 247–52
23. Zaneveld, L. J. and Williams, W. L. (1970). A sperm enzyme that disperses the corona radiata and its inhibition by decapacitation factor. *Biol. Reprod.*, **2**, 363–8
24. Sathananthan, A. H., Trounson, A. O., Wood, C. and Leeton, J. F. (1982). Ultrastructural observations on the penetration of human sperm into the zona pellucida of the human egg in vitro. *J. Androl.*, **3**, 356–64
25. Baltz, J. M., Katz, D. F. and Cone, R. A. (1988). Mechanics of sperm egg interaction at the zona pellucida. *Biophys. J.*, **54**, 643–54
26. Trounson, A. O., Mohr, I. R., Wood, C. and Leeton, J. F. (1982). Effect of delayed insemination on *in vitro* fertilization, culture and transfer of human embryos. *J. Reprod. Fertil.*, **64**, 285–94
27. Tesarik, J., Pilka, L. and Travnik, P. (1988). Zona pellucida resistance to sperm penetration before the completion of human oocyte maturation. *J. Reprod. Fertil.*, **83**, 487–95
28. Tesarik, J. and Kopecny, V. (1986). Late preovulatory synthesis of proteoglycans by the human oocyte and cumulus cells and their secretion into the oocyte–cumulus-complex extracellular matrices. *Histochemistry*, **85**, 523–8
29. Chen, C. and Sathananthan, A. H. (1986). Early penetration of human sperm through the vestments of human eggs *in vitro*. *Arch. Androl.*, **16**, 183–97
30. Bliel, J. D. and Wassarman, P. M. (1980). Mammalian sperm–egg interaction: Identification of a glycoprotein in mouse egg zonae pellucidae possessing receptor activity for sperm. *Cell*, **20**, 873–82
31. Dandekar, P. and Talbot, P. (1992). Perivitelline space of mammalian oocytes: Extracellular matrix of unfertilized oocytes and formation of a cortical granule envelope following fertilization. *Mol. Reprod. Dev.*, **31**, 135–43
32. Fusi, F. M. and Bronson, R. A. (1992). Sperm surface fibronectin. Expression following capacitation. *J. Androl.*, **13**, 28–35
33. Bronson, R. A., Fleit, H. B. and Fusi, F. (1990). Identification of an oolemmal IgG Fc receptor: Its role in promoting binding of antibody-labelled

human sperm to zona free hamster eggs. *Am. J. Reprod. Immunol.*, **23**, 87–92
34. Bronson, R. A., Fusi, F. M. and Fleit, H. B. (1992). Monoclonal antibodies identify Fcτ receptors on unfertilized human oocytes but not spermatozoa. *J. Reprod. Immunol.*, **21**, 293–307
35. Fusi, F. and Bronson, R. A. (1991). Failure to detect integrins of the Beta-2 Subclass on the human sperm surface. *Am. J. Reprod. Immunol.*, **25**, 143–5
36. Anderson, D. J., Wang, H. and Jack, R. M. (1990). A possible role of the complement component C_3 and its receptors, membrane cofactor protein in human sperm/egg interaction. *37th Annual Meeting, Society for Gynecologic Investigation*, St. Louis, Missouri, 21–24 March
37. Blobel, C. P., Wolfsberg, T. G., Turek, C. W., Myles, D. G., Primakoff, P. and White, J. M. (1992). A potential fusion peptide and an integrin ligand domain in a protein active in sperm-egg fusion. *Nature*, **356**, 248–52
38. Wassarman, P. (1987). The biology and chemistry of fertilization. *Science*, **235**, 553–60
39. Wassarman, P. M. (1983). Cellular interactions and development: molecular mechanisms. In Yamada, K. M. (ed.) pp. 1–28. (New York: Wiley-Interscience)
40. Wassarman, P. M., Bliel, J. D., Florman, H. M., Greve, R. T. and Salvmann, G. S. (1986). The mouse eggs' extracellular coat: synthesis, structure and function. In Gall, J. G. (ed.) *Gametogenesis and the Early Embryo*, pp. 371–88. (New York: Liss)
41. Yanagimachi, R. (1989). Sperm capacitation and gamete interaction. *J. Reprod. Fertil.* (Suppl), **38**, 27–33
42. Tesarik, J. and Kopecny, V. (1989). Developmental control of the human male pronucleus by ooplasmic factors. *Hum. Reprod.*, **4**, 962–8
43. Tesarik, J. and Kopecny, V. (1989). Nucleic acid synthesis and development of human male pronucleus. *J. Reprod. Fertil.*, **86**, 549–58
44. Thibault, C. and Girard, M. (1970). Facteur cytoplasmique necessaire à la formation du pronucleus mâle dans l'ovocyte de lapine. *C. R. Acad. Sci.*, **270**, 2025–6
45. Yanagimachi, R. (1981). Mechanisms of fertilization in mammals. In Mastroianni, L. and Biggers, J. D. (eds.) *Fertilization and Embryonic Development* In Vitro, pp. 81–192. (New York: Plenum Press)
46. Schmiady, H., Sperling, K., Kentenich, H. and Stauber, M. (1986). Prematurely condensed human sperm chromosomes after *in vitro* fertilization (IVF). *Hum. Genet.*, **74**, 441–3
47. Zenzes, M. T., Belkien, L., Bordt, J., Kan, I., Schneider, H. P. G. and Nieschlag, E. (1985). Cytologic investigation of human *in vitro* fertilization failures. *Fertil. Steril.*, **43**, 883–91
48. Zenzes, M. T., deGeyter, C., Bordt, J., Schneider, H. P. G. and Nieschlag, E. (1990). Abnormalities of sperm chromosome condensation in the cytoplasm of immature human oocytes. *Hum. Reprod.*, **5**, 842–6
49. Tesarik, J. and Kopecny, V. (1989). Development of human male pronucleus: ultrastructure and timing. *Gamete Res.*, **24**, 135–49
50. Lassalle, B. and Testart, J. (1991). Sequential transformations of human sperm nucleus in human egg. *J. Reprod. Fertil.*, **91**, 393–401
51. Brandiff, B. F., Gordon, L. A., Segraves, R. and Pinkel, D. (1991). The male-derived genome after sperm–egg fusion: spatial distribution of chromosomal DNA and paternal–maternal genomic association. *Chromosoma*, **100**, 262–6

Section 2

Male factor diagnosis

The concept of male factor in assisted reproduction

5

A. A. Acosta

INTRODUCTION

Establishing a clear concept of male factor in assisted reproduction is critical. No matter what definition we adopt, we need to strive for a common one that allows the establishment of clear diagnostic guidelines, therapeutic proposals and, overall, to compare results in a meaningful way.

DEFINITIONS OF MALE FACTOR

Since the very beginning of assisted reproduction the treatment of the male factor was rapidly incorporated into the indications but, for the most part, an abnormal semen analysis judged by the World Health Organisation (WHO) criteria was the fundamental factor which lead to the inclusion of these patients in this therapeutic modality. More recent publications have not clarified the issue. A few examples will suffice. Pool *et al.*[1], revisiting reinsemination with donor sperm after failed fertilization with husbands' gametes, list the reasons for suggesting donor backup in four couples as: (1) status-post varicocelectomy; (2) poor sperm penetration assay (SPA), failed gamete intrafallopian transfer (GIFT); (3) male factor with secondary infertility; and (4) antisperm antibodies. If we use these criteria then a large number of patients will be diagnosed as severe male factor when they do not fulfill those criteria. On the other hand, failed fertilization is certainly an excellent decisive factor in a well established laboratory, but unless we can predict it, by the time we learn about it, it is too late. Fakih and Vijayakumar[2], recommending the use of follicular fluid as a sperm capacitation and gamete transfer medium in GIFT in patients with oligo-asthenospermia, define the male factor as a combination of any two abnormal characteristics, namely, concentration $<20\times10^6$ sperm/mL, motility <40%, normal morphology <40%, Penetrak results <40 mm, hamster egg penetration assay <10% or penetration index <1% and agglutination >10%. These criteria do not fit with the WHO criteria for normality, and some of these people may even fertilize normally in *in vitro* fertilization (IVF). Hammitt *et al.*[3] diagnose male factor infertility when the concentration was $<20\times10^6$ sperm/mL, motility <40% (speed of 1+ or 2++), or when the test for ASA (immunobead technique) revealed ≥20% IgG or IgA binding to any region other than the tail tip. Hinting *et al.*[4] state only that spermatozoa were classified into four motility categories according to the WHO classification of 1987 (grades A, B, C and D); sperm morphology was also categorized using the criteria of the WHO, and antisperm antibodies utilizing the sperm mixed antiglobulin reaction (MAR) test (direct and indirect), and the adenosine triphosphate (ATP) release cytotoxicity test in serum. They defined oligozoospermia as $<20\times10^6$ sperm/mL, asthenozoospermia <25% spermatozoa with grade A motility, teratozoospermia <25%, spermatozoa with normal morphology and immunological factor >40% of motile spermatozoa reacting positively in the sperm MAR test.

Diedrich *et al.*[5] do not give any criteria but, judging by the characteristics of the sperm in the patients treated, patients with oligozoospermia seem to have <20 million sperm/mL concentration, patients with asthenozoospermia have a motility <35% and patients with teratozoospermia have a morphology <35%. Tucker *et al.*[6], trying to define the application of partial zona dissection in male infertility, define this factor as counts $<10\times10^6$ sperm/mL, motility of <21%, and/or morphological abnormalities of >89%, besides including patients that have failed to fertilize in previous cycles.

Tournaye *et al.*[7] applied zygote intrafallopian transfer (ZIFT) and *in vitro* fertilization to patients with male factor infertility. They defined the following inclusion criteria:

(1) Couples suffering from primary infertility for at least 3 years;

(2) Male partner's best semen analysis subnormal, using the WHO criteria for normality (sperm count $>20\times10^6$ sperm/mL, type A motility >25%, or type A+type B motility >50% and normal morphology >50%). Sperm index (density×percentage progressive motility×percentage normal forms) $<5\times10^6$ sperm/mL, and a swim-up result of at least 0.1×10^6 sperm/mL with progressive motility.

Enginsu *et al.*[8], studying the male factor as determinant of *in vitro* fertilization outcome, excluded semen samples with a concentration of $<20\times10^6$ sperm/mL and/or progressive motility <30% in order to study the contribution of morphology, *per se*, into the results and used strict criteria to study morphological characteristics of the sample. They concluded that morphology evaluation by strict criteria was the best predictor for IVF outcome.

Wolf *et al.*[9] considered normal sperm samples those with a concentration $>40\times10^6$ sperm/mL, with motility and normal forms >40%. If one or several of these parameters were below those limits, they were included in the group with subnormal sperm. The patient had no presence of antisperm antibodies, the sperm showed a good ability to penetrate a column of human ovulatory cervical mucus, and to stay motile after 4 h of contact. The sperm movement pattern, using a computerized system, was normal and the sperm were able to survive at least 24 h at 20°C after selection through a 2-density Percoll gradient. The human sperm hamster zona-free penetration assay was positive (sperm decondensing in >40% of zona-free hamster oocytes).

Lippi *et al.*[10] reviewed the result of subzonal insemination in cases of 'extreme male factor infertility'. The definition for this extreme male factor infertility was either fertilization failure in previous IVF cycles, or <50,000 motile spermatozoa recoverable after semen preparation; different from severe male factor, in whom sufficient motile spermatozoa (>50,000) can be recovered from that preparation.

Sakkas *et al.*[11], evaluating the IVF treatment of moderate male factor infertility, defined it as oligozoospermia, asthenozoospermia or teratozoospermia, alone or in combination, according to the WHO guidelines of 1987.

This brief list of examples suffice to point to the complete lack of uniformity to define a male factor in assisted reproduction and furthermore to identify the categories of severe male factor and extreme male factors as proposed by us and others.

THE NEED FOR UNIFORMITY

In a previous publication[12] we addressed the issue of the definition of male factor in assisted reproduction. Since we started working in the field of male factor using the different techniques of assisted reproduction (IVF, GIFT, ZIFT) and assisted fertilization, the complete lack of uniformity in the understanding and defining this group of patients, as previously stated, was apparent. We proposed several questions in that publication[12] that are still pertinent for reproductive endocrinologists, infertility specialists, andrologists, urologists, scientists and laboratory personnel working with male factor patients. In our daily clinical work and after a patient has had preliminary investigations, the first question asked by those patients is: 'Is my sperm normal?' The criteria established by the WHO[13] allow categorization of normal and subnormal samples. When the male fulfills the WHO criteria for normal semen analysis then we assume that he is normal and, therefore, fertile. Nevertheless, it was a consensus in 1994 that a plain semen analysis is not enough to judge sperm fertilizing ability, even when it is normal, and that some of these people may have specific defects that may not be picked up by these very simple tests. Therefore, a battery of tests needs to be done in order to determine the real sperm capabilities for fertilization and establishment of a pregnancy.

If the man is in the subnormal category, his second question is: 'Am I ever going to be able to father a child?' This question is much more difficult to answer because one has to take into account the fertility of the wife, which is another unknown factor. Even when the wife is fully investigated, the programs for therapeutic insemination donor (TID) indicate that approximately 15% will become pregnant in those programs (unexplained female infertility). Furthermore, the normal values recommended by the WHO do not intend to answer that question and very few references have been published in the literature in that specific regard. The criteria from Tygerberg[14] are among the few published in the literature trying to distinguish between males capable of establishing a pregnancy in natural reproduction, and those who most probably will not be able to establish a pregnancy, or who are unlikely to establish a pregnancy. When a patient falls into the subnormal category, the clinician may resort to medical or surgical treatments according to the etiologic factor found, to try to improve the sperm quality and the fertilization potential. In terms of medical treatment, gonadotropins, antiestrogens, androgens, aromatase inhibitors, stimulators of motility and other agents have been tried with very little proven success (see Chapter 32). Furthermore, the high success rate obtained with assisted fertilization (see Chapter 29) seems to render these treatments irrelevant; on the other hand, the key question of understanding testicular physiology and pathophysiology in unexplained oligo-astheno-teratozoospermia remains widely open. These treatments should be attempted if the clinician considers them feasible, because the cost will be much less and pregnancy may be obtained without resorting to the much more sophisticated and more expensive procedures offered by assisted reproduction and assisted fertilization.

When all conventional methods of treatment in the male have failed and pregnancy does not occur, the clinician is left with the procedures of assisted reproduction to complete the diagnostic testing of sperm function, and to attempt to solve the therapeutic problem.

A third question that is rapidly raised by patients when we propose treatment by assisted reproduction is even more difficult to answer. Is the semen quality enough to allow normal fertilization and pregnancy, or can the patient expect problems even with the use of this modern technology? It is important, therefore, in those cases to try to be able to correlate the quality of the sperm available with the possible outcome of assisted reproduction in terms of fertilization rate, implantation rate, total pregnancy rate per cycle (retrieval) and per transfer, term pregnancy rate per cycle (the most important information in programs of assisted reproduction) and per transfer. In order to determine which is or can be considered normal in terms of gamete interaction and fertilization rates in each embryology laboratory, clearcut information should be obtained in regard to fertilization success when normal gametes are used. If the mean and standard deviations are determined for the fertilization rate of preovulatory oocytes, then anything below 2SD of that mean should be considered abnormal (low) fertilization for that laboratory. A differential diagnosis between oocyte defects, sperm defects and combined factors, should be attempted. In the Norfolk program, using information obtained during the years 1989–91, when all female *in vitro* fertilization (IVF) patients classified as tubal factor, having a normal follicle-stimulating hormone (FSH)/luteinizing hormone (LH) ratio on day 3 of the menstrual cycle, and producing three or more preovulatory oocytes at retrieval that were inseminated with perfectly normal sperm were analyzed (173 cycles and 1305 oocytes), the total fertilization rate (total number of oocytes fertilized/total number of oocytes inseminated) was 89.3 ± 20.3% (mean ± SD), and the normal fertilization rate (total number of oocytes with normal fertilization over total number of oocytes inseminated) was 78.7 ± 22.3% (mean ± SD). The minimum total fertilization rate that can be considered normal in the Norfolk program is therefore 48.7%; the normal fertilization rate is 34.1%. In other words, fertilization values below 50% and 35%, respectively, should be considered abnormal and in the presence of normal stimulation and morphologically normal oocytes with sperm abnormalities present, the reduced fertility should be ascribed to a male factor in assisted reproduction. Similar investigations performed in the embryology laboratory at the Tygerberg program in South Africa revealed very similar figures[15] indicating that perhaps these values are valid for most well-established embryology laboratories.

Unfortunately, the regular parameters investigated in a routine semen analysis or even in sperm function tests do not allow us to predict which patient is going to fall into which category; therefore, the IVF attempt becomes a diagnostic test to certify the existence of a male factor in assisted reproduction.

Subfertile sperm falling below the level of normality defined by the WHO and, therefore, suspected of being subfertile, that produce fertilization rates in the *in vitro* system above the 50% and 35% total fertilization and normal fertilization rates previously mentioned, should not be included in the category of male factor in assisted reproduction, because although they are subnormal and potentially subfertile, they behave in the *in vitro* system as normal sperm; the inclusion of these patients within the male factor in assisted reproduction category will certainly improve the results obtained in those patients substantially.

In some cases, the diagnosis of the etiology of low fertilization or lack of fertilization is easy, and clear abnormalities are found in one of the gametes or both. On the other hand, if no detectable problems can be observed in oocytes or sperm, I believe that a cross-matched test should be performed if the laboratory is prepared to do so, to determine where the main responsibility for the problem lies. Immature oocytes (prophase I) that have matured *in vitro*, obtained from the patient in question and having a known fertilization rate for that category of oocytes in each embryology laboratory should be inseminated with the sperm of the husband, which may have already been done, and that of a donor, and allowed to reach only the pronuclear stage without being permitted to proceed unless the patient decides otherwise. The same procedure is done using immature oocytes from a consenting available female donor, which should be inseminated with sperm from the original patient's husband, and from a donor. This extensive procedure will be extremely useful to clarify the issue of unexplained lack of fertilization when a laboratory error can be excluded.

Other tests that have already been described in other chapters of this book, such as sperm fusion, penetration and decondensation in the hamster zona-free oocyte system (sperm penetration assay, or SPA), the human zona pellucida sperm binding assay (hemizona assay), the acrosine content and test for human zona pellucida receptors on the sperm surface can be used as complementary investigation and can help in the determination of the sperm fertilizing ability.

SEVERE MALE FACTOR THRESHOLD

The last, and equally important question that the patient poses and which the clinician should be able to consider is the minimum sperm quality that can be used in assisted reproduction with reasonable chances of fertilization. This characterization is vital because it will allow the clinician to discourage patient participation in assisted reproduction when semen parameters are below threshold, or will indicate the need for systemic treatment, sperm improvement using laboratory techniques or assisted fertilization. This threshold represents what we call a severe male factor in assisted reproduction and criteria need to be established for the prediction of no fertilization.

With the present success of intracytoplasmic sperm injection (ICSI) (Chapter 29), it seems that one of the most important questions that we will need to answer in the immediate future will be which patients should be put on that procedure. Nonetheless, and if the results obtained in Belgium can be repeated in other centers, it is quite possible that all male factors should go directly to ICSI, because regular insemination for *in vitro* fertilization and embryo transfer, even when fertilization occurs and when the number of embryos transferred is adequate, cannot match the results obtained by that technique.

References

1. Pool, T. B., Martin, J. E., Ellsworth, L. R., Perez, J. B. and Atiee, S. H. (1990). Zygote intrafallopian transfer with 'donor rescue': a new option for severe male factor infertility. *Fertil. Steril.*, **54**, 166–8
2. Fakih, H. and Vijayakumar, R. (1990). Improved pregnancy rates and outcome with gamete intrafallopian transfer when follicular fluid is used as a sperm capacitation and gamete transfer medium. *Fertil. Steril.*, **53**, 515–20
3. Hammitt, D. G., Syrop, C. H., Hahn, S. J., Walker, D. L., Butkowski, C. R. and Donovan, J. F. (1990). Comparison of concurrent pregnancy rates for *in vitro*

fertilization–embryo transfer, pronuclear stage embryo transfer and gamete intrafallopian transfer. *Hum. Reprod.*, **5**, 947–54

4. Hinting, A., Comhaire, F., Vermeulen, L., Dhont, M., Vermeulen, A. and Vandekerckhove, D. (1990). Possibilities and limitations of techniques of assisted reproduction for the treatment of male infertility. *Hum. Reprod.*, **5**, 544–8
5. Diedrich, K., Bauer, O., Werner, A., van der Ven, H., al Hasani, S. and Krebs, D. (1991). Transvaginal intratubal embryo transfer: a new treatment of male infertility. *Hum. Reprod.*, **6**, 672–5
6. Tucker, M. J., Bishop, F. M., Cohen, J., Wiker, S. R. and Wright, G. (1991). Routine application of partial zona dissection for male factor infertility. *Hum. Reprod.*, **6**, 676–81
7. Tournaye, H., Devroey, P., Camus, M., Valkenburg, M., Bollen, N. and Van Steirteghem, A. C. (1992). Zygote intrafallopian transfer or *in vitro* fertilization and embryo transfer for the treatment of male factor infertility: a prospective randomized trial. *Fertil. Steril.*, **58**, 344–50
8. Enginsu, M. E., Pieters, M. H., Dumoulin, J. C., Evers, J. L. and Geraedts, J. P. (1992). Male factor as determinant of *in vitro* fertilization outcome. *Hum. Reprod.*, **7**, 1136–40
9. Wolf, J. P., Ducot, B., Kunstmann, J. M., Frydman, R., Jouannet, P. (1992). Influence of sperm parameters on outcome of subzonal insemination in the case of previous IVF failure. *Hum. Reprod.*, **7**, 1407–13
10. Lippi, J., Mortimer, D. and Jansen, R. P. (1993). Subzonal insemination for extreme male factor infertility. *Hum. Reprod.*, **8**, 908–15
11. Sakkas, D., Gianaroli, L., Diotallevi, L., Wagner, I., Ferraretti, A. P. and Campana, A. (1993). IVF treatment of moderate male factor infertility: a comparison of mini-Percoll, partial zona dissection and sub-zonal sperm insertion techniques. *Hum. Reprod.*, **8**, 587–91.
12. Acosta, A. A. (1992). Male factor in assisted reproduction. *Fertil. Reprod. Med. Clin. N. Am.*, **3**, 487–503
13. World Health Organization (1992). *WHO Laboratory Manual for the Examination of Human Semen and Sperm Cervical Mucus Interaction*, pp. 43–4. (Cambridge: Cambridge University Press)
14. Van Zyl, J. A., Menkveld, R., Kotze, T. J. N. and Van Nickerk, J. A. (1976). *Proceedings of the 17th International Urology Conference, Johannesburg*, 25–30 July, 1976, Vol. 2, 263–71. (Paris: Diffusion Doin)
15. Franken, D. R., Acosta, A. A., Kruger, T. F., Lombard, C. J., Oehninger, S. and Hodgen, G. D. (1993). The hemizona assay: its role in identifying male factor infertility in assisted reproduction. *Fertil. Steril.*, **59**, 1075–80

Basic semen analysis 6

R. Menkveld and T. F. Kruger

INTRODUCTION

In 1866 the importance of the presence of spermatozoa for fertilization was stressed by Sims[1], who performed post-coital examinations on fluids of the vagina and the endocervix and stated that spermatozoa had to be present in the endocervical mucus for conception to occur. It is only since the turn of this century that a more scientific approach for semen analysis was adopted and, according to Ross[2], it was only in the 1940s that Wiesman stated that a semen analysis was not complete unless the volume, motility, concentration and morphology were determined. This was further supported by the work of Hotchkiss in 1945[3].

Minimum requirements for semen analysis and semen parameter standards were established in 1951 by the American Fertility Association[4], in 1966 by Freund[5], and in 1971 by Eliasson[6]. The minimum requirements for a complete semen analysis are still being extended with time, and today must also include so-called screening tests for the presence of antispermatozoa antibodies, such as the mixed antiglobulin reaction (MAR) test[7], and can also include a peroxidase test[8] for the presence of leukocytes, sperm penetration tests[9] or its replacements, such as bovine mucus[10] or hyaluronic acid[11], while the sperm–cervical mucus contact test[12] is also included by some authors[13].

Functional tests, such as the zona-free hamster ova penetration test[14,15], tests for the acrosome reaction, the determination of the sperm acrosin activity[16] and the hemizona assay[17], can be performed when indicated by unexplained poor fertilization on subsequent semen samples.

A complete semen analysis can therefore be divided into the following five categories: (1) background data; (2) physical data; (3) quantitative and qualitative analysis; (4) biochemical analysis; and (5) screening tests.

These components cannot be seen as isolated aspects; it is therefore important to regard all these aspects with equal importance, as all these factors are interrelated. For example, the results of a semen analysis are greatly influenced by days of abstinence, method of production and previous health conditions, so that the results cannot be interpreted if these basic facts are not known.

Semen analysis has and will be the most important factor in the initial investigation of male fertility potential. It is, therefore, extremely important that a semen analysis be performed skillfully and properly. If the necessary background data are obtained and the results interpreted correctly and intelligently a wide spectrum of information can be obtained, especially if a short personal and medical history is also taken on the day of the first semen analysis.

BASIC SEMEN ANALYSIS

Specimen handling

Semen samples present a possible biohazard as they may contain harmful viruses, e.g. human immunodeficiency virus (HIV), hepatitis and herpes. Therefore, semen samples should be handled with care and the wearing of protective gear is advised (gloves, masks, spectacles). Further information is given in the new WHO manual[18].

Background data

A semen analysis cannot be interpreted unless certain basic facts are known. The method by which the sample was produced, the time lapse between the production and analysis, days of abstinence and type of container used are all factors that can have an influence on the results, as will be discussed below.

Methods for the production of semen

Today it is becoming increasingly important that the semen sample be produced in a specially equipped and, if necessary, air conditioned room at the laboratory[19,20], especially where special tests are involved[21]. This method has the advantage that observations such as the presence of coagulation and the occurrence of liquefaction can be made and control can be exercised over environmental conditions, the time lapsed between ejaculation and investigation and the way in which the sample is produced because, although specified, many patients still produce samples by coitus interruptus or using a condom if the sample is brought to the laboratory. Coitus interruptus has the disadvantage that the first part of the sample may be lost. An indication that the sample may have been produced by coitus interruptus will be the presence of vaginal epithelium cells[20].

When the patient produces the sample at the laboratory a relationship can be built with him; information is easy to obtain and his inquiries can be answered. It often happens that a sample is brought to the laboratory and left on a counter without any information. The analysis results of such semen cannot be evaluated or interpreted because the method of production, days of abstinence and time of ejaculation are not known.

Patients having problems in producing a semen sample by masturbation can use a vibrator[22] which will give similar results to a masturbation sample[23], or a special plastic condom (Milex^{R})[24] can be used. However, better results have been obtained with the use of the new seminal collective device[25] (HDC Corporation, Mountain View CA, USA).

Semen samples should thus be produced by masturbation into a clean plastic container which is either sterile-packed at shipment, or sterilized. The patient is instructed to urinate and then to wash his hands with soap and the glans of the penis without soap.

The patient should be asked for the precise period of abstinence, as well as the occurrence of any infections or illnesses in the last 3 months, if it is his first visit, or since his previous semen analysis. Questions included in his medical history should be: has he had any medication or anesthesia in the past 3 months, any history of operations of the urogenital tract, especially a Y–V operation, an orchidopexy, orchiectomy, varicocelectomy or testicular biopsy, or if he had any severe injuries of the testicles or orchitis. A note should also be made about his smoking and drinking habits.

Containers

In the early years glass containers were used, but they had the disadvantage that they had to be washed and sterilized after use and may have broken[19]. The ideal container is a 60–100 mL wide-mouth plastic jar made of polypropylene with a screw-cap that fits tightly to prevent any loss of semen when it is transported. In our experience, some types of plastics (such as polystyrene) have the disadvantage that they may cause increased viscosity, or may be toxic to the spermatozoa and influence the motility. Check *et al.*[26] found that glass was slightly superior to polypropylene, but especially to polystyrene with regard to certain motility parameters. It is, therefore, important to test any new kind of container before use.

Abstinence

Since the 1930s, it has been well known that the period of abstinence can have a significant effect on semen volume and sperm concentration[27,28]. It is therefore important that a fixed period of abstinence should be prescribed, so that semen analyses are performed according to more standardized conditions, and so that the results of different semen analyses can be compared with each other. If this is not done, it is impossible to know if the differences between the parameters of different semen samples from the same patient are due to a normal variation, the difference in days of abstinence, or both. In a study performed on 1808 men, Menkveld *et al.*[27,28] found that the optimal period of abstinence obtaining maximal semen parameters was 3–5 days and today this is the most generally prescribed period of abstinence.

Physical parameters

Parameters describing the appearance of the sample are classified by Freund[29] and Zaneveld and Polakoski[30] as physical parameters and include color, liquefaction and viscosity, while coagulation and odor can also be added to this category, although, strictly speaking, a biochemical characteristic pH is also included in this group. All these parameters are simple to perform and are mainly executed by eye.

Coagulation

This is an important aspect of semen analysis which is ignored by many investigators, mainly because many semen samples are still produced at home instead of in the laboratory. Human semen is ejaculated in a liquefied state but is quickly transformed into a semisolid state or coagulum, probably under the influence of the enzyme protein kinase[31] secreted by the vesicula seminalis. In a normal situation almost the entire sample is transformed into the coagulated state and only a very small part remains liquid. This is generally regarded as the first portion of the ejaculate, containing the major part of the motile sperm fraction. In cases where coagulation does not occur, it may be the result of a congenital absence of the vas deferens and the seminal vesicula, as the coagulating enzymes originate from the seminal vesicles, and are then also associated with the absence of fructose in the seminal plasma.

Liquefaction

In a normal sample liquefaction occurs within 10–20 min. This is caused by a proteolytic enzyme fibrinolysin, which is secreted by the prostate[32], as well two other proteolytic enzymes, fibrinogenase and aminopeptidase[33]. Liquefaction, therefore, serves as an indicator of normal prostate function.

After complete liquefaction the sample will appear homogeneous in composition and color[34]. Small roundish particles may still be present in some samples; however, these can be regarded as normal and will usually dissolve within an hour. If liquefaction takes more than 20 min or does not occur at all it is a sign that the prostate is not functioning normally, usually as a result of a previous prostatitis. In some cases this non-liquefaction of semen may be a cause of infertility, as the spermatozoa are not released from the coagulum.

Viscosity

In 1934 Cary and Hotchkiss[35] described the consistency of semen as slightly more viscous than water, a parameter that could easily be determined by forcing the semen slowly through a pipette. The most convenient way to determine viscosity is by means of a modified pipette method[19]. Semen is drawn into a Pasteur pipette and slowly released in a dropwise fashion. Viscosity is regarded as normal when single drops are formed that are released within a distance of 20 mm from the point of the pipette. If threads of between 20 and 40 mm are formed, viscosity is regarded as slightly increased, between 40 and 80 mm as increased, and >80 mm as grossly increased.

It is also important to distinguish between a delayed period of liquefaction (non-homogeneous appearance) and an increase in the viscosity (homogeneous but 'sticky'). Increased viscosity may be the result of an abnormal prostate function due to an infection in the genital tract, prostate or seminal vesicula[36], or an artifact as a result of the use of an unsuitable type of plastic container, frequent ejaculation and the psychological state of the patient. An increase in viscosity is, according to Amelar[22], not a cause of infertility, but can have an adverse effect on the determination of spermatozoa concentration and motility.

To reduce the viscosity the semen can be drawn into a 10 mL or 5 mL syringe and forced out several times through a number 18 or 19 needle. This can be repeated several times until viscosity is normal. This method will produce an increase in air bubbles, but this will disappear after some time. Biochemical means are now available, such as α-amylase[37] and chymotrypsin[38], to reduce high viscosity.

Volume

The most common method still used today to determine the volume is by transferring the sample to a 15 mL graduated conical tube and read the volume to the nearest 0.1 mL.

The normal volume of an ejaculate after 3–5 days of sexual abstinence is 2–6 mL. Hotchkiss[3] stressed the importance of a normal volume, as this is needed for a good buffering function of the seminal pool against the acid secretions of the vagina. If the volume of a semen sample is smaller than 1.0 mL it is important to establish if the sample was complete. This is important, as the first portion containing the major amount of sperm with the best motility is often lost. A low volume may, however, also be the result of an obstruction due to a previous infection of the genital tract or of a congenital absence of the seminal vesicula and vas deferens. This condition will be associated with the absence of fructose[30]. A small volume may also be due to retrograde ejaculation, especially if the patient had any previous surgery of the prostate or the bladder neck. Retrograde ejaculation can be diagnosed by investigation of the urine after an ejaculation.

Color

By paying attention to the color of the semen sample an indication of possible pathology of the semen can be readily obtained. Cary and Hotchkiss[35] described the color of normal semen as opaque and grayish, which will change to yellowish with an increase in the days of abstinence. Hotchkiss[3] noticed that fresh blood will give semen a reddish color and old blood a brownish color, which may be caused by an inflammation. In cases of inflammation a more yellowish color may exist, while samples with a low concentration will usually have a transparent and watery consistency. Schirren[34] found that certain types of medicine, such as antibiotics, can discolor the semen.

Odor

Although semen has a strong distinctive odor derived from the prostatic secretions, the parameter is seldom used. The odor is compared to that of the flowers of the chestnut or the St John's bread tree. It is thought that the odor is caused by oxidation of the spermine secreted by the prostate. Only with the absence of odor or when an uncharacteristic odor is present should a note be made, as this is usually associated with an infection[30] or a long period of abstinence[19].

pH

Both colormetric and glass electrode methods are used to determine the pH of semen[34]. Although the electronic method is more accurate[34], preference should be given to pH measurement by the colorimetric method, using a special indicator paper (range 6.4–8.0; Merck #9557), due to hygienic reasons and the possibility of transferring sexually transmitted disease (STD). After liquefaction, a drop of semen is placed on the indicator strip and immediately compared against a color scale. The pH of a normal ejaculate may vary between 7.2 and 7.8.

Schirren[34] stressed the importance of pH measurements, as in cases of an acute prostatitis, vesiculitis or bilateral epididymitis pH will always be more than 8.0. In cases of a chronic infection of the mentioned organs pH will always be below 7.2 and can be as low as 6.6. With an obstruction of the ejaculatory duct, or in cases where only prostatic fluids are secreted, pH will be less than 7.0.

Wet preparation examination

After completion of the physical examination the centrifuge tubes are placed on a laboratory rotator (e.g. Hetorotator, Instruments AB, Sweden) for the duration of all subsequent procedures. After 10 min rotation, a drop of semen is taken and placed on a precleaned slide kept at 37°C until use. The drop is covered with a 20×40 mm coverslip and left for a few minutes to stabilize before examination.

General appearance

All examinations of wet preparations are done with phase contrast optics with a 100× or 150× (low power field, LPF) and 400× (high power field, HPF) magnification. The examination starts with scanning through 10 LPF to gain an impression of the general appearance of the sample. The impression obtained here will dictate all the subsequent procedures. For instance, the performance of a MAR test[7] or a supravital staining test[39] will depend on the presence of enough motile spermatozoa or enough spermatozoa to make an accurate determination of the motility and speed of forward progression. An estimation of the number of spermatozoa per HPF will determine the dilution of the sample for the determination of the sperm concentration and drop size for the morphology smears.

Agglutination and cells

The sample is also examined for the presence of agglutinated sperm. Two types of agglutination are possible. In the first instance this can be due to non-specific agglutination where sperm adhere to cells present in the seminal plasma. The second is specific agglutination which is caused by antispermatozoa antibodies[40]. Agglutination is described as negative (–), occasional (±), slight (+), moderate (++) or severe (+++). A note is also made of the presence of other cells, such as round cells, and the presence of spermine phosphate crystals which are recorded in the same way as for agglutination. The presence of any organisms is also recorded.

The slides can be kept at room temperature in a Petri dish on a moist gauze and re-examined after 90 min. After this, the Petri dish with slides can be incubated at 37°C and examined every 2–4 h. Although not physiological, the purpose of this step is twofold. The first is to monitor motility and forward progression as a function of time under laboratory conditions. Normal spermatozoa will show a gradual loss of motility and speed of forward progression, but will still exhibit some motility after 8 h. In the presence of metabolic abnormalities or the presence of antispermatozoal antibodies, the motility loss will be exhibited much sooner. The second is that certain aspects such as agglutination, the forming of spermine phosphate crystals and the presence of organisms can be better observed.

Analysis of quantitative and qualitative parameters

Parameters that are classified under this heading are those that are regarded by many laboratories to comprise a complete or standard semen analysis and include the estimation of the quantitative (percentage of motile spermatozoa) and qualitative (speed of forward progression) motility, the supravital staining procedure to determine vitality, spermatozoa concentration and the morphology of the spermatozoa. The MAR test[7] should also be included as a routine procedure.

Motility and forward progression

Over the years, the development of the motility evaluation has been such that three aspects or categories are now established. These were identified in 1938 by Hotchkiss *et al.*[41], who made the statement that motility should be evaluated according to three factors:

(1) The kind and aggressiveness of movement or qualitative motility (speed of forward progression);

(2) The quantitative motility expressing the percentage of (un)active spermatozoa (% motile); and

(3) The duration of motility (*in vitro*).

Motility

Motility is now usually determined by one of two methods. The first is by manual observation of the sample with phase contrast optics. More recently automated semen analysis (CASA) techniques have been introduced with varying degrees of success[18,42].

For the manual method a small drop of semen is placed on a clean microscope slide and covered with a coverslip. The drop should completely fill the area under the coverslip, with no empty edges and no floating of the specimen. About 10 HPF are examined and the motility is expressed as the percentage of live spermatozoa to the nearest 5% or 10%[43,44], although today the estimation of the percentage motile is made to the nearest 10%.

Forward progression

The grading of the type of movement or aggressiveness or speed of forward progression (FP) is usually done according to an arbitrary grading system on a scale from 0–4[41], 1–5 or 0–10[43], 0 meaning no FP and 4 or 10 meaning excellent FP. If this method is used, the FP is most commonly expressed on a scale 0–4, as follows:

- 0 no movement
- 1 movement – none forward
- 1+ movement – a few now and then
- 2 movement – undirected, slow
- 2+ movement – slowly but directly forward
- 3– movement – fast but undirected
- 3 movement – fast and directly forward
- 3+ movement – very fast and directly forward
- 4 movement – extremely fast and directly forward (wave-like)

The World Health Organization[18] prescribes a more descriptive evaluation where percentages are allocated to the type of movement graded from a to d as follows:

Grade a = rapid progressive motility

Grade b = slow or sluggish progressive motility

Grade c = non-progressive motility

Grade d = immotile

The number of spermatozoa in each category can be counted for 100 spermatozoa. The count should be repeated and the average taken; percentages for the different categories count up to 100%. A second drop should be checked. The results of the two counts are then averaged, provided that there is less than 10% discrepancy[18].

Duration of motility

The estimation and relevance of the estimation of the duration of motility continues to be a controversial aspect. MacLeod[45] pointed out that the seminal plasma is only a temporary transport medium and that it is unphysiological to assess the duration of sperm motility in this way. However, it is known that motile spermatozoa can still be present in a semen sample after 24 h at room temperature. Therefore, we believe that valuable information can be obtained by regular examinations of a wet preparation as stated before.

Poor motility or asthenozoospermia (Table 1 explains further terminology) can be caused by several factors. These factors can be divided into four categories as follows: (1) artefacts; (2) morphological abnormalities; (3) inherent factors; and (4) other factors.

Artefacts can be caused by the wrong method of collection, such as the use of a condom which may be sperm toxic, the sample may be contaminated by vaginal secretions, the use of lubricants[46], an incomplete sample, a long delay in transferring the sample to the laboratory, or exposure to extreme temperatures. Artefacts can also be caused by technical factors, such as cold shock as a result of the use of cold containers in the laboratory, slides and pipettes, the use of unsuitable, contaminated or wet containers, storage of the sample at adverse temperatures[47,48] and the wrong thickness of the wet preparation[49].

Table 1 Terminology used in andrology to describe semen deviations*

Term	*Meaning*
-spermia	Refers to the ejaculate
Aspermia	No semen ejaculated
Hematospermia	Blood present in ejaculate
Leukocytospermia	Leukocytes present in ejaculate
-zoospermia	Refers to spermatozoa in ejaculate
Azoospermia	No spermatozoa in semen
Normozoospermia	Normal semen parameters
Oligozoospermia	Low spermatozoa concentration
Asthenozoospermia	Poor motility and/or forward progression
Teratozoospermia	Reduced percentage of morphologically normal spermatozoa
Necrozoospermia	All spermatozoa dead as seen with supravital staining
Globozoospermia	Round-headed acrosomeless spermatozoa

Since it is often the practice to describe all deviations from normal semen variables with words the above international nomenclature was introduced. As these terms may have different values allocated to them in different laboratories it is very important that, when used for the first time in a publication, the numerical value of each term should be specified. *Adapted with permission of *World Health Organisation*[18]

Morphological abnormalities can include structural abnormalities of the midpiece[50], the short tail[51] and immotile-cilia or Kartagener syndromes[52].

Inherent factors are those caused as a result of a fault during forming and maturation of the spermatozoa before they are released from the Sertoli cells[53,54] or during transport through the epididymis[55] and ductal system, or through abnormal functions of the prostate or seminal vesicula.

Other factors that can cause a poor motility are the presence of hematospermia, a varicocele, chromosomal aberrations, bacterial infections, abnormal pH[48,56] and the presence of certain metals or metal ions[57].

The mixed antiglobulin reaction (MAR) test

A MAR test, as described by Jager *et al.*[7], must be included in all semen analyses as a routine procedure as a screening test for the possible presence of antisperm antibodies if a sufficient number of motile spermatozoa are present.

For the MAR test a suspension of sensitized R_1R_2 erythrocytes is needed. The erythrocytes are sensitized by washing these O Rh positive erythrocytes three times with a phosphate buffered saline (PBS) solution, pH 7.5. This suspension is mixed 5:1 with a strong incomplete anti-D serum (Behring ORRA 20/21) and incubated at 37°C for 30 min. After incubation the suspension is again washed three times in PBS and suspended to a hematocrit of 5–10%[7]. This suspension can be kept at 4°C for a few days.

For the MAR test, a drop of semen is placed on a clean glass slide followed by a drop of undiluted monospecific antisera to human IgG (Behring ORCM 04/05) and a drop of sensitized R_1R_2 erythrocytes suspension. Care should be taken that the drops do not touch each other, as this can influence the outcome of the test. The drops are thoroughly mixed with a coverslip and then covered by the same coverslip. The test is read after 10 min at room temperature. No interpretation is made if no red blood cell agglutinates are observed. The test is reported as negative if no motile spermatozoa are incorporated in the red cell agglutinates. The test is doubtful when <10% of motile sperm are incorporated in the red cell agglutinates, positive if ⩾10–90% of motile spermatozoa are incorporated in the red cell agglutinates, and strongly positive if >90% of motile spermatozoa are incorporated. In all cases of a positive MAR test (⩾10%) blood and seminal plasma should be obtained for subsequent testing of antisperm antibody titers with the micro-agglutination[58] and immobilization[59] tests at a later stage. The immunobead test[60] should be done with the next semen analysis to determine the isotypes of antibody present, i.e. IgA, IgG and IgM[61].

Sperm concentration

In 1929 the well-known paper by Macomber and Sanders[62] was published, describing their sperm counting technique which forms the basis for most of the techniques used today. A 1:20 dilution was made with the aid of a white blood cell pipette and the count performed on a hemocytometer. The diluting fluid consisted of a 5% $NaHCO_3$ to which 1% formalin was added.

Instead of the white blood cell pipette, Eliasson[24] used micropipettes to make a 1:50, 1:100 or a 1:200 dilution. Van Zyl[63] introduced the use of a glass tuberculin syringe instead of the white blood cell pipette. With this method it is possible to make a 1:10, 1:20 or a 1:100 dilution. Menkveld *et al.*[64] demonstrated that the results of the tuberculin syringe (TS) method compared well with the results of the white blood cell pipette (WCP) method. Makler introduced a special sperm counting chamber in 1979 which was improved in 1980[65]. With this method, it is possible to do sperm counts directly on undiluted semen samples, after immobilization of the spermatozoa in a hot water bath at ±60°C. In cases of a low sperm concentration the method has a high coefficient of variation and several drops must be counted[65]. Menkveld *et al.*[64] compared their TS method with the Makler Chamber (MC) and WCP methods and found that, in their hands, the TS method had the best relative accuracy followed by the MC method and then the WCP method[27,28,66]. Today, the counting of spermatozoa with the aid of computerized equipment (CASA) is gaining ground and is now the standard method in many laboratories[18,42].

The method described by Van Zyl *et al.*[63] and Menkveld *et al.*[64,66] is a simple technique for the determination of the sperm count. According to the estimated number of spermatozoa per LPF, a 1:10, 1:20 or 1:100 dilution is prepared. An aliquot of 0.2 mL semen is transferred to a small Wassermann tube (75×13 mm φ). In a separate tube 1.5 mL of dilution fluid is placed. The semen is drawn to the 0.05 or 0.1 mL mark for a 1:20 or 1:10 dilution, respectively. Then the syringe is filled to the 1.0 mL mark with the dilution fluid. The syringe is emptied into a clean tube. The suspension is left for 5 min at room temperature so that the sperm can become immobilized. For a 1:100 dilution, a 1:10 dilution is diluted 1:10. After standing for the desired time, the suspension is again thoroughly mixed and transferred to an improved Neubauer hemocytometer with double rulings (Assistent, Germany) by means of a Pasteur pipette. One white blood cell block comprising 16 small blocks are counted on opposite locations on each side of the chamber to compensate for possible filling defects[67,68]. Counts are performed in the standard fashion. Sperm concentration is calculated using the formula published by Freund[29]. Two dilutions are made for every sample and the average concentration calculated and taken as the concentration for the specific sample[66]. If the difference between the two samples is more than 10% for concentration of $<60\times10^6$/mL and >20% for concentration of $\geqslant 60\times10^6$/mL the dilutions are repeated[6]. The TS method has one disadvantage, in that a correction must be made for the extra volume that is drawn up in the tip of the syringe. The result must be multiplied by 0.8, 0.7 and 0.64 for 1:10, 1:20 and 1:100 dilutions, respectively. Despite this disadvantage, very accurate determinations are obtained as compared with the WCP and MC methods[64].

Differences still exist as to what can be regarded as a normal sperm concentration, and many different so-called normal counts have been proposed: i.e. $\geqslant 60\times10^6$/mL by Macomber and Sanders[62], $\geqslant 20\times10^6$/mL by Eliasson[24], and by MacLeod and Gold[69], and $\geqslant 10\times10^6$/mL by Van Zyl[63] and by Van Zyl *et al.*[70,71].

Supravital staining

A supravital staining test should be performed on every sample with a sperm concentration of $>1.0\times10^6$/mL. The method as described by Eliasson[39] is recommended. A drop of semen is placed on a spotplate and mixed with one drop of a 1% aqueous Eosin Y solution; after 15 s two drops of a 10% aqueous Nigrosin solution are added and thoroughly mixed. A drop of this mixture is transferred to a clean glass slide and a thin smear made and air-dried. The smears are examined with a 100× oil magnification. Any red or not totally white sperm cells are regarded as dead. The results are expressed as the percentage of live (white) sperm.

The performance of a supravital technique is important to distinguish between live and dead spermatozoa, as spermatozoa can still be alive but immotile due to several factors, such as cold shock. In practice, the supravital staining results should always be some percentage points higher than the estimated motility. A diagnosis of necrozoospermia (all spermatozoa dead) can only be made if supported by the supravital staining results.

Morphology

Morphology evaluation can be divided into two categories, i.e. the morphological evaluation of spermatozoa and the evaluation of semen cytology. Therefore two slides are prepared, one thicker smear for cytology and one thin smear for the morphology evaluation.

Morphological evaluation of spermatozoa

The morphological evaluation of spermatozoa as discussed here is based on the methodology as described by Menkveld[27], Kruger *et al.*[72,73] and Menkveld *et al.*[74]. Slides are thoroughly cleaned before use by washing in a detergent, rinsing in clean water and then rinsing in alcohol and dried[75]. Coverslips are also washed with alcohol. For the morphology evaluation smear, a small drop of semen is used to make a very thin smear. All the spermatozoa will be at one focus level and each sperm can be visualized separately; no more than 5–10 spermatozoa will be present per visual field at oil magnification (1000 or 1250×). The thickness of the smear can also be controlled by altering the size of the semen drop and by adjusting the angle and speed of the slide used to make the smear[3,6]. The slides are left to air dry, immediately fixed in alcohol, and then stored for later reference or until staining. A modified Papanicolaou method should be used for staining of the smears[18,74,76]. Alternative staining methods do exist, and these can be used depending on the laboratory's requirements: Shorr[77], Spermac[78,79], and Diff-Quik[80] staining.

According to the strict Tygerberg criteria[27,74], a normal spermatozoon is defined as having an oval form with a smooth contour, an acrosome comprising between 40% and 70% of the distal part of the sperm head and without any abnormalities of the neck, midpiece or tail, and no cytoplasmic droplets of more than half of the sperm head, as described by Eliasson[6]. The dimensions for normality and abnormalities of spermatozoa have been described by Eliasson in the same article and are slightly different than those proposed by the WHO[18].

The morphological classification system as proposed by the strict Tygerberg criteria is based on the methods described by MacLeod[81] and Eliasson[6]. To be classified as normal, the whole spermatozoon must be normal. The other classes used are too large, too small, tapering and duplications. Spermatozoa that cannot be placed in one of these groups are classified as amorphous. The strict Tygerberg criteria system[27,74] added one class: normal head with other abnormalities, such as abnormalities of the tail and/or neck, and/or sperm with a cytoplasmic droplet. These abnormalities are also recorded for abnormal spermatozoa when present and are recorded per 100 spermatozoa. Precursors are also included into this group and all are counted on a separate tally.

Where possible, 200 spermatozoa should be evaluated with the highest magnification possible, preferably 1250×. In case of any doubt about the dimensions of a sperm the size is measured with a micrometer. All the spermatozoa should not be evaluated in one, but in several areas: the corner areas and an area in the middle of the slide. This will increase the accuracy of the evaluation.

Evaluation of semen cytology

For the evaluation of the semen cytology, by which is meant the investigation of the sample for the presence of different cells and organisms, a thicker smear is prepared. A small drop of egg albumen is added to ensure a better adherence of the cells to the slide. The slide is fixed immediately in 1:1 ether : alcohol for 30 min and stained together with the slides for morphology evaluation.

The slides are screened at a low magnification (15×) and if any cells or organisms are observed, a 40× objective is used to make a better diagnosis. Cells looked for are especially white blood cells (polymorphs), epithelium cells, histiocytes and ghost cells (cytoplasma without a nucleus). The presence of these cells are recorded separately as: – = no cells; ± = occasional; + = 1–5/HPF; ++ = 5–10/HPF; and +++ = >10/HPF.

Additional procedures

Azoospermia

On the identification that the semen sample contains no spermatozoa, i.e. azoospermia, the following steps are performed. The sample is concentrated on a glass slide in a cytospin centrifuge by first mixing 0.5 mL semen with 1.0 mL of saline and centrifuged for 10 min at 1500 rpm. The slide is air-dried and stained by the Papanicolaou method. The results are interpreted as follows:

No sperm – azoospermia

Sperm present – severe oligozoospermia

Vasectomy patients are similarly treated to confirm azoospermia.

Moderate oligozoospermia ($<5.0 \times 10^6$/mL)

In cases were the spermatozoa concentration is $<5.0\times10^6$/mL the remaining semen, after completion of all the procedures, is centrifuged at ±200***g*** for 10 min. The pellet is suspended in a small volume of medium and a small drop used to make a standard smear. The smear is air-dried and stained for use in cases were there are too few sperm present on the original morphology smear.

Semen biochemistry

If the volume of a semen sample is ⩾2 mL, an aliquot of 0.5 to 1.0 mL semen is taken from the sample directly after the determination of the physical parameters, placed in a Wassermann tube and stored at 4–8°C until all the samples are received. The samples are then centrifuged at 3000***g*** for 30 min to obtain clean seminal plasma without spermatozoa. The seminal plasma can then be used for the determination of zinc, acid phosphatase, fructose, etc.

Semen cultures

In all cases where a semen analysis is done for the first time, swabs should be sent away for culturing of aerobic bacteria and for *Ureaplasma* and *Mycoplasma*. The same is done if more than 1+ white blood cells are found. The patient should be instructed to pass urine, then to wash his hands with soap and water and the glans penis with water alone. The semen is produced in individually packed and sterilized containers.

The Kremer test

The sperm penetration meter test, originally described by Kremer in 1965[9], quantifies the penetration capacity of spermatozoa in glass capillary tubes filled with either cervical mucus or blood serum, thus giving information about a possible immunoreaction in cervical mucus and progressive motility in cervical mucus or blood serum.

An appropriate chamber is required with one to three small containers(s) at the lower end of a glass slide to receive the semen, and marked with centimeter graduations. The mucus or serum-filled capillary tubes are then placed in these semen-filled containers and secured with putty. The entire chamber is placed in a humidified container and incubated at 37°C for up to 24 h. Readings can then be taken at predetermined time points, for example 2, 4, 8 and 24 h. The readings taken are the penetration depth, the number of spermatozoa penetrating to the 5 cm mark, and the degree of motility in the upper third of the capillary.

Instead of human cervical mucus or blood serum bovine mucus[10], commercially available as Penetrak®[82], or hyaluronic acid[11], also commercially available as Sperm Select®[83], can also be used for penetration studies.

Fructose determination (colorimetric bench method)

Fructose is *inter alia* an indicator of the secretory function of the seminal vesicles. The estimation of fructose is particularly important in cases of azoospermia as low fructose levels may indicate congenital dysgenesis (absence) of the seminal vesicles and vas deferens.

A bench method for the quick determination of fructose has been described by Amelar, based on the Selivanoff method[22]. Five mg of Resorcinol is added to 33 mL of concentrated HC1 and then diluted to a total of 100 mL with distilled water; 0.5 mL semen is added to 5 mL of the reagent in a heat-resistant glass tube, and the glass tube placed in boiling water for at least 1 min.

The presence of fructose will be indicated by a red coloring, the intensity reflecting the concentration of fructose in the seminal plasma.

Peroxidase test for leukocytes

The ejaculate usually contains cells other than spermatozoa, sometimes called round cells. Of importance is the presence of leukocytes, which may be an indication of the presence of an inflammation. A specific stain[8] is available to distinguish the peroxidase-positive leukocytes from other cells, especially germinal epithelium cells or precursors.

A stock solution is prepared by dissolving 125 mg benzidine and 150 mg cyanosine (Phloxine) in 50 mL 95% alcohol and is then further diluted with 50 mL distilled water. This solution can be stored in a light-protected bottle. A 3% hydrogen peroxide solution is also prepared[8].

Before the test is performed 250 μL of the stock solution is mixed with 20 μL of the peroxide solution. For the test itself, one drop of semen is mixed with one drop of the above working solution on a clean glass slide and covered with a coverslip, examined microscopically after 2 min and the number of brown cells per HPF estimated. Neutrophil granulocytes (leukocytes) stain brown, granules of basophil and eosinophil granulocytes stain reddish brown to violet, while lymphocytes and precursors stain light pink as they are peroxidase negative. The concentration of peroxidase positive cells can be counted with the aid of a hemocytometer and expressed as 10^6/mL semen.

Computer-assisted analysis (CASA)

The last decade has seen the development of many computer-based systems to analyze semen samples more accurately, objectively and efficiently. Although systems for the measurement of sperm concentration[18,42,76,84] and normal morphology[85] exist, the motility parameter has received the most attention[18,84]. These systems have primarily enabled the critical analysis of sperm head kinematics; flagellar kinematics remains a future challenge. To date numerous parameters of sperm head motion have been identified, of which 11 have been officially accepted and standardized. CASA has also been invaluable in the characterization of hyperactivated motility[18].

Three of the most generally used CASA parameters are:

(1) Curvilinear velocity (VCL), i.e. the measure of the rate of travel of the centroid of the sperm head over a given time period. This is calculated from the sum of the straight lines joining the sequential positions of the sperm head along the sperm's track.

(2) Straight line velocity (VSL) is the straight line distance between the first and last centroid positions for a given time period.

(3) Linearity of forward progression (LIN) is reported as the ratio of VSL to VCL and expressed as a percentage. A value of 100 represents cells swimming in a perfectly straight line[18,76,84].

INTERPRETATION OF SEMEN ANALYSIS RESULTS

Source of variations affecting semen parameters

Many sources of variation are known, but only some of those that can cause large variations in semen parameters, such as abstinence or illness, will be discussed.

Abstinence

Today it is an accepted fact that abstinence has a pronounced effect on the semen parameters[19,27,28,30]. This is due to the fact that production of spermatozoa and the secretions of the accessory glands that form the seminal plasma are continuous processes. It has been demonstrated[19,27,28,30] that abstinence can have a varied effect, from small or no influence to statistically significant differences, on the morphology, vitality, motility, sperm concentration and volume.

Menkveld[27] and Menkveld *et al.*[66] found similar effects. They found a nearly linear increase of 0.34 mL/day in the volume, from 2.53 ± 1.8 mL with 1 day to 3.98 ± 1.9 mL with 5 days of abstinence. The influence on the sperm concentration was also marked; although there was a small decrease from 1 to 2 days of abstinence, the sperm concentration thereafter increased with every day that the abstinence increased up to the period of between 6 and 9 days. There was a decrease in the percentage of motile spermatozoa. The best motility of 50.6 ± 13.3% motile spermatozoa was found in the group of men with 1 day of abstinence and decreased to 40.7 ± 14.9% motile spermatozoa for a group of men with ⩾21 days of abstinence. There was no change in the speed of forward progression. The percentage of morphologically normal spermatozoa followed an unexpected pattern. There was a drop in the percentage of normal forms if the abstinence increased from 1 to 2 days. After that the percentage of normal forms increased when the abstinence increased to 3 and 4 days where the highest values of 44.8±18.2% morphologically normal forms were found. With every extra day of abstinence thereafter the percentage of normal forms showed a decrease. It can, therefore, be concluded that the optimal semen parameter values are obtained with a period of abstinence of between 3 and 5 days. This is in agreement with the 2–5 days suggested by Mortimer[19].

Seasonal influences

It is generally accepted that the human is not a seasonal breeder, and that spermatogenesis is a continuous and active process throughout the year. A few articles, however, have been published where a possible seasonal influence has been investigated[86–88]. From the literature it appears that this influence is the result of increased summer temperatures and mainly has an influence on the sperm concentration and/or the sperm morphology. The article of Tjoa *et al.*[87] is the only one where distinct differences were found. The study was done in an area known for its high daytime temperatures with an average of up to 28.9°C. Bornman *et al.*[89] also found a decrease due to a rise in temperature, but only in the percentage of normal forms. Their study was done in the Pretoria area of South Africa, where summer daytime temperatures can reach up to 34°C. Menkveld *et al.*[27,66] only found that there was a small tendency for a higher median sperm concentration in the late winter and early spring with the highest median concentration of 40.16×10^6/mL in September. The temperatures in the Cape Town area of South Africa area are very mild, with an average maximum summer temperature of 26.3°C in January.

Occupational influences

The first report was that of Lancranjan et al.[90], who found a decreased fertility of men exposed to lead. The higher the exposure, the more severe the impairment. The impairment was noted for all semen parameters. Other investigations were performed on men working in dibromochloropropane (DBCP) plants[91] and on lorry drivers[92]. Higher incidences of impaired semen parameters were found in all these groups.

Menkveld et al.[27,66] found that lorry drivers, metal workers, electricians and men in the armed forces had a lower incidence of fertile males based on their criteria[66,70] for normality (Table 2). The incidences were 59.1%, 56.4%, 58.3% and 58.6%, respectively, as against an overall mean incidence of 64.5% fertile males. It was also interesting to note that couples in the lower socio-economic groups had a higher incidence of primary infertility of between 80.0% and 86.4% against an overall incidence of 77.0%. Couples in the higher socio-economic groups, especially clergymen, engineers and attorneys, had a higher incidence of secondary infertility, i.e. 38.5%, 31.1% and 48.6%, respectively, as against an overall mean incidence of 23.0%. The incidence of infertile males in this group, however, was no higher than the overall average incidence. Menkveld et al.[27,66] expressed the thought that increased environmental stress with increasing job demands may play a substantial role in this phenomenon as observed in these professional groups.

Influence of illness

Mention is often made in articles or chapters on male infertility that a common cold, a bout of influenza or some other febrile illness will have an effect on the sperm concentration and that questions on this should be included in the questionnaire to be completed with every semen analysis[19,34].

MacLeod published several articles[93,94] demonstrating the effect of a viral infection with an increased body temperature as well as the effect of chickenpox on semen quality. He found that the sperm concentration, motility, forward progression and morphology were all impaired.

Table 2 Summary of lower old international normal parameters and normal values used at Tygerberg Hospital

Semen parameters	Semen values	
	International	Tygerberg Hospital*
Volume (mL)	2–6	1–6
Count (×10⁶/mL)	⩾20.0	⩾10.0
Motility (% motile)	⩾40	⩾30
Forward progression (1–4)	⩾3.0	⩾2.0
Morphology (% normal)	⩾60	⩾20

*Adapted from references[27,70]

The same effect was observed by Menkveld et al.[27,66]. The effect can be quite drastic and is an important factor when evaluating semen analysis results. Two cases presented by Menkveld et al.[27,66] illustrated that the motility, speed of forward progression and the percentage of morphological normal spermatozoa were the first parameters to show negative effects of illness. Sperm concentration was not immediately negatively affected, probably due to storage of spermatozoa in the genital tract. This would also suggest that sperm morphology and movement can be altered while in the genital tract, especially the epididymis[55]. The negative effect of illness is reflected longest in the sperm morphology, which may indicate that spermatogenesis and spermiogenesis are very sensitive as far as the whole process of morphogenesis is concerned.

Decreasing semen parameters

Although not directly related to fluctuations in semen parameters, the possibility of decreasing semen parameters is a factor that should be kept in mind when studies performed in different time periods or decades are used for comparative analysis. The aspect of decreasing semen parameters first received attention in a publication by Nelson and Bunge[95]. Since this paper many others have been published, discussing whether the overall sperm counts of fertile and infertile populations are indeed decreasing or not. The thought of decreasing semen parameters is supported by many researchers[96,97] and opposed by others[98,99]. Mortimer[19] warns that one must be cautious in making such a statement, as numerous factors other than an evolutionary biological shift may be involved, not the least being technical error, statistical analysis of data and the difference in reference populations. Menkveld *et al.*[27,66,100] found no decrease in the sperm concentration, motility and speed of forward progression over a 15-year period. However, they did find a decrease in the percentage of morphological normal spermatozoa from 61.3% and 68.5% for Caucasian and Black populations, respectively, in 1968, to 28.7% and 29.0%, respectively, in 1982. Negative Pearson correlation coefficients of –0.3403 and –0.4156 found between years and morphology for the Caucasian and Black populations were statistically significant. The decrease was attributed to the incorporation of stricter morphology evaluation criteria[27,74] and to a real decrease due to possible environmental and socio-economic changes, as the decline was much stronger in the Black group where bigger socio-economical changes occurred over the 15-year period[100].

Conclusions

The adverse environmental effects investigated above seem to have their most pronounced effects on sperm morphology[27,66,100]. Menkveld *et al.*[27,66,100], like MacLeod[81,93,94], came to the conclusion that sperm morphology is a very sensitive parameter that will reflect any adverse influence on the body/testes in a short time. Menkveld *et al.*[27,66] speculated that any illness or infection will cause a temporary decrease in the percentage of morphological normal forms after which it will return to its original value. However, if the testes are repeatedly attacked by adverse influences or conditions this may start to cause histological changes in the lamina propria and basal membrane or Sertoli cell function, which will then adversely influence spermatogenesis and will first be reflected in a gradual lowering of the percentage of morphological normal spermatozoa[100,101], with an increase in the percentage of elongated sperms as well as an increase in the number of immature forms. This will then be followed by a decrease in the sperm concentration[27,66,101].

Number of semen analyses to be performed

Zaneveld and Polakoski[30] advocated that if a patient produced a normal sample with the first semen analysis, then no necessity existed to perform any further semen analysis. However, if the sample was a borderline case or classified as abnormal according to the specific laboratory's standards, it would be necessary to do more semen analyses before a final diagnosis could be made. In these cases, they recommend that three semen analyses with 3–5-week intervals should be carried out.

Ross[2] stipulated that three semen samples must be analyzed with 2–6-week intervals before a diagnosis of an abnormal semen profile can be made. Some authors feel that there will always be some variation from sample to sample and that it is, therefore, necessary to perform at least two semen analyses before a diagnosis can be made[25,102,103], while others[24] state that several, or 3–4 semen analyses[19,70] over a period of 3 months, are required to estimate a patient's fertility potential.

In cases where the first semen analysis showed doubtful results, Sherins *et al.*[104] found that it may be necessary to do 6–9 semen analyses before a reliable interpretation could be made. From the studies by Menkveld *et al.*[27,66,105] where the results of four consecutive semen analyses of 1199 men were compared, it was concluded that in normal circumstances and comparable days of abstinence, the first semen sample can be regarded as representative of the other three semen samples[105].

An aspect that must now seriously be considered is the cost factor. Due to increasing costs, the tendency is to keep the number of semen samples to a minimum. A good policy will therefore be that, in cases where the first semen sample is classified as normal according to the specific laboratory's standards, the semen analysis should be repeated on a later occasion if necessary, and in cases where the semen analysis was abnormal, the analysis should be repeated two or three times within a period of 3 months so that a good semen profile of the patient can be obtained.

Interpretation of results

The evaluation of a semen specimen must be based on an overall picture that relates seminal volume,

Table 3 New World Health Organization normal semen variables values*

Semen parameters	*Normal values*
Volume	≥2.0 mL
pH	7.2–8.0
Sperm concentration	≥20 × 10^6 spermatozoa/mL
Total sperm count	≥40 × 10^6 spermatozoa
Motility	≥50% with forward progression (categories (a) and (b)) or ≥25% with rapid linear progression (category (a))
Morphology	≥30% with normal morphology
Viability	≥75% alive
Fructose	≥13 μmol per ejaculate
MAR test	<10% with adherent particles
Immunobead test	<20% spermatozoa with adherent beads

WHO classification of forward progression: (a) rapid linear progressive motility; (b) slow or sluggish linear or non-linear movement; (c) non-progressive motility; and (d) all immotile. Adapted from 1992 *WHO Manual*[18]

spermatozoa concentration, quantitative and qualitative motility, morphological evaluation and the results of additional tests, such as the MAR test[7] and biochemical results. It must be kept in mind that even when results are far below the normal values of a laboratory conceptions can still occur, although the time to reach this goal may take longer in these cases[74,106].

A distinction should also be made according to the reason for which the semen analysis was requested. Results of a semen analysis which may give a bad prognosis for *in vivo* fertilization may still be adequate for *in vitro* fertilization. Calculating an index of total concentration of morphological normal motile spermatozoa[17] may be of use for *in vitro* fertilization, but is of little relevance for *in vivo* fertilization as volume plays an important part in these calculations. It is known that oligozoospermia is frequently associated with large semen volumes, which must be regarded as an abnormal parameter, and this abnormal factor can therefore not be used to calculate such an index and compensate for the low count. These large semen volumes are associated with semen loss from the vagina after intercourse, resulting in a large percentage of the available spermatozoa also being lost.

Much has been written about interrelationships between semen parameters[19,107] and the compensating interaction of semen parameters. Although there may be a general tendency[108] that high sperm concentrations are associated with higher percentages of motility and normal morphology, Menkveld *et al.*[27,74,101] have shown that there are exceptions, particularly as far as the morphology is concerned[72,101]. As far as the compensating interaction of semen parameters is concerned, the above-mentioned argument also holds true. In cases where the volume is within the normal range a certain degree of compensating interaction may occur, but this will be limited. It was observed[28,70] while calculating normal values and minimal values for conception based on the occurrence of conceptions in an infertile population (which incidentally should be used, not so-called 'normal populations') that a single, constantly very abnormal semen parameter could be associated with only sporadic or no occurrence of conception in apparently normal women[66,109].

Standards for normal semen parameters

Normal standards or values for so-called normal or fertile semen based on the use of the basic semen parameters, i.e. volume, motility, speed of forward progression and morphology, have from time to time been published (Table 3, new WHO normal values)[18]. These values were mostly obtained through studies performed on so-called fertile populations[14,18]. This means that pregnancies were also obtained with lower values, as indicated in the manual. Many people, especially those not working in the field, do not take this fact into consideration and confuse normality with fertility. This results in the situation that, if the semen parameters (variables) are not within the normal range as given in the publications[14,18], the male is regarded as infertile or not capable of fertilizing his spouse. This can lead to social problems and stress among couples; for example, in cases where spontaneous pregnancies occur after such a pronouncement has been made.

The difference between standards for normality and fertility has been demonstrated by van Zyl *et al.*[70], Menkveld[27] and Menkveld *et al.*[28,66]. Results of semen analyses of males who had recently impregnated their wives were classified according to old WHO[14,75] values for normality (Table 2) and the values for fertility used at Tygerberg hospital[27,28,66,70]. Only 18.8% of the men were classified as normal or fertile according to the WHO criteria, as against 68.4% with the Tygerberg values. The Tygerberg normal values were based on comparison of the values of each separate semen parameter with pregnancies obtained, and the lowest value for each semen parameter above which no significant increase in the pregnancy rate per interval group occurred was taken as the normal value for fertility[28,70–73].

Studies on IVF results[110] have also indicated that fertilization and pregnancies can be obtained with semen parameters values which are well below the normal WHO limits[14,18]. This was true for sperm concentration and especially morphology[110,111], even when evaluated according to WHO criteria and not the strict Tygerberg criteria[74] where even lower limits may be expected[72,73,111].

Therefore, as semen analyses are used mainly to investigate male fertility potential of an infertile population, the datum point for establishing standards for fertility evaluation should not be based on what is average in a normal population, but rather

Table 4 Proposed interval groups for the classification of a male's fertility potential as used at Tygerberg Hospital*

Semen parameters	*Infertile*	*Subfertile*	*Fertile*
Concentration ($\times 10^6$/mL)	<2.0	2.0–9.9	⩾10.0
Motility (% motile)	<10	10–29	⩾30
Forward progression (0–4)	<1.0	1.0–1.9	⩾2
Motility index	<20.0	20.0–49.9	<50
Morphology (% normal)	0–4	5–14	⩾15
Volume (mL)	—	<1.76	1–6

Fertile = optimal chance for conception; subfertile = reduced chance for conception; Infertile = very small chance for conception; and sterile = azoospermia or globozoospermia. *Adapted from Menkveld *et al.*[66] and Van Zyl *et al.*[70]

on what minimum semen parameters values are needed to give a reasonable chance for conception. These values will be much lower than the mean values for normality of a population with proven fertility. For this the WHO[18] manual does not provide guidelines.

On these grounds, the following values are proposed (Table 4) for the classification of male fertility potential based on results of fertilization *in vivo*[27,66,70,71,109] or *in vitro*[72,73] obtained from an infertile population. Semen parameters should be reclassified for diagnostic and prognostic purposes, for example fertile, subfertile, infertile and sterile, when azoospermia is present.

The classification is based on the male's poorest semen parameter[66]. In the subfertile group, some compensating interaction between the different semen parameters may occur, but if a specific semen falls in the infertile category, the impairment is so severe that even one or more good semen parameters cannot compensate for the single poor parameter[66,72,73].

References

1. Sims, J. M. (1869). On the microscope as an aid in the diagnosis and treatment of sterility. *N. Y. Med. Bull.*, **8**, 393–413
2. Ross, L. S. (1983). Diagnosis and treatment of infertile men: A clinical perspective. *J. Urol.*, **130**, 847–54
3. Hotchkiss, R. S. (1945). *Fertility in Men.* (London: William Heinemann Medical Books)
4. Abarbanel, A. R., Brown, W. E., Greulich, W. W., Pommerenke, W. T., Simmons, F. A. and Sturgis, S. (1951). Evaluation of the barren marriage. Minimal

procedures. *Fertil. Steril.*, **2**, 1–14
5. Freund, M. (1966). Standards for the rating of human sperm morphology. A cooperative study. *Int. J. Fertil.*, **11**, 97–118
6. Eliasson, R. (1971). Standards for investigation of human semen. *Andrologie*, **3**, 49–64
7. Jager, S., Kremer, J. and Van Slochteren-Draaisma, T. (1978). A simple method of screening for anti-sperm antibodies in the human male – detection of spermatozoal surface IgG with the direct Mixed Antiglobulin Reaction carried out on untreated fresh human semen. *Int. J. Fertil.*, **23**, 12–21
8. Ludwig, G. and Fick, J. (1990). *Spermatology, Atlas and Manual*, pp. 32–3. (Berlin: Springer-Verlag)
9. Kremer, J. (1965). A simple sperm penetration test. *Int. J. Fertil.*, **10**, 209–14
10. Zavos, P. M. and Cohen, M. R. (1980). Bovine mucus penetration test: an assay for fresh and cryopreserved human spermatozoa. *Fertil. Steril.*, **34**, 175–6
11. Wikland, M., Wik, O., Steen, Y. and Qvist, K. (1987). A self-migration method for preparation of sperm for *in-vitro* fertilization. *Hum. Reprod.*, **2**, 191–5
12. Kremer, J. and Jager, S. (1976). The sperm–cervical mucus contact test: A preliminary report. *Fertil. Steril.*, **27**, 335–40
13. Mortimer, D. (1985). The male factor in infertility. Part II: Sperm function testing. *Curr. Probl. Obstet. Gynecol. Fertil.*, **8**, 4–75
14. Word Health Organization (1987). *WHO Laboratory Manual for the Examination of Human Semen and Semen–Cervical Mucus Interaction*, 2nd edn. (Cambridge: Cambridge University Press)
15. Yanagimachi, R., Yanagimachi, H. and Rogers, B. J. (1976). The use of zona-free hamster ova as a test-system for the assessment of the fertilizing capacity of human spermatozoa. *Biol. Reprod.*, **15**, 471–6
16. Schill, W.-B. and Feifel, M. (1984). Low acrosin activity in Polyzoospermia. *Andrologia*, **16**, 589–91
17. Franken, D. R., Kruger, T. F., Menkveld, R., Oehninger, S., Coddington, C. C. and Hodgen, G. D. (1990). Hemizona assay and teratozoospermia: increasing sperm insemination concentrations to enhance zona pellucida binding. *Fertil. Steril.*, **54**, 497–503
18. Word Health Organization. (1992). *WHO Laboratory Manual for the Examination of Human Semen and Sperm–Cervical Mucus Interaction*, 3rd edn. (Cambridge: Cambridge University Press)
19. Mortimer, D. (1985). The male factor in infertility. Part I: Semen analysis. *Curr. Prob. Obstet. Gynecol. Fertil.*, **8**, 4–87
20. Alexander, N. J. (1982). Male evaluation and semen analysis. *Clin. Obstet. Gynecol.*, **25**, 463–82
21. Hendry, W. F. (1979). Male infertility. *Br. J. Hosp. Med.*, **22**, 47–60
22. Amelar, R. D. (1966). *Infertility in Men*, pp. 13–15. (Philadelphia: F. A. Davies Co.)
23. Toussaint, D. N., Roth, E. J., Chen, D., Ling, E. A. and Jeyendran, R. S. (1993). Comparison of semen quality obtained by vibratory stimulation and masturbation. *Hum. Reprod.*, **8**, 1067–9
24. Eliasson, R. (1975). Analysis of semen. In Behrman, S. J. and Kistner, S. W. (eds.) *Progress in Infertility*, 2nd edn, pp. 691–713. (Boston: Little, Brown Co.)
25. Mehan, D. J. and Chehval, M. J. (1977). A clinical evaluation of a new silastic seminal fluid collection device. *Fertil. Steril.*, **28**, 689–91
26. Check, J. H., Shanis, B. S., Wu, C. H. and Bollendorf, A. (1988). Evaluating glass, polystyrene, and polypropylene containers for semen collection and sperm washing. *Arch. Androl.*, **20**, 251–5
27. Menkveld, R. (1987). An investigation of environmental influences on spermatogenesis and semen parameters. *Ph.D. Dissertation, Faculty of Medicine, University of Stellenbosch, South Africa*
28. Menkveld, R. and Kruger, T. F. (1990). Basic semen analysis. In Acosta, A. A., Swanson, R. J., Ackerman, S. B., Kruger, T. F., van Zyl, J. A. and Menkveld, R. (eds.) *Human Spermatozoa in Assisted Reproduction*, pp. 68–84. (Baltimore: Williams and Wilkins)
29. Freund, M. (1968). Performance and interpretation of the semen analysis. In Rolands, M. (ed.) *Management of the Infertile Couple*, p. 48. (Springfield: Charles C. Thomas)
30. Zaneveld, L. J. D. and Polakoski, K. L. (1977). Collection and the physical examination of the ejaculate. In Hafez, E. S. E. (ed.) *Techniques of Human Andrology*, pp. 147–72. (Amsterdam: Elsevier/North-Holland Biomedical Press)
31. Mandal, A. and Bhattacharyya, A. K. (1985). Studies on the coagulational characteristics of human ejaculates. *Andrologia*, **17**, 80–6
32. Amelar, R. D. (1962). Coagulation, liquefaction and viscosity of human semen. *J. Urol.*, **87**, 187–90
33. Mann, T. (1971). Biochemical appraisal of human semen. In Joël, C. A. (ed.) *Fertility Disturbances in Men and Women*, pp. 146–61. (Basel: Karger)
34. Schirren, C. (1972). *Practical Andrology*, pp. 10–11. (Berlin: Verlag Brüder Hartman)
35. Cary, H. W. and Hotchkiss, R. S. (1934). Semen appraisal. A differential stain that advances the study of cell morphology. *J.A.M.A.*, **102**, 587–90
36. Portnoy, L. (1946). The diagnosis and prognosis of male infertility: A study of 44 cases with special reference to sperm morphology. *J. Urol.*, **48**, 735–46
37. Vermeiden, J. P. W., Bernardus, R. E., ten Brug, C. S., Statema-Lohmeijer, C. H., Willemsen-Brugma, A. M. and Schoemaker, J. (1989). Pregnancy rate is significantly higher in *in vitro* fertilization procedure with spermatozoa isolated from nonliquefying semen in which liquefaction is induced by α-amylase. *Fertil. Steril.*, **51**, 149–52
38. Tucker, M., Wright, G., Bishop, F., Wiker, S., Cohen, J., Chan, Y. M. and Sharma, R. (1990). Chymotrypsin in semen preparation for ARTA. *Mol. Androl.*, **2**, 179–86

39. Eliasson, R. (1977). Supravital staining of human spermatozoa. *Fertil. Steril.*, **28**, 1257
40. Rose, N., Hjort, T., Rümke, P., Harper, M. J. K. and Vyazox, O. (1976). Techniques for detection of iso- and auto-antibodies to human spermatozoa. *Clin. Exp. Immunol.*, **23**, 175–99
41. Hotchkiss, R. S., Brunner, E. K. and Grenley, P. (1938). Semen analysis of two hundred fertile men. *Am. J. Med. Sci.*, **196**, 362–84
42. Knuth, U. A., Yeung, C.-H. and Nieschlag, E. (1987). Computerized semen analysis: objective measurement of semen characteristics is biased by subjective parameter setting. *Fertil. Steril.*, **48**, 118–24
43. Freund, M. and Peterson, R. N. (1976). Semen evaluation and fertility. In Hafez, E. S. E. (ed.) *Human Semen and Fertility Regulation in Men*, pp. 344–54. (St Louis: Mosby Co.)
44. MacLeod, J. and Heim, L. M. (1945). Characteristics and variation in semen specimens in 100 normal young men. *J. Urol.*, **54**, 474–82
45. MacLeod, J. (1965). The semen examination. *Clin. Obstet Gynecol.*, **8**, 115–27
46. Goldenberg, R. L. and White, R. (1975). The effect of vaginal lubricants on sperm motility *in vitro*. *Fertil. Steril.*, **26**, 872–3
47. Carruthers, G. B. (1981). Assessment of the semen. In Philipp, E. E. and Carruthers, G. B. (eds.) *Infertility*, p. 195. (London: William Heinemann Medical Books)
48. Appell, R. A. and Evans, P. R. (1977). The effect of temperature on sperm motility and viability. *Fertil. Steril.*, **28**, 1329–32
49. Makler, A. (1978). The thickness of microscopically examined seminal samples and its relationship to sperm motility estimation. *Int. J. Androl.*, **1**, 213–19
50. Folgerø, T., Bertheussen, K., Lindal, S. and Torbergson, T. (1993). Mitochondrial disease and reduced sperm motility. *Hum. Reprod.*, **8**, 1863–8
51. Barthelemy, C., Tharanne, M. J., Lebos, C., Lecomte, P. and Lansac, J. (1989). Tail stump spermatozoa: Morphogenesis of defect. An ultrastructural study of sperm and testicular biopsy. *Andrologia*, **22**, 417–25
52. Eliasson, R., Mossberg, B., Cammer, P. and Afzelius, A. (1977). The immotile-cilia syndrome. A congenital ciliary abnormality as an etiologic factor in chronic airway infection and male sterility. *N. Engl. J. Med.*, **297**, 1–6
53. Atherton, R. W. (1977). Evaluation of sperm motility. In Hafez, E. S. E. (ed.) *Techniques of Human Andrology*, pp. 173–87. (Amsterdam: Elsevier/North-Holland Biomedical Press)
54. MacLeod, J., Pazianos, A. and Ray, B. S. (1964). Restoration of human spermatogenesis by menopausal gonadotrophins. *Lancet*, **1**, 1196–79
55. Purvis, K., Brekke, I. and Tollefsrud, A. (1991). Epididymal secretory function in men with asthenoteratozoospermia. *Hum. Reprod.*, **6**, 850–3
56. Bar-Sagie, D., Mayevsky, A. and Bartoov, B. (1981). A fluorometric technique for simultaneous measurement of pH and motility in ram semen. *Arch. Androl.*, **7**, 27–33
57. Kesserü, E. and León, F. (1974). Effect of different solid metals and metallic pairs on human sperm motility. *Int. J. Fertil.*, **19**, 81–4
58. Friberg, J. (1974). A simple and sensitive micromethod for demonstration of sperm-agglutinating activity in serum from infertile men and women. *Acta. Obstet Gynecol. Scand.* (Suppl), **36**, 21–9
59. Isojima, S., Shun, T. and Ashitaka, Y. (1968). Immunologic analysis of sperm-immobilizing factor found in sera of women with unexplained sterility. *Am. J. Obstet. Gynecol.*, **101**, 677–83
60. Clarke, G. N., Stojanoff, A. and Cauchi, M. N. (1982). Immunoglobulin class of sperm-bound antibodies in semen. In Branatov, K. (ed.) *Immunology of Reproduction. Proceedings of the Fifth International Symposium on Immunology of Reproduction*, pp. 482–5. (Sofia: Bulgarian Academy of Sciences Press)
61. Menkveld, R., Kruger, T. F., Kotze, T. J. vW., Windt, M-L. and Pretorius, E. (1991). Detection of sperm antibodies on unwashed spermatozoa with the immunobead test: A comparison of results with the routine method and seminal plasma TAT and SCMC test. *Am. J. Reprod. Immunol.*, **25**, 88–91
62. Macomber, D. and Sanders, M. B. (1929). The spermatozoa count. Its value in the diagnosis, prognosis and treatment of sterility. *N. Engl. J. Med.*, **200**, 981–4
63. Van Zyl, J. A. (1972). A review of the male factor in 231 infertile couples. *S. Afr. J. Obstet. Gynecol.*, **10**, 17–23
64. Menkveld, R., Van Zyl, J. A. and Kotze, T. J. vW. (1984). A statistical comparison of three methods for the counting of human spermatozoa. *Andrologia.*, **16**, 554–8
65. Makler, A. (1980). The improved ten-micrometer chamber for rapid sperm count and motility evaluation. *Fertil. Steril.*, **33**, 337–8
66. Menkveld, R. and Kruger, T. F. (1990). Basic semen analysis: The Tygerberg experience. In Acosta, A. A., Swanson, R. J., Ackerman, S. B., Kruger, T. F., van Zyl, J. A. and Menkveld, R. (eds.). *Human Spermatozoa in Assisted Reproduction*, pp. 164–76. (Baltimore: Williams and Wilkins)
67. Chamberlain, A. C., Turner, F. M. (1952). Errors and variations in the white-cells counts. *Biometrics*, **8**, 55–65
68. Berkson, J., Magath, T. B. and Hurn, M. (1940). Error of estimate of the blood cell count as made in the hemocytometer. *Am. J. Physiol.*, **128**, 309–23
69. MacLeod, J. and Gold, R. Z. (1951). The male factor in fertility and infertility. II. Spermatozoa counts in 1,000 men of known fertility and in 1,000 cases of infertile marriage. *J. Urol.*, **66**, 436–9
70. Van Zyl, J. A., Menkveld, R., Kotze, T. J. vW. and van Niekerk, W. A. (1976). The importance of spermiograms that meet the requirements of inter-

national standards and the most important factors that influence semen parameters. *Proceedings of the 17th Congress of the International Urological Society*, Vol. 2, pp. 263–71. (Paris: Diffusion Dion Editeurs)
71. Van Zyl, J. A., Menkveld, R., Kotze, T. J. vW., Retief, A. E. and Van Niekerk, W. A. (1975). Oligozoospermia: A seven-year survey of the incidence, chromosomal aberrations, treatment and pregnancy rate. *Int. J. Fertil.*, **20**, 129–32
72. Kruger, T. F., Menkveld, R., Stander, F. S. H., Lombard, C. J., van der Merwe, J. P., van Zyl, J. A. and Smith, K. (1986). Sperm morphologic features as a prognostic factor in *in vitro* fertilization. *Fertil. Steril.*, **46**, 1118–23
73. Kruger, T. F., Acosta, A. A., Simmons, K. F., Swanson, R. J., Matta, J. F. and Oehninger, S. (1988). Predictive value of abnormal sperm morphology in *in vitro* fertilization. *Fertil. Steril.*, **49**, 112–17
74. Menkveld, R., Stander, F. S. H., Kotze, T. J. vW., Kruger, T. F. and van Zyl, J. A. (1990). The evaluation of morphological characteristics of human spermatozoa according to stricter criteria. *Hum. Reprod.*, **5**, 586–92
75. World Health Organization. (1980). *WHO Laboratory Manual for the Examination of Human Semen and Semen–Cervical Mucus Interaction.* (Singapore: Press Concern)
76. Mortimer, D. (1994). *Practical Laboratory Andrology.* (Oxford: Oxford University Press)
77. Jeulin, C., Feneux, D., Serres, C., Jouannet, P., Guillet-Rosso, F., Belaisch-Allart, J., Frydman, R. and Testart, J. (1986). Sperm factors related to failure of human *in vitro* fertilization. *J. Reprod. Fertil.*, **76**, 735–44
78. Oettlé, E. E. (1986). Using a new acrosome stain to evaluate sperm morphology. *Vet. Med.*, **81**, 263–6
79. Menkveld, R. (1991). Appendices. In Menkveld, R., Oettlé, E. E., Kruger, T. F., Swanson, R. J. and Oehninger, S. (eds.) *Atlas of Human Sperm Morphology*, pp. 115–18. (Baltimore: Williams and Wilkins)
80. Kruger, T. F., Ackerman, S. B., Simmons, K. F., Swanson, R. J., Brugo, S. S. and Acosta, A. A. (1987). A quick, reliable staining technique for human sperm morphology. *Arch. Androl.*, **18**, 275–7
81. MacLeod, J. and Gold, R. Z. (1952). The male factor in fertility and infertility. IV. Sperm morphology in fertile and infertile marriage. *Fertil. Steril.*, **2**, 394–414
82. Schütte, B. (1986). Penetration ability of human spermatozoa into standardized bovine cervical mucus (Penetrak[R]) in patients with normal and pathological semen samples. *Andrologia*, **19**, 217–24
83. Huszar, G., Willetts, M. and Corrales, M. (1990). Hyaluronic acid (Sperm Select®) improves retention of sperm motility and velocity in normospermic and oligospermic specimens. *Fertil. Steril.*, **54**, 1127–34
84. Mortimer, D., Goel, N. and Shu, M. A. (1988). Evaluation of the CellSoft automated semen analysis system in a routine laboratory setting. *Fertil. Steril.*, **50**, 960–8
85. Kruger, T. F., Du Toit, T. C., Franken, D. R., Acosta, A. A., Oehninger, S. C., Menkveld, R. and Lombard, C. J. (1993). A new computerized method of reading sperm morphology (strict criteria) is as efficient as technician reading. *Fertil. Steril.*, **59**, 202–9
86. Mortimer, D., Tempelton, A. A., Lenton, E. A. and Coleman, R. A. (1983). Annual patterns of human sperm production and semen quality. *Arch. Androl.*, **10**, 1–5
87. Tjoa, W. S., Smolensky, M. H., Hsi, B. P., Steinberger, E. and Smith, K. D. (1982). Circannual rhythm in human sperm count revealed by serially independent sampling. *Fertil. Steril.*, **38**, 454–9
88. Hotchkiss, R. S. (1941). Factors in stability and variability of semen specimens – observations on 640 successive samples from 23 men. *J. Urol.*, **45**, 875–88
89. Bornman, M. S., Schullenburg, G. W., Boomkar, D., Van der Merwe, C. A. and Reif, S. (1990). Ambient temperature and semen quality. *Abstract, Reproductive Biology Workshop*, Faculty of Medicine, University of Pretoria, Pretoria
90. Lancranjan, I., Popescu, H. I., Gavanescu, O., Klepsch, I. and Estranges, M. (1975). Reproductive ability of workmen occupationally exposed to lead. *Arch. Environ. Hlth*, **30**, 396–401
91. Whorton, J. D. and Meyer, C. R. (1984). Sperm count results from 861 American chemical/agricultural workers from 14 separate studies. *Fertil. Steril.*, **42**, 82–6
92. Sas, M. and Szöllösi, J. (1979). Impaired spermiogenesis as a common finding among professional drivers. *Arch. Androl.*, **3**, 57–60
93. MacLeod, J. (1966). The clinical implications of deviations in human spermatogenesis as evidenced in seminal cytology and experimental production of these deviations. *Excerpta Medica International Congress*, Series No. 133, pp. 563–74. *Proceedings of the Fifth Congress on Fertility and Sterility*, Stockholm, 16–22 June
94. MacLeod, J. (1951). Effect of chickenpox and of pneumonia on semen quality. *Fertil. Steril.*, **2**, 523–33
95. Nelson, C. M. K. and Bunge, R. G. (1974). Semen analysis: Evidence for changing parameters of male fertility potential. *Fertil. Steril.*, **25**, 503–7
96. James, W. H. (1980). Secular trend in reported sperm counts. *Andrologia*, **12**, 381–8
97. Leto, S. and Frensilli, F. J. (1981). Changing parameters of donor semen. *Fertil. Steril.*, **36**, 766–70
98. MacLeod, J. and Wang, Y. (1979). Male fertility in terms of semen quality: a review of the past, a study of the present. *Fertil. Steril.*, **31**, 103–16
99. David, G., Jouannet, P., Martin-Boyce, A., Spira, A. and Schwartz, D. (1979). Sperm counts in fertile and infertile men. *Fertil. Steril.*, **31**, 453–5
100. Menkveld, R., van Zyl, J. A., Kotze, T. J. vW. and Joubert, G. (1986). Possible changes in male fertility

over a 15-year period. *Arch. Androl.*, **17**, 143–4

101. Menkveld, R., Kotze, T. J. vW. and Kruger, T. F. (1992). Relationship of human sperm morphology with other semen parameters as seen in different reference populations. *Hum. Reprod.*, **6**, Suppl., 1, 96–7
102. Amelar, R. D., Dubin, L. and Schoenfeld, C. (1973). Semen analysis: An office technique. *Urology*, **2**, 605–11
103. Taylor, P. J. and Martin, R. H. (1981). Semen analysis in the investigation of infertility. *Can. Fam. Phys.*, **27**, 113–16
104. Sherins, R. J., Brightwell, D. and Sternthal, P. M. (1977). Longitudinal analysis of semen of fertile and infertile men. In Troen, P. and Nankin, H. R. (eds.) *The Testis in Normal and Infertile Men*, pp. 473–88. (New York: Raven Press)
105. Menkveld, R., Kotze, T. J. vW. and Kruger, T. F. (1992). An investigation to determine if the first semen analysis is representative of consecutive semen analyses. *Hum. Reprod.*, **6**, Suppl. 1, 93–4
106. Jouannet, P., Ducot, B., Feneux, D. and Spira, A. (1988). Male factors and the likelihood of pregnancy in infertile couples. 1. Study of sperm characteristics. *Int. J. Androl.*, **11**, 379–94
107. MacLeod, J. and Gold, R. Z. (1952). The male factor in fertility and infertility. VIII. A study of variation in semen quality. *Fertil. Steril.*, **7**, 387–410
108. MacLeod, J. (1962). A possible factor in etiology of human male infertility. *Fertil. Steril.*, **13**, 29–33
109. Van Zyl, J. A., Kotze, T. J. vW. and Menkveld, R. (1990). Predictive value of spermatozoa morphology in natural fertilization. In Acosta, A. A., Swanson, R. J., Ackerman, S. B., Kruger, T. F., van Zyl, J. A. and Menkveld, R. (eds.) *Human Spermatozoa in Assisted Reproduction*, pp. 319–24. (Baltimore: Williams and Wilkins)
110. Hinting, A., Comhaire, F., Vermeulen, L., Dhont, M., Vermeulen, A. and Vandekerckhove, D. (1990). Value of sperm characteristics and results of *in-vitro* fertilization for predicting the outcome of assisted reproduction. *Int. J. Androl.* **13**, 59–66
111. Enginsu, M. E., Dumoulin, C. J. M., Pieters, M. H. E. C., Bras, M., Evers, J. L. H. and Geraedts, J. P. M. (1991). Evaluation of human sperm morphology using strict criteria after Diff-Quik staining: correlation of morphology with fertilization *in vitro*. *Hum. Reprod.*, **6**, 854–8

Evaluation of sperm motility in assisted reproduction

7

K. Kaskar and D. R. Franken

INTRODUCTION

The importance of human sperm motility during the fertilization process has received considerable attention over the past decade. Not only have new methods been developed to evaluate motion characteristics of human spermatozoa, but pharmacological treatment for impaired sperm motility has also been applied.

Male factor disorders affect more than 30% of infertile couples. Thus, it has become important to perform a complete andrological consultation and a basic semen evaluation in all male partners of couples consulting for infertility. The advent and development of assisted reproductive technologies have not only improved clinical results, but also have enhanced our basic understanding of the physiology of sperm and sperm preparation methods. Assisted reproduction has become one of the more successful therapeutic modalities for a wide variety of sperm function disorders, e.g. artificial insemination and *in vitro* fertilization (IVF)[1].

The association of specific seminal characteristics (sperm concentration, percentage of motile cells and percentage normal sperm forms) with the success rate of assisted reproductive techniques, and IVF in particular, has been under great scrutiny[2,3]. The analysis of the relationships between conventional semen parameters and fertilization rates *in vitro* has shown that sperm motility, concentration and morphology must be considered in estimating opportunities for successful intervention, as in the case of IVF and gamete intrafallopian transfer (GIFT)[4]. A reduction in the percentage of progressive motility alone does not seem to have a significant impact on IVF results unless it is below a threshold value of 10%. The semen sample should have an acceptable sperm concentration and morphology and/or that at least 1.5×10^6 motile spermatozoa can be recovered after swim-up separation[1].

Computer-assisted analysis of sperm motion characteristics is a valuable tool which may aid in diagnosis of disordered sperm function in subfertile males[5,6]. Objective analysis of sperm motion parameters by Computer Assisted Semen Analyzer (CASA) has resulted in positive and significant correlations between the amplitude of lateral head displacement[7], curvilinear velocity[8], linearity and straight line velocity[9], and fertilization rates *in vitro*. Other sperm motion parameters have not yet been correlated with failure/success of fertilization of human oocytes under *in vitro* conditions.

HYPERACTIVATION

Prerequisite pre-fertilization changes by sperm, termed 'capacitation'[10], provide sperm with the ability to fertilize eggs. These processes are generally regarded as encompassing all pre-fertilization changes occurring in sperm up to, but not including, loss of the acrosome[11]. The endpoints of capacitation are often described as the acrosomal loss, as well as changes in the motion characteristics. Capacitation alters the pattern of motility exhibited by freely swimming sperm, changing from a fairly rigid flagellar beat pattern to one of extreme flexure, often associated with increased thrust[12], which is referred to as hyperactivated motility[13]. Without the transition to hyperactivated motility sperm are unable to penetrate the zona pellucida[14], and possibly unable to fertilize eggs. Hyperactivation, *per se*, is marked by increased curvature in swimming trajectories and/or increased lateral displacement of the sperm head along their path[15]. However, the physiological role of this change in motility is not clearly understood because almost all relevant data have been obtained under *in vitro* conditions.

First observed in 1969 by Yanagimachi[16], sperm hyperactivation is a distinctive, vigorous motility which has been described for mammals and for the human[15]. Early reports described hyperactivated motility in terms of sperm flagellar motion, sperm vigor and trajectory. These hyperactivated sperm were said to be extremely vigorous; their principal feature was a repeated pattern of high-curvature undulations of the flagellum. Subjective visual assessments have led to a remarkable set of metaphors used to characterize the swimming trajectories of hyperactivated sperm. Such motions have been referred to as 'bobbing'[17], 'high amplitude'[18], 'serpentine'[18], 'whiplash'[19], 'figure-of-eight'[20] and 'darting'[21]. Clearly, these terms did not permit the standardization in the identification of hyperactivation.

Recently, the sperm have been divided according to their swimming patterns as follows[22]:

(1) *Circular high-curvature:* previously called wide amplitude, this is seen as relative planar beating of the flagellum, marked side-to-side head movements, and a beat envelope of $\geqslant 19\ \mu m$[22].

(2) *Thrashing:* an extremely erratic trajectory, at least three rapid U-shaped flexions, and a change in the plane of the flagellar beat with each flexion.

(3) *Star-spin:* rapidly spinning in one place, with no forward progression.

(4) *Helical:* a highly three-dimensional trajectory with regular repeats.

(5) *Non-hyperactivated:* a fairly straight trajectory, an even roll of the head about the central axis, and a minimal curvature of the flagellum.

In general, the flagella of hyperactivated spermatozoa generate beats of decreased symmetry, involving bends of increased curvature in the midpiece and proximal principal piece. Many studies have indicated that the movements of at least some hyperactivated sperm are intermittent (as in the rabbit) with phases of relatively lesser or greater progressiveness. The less progressive phase is the classic high-curvature motion and is most commonly described subjectively as whiplash and as figure-of-eight motion. The more progressive movements are sometimes called darting motion[21], because of the jerky but progressive swimming trajectories observed. Suarez[23] described, in golden hamster sperm, a discrete intermediate state immediately preceding whiplash motion. This state, termed helical motion, relates to that described by Burkman[22] and consists of a more three-dimensional but relatively progressive swimming trajectory through which the sperm head traces a helix.

Robertson *et al.*[24] developed an automated method to identify and count two subpopulations of hyperactivated cells. One population of cells displayed the star-shaped trajectories which correspond to those identified by Burkman[22]; a second population, which was termed transitional, more closely approximated hyperactivation as originally described by Yanagimachi[18]. This transition phase is similar to sperm with forward progression, except that the proximal flagellar waves were much larger in amplitude and less regular in their rate of development and propagation.

Because of the great variability that exists between the methods that are employed to measure sperm motility, large differences have occurred in the assignment of values for the motion parameters for the above states of hyperactivation. Nonetheless, whichever method is applied to describe hyperactivation, this phenomenon has been shown to be of increasing importance in human fertilization, its use being directed as a biomarker of fertilizing ability in the *in vitro* situation. Chan *et al.*[25] have shown that the percentage of hyperactivated sperm increases from the raw semen (5.2 ± 1.0), to immediately after washing (16.3 ± 1.8), and after 6 h incubation (29.2 ± 4.0) (mean $\pm$ SEM). A positive correlation between sperm hyperactivation and fertile males has been reported[15]. Chan *et al.*[25] have shown positive correlations between hyperactivation and sperm penetration of oocytes as measured by the sperm penetration assay.

Sperm penetration is dependent not only on factors such as sperm concentration, motility and morphology[26,27], but also on the capacitational status of sperm[28]. *In vitro* studies of sperm mucus penetration have shown that movement characteristics account for 85% of the variability in penetration[26], with the concentration of motile sperm and linear velocity of progression being the two most important functions determining the number of sperm penetrating per unit time. Many morphologically abnormal sperm are excluded from penetration of cervical mucus which is due to the associated abnormality in flagellar activity, slower swimming speed and greater sperm head–mucus resistance experienced than normal sperm[29]. There are remarkable variations in velocity of sperm motility and dimensions of the sperm head. This variability has both physiological and morphological significance, and seems to play a major role in the selection process during the development, maturation and transport in the female reproductive tract.

METHODS EMPLOYED IN ASSESSING SPERM MOTILITY

The importance of sperm motility for successful fertilization of oocytes[30] has led to the development of sophisticated laboratory equipment for motility determinations.

The methods evolved through the years include:

Subjective methods

(1) Estimations of percentages of progressively motile, weak motile and immotile spermatozoa[31].

(2) Assessment of quantitative motility by counting motile and immotile spermatozoa in 10 different microscopic view-fields.

(3) Qualitative evaluation of forward movement[32].

(4) Determination of the motility index[33].

Objective methods

(1) Multiple-exposure photography (MEP)[34,35].

(2) Laser–Doppler spectroscopy[36,37].

(3) Videomicrography[38].

(4) Semi-automated computer assisted[39–41].

(5) Automated computer assisted[42].

The advent of computerized digital analysis systems has made the task of measuring sperm motility parameters much easier. The biggest advantage of these systems is that they allow for rapid and accurate analysis of sperm movement. It also allows a large number of sperm to be analyzed on a per-sperm basis in a short period of time. The user can specify the tracking interval, the number of points needed for velocity and lateral head calculations, and criteria for recognition of motile cells. Comparison of results obtained by digital and manual analyses of the same sperm sample shows no significant differences[43].

Various parameters have been described in the literature to express the motility patterns of spermatozoa. Many of these parameters were synonymous and described the same characteristics, but sometimes the same term was used to describe different characteristics. Consensus on these parameters was reached at the 'Automated Sperm Motility Analysis' workshop held at the American Society of Andrology's Annual Meeting in Houston (TX, USA) during March 1988[44]. These parameters have now been standardized and are currently used in motion analysis[45,46]. These parameters include the following.

Curvilinear velocity (VCL) VCL (μm/s) is the measure of the rate of travel of the centroid of the sperm head over a given period of time, i.e. the local speed along the curvilinear path traced by the sperm head. This is calculated from the sum of the straight lines joining the sequential positions of the sperm head along the spermatozoon's track (Figure 1).

Straight-line velocity (VSL) VSL (μm/s) (formerly known as the progression velocity) is the straight-line distance between the first and last centroid positions for a given period of time rather than the sum of all intermediate distances (Figure 1).

Average path velocity (VAP) VAP (μm/s) is the spatially averaged path that eliminates the wobble of the sperm head, while preserving the basic curvature of the path. Since this is derived using visual interpolation, various mathematical smoothing techniques or geometric construction, the precise method of derivation should be stipulated (Figure 1).

Linearity of forward progression (LIN) LIN is reported as a ratio of VSL to VCL, expressed as a percentage. The values range from 0 to 100 with a value of 100 representing cells swimming in a straight-line

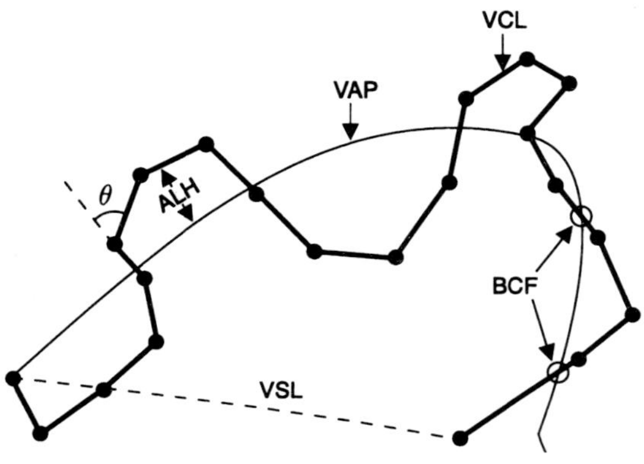

Figure 1 Motion parameters of a single sperm track. VSL: straight line velocity; VCL: curvilinear velocity; VAP: average path velocity; ALH: beat cross frequency; θ: angle of deviation

pattern. The value decreases as the non-linearity of the swimming pattern increases.

Wobble (WOB) WOB (formerly known as the curvilinear progressiveness ratio) is the ratio of VAP to VCL. This measures the wobble of the sperm head about the average path.

Straightness (STR) STR (formerly known as the linear index) is the ratio of VAP to VSL. This measures the straightness of the average path.

Maximum amplitude of lateral head displacement (maxALH) The centroid positions are recorded and a mean trajectory, based on each of these positions, is generated. For each point, the two adjacent points on either side (total of five points) are averaged and a least-squares curve fit is applied. Values for maxALH, calculated from the computer generated mean trajectory, are multiplied by 2 and expressed in μm (Figure 1).

Mean amplitude of lateral head displacement (meanALH) The central positions for a cell and the mean trajectory are established in the same way as for maxALH. All ALH values for a given sperm during the analysis time are used to generate a mean value (Figure 1).

Beat cross frequency (BCF) BCF is defined as the number of times the centroid of the sperm head crosses the computer-generated mean trajectory for that cell in Hz (beats/s). This parameter provides an estimate of flagellar beat frequency based on the movement of the sperm head (Figure 1).

Dance This is defined by the product of VCL and meanALH and is expressed in $\mu m^2/s$.

Dancemean This is defined as the product of the meanALH and the ratio of the VCL and the VSL, and is expressed in μm.

Mean angle of deviation (MAD) The time-average of absolute values of the instantaneous turning angle of the sperm head along its curvilinear trajectory. MAD is a measure of the curvature of the sperm track (Figure 1).

Curvature (CURV) The curvature of the sperm path based on a scale of 0–1.

Riser displacement (RIS) The point-to-point distance of the actual sperm-head trajectory to its average path.

Frequency of the fundamental harmonic (HAR) The fundamental frequency of the oscillation of the curvilinear trajectory around its average path.

Magnitude of the fundamental harmonic (MAG) The measure of the peak-to-peak dispersion of the curvilinear trajectory about its average path at the fundamental frequency (amplitude squared height of the HAR).

Area of the fundamental harmonic (PBW) The area under the fundamental harmonic peak in the magnitude spectrum. This parameter is a measure of the power-bandwidth of the signal.

Values for motility parameters should not exceed one decimal place, with the exception of three progression ratios (LIN, WOB, STR) which are expressed as integer percentages in the range 0–100.

All these motility parameters give a clear indication of movement characteristics of sperm. Sperm can be categorized into hyperactivated and non-hyperactivated on the basis of their motility parameters. These parameters show great promise as indicators for outcome of *in vitro* fertilization, since motility has been linked to fertilization[47].

It should be noted that measurement of sperm head motion is sensitive to the experimental technique, i.e.

(1) Accuracy in spatial measurement, which relates to magnification and spatial resolution of magnification systems and to size of sperm heads;

(2) Time resolution of systems (framing rate in relation to speed of the sperm head); and

(3) Mathematical algorithms used to calculate average sperm path and amplitude of lateral head displacement[47].

BASIC PRINCIPLES OF MEASUREMENT

Motility is a vitally important characteristic of sperm which needs to be measured objectively and accurately[44], thus the conditions under which it is evaluated are of utmost importance.

Preparation depths

Specimen chambers of 10 μm depth do not influence motility of human sperm in semen, but do influence motility of sperm in medium or prepared from swim-up migration, since these show greater lateral movements of the head. Thus, the use of deeper preparations (20 μm) is required for washed sperm. Volumes of 10 μL under 22×22 mm coverslips give preparations of 20 μm depth[49,50]. Studies on hyperactivation require a depth of 32 μm[24,43]. The deeper the preparation depth, the less will be the artifactual biasing of the results due to constraining of sperm.

The 'sticking-to-glass' phenomenon

Spermatozoa in seminal plasma do not show a tendency to attach to glass surfaces. However, washed sperm populations do show this affinity for glass. This 'sticking-to-glass' phenomenon may be reduced by addition of either serum albumin[51] or polyvinyl alcohol[52] in the medium or by the use of glass coating agents, such as nitrocellulose[53]. Since this affinity for glass is time-dependent, studies on washed sperm should be done as quickly as possible.

Temperature

Sperm motility is dependent upon cellular metabolism and is, therefore, temperature sensitive. While the percentage of motile and immotile sperm, or progressively and non-progressively motile sperm may not change significantly between 37°C and 20°C[32], the actual sperm movement characteristics will be affected. Velocity is extremely temperature sensitive and may increase by 60–100% when the temperature is increased from 25°C to 37°C[54]. Thus, all studies on human sperm motility should be carried out at 37°C. All chambers, sample via, and pipette tips must be preheated at 37°C before use and the microscope must be equipped with a heated stage.

Dilution

A sperm sample may have to be diluted if the suspension is too concentrated for motility evaluation. Seminal spermatozoa should be diluted with homologous seminal plasma prepared from another aliquot of the same semen sample by centrifugation[44]. The reason for this is that culture medium will cause substantial changes in the movement patterns. For dilution of washed sperm, culture medium can be used.

Mixing

Thorough mixing of a semen sample or sperm suspension is essential before an aliquot is taken for any quantitative procedure. Suitable mixing procedure includes fairly vigorous swirling of the sample, very gentle vortex mixing, automatic cradling, or stirring with a glass or plastic rod[55]. High-speed vortex mixing should not be used since it may damage sperm cells and affect motility.

Microscope optics

For manual track reconstruction, both positive-low and negative-high contrast optics and Nomarski differential interference optics have been used. However, for digital image analysis, negative-high phase contrast optics provides better images and should probably be used for all recordings to be analyzed automatically. It has also been suggested that recordings be made using the lowest power objective possible, since this gives brighter images and greater depth of field[44].

Video standards

Various VCR standards exist depending upon the purpose of the recording. The U-Matic system has been restricted to broadcast and serious research applications, whereas the Beta system is widely used domestically. Three speeds are obtainable in the Beta format (I, II and III), Beta I being used more professionally. The Video 8 and VHS systems are also restricted to domestic camcorders. The VHS system has two speeds: standard play and long play. For image analysis purposes, the tape with the fastest speed available should be used to give the highest quality image for digitization, i.e. Beta I or II, or VHS in standard play mode[44].

Television standards

The different television broadcasting and recording systems around the world play a confounding role in videomicrographical analysis of sperm motility. The National Television Standards Committee (NTSC) system has 525 lines and scans at 60 Hz with images running at 30 frames. The phase alternating line (PAL) and sequential *couleur avec mémoire* (SECAM) systems operate with 625 lines and 50 Hz giving 25 frames, the only difference being in the color-encoding of the signal which plays no role in the monochrome images used for motility analysis. The frame-by-frame analysis used in different countries will be at either 25 or 30 frames. This will cause no major differences in movement characteristics but will, however, cause differences in the VCL measurements[44]. Also, the resolution of images obtained using the PAL system are higher than those obtained with the NTSC format.

Frame rate

The frame rate plays a major role in the movement characteristics of swimming spermatozoa[41]. While VSL remains relatively constant, VCL is extremely frame rate dependent, limiting its use to define subpopulations of cells (motile and immotile). However, VAP remains more or less constant if derived geometrically. Standardization of the image sampling frequency, or the use of different frame rates, must be used to avoid discrepancies between analyses. Basic measurements of human semen should be made at 30 frames/s since the average VCL is <70 μm/s. However, processed human specimens that contain significantly faster sperm should be evaluated at 60 frames/s or higher[56]. Failure to use the appropriate video framing rate will result in significant errors in VCL, BCF, ALH, LIN, WOB and STR.

SPERM MOTILITY AND ASSISTED REPRODUCTION

Sperm motility and its importance for successful fertilization of the oocyte[30] has led to the development of sophisticated laboratory equipment for motility determinations. Progress in the field of *in vitro* fertilization and embryo transfer resulted in additional efforts to improve the understanding of the relationship between motility and fertilization[57–59]. For *in vitro* fertilization purposes, the role of sperm density is of less importance[60], but sperm motility[61] and morphological quality[58] have been receiving increasing attention.

Sperm motility and forward progression

Work done thus far has focused on assigning motility values for sperm according to their forward progression (0–4) but very little has been done on linking these values to morphology. Bongso *et al.*[62] have compared visual assessments of motility (0–3) with computerized motility analysis. Cut-off points of ⩾ grade 2 motility (moderate forward progression) determine the actual potential and likely success of IVF. Fertilization rate per patient was virtually an 'all-or-none' phenomenon in which >80% of eggs fertilized with ratings ⩾2 and <21% fertilized with ratings below 2[63]. Quigley[64] has also been unsuccessful in obtaining fertilization unless a minimum motility grade of 2+ or better was present.

Using the cut-off point of 2+ forward progres-

Table 1 Motility characteristics of sperm from P, G and N patterns of 37 patients

Parameter	*P pattern (<4% normal) (n=10)*	*G pattern (5–14% normal) (n=8)*	*N pattern (>14% normal) (n=19)*
VCL (μm/s)	72.9±7[a,b]	86.3±16[a]	91.0±16[b]
VSL (μm/s)	19.7±7[c]	26.5±18	32.6±15[c]
LIN (%)	26.2±9	26.2±13	31.8±13
Conc. (×10^6 sperm/mL)	37.9±35[d,e]	80.8±39[d]	89.7±72[e]
Motility (%)	38.0±21[f,g]	43.7±9[f,h]	52.1±8[g,h]
FP (0–4)	2.0±0.6[i]	2.5±0.3	2.7±0.3[i]

Values are expressed as mean±SD. [a]P=0.04; [b]P=0.002; [c]P=0.02; [d]P=0.03; [e]P=0.05; [f]P=0.03; [g]P=0.02; [h]P=0.04; [i]P<0.001

sion, average values for straight-line velocity were allocated as 34.29 μm/s[65] and 35.05 μm/s[66]. It was then recommended by Bongso *et al.*[62] that ratings of ⩾55 μm/s will safely predict the success of fertilization, since this coincides with the grade 2 motility. Mathur *et al.*[67] postulated that the number of sperm moving at a speed of 31–50 μm/s was higher in a fertile group than in an infertile group.

Sperm motility and morphology

Morphological aberrations may be markers of other functional defects. Morphologically normal sperm have significantly higher VSL and LIN values and can exhibit higher flagellar frequencies and high straight-line velocities when compared with morphologically abnormal spermatozoa[68,69]. We have shown that the P pattern men (<4% normal forms) have significantly lower straight-line velocity than the N pattern men and that VCL differs significantly among the P, G and N patterns (Table 1). Other semen parameters that appear to differ with the percentage normal morphology are the sperm concentration and the percentage motile sperm.

Using strict criteria, sperm morphology has been shown to be an excellent predictor of IVF outcome[70,71]. Teratozoospermic semen with sperm of abnormal head morphology may have a disproportionate number of non-functional cells[69,72]. Patients with a poor prognosis pattern (P pattern) have an impaired capacity to bind to the zona under hemizona assay (HZA) conditions[73,74] and this correlates well with their poor IVF rates under standard conditions[70]. Clinical testing has demonstrated a positive correlation between the number of sperm bound to the hemizona and success during *in vitro* fertilization[74,75]. Morphologically abnormal sperm from fertile and infertile men are likely to be immotile or sluggishly motile. Abnormal spermatozoa seem to have impaired forward progression characteristics when compared with normal spermatozoa.

The associated abnormalities of sperm flagellar activity may be responsible for fertilization dysfunction[68]. Chan *et al.*[8] have shown that sperm morphology and movement characteristics have a predictive value of 74.1% accuracy in the outcome of *in vitro* fertilization.

We did not assign values according to the forward progression groups, but rather to the morphological groups as outlined by Kruger *et al.*[70]. Using 'strict criteria', patients were divided into P (<4% normal), G (5–14% normal) and N patterns (>14% normal forms). Findings indicate that sperm motility is related to the percentage normal sperm in the semen sample. Whether abnormal head shapes hinder the hydrodynamic movement is still unclear, but a decrease in motility was observed in abnormal sperm[68,69]. Furthermore, sperm morphology has been correlated to fertilization success[70,76]. We have assigned average motility values for the different morphological groups (Table 1)[77]. Results show that, for fertile men classified according to the >14% normal sperm criteria, the minimum straight-line velocity should be 32.6 μm/s. This stands in accordance to the literature cited above for the forward progression group of 2+. In addition to the above requirement, the average value for VCL and LIN for fertile men should be 91.0 μm/s and 31.8%, respectively. According to Table 1, VSL has little

Table 2 Relationship between semen parameters and hemizona binding potential of human sperm from 144 men

Parameter	*P pattern (<4%) (n=41)*	*G pattern (5–14%) (n=61)*	*N pattern (>14% normal) (n=42)*
Conc (×10^6 sperm/mL)	32.8±29^{a,b}	76.1±54^{b}	95.4±61^{a}
Motility (%)	41.2±17^{c,d}	50.9±11^{c}	53.4±11^{d}
Morph. (% normal)	2.4±1.2^{e,f}	9.2±3^{e,g}	18.9±4^{f,g}
Bound sperm (hemizona assay)	22.4±16^{h,i}	43.1±40^{h,j}	61.9±36^{i,j}
Hemizona index (%)	29.3±26^{k,l}	57.6±62^{k,m}	102.4±80^{l,m}

Values are expressed as mean±SD. $^{a}P<0.001$; $^{b}P<0.01$; $^{c}P=0.002$; $^{d}P=0.001$; $^{e-j}P<0.05$; $^{k}P=0.01$; $^{l}P<0.001$; $^{m}P=0.005$

significance in distinguishing between the P, G and N patterns, since significant differences were only noted when comparing the P and N patterns. However, VCL differentiates between the P and both the G and N patterns. On the other hand, none of the three motion characteristics (VCL, VSL and LIN) could differentiate between samples from the G pattern population versus the N pattern. Therefore, only in severe teratozoospermia (<4% normal forms) do motion characteristics play a differentiating role.

The fact that no significant differences are obtained between the G and N patterns eliminates the possibility of inadequate motility or velocity as a contributing factor for the impaired fertilization rates. However, in cases where teratozoospermia exists in combination with other abnormalities, such as oligo- or asthenozoospermia, motility will play a significant contributing role.

Teratozoospermia has also been correlated to poor zona pellucida binding. Franken *et al.*[78] have shown that teratozoospermic patients have a hemizona index (HZI) of 30.5% as compared to the normozoospermic men (HZI=69.4%). According to Table 2, the mean hemizona indices for P, G and N pattern men were 29.3%, 57.6% and 102%, respectively. The number of sperm bound to the hemizonae for these P, G and N pattern men were 22.4, 43.1 and 61.9 sperm, respectively. This stands in accordance with the results of Franken *et al.*[79], who showed that the number of sperm bound to the zona for teratozoospermic men is significantly lower than that of fertile men (44.6±23 versus 103.3±58; mean ±SEM).

Use of stimulants in assisted reproduction

The use of stimulants to improve sperm motility has recently become very widespread. Discrepancies still occur as to clinical importance of stimulants, since standardization, as far as concentrations and methodologies used, is still lacking. Literature suggests that methyl xanthines, such as pentoxifylline and caffeine, show stimulation of sperm motility and may have potential use in an IVF program.

Pentoxifylline

Pentoxifylline has been shown to increase the *in vitro* motility of ejaculated sperm from both normo- and asthenozoospermic men[80], and also the successful fertilization rates in normo- and oligozoospermic men[81]. However, Yovich *et al.*[81] showed an improvement of sperm motility of oligozoospermic samples treated with pentoxifylline, but no difference in motility was noted when pentoxifylline was added to normozoospermic samples. Using normozoospermic samples, Mbizvo[82] showed significant stimulation of hyperactivation when using pentoxifylline at 1–2 h incubation, after which the percentage of hyperactivated sperm declined within the following 4 h to that of the control sample.

Lewis[83] has shown that pentoxifylline-treated sperm did not increase the straight-line velocity but did, however, significantly increase the curvilinear velocity up to 4 h incubation. In contrast, Tesarik *et al.*[84] showed that pentoxifylline reaches its maximum stimulatory effect on normo- and

Table 3 Effect of pentoxifylline on movement characteristics of spermatozoa from teratozoospermic samples under test-tube conditions

	VCL (μm/s)	*VSL (μm/s)*	*LIN (%)*	*MOT (%)*
Control (0 h)	84.60 ± 10[a]	23.35 ± 12	22.83 ± 9	91.1 ± 7
Pentox (0 h)	102.77 ± 14[ac]	27.20 ± 10[d]	23.65 ± 7[e]	89.5 ± 6
Control (4 h)	85.47 ± 12[b]	19.81 ± 14	17.62 ± 9	70.6 ± 4
Pentox (4 h)	73.16 ± 4[bc]	10.66 ± 2[d]	11.86 ± 1[e]	64.9 ± 7

All values expressed as mean ± SD. Values with corresponding letters show significant differences: [a]*P*=0.005; [b]*P*=0.01; [c]*P*=0.003; [d]*P*=0.001; [e]*P*=0.001

Table 4 Effect of pentoxifylline on movement characteristics of spermatozoa from teratozoospermic samples under hemizona assay (HZA) conditions

	VCL (μm/s)	*VSL (μm/s)*	*LIN (%)*	*MOT (%)*
Control (0 h)	83.91 ± 10[a]	21.51 ± 10	22.30 ± 9	92.8 ± 7
Pentox (0 h)	100.04 ± 13[ab]	26.40 ± 80[c]	26.2 ± 12[d]	88.9 ± 4
Control (4 h)	76.64 ± 11	13.16 ± 8	14.43 ± 5	69.3 ± 8
Pentox (4 h)	76.00 ± 7[b]	9.14 ± 4[c]	11.05 ± 4[d]	66.1 ± 6

All values expressed as mean ± SD. Values with corresponding letters show significant differences: [a]*P*=0.007; [b]*P*=0.0003; [c]*P*=0.0001; [d]*P*=0.004

asthenozoospermic samples within 10 min of treatment and lasts for at least 2 h. We have shown that teratozoospermic sperm treated with pentoxifylline showed an initial stimulation of VCL at 0 h incubation, but a decline of this parameter after 4 h incubation when compared to the control samples, under test-tube conditions (Tables 3,4)[85]. These findings are in accord with those of Tesarik *et al.*[84], in which a maximal effect of pentoxifylline was reached within 10 min of exposure. The time delay in this study from the point of pentoxifylline exposure to the point of motility recording was also within 10 min, thus the 0 h incubation time period in our study can be compared to the 10 min time interval described by Tesarik *et al.*[84]. Also in their study, the VCL of pentoxifylline treated sperm declined to that of the control sperm after 4 h incubation. Kay *et al.*[86] have produced similar results where the percentage hyperactivated motility of sperm washed free of pentoxifylline remained elevated compared to the control for a period of 1 h, but this effect became insignificant after 3 h incubation. Thus, from these results, it is clear that pentoxifylline has a short-lived effect on sperm movement characteristics. However, under hemizona assay conditions no difference was found in sperm motility between samples with or without pentoxifylline at 4 h incubation (Table 4)[85].

With regard to the change in motility from 0 to 4 h incubation, sperm samples treated with pentoxifylline showed significantly lower motility values (VCL, VSL, LIN) when compared to the control samples. Reports have suggested a toxic effect of methyl xanthines on the sperm ultrastructure, especially damage to the sperm plasma membrane[87], although additional studies in this field are needed. Other reports attribute the rapid decline in sperm motility to an accelerated rate of capacitation[88], since on completion of capacitation sperm undergo the acrosome reaction and have a shorter life span than non-reacted sperm[89]. Prolonged exposure may, therefore, be detrimental to sperm function, and its use in assisted reproductive programs should be limited to short incubation periods. Applications could include the use of pentoxifylline to increase the swim-up yield.

Caffeine

Caffeine is a methyl xanthine and is known to inhibit the action of phosphodiesterase, thereby preventing the destruction of adenosine 3′, 5′-cyclic monophosphate (cAMP) into 5-AMP. This causes an increase in the endogenous concentration of cAMP, thereby maintaining its activity in various physiological responses, of which muscle contraction is one. It has been shown that caffeine stimulates the motility of normozoospermic sperm significantly at concentrations between 3 and 6 mM. As the concentration of caffeine increases to a maximum of 60–120 mM, its effect changes from stimulatory to inhibitory[90,91]. We have shown that caffeine has a stimulatory effect on the motility of sperm from the normozoospermic donor (control)[85]. However, the data suggest that caffeine appears to exert no effect on the motility of sperm from teratozoospermic patients[85]. Lack of the teratozoospermic semen sample's motility to respond to the stimulatory effect of caffeine might be manifested in the inability of these spermatozoa to react to such stimulation. Whether this difference is due to functional defects of teratozoospermic samples related to structural defects is unclear. Although incubation for 1 h with caffeine to a final concentration of 6 mM stimulated motility, greater surface morphological damage appeared to occur than in placebo-treated controls[92]. These detrimental changes were greater in infertile asthenozoospermic samples than in normal fertile controls. Sperm from normal fertile men may therefore be better equipped to withstand the adverse effects of caffeine for longer periods. Harrison *et al.*[87] showed that the sperm plasma membrane in infertile patients was less able to cope with the changes in the environmental situation, damaging earlier and more severely in comparison to the controls. Not only does the damage caused make the incubation of semen with caffeine unwise, but the time restraints, especially in asthenozoospermic patients, show that it is also an impractical method of increasing pregnancy potential in such cases.

Follicular fluid

Follicular fluid (FF) is a dynamic medium that is rich in steroids, peptide hormones and growth factors[93]. Lipid derivatives, glycosaminoglycans and albumin found in FF have been shown to stimulate sperm capacitation[94] and the acrosome reaction[95,96]. The steroidal fraction of FF has been shown to be a stimulator of human sperm capacitation, acrosome reaction[95,97] and also hyperactivated motility[98]. Progesterone within FF causes an influx of extracellular Ca^{2+} by acting at the sperm cell surface level. Evidence suggests that the action of Ca^{2+} is mediated through cyclic nucleotide metabolism since Ca^{2+} involves a rise in sperm cAMP concentration and can be shown to activate adenyl cyclase activity in broken cell preparations of spermatozoa[99]. However, Ca^{2+} does have a more direct effect on the phosphorylation of motility associated proteins in both actin-[100] and tubulin-[101] based systems. Wishart and Ashizawa[102] observed an effect of calcium on motility with no demonstrable change in cyclic nucleotide metabolism.

Follicular fluid may also be toxic to sperm or may impair motility[94,95,103]. Acrosome reacting sperm are thought to lose their motility rapidly[104,105], and this could explain the decrease in motility observed after 8 h incubation, since FF is known to stimulate the acrosome reaction.

Contrary to previous literature[98], our findings show that human FF under our test-tube conditions has an inhibitory effect on the motility of human sperm after 8 h incubation, as evidenced by the motility parameters investigated[106]. Semen samples incubated with FF show a higher population of sperm bound to the hemizona (at 8 h). The initial decrease in binding could be attributed to lower motility values at 4 h incubation. After 8 h, the samples in the presence of FF showed a higher binding potential than the control. Corresponding motility values were significantly lower than those of the sample incubated without FF[106].

Reports on the effect of FF on sperm motility have been conflicting. Mortimer and Camenzind[103] showed an inhibitory effect, while Falcone *et al.*[107] and Kamijo and Bastias[108] showed stimulatory effects of FF on sperm motility. Mendoza and Tesarik[104] have shown that prolonged exposure of sperm to FF changes the motility patterns, whereas short exposure does not. The discrepancies that exist could be due to differences in the techniques used for recovery, treatment and storage of FF, and methods used for the preparation of sperm suspensions and the evaluation of sperm motility. Mbizvo *et al.*[98] have reported that FF induces hyperactivated motility of human spermatozoa, and that progesterone could be one of the active components responsible for this induction. Hong *et al.*[109] observed an increase in hyperactivated motility from 5±5% to 27±14% after incubation with FF, but only during the first 3 h of incubation. In contrast to previous findings, our observations show that FF exhibits inhibitory effects on the motility of sperm from normozoospermic men. However, the role of the progesterone within the FF was neglected in this study, and future protocols regarding this dynamic fluid should incorporate analysis of steroid content. Also, the concentration of FF used in this study was 50%, which may be too high, since Mbizvo *et al.*[98] recommended a concentration of 20% to be optimal, and at higher concentrations may have no or inhibitory effects on sperm hyperactivation.

The use of these stimulants may not be of practical value for assisted reproduction and should be used with caution, since not much is understood about their mode of action, and more importantly their detrimental effects on sperm structure and function.

Sperm motility and zona pellucida

We have shown that sperm motility in the presence of the zona pellucida appears to be significantly higher than in its absence[106]. This provides evidence supporting a physiologically important role of the zona pellucida in sperm motility. Reports indicate that the zona pellucida plays a role in selecting normal sperm in the binding process of sperm preceding fertilization[110].

Katz and Yanagimachi[111] have described the flagellar movements of hyperactivated hamster sperm on the cumulus-free zona pellucida as being of high amplitude and more symmetrical than those of free swimming hyperactivated sperm. Tightly bound sperm displayed intermittent episodes of higher frequency, low amplitude beating[48]. These apparent changes in flagellar motion could be related to the occurrence of the acrosome reaction and/or tight binding of the sperm head to the zona pellucida.

CONCLUSION

Before any motility studies can be used or applied to the clinical practice, methods and criteria for measurement must be standardized to eliminate interlaboratory differences in order to compare results and values. Among the numerous factors that play a role in motion analysis of sperm, frame rate is of importance since it directly influences the results obtained. As described by Davis and Katz[59], the frame rate markedly influences the measurement of sperm motion characteristics, especially VCL. Computer-assisted analysis performed at 25 frames/s (50 Hz) and manual analysis at 10 frames/s (20 Hz) have shown the former to yield higher VCL values and lower LIN values (K. Kaskar *et al.*, unpublished). The difference is due to the increased number of track points obtained at a higher frequency, resulting in a more sinusoidal track. At lower frequencies, the path obtained is smoother due to fewer track points, leading to the higher linearity obtained. Therefore, by decreasing the frame rate, useful information regarding the rapid side-to-side movements of the sperm head is eliminated. In sperm samples with high curvilinear velocity, this could lead to inaccurate interpretation of results. Therefore, for faster moving sperm, it would be ideal to use a higher framing rate.

Since computer-assisted semen analysis provides values for sperm concentration and motility more rapidly and accurately than traditional methods, this is ideal for small and non-specialized laboratories. Mortimer[44] suggested that, in centers providing tertiary level infertility services and following WHO recommended methods with appropriate standardization and quality control, computer-assisted semen analysis systems may not yet be sufficiently accurate to replace the traditional methods.

In conclusion, our results emphasize the importance of sperm motility, in conjunction with sperm morphology, in human fertilization *in vitro*. Thus, the scope within the field of sperm motility as a predictor of male factor infertility seems to be of great potential, especially if employed in conjunction with other seminal characteristics.

References

1. Acosta, A. A., Oehninger, S., Morshedi, M., Swanson, R. J., Scott, R. and Irianni, F. (1989). Assisted reproduction and treatment of the male-factor. *Obstet. Gynecol. Surv.*, **44**, 1–18
2. Mahadevan, M. M. and Trounson, A. T. (1984). The influence of seminal characteristics on the success rate of human *in vitro* fertilization. *Fertil. Steril.*, **42**, 400–5
3. Rodriguez-Rigau, L. J., Ayala, C., Grunert, G. M., Woodward, R. M., Lotze, E. C., Feste, J. R., Gibbons, W., Smith, K. D. and Steinberger, E. (1989). Relationship between the results of sperm analysis and GIFT. *J. Androl.*, **10**, 139–44
4. Oehninger, S. C. and Hodgen, G. D. (1991). How to evaluate human spermatozoa for assisted reproduction. In De Cherney, A. N. (ed.) *Assisted Reproductive Reviews*, pp. 15–27. (Baltimore: Williams and Wilkins)
5. Mortimer, S. T. and Mortimer, D. (1990). Kinetics of human spermatozoa incubated under capacitating conditions. *J. Androl.*, **11**, 195–203
6. Ginsburg, K. A., Sacco, A. G., Ager, J. W. and Moghissi, K. (1990). Variation of movement characteristics with washing and capacitation of spermatozoa. II. Multivariate statistical analysis and prediction of sperm penetrating ability. *Fertil. Steril.*, **53**, 704–8
7. Jeulin, C., Feneux, D., Serres, C., Jouannet, P., Guillet-Rosso, F., Belaisch-Allart, J., Frydman, J. and Testart, J. (1986). Sperm factors related to failure of human IVF. *J. Reprod. Fertil.*, **70**, 735–44
8. Chan, S. Y. W., Wang, C., Chan, S. T. H., Ho, P. C., So, W. W. K., Chau, Y. F. and Ma, H. K. (1989). Predictive value of sperm morphology and movement characteristics in the outcome on *in vitro* fertilization of human oocytes. *J.* In Vitro *Fertil Embryo Transf.*, **6**, 142–7
9. Liu, D. Y., Clarke, G. N. and Baker, H. W. G. (1990). Relationships between sperm motility assessed with Hamilton–Thorn motility analyzer and fertilization rates *in vitro*. *J. Androl.*, **12**, 231–9
10. Austin, C. R. (1952). The 'capacitation' of the mammalian sperm. *Nature*, **170**, 326
11. Bedford, J. M. (1970). Sperm capacitation and fertilization in mammals. *Biol. Reprod.* Suppl., **2**, 128–58
12. Johnson, L. L., Katz, D. F. and Overstreet, J. W. (1981). The movement characteristics of rabbit spermatozoa before and after activation. *Gamete Res.*, **4**, 275–82
13. Yanagimachi, R. (1981). Mechanisms of fertilization in mammals. In Mastroianni, L. and Roberts, K. D. (eds.) *Fertilization and Embryonic Development* In Vitro, pp. 81–187. (New York: Plenum Press)
14. Fraser, L. R. (1981). Dibutyryl cyclic AMP decreases capacitation time *in vitro* in mouse spermatozoa. *J. Reprod. Fertil.*, **62**, 63–72
15. Burkman, L. J. (1984). Characterization of hyperactivated motility by human spermatozoa during capacitation: comparison of fertile and oligozoospermic sperm populations. *Arch. Androl.*, **13**, 153–65
16. Yanagimachi, R. (1969). *In vitro* acrosome reaction and capacitation of golden hamster spermatozoa by bovine follicular fluid and its fractions. *J. Exp. Zool.*, **170**, 269–80
17. Gwatkin, R. B. L. and Anderson, O. F. (1969). Capacitation of hamster spermatozoa by bovine follicular fluid. *Nature*, **224**, 1111–12
18. Yanagimachi, R. (1970). The movement of golden hamster spermatozoa before and after capacitation. *J. Reprod. Fertil.*, **23**, 193–6
19. Cooper, G. W., Overstreet, J. W. and Katz, D. F. (1979). Sperm transport in the reproductive tract of the female rabbit: motility patterns and the flagellar activity of spermatozoa. *Gamete Res.*, **2**, 35–42
20. Fraser, L. R. (1977). Motility pattern in mouse spermatozoa before and after capacitation. *J. Exp. Zool.*, **197**, 439–44
21. Corselli, J. and Talbot, P. (1986). An *in vitro* technique to study penetration of hamster–oocyte–cumulus complexes by using physiological numbers of sperm. *Gamete Res.*, **13**, 293–308
22. Burkman, L. J. (1991). Discrimination between nonhyperactivated and classical hyperactivated motility patterns in human spermatozoa using computerized analysis. *Fertil. Steril.*, **55**, 363–71
23. Suarez, S. S., Vincenti, L. and Ceglia, M. W. (1987). Hyperactivated motility induced in mouse sperm by calcium A23187 is reversible. *J. Exp. Zool.*, **244**, 331–6
24. Robertson, L., Wolf, D. P. and Tash, J. S. (1988). Temporal changes in motility parameters related to acrosomal status: identification and characterization of populations of hyperactivated human sperm. *Biol. Reprod.*, **39**, 797–805
25. Chan, P. J., Tredway, D. R., Su, B. C., Corselli, J., Davidson, B. J. and Sakugawa, M. (1992). Sperm hyperactivation as quality control for sperm penetration assay. *Urology*, **39**, 63–6
26. Aitken, R. J., Warner, P. E. and Reid, C. (1986). Factors influencing the success of sperm–cervical mucus interaction in patients exhibiting unexplained infertility. *J. Androl.*, **7**, 3–10
27. Mortimer, D., Pandya, I. J. and Sawers, R. S. (1986). Relationship between human sperm motility characteristics and sperm penetration into human cervical mucus *in vitro*. *J. Reprod. Fertil.*, **78**, 93–102
28. Barratt, C. L. R. and Cooke, D. (1991). Sperm transport in the human female reproductive tract – a dynamic interaction. *Int. J. Androl.*, **14**, 394–441
29. Katz, D. F., Morales, P., Samuels, S. J. and Overstreet, J. W. (1990). Mechanisms of filtration of morphologically abnormal human sperm by cervical mucus. *Fertil. Steril.*, **54**, 513–16

30. Bostofte, E., Serup, J. and Rebbe, H. (1983). Relation between spermatozoa motility and pregnancies obtained during a twenty-year follow up period. Spermatozoa Motility and Fertility. *Andrologia*, **15**, 682–6
31. Schirren, C. (1982). Motilitatsbestimmung der Spermatazoen. *Andrologia*, **14**, 548–50
32. World Health Organization. (1987). *Laboratory Manual for the Examination of Human Semen and Semen–Cervical Mucus Interaction*, 2nd edn, p. 7. (Cambridge: The Press Syndicate of the University of Cambridge)
33. Ischii, N., Mitsukawa, S. and Shirai, M. (1977). Sperm motile efficiency. *Andrologia*, **9**, 55–62
34. Makler, A. (1978). A new multiple exposure photography method for objective human spermatozoal motility determination. *Fertil. Steril.*, **30**, 192–9
35. Kamidono, S., Hazama, M., Matsumoto, O., Takada, K., Tomioka, O. and Ishigami, J. (1983). Study on human spermatozoal motility: Preliminary report on newly developed multiple exposure photography method. *Andrologia*, **15**, 111–19
36. Steiner, R., Baumeister, T. H., Buhl, A. and Kaufman, R. (1982). Motility measurements of human spermatozoa: Comparison of dynamic light scattering and microphotographs. In Satelle D. B., Lee, W. I. and Ware, B. R. (eds.) *Biomedical Applications of Laser Light Scattering*, pp. 221–30. (Amsterdam: Elsevier Biomedical Press)
37. Hartmann, R., Steiner, R., Hofmann, N. and Kaufmann, R. (1983). Human sperm motility – enhancement and inhibition measured by laser Doppler spectroscopy. *Andrologia*, **15**, 120–34
38. Katz, D. F. and Overstreet, J. W. (1981). Sperm motility assessment by videomicrography. *Fertil. Steril.*, **35**, 188–93
39. Holt, W. V., Moore, H. D. M. and Hillier, S. G. (1985). Computer assisted measurement of sperm swimming speed in human semen: correlation of results with *in vitro* fertilization assays. *Fertil. Steril.*, **44**, 112–19
40. Samuels, J. S. and Van der Horst, G. (1986). Sperm swimming velocity as evaluated by frame-lapse videography and computer analysis. *Arch. Androl.*, **17**, 151–5
41. Mortimer, D., Curtis, E. F. and Ralston, A. (1988). Semi-automated analysis of manually reconstructed tracks of progressively motile human spermatozoa. *Hum. Reprod.*, **3**, 303–9
42. Katz, D. F. and Davis, R. O. (1987). Automatic analysis of human sperm motion. *J. Androl.*, **8**, 170–81
43. Mack, S. O., Wolf, D. P. and Tash, J. S. (1988). Quantitation of specific parameters of motility in large numbers of human sperm by digital image processing. *Biol. Reprod.*, **38**, 270–81
44. Mortimer, D. (1990). Objective analysis of sperm motility and kinematics. In Keel B. A. and Webster B. W. (eds.) *The CRC Handbook of Laboratory Diagnosis and Treatment of Infertility*, pp. 97–133. (Baca Raton, FL: CRC Press)
45. Davis, R. O., Niswander, P. W. and Katz, D. F. (1992). New measure of sperm motion: I. Adaptive smoothing and harmonic analysis. *J. Androl.*, **13**, 139–52
46. Owen, D. H. and Katz, D. F. (1993). Sampling factors influencing accuracy of sperm kinematic analysis. *J. Androl.*, **14**, 210–21
47. Edvinsson, A., Bergman, B., Steen, Y. and Nillson, S. (1983). Characteristics of donor semen and cervical mucus at the time of conception. *Fertil. Steril.*, **39**, 327–32
48. Katz, D. F., Drobnis, E. Z. and Overstreet, J. W. (1989). Factors regulating mammalian sperm migration through the female reproductive tract and oocyte vestments. *Gamete Res.*, **22**, 443–69
49. Mortimer, D., Courtot, A. M., Giovangrandi, Y., Jeulin, C. and David, G. (1984). Human sperm motility after migration into, and after incubation in, synthetic media. *Gamete Res.*, **9**, 131–44
50. Overstreet, J. W., Katz, D. F., Hanson, F. W. and Fonseca, J. R. (1979). A simple inexpensive method for objective assessment of human sperm movement characteristics. *Fertil. Steril.*, **31**, 162–72
51. Harrison, R. A. P., Dott, H. M. and Foster, G. C. (1978). Effect of ionic strength, serum albumin and other macromolecules on the maintenance of motility and the surface of mammalian spermatozoa in a simple defined medium. *J. Reprod. Fertil.*, **52**, 65–73
52. Neill, J. M. and Olds-Clarke, P. (1987). A computer-assisted assay for mouse sperm hyperactivation demonstrates that bicarbonate but not bovine serum albumin is required. *Gamete Res.*, **18**, 121–40
53. Chapeau, C. and Gagnon, C. (1987). Nitrocellulose and polyvinyl coatings prevent sperm adhesion to glass without affecting the motility of intact and demembranated human spermatozoa. *J. Androl.*, **8**, 34–40
54. Milligan, M. P., Harris, S. J. and Dennis, K. J. (1978). The effect of temperature on the velocity of human spermatozoa as measured by time lapse photography. *Fertil. Steril.*, **30**, 592–4
55. Mortimer, D. (1985). The Male Factor in Infertility. Part I. Semen Analysis. *Current Problems in Obstetrics, Gynaecology and Fertility*, Vol. III, No. 7, pp. 1–75. (Chicago: Year Book Medical Publishers)
56. Davis, R. O. and Katz, D. F. (1993). Operational standards for CASA instruments. *J. Androl.*, **14**, 385–94
57. Aitken, R. J., Best, F. S., Warner, P. and Templeton, A. (1984). A prospective study of the relationship between semen quality and fertility in cases of unexplained infertility. *J. Androl.*, **5**, 297–303
58. Pusch, H. H., Leitinger, S., Winter R. and Urdl, W. (1986). Evaluation of sperm motility by laser-Doppler spectroscopy in an *in vitro* fertilization programme. *Hum. Reprod.*, **1**, 233–5
59. Van Uem, J. F. H. M., Acosta, A. A., Swanson, J. R., Mayer, J., Ackerman, S., Burkman, L. J., Veeck, L., McDowell, J. S., Bernardus, R. E. and Jones, H. W. Jr.

(1985). Male factor evaluation in *in vitro* fertilization: the Norfolk experience. *Fertil. Steril.*, **44**, 375–83

60. Trounson, A., Leeton, I., Wood, C., Webb, J. and Kovacs, C. (1980). The investigation of idiopathic infertility by *in vitro* fertilization. *Fertil. Steril.*, **34**, 431–7
61. Battin, D., Vargyas, J. M., Sato, F., Brown, J. and Marrs, R. P. (1985). The correlation between *in vitro* fertilization of human oocytes and semen profile. *Fertil. Steril.*, **44**, 835–8
62. Bongso, T. A., Ng, S. C., Mok, H., Lim, M. N., Teo, H. L., Wong, P. C. and Ratnam, S. S. (1989). Effect of sperm motility on human *in vitro* fertilization. *Arch. Androl.*, **22**, 185–90
63. Grunfeld, L. and Richardson, K. (1987). Linear sperm motion does not predict human oocyte fertilization. *The American Fertility Society, 43rd Annual Meeting*, Abstr. 040, p. 18
64. Quigley, M. M. (1984). Patient screening and selection. In Wolf, D. P. and Quigley, M. M. (eds.) *Human* In Vitro *Fertilization and Embryo Transfer*, pp. 39–51. (New York: Plenum Press)
65. Janick, J. and MacLeod, J. (1970). The measurement of human spermatozoan motility. *Fertil. Steril.*, **21**, 140–6
66. Franken, D. R., Slabber, C. F., Maas, D. A. and Giesteira, M. V. K. (1973). Forward progression of spermatozoa: Standardization of results. *S. Afr. Med. J.*, **54**, 438–40
67. Mathur, S., Carlton, M. and Ziegler, J. (1986). A computerized sperm motion analysis. *Fertil. Steril.*, **46**, 484–8
68. Morales, P., Katz, D. F., Overstreet, J. W., Samuels, S. J. and Chang, R. J. (1988). The relationship between the motility and morphology of spermatozoa in human semen. *J. Androl.*, **9**, 241–7
69. Katz, D. F., Diel, L. and Overstreet, J. W. (1982). Differences in the movement of morphologically normal and abnormal human seminal spermatozoa. *Biol. Reprod.*, **26**, 566–70
70. Kruger, T. F., Acosta, A. A., Simmons, K. F., Swanson, R. J., Matta, J. F. and Oehninger, S. (1988). Predictive value of abnormal morphology in *in vitro* fertilization. *Fertil. Steril.*, **49**, 112–17
71. Oehninger, S. C., Acosta, A. A., Morshedi, M., Veeck, L., Swanson, R. J., Simons, K. F. and Rosenwaks, Z. (1988). Corrective measurements and pregnancy outcomes in IVF in patients with severe sperm morphology abnormalities. *Fertil. Steril.*, **50**, 283–7
72. Overstreet, J. W., Price, M. J., Blazak, W. F., Lewis, E. L. and Katz, D. F. (1981). Simultaneous assessment of human sperm motility and morphology by videomicrography. *J. Urol.*, **126**, 357–60
73. Burkman, L. J., Coddington, C. C., Franken, D. R., Kruger, T. F., Rosenwaks, Z. and Hodgen, G. D. (1988). The hemizona assay (HZA): development of a diagnostic test for the binding of human spermatozoa to the human hemizona pellucida to predict fertilization potential. *Fertil. Steril.*, **49**, 688–97
74. Franken, D. R., Burkman, L. J., Oehninger, S., Coddington, C. C., Veeck, L., Kruger, T. F., Rosenwaks, Z. and Hodgen, G. D. (1989). The hemizona assay: a predictor of human sperm fertilizing potential in IVF treatment. *J.* In Vitro *Fertil. Embryo Transf.*, **6**, 44–50
75. Oehninger, S. C., Coddington, C. C., Scott, R., Franken, D. R., Burkman, L. J., Acosta, A. A. and Hodgen, G. D. (1989). Hemizona assay: assessment of sperm dysfunction and prediction of IVF outcome. *Fertil. Steril.*, **51**, 665–70
76. Liu, D. Y. and Baker, H. W. G. (1990). Relationships between human sperm acrosin, acrosomes, morphology and fertilization *in vitro*. *Hum. Reprod.*, **5**, 298–303
77. Kaskar, K., Franken, D. R., Van der Horst, G., Oehninger, S. C., Kruger, T. F. and Hodgen, G. D. (1994). The relationship between morphology, quantitative motility and zona pellucida binding potential of spermatozoa in human semen. *Andrologia*, **26**, 1–4
78. Franken, D. R., Acosta, A. A., Kruger, T. F., Lombard, C. J., Oehninger, S. and Hodgen, G. D. (1993). The hemizona assay: its role in identifying male factor infertility in assisted reproduction. *Fertil. Steril.*, **59**, 1075–80
79. Franken, D. R., Coddington, C. C., Burkman, L. J., Oosthuizen, W., Oehninger, S. C., Kruger, T. F. and Hodgen, G. D. (1991). Defining the valid hemizona assay: accounting for binding variability within zonae pellucidae and within semen samples from fertile males. *Fertil. Steril.*, **56**, 1156–61
80. Shen, M. R., Chiang, P. H., Yang, R. C., Hong, C. Y. and Chen, S. S. (1991). Pentoxifylline stimulates human sperm motility both *in vitro* and after oral therapy. *Br. J. Clin. Pharmacol.*, **31**, 711–14
81. Yovich, J. M., Edirisinghe, W. R., Cummins, J. M. and Yovich, J. L. (1988). Preliminary results using pentoxifylline in a pronuclear stage tubal transfer (PROST) program for severe male factor infertility. *Fertil. Steril.*, **50**, 179–81
82. Mbizvo, M. T., Johnston, R. C. and Baker, G. H. W. (1993). The effect of the motility stimulants, caffeine, pentoxifylline, and 2-deoxyadenosine on hyperactivation of cryopreserved human sperm. *Fertil. Steril.*, **59**, 1112–17
83. Lewis, S. E. M., Moohan, J. M. and Thompson, W. (1993). Effects of pentoxifylline on human sperm motility in normozoospermic individuals using computer-assisted analysis. *Fertil. Steril.*, **59**, 418–23
84. Tesarik, J., Thebault, A. and Testart, J. (1992). Effect of pentoxifylline on sperm movement characteristics in normozoospermic and asthenozoospermic specimens. *Hum. Reprod.*, **7**, 1257–63
85. Kaskar, K., Franken, D. R., van der Horst, G. and Kruger, T. F. (1994). The effect of pentoxifylline on the movement characteristics and zona binding

potential of teratozoospermic men. *Hum. Reprod.*, **9**, 477–81
86. Kay, V. J., Coutts, J. R. T. and Robertson, L. (1993). Pentoxifylline stimulates hyperactivation in human spermatozoa. *Hum. Reprod.*, **8**, 727–31
87. Harrison, R. F., Sheppard, B. L. and Kaliszer, M. (1980). Observations on the motility, ultrastructure and elemental composition of human spermatozoa incubated with caffeine. *Andrologia*, **12**, 34–42
88. Rogers, B. F. (1981). Factors affecting mammalian *in vitro* fertilization. In Jagiello, G. and Vogel, H. J. (eds.) *Bioregulators of Reproduction*, pp. 459–86. (New York: Academic Press)
89. Hammitt, D. G., Bedia, E., Rogers, P. R., Syrop, C. H., Donovan, J. F. and Williams, R. A. (1989). Comparison of motility stimulants for cryopreserved human semen. *Fertil. Steril.*, **52**, 495–502
90. Moussa, M. M. (1983). Caffeine and sperm motility. *Fertil. Steril.*, **39**, 845–48
91. Levin, R. M., Greenberg, S. H. and Wein, A. J. (1981). Quantitative analysis of the effects of caffeine on sperm motility and cyclic adenosine 3′,5′-monophosphate (AMP) phosphodiesterase. *Fertil. Steril.*, **36**, 798–802
92. Harrison, R. F., Sheppard, B. L. and Kaliszer, M. (1980). Observations on the motility, ultrastructure and elemental composition of human spermatozoa incubated with caffeine. II. A time-based study. *Andrologia*, **12**, 434–43
93. Chao, H. T., Ng, H. T., Kao, S. H., Wei, Y. H. and Hong, C. Y. (1991). Human follicular fluid stimulates the motility of washed human sperm. *Arch. Androl.*, **26**, 61–5
94. Mukherjee, A. B. and Lippes, J. (1972). Effect of human follicular and tubal fluids on human, mouse and rat spermatozoa *in vitro*. *Can. J. Genet. Cytol.*, **14**, 167–74
95. Suarez, S. S., Wolf, D. P. and Meizel, S. (1986). Induction of the acrosome reaction in human spermatozoa by a fraction of human follicular fluid. *Gamete Res.*, **14**, 107–21
96. Siegel, M. S., Pauon, R. J. and Graczykowski, J. W. (1990). The influence of human follicular fluid on the acrosome reaction, fertilizing capacity and proteinase activity of human spermatozoa. *Hum. Reprod.*, **5**, 975–80
97. Tesarik, J. (1985). Comparison of acrosome reaction-inducing activities of human cumulus oophorus, follicular fluid and ionophore A23187 in human sperm populations of proven fertilizing ability *in vitro*. *J. Reprod. Fertil.*, **74**, 383–8
98. Mbizvo, M. T., Burkman, L. J. and Alexander, N. J. (1990). Human follicular fluid stimulates hyperactivated motility in human sperm. *Fertil. Steril.*, **54**, 708–12
99. Lindemann, C. B. and Kanous, K. S. (1989). Regulation of sperm motility. *Arch. Androl.*, **23**, 1–22
100. Aldestein, R. S. and Eisenberg, E. (1980). Regulation and kinetics of the actin–myosin–ATP interaction. *Annu. Rev. Biochem.*, **19**, 921–56
101. Schulman, H. (1985). Phosphorylation of microtubule-associated proteins by a Ca^{2+}/calmodulin dependent protein kinase. *J. Cell Biol.*, **99**, 11–19
102. Wishart, G. J. and Ashizawa, K. (1987). Regulation of the motility of fowl spermatozoa by calcium and cAMP. *J. Reprod. Fertil.*, **80**, 607–11
103. Mortimer, D. and Camenzind, A. R. (1989). The role of follicular fluid in inducing the acrosome reaction of human spermatozoa incubated *in vitro*. *Hum. Reprod.*, **4**, 169–74
104. Mendoza, D. and Tesarik, J. (1990). Effect of follicular fluid on sperm movement characteristics. *Fertil. Steril.*, **54**, 1135–39
105. Bedford, J. M. (1983). Significance of the need for sperm capacitation before fertilization in eutherian mamma. *Biol. Reprod.*, **28**, 108–20
106. Kaskar, K., Franken, D. R., van der Horst, G., Kruger, T. F., Oehninger, S. C. and Hodgen, G. D. (1993). The effect of follicular fluid on sperm motility and zona pellucida binding potential of normozoospermic men. *Assist. Reprod. Technol./Androl.*, **4**, 285–93
107. Falcone, L., Gianni, S., Piffaretti-Yanez, A., Marchini, M., Eppenberger, U. and Balerna, M. (1991). Follicular fluid enhances sperm motility and velocity *in vitro*. *Fertil. Steril.*, **55**, 619–23
108. Kamijo, H. and Bastias, M. C. (1991). Effect of human follicular fluid and maternal serum on human sperm motility and acrosome reaction. *Assist. Reprod. Technol./Androl.*, **2**, 299–313
109. Hong, C. Y., Chao, H. T., Lee, S. L. and Wei, Y. H. (1993). Modification of human sperm function by human follicular fluid: a review. *Int. J. Androl.*, **16**, 92–7
110. Cross, N. L., Morales, P., Overstreet, J. W. and Hanson, F. W. (1988). Induction of the acrosome reaction by the human zona pellucida. *Biol. Reprod.*, **38**, 235–44
111. Katz, D. F. and Yanagimachi, R. (1981). Movement characteristics of hamster and guinea pig spermatozoa upon attachment to the zona pellucida. *Biol. Reprod.*, **25**, 785–91

Evaluation of sperm morphology by light microscopy

8

R. Menkveld and T. F. Kruger

INTRODUCTION

After van Leeuwenhoek's first letter to the Royal Society in London with detailed descriptions and drawings of the morphology of the human spermatozoon, little attention was paid to morphology evaluation. It was only as recently as the turn of this century that the evaluation of sperm morphology became a focus of interest, and it was accepted that normal and pathological forms could appear simultaneously in a semen sample[1,2]

It has only been since the 1930s that the role of sperm morphology in fertilization received more attention. Even at that early stage, contradictory reports were published on the importance and role of sperm morphology. In 1930, Cary[3] stated that morphology of human spermatozoa bears a definite relation to their success of migration through cervical mucus. This statement was repeated by Cary and Hotchkiss[4] when they wrote, 'Abnormal forms may process motility, but are rarely, if ever, found in the upper levels of cervical mucus and we must consider them ineffectual for fertilization'. As far as the investigation of semen samples was concerned, it was stated by Moench and Holt[5] in 1932 that 'Morphology of the sperm head seems to be the most reliable indicator of fertilizing power of these cells'. This was in contrast to the statement made by Huhner[6] in 1921 that 'If there are many active moving spermatozoa per microscopic field present, sperm morphology is of no importance and the presence of many abnormal spermatozoa will have no influence on the outcome of the post-coital test.'

Since that period, very little attention was paid to sperm morphology and its role in fertilization. Most references were made to the sperm count only and occasionally to sperm motility. If reference was made to sperm morphology it was usually to point out that sperm morphology played little or no role in natural fertilization[7–9]. Van Zyl *et al.*[10] stated that no references could be found in the British literature in the previous 10-year period reporting on a positive relationship between sperm morphology and natural *in vivo* fertilization.

It is, therefore, clear that sperm morphology remains one of the most controversial semen parameters in terms of its role in establishing a male's fertility potential[11–13], and as a prognostic parameter for fertilization in natural *in vivo* conception, *in vitro* fertilization (IVF), the hamster test[14], artificial insemination by husband (AIH) and gamete intrafallopian transfer (GIFT)[15–17]. This controversy can be ascribed mainly to the fact that, until recently, no clear and standardized criteria existed for a normal spermatozoon based on biological evidence[18]. The consequence was and is that diverse results are found in different laboratories and even within the same laboratory, as has been shown by the classic work of Freund[19], and more recently by Fredricsson[20] and Jequier and Ukombe[21].

With the introduction of the strict Tygerberg criteria[18] based on biological evidence for normality and the World Health Organization (WHO) manual (1992)[22] accepting in principle the basic criteria set forth by the strict Tygerberg criteria, we have moved closer to this objective.

Recently, much emphasis has been placed on sperm functional tests such as the hemizona assay, acrosin activity, sperm nuclear maturity, acrosomal status, the acrosome reaction, the hamster ovum penetration test, sperm–zona pellucida and sperm–oolemma binding tests and the zona pellucida (ZP) penetrating test. Of these, Liu and Baker[23] regard the sperm–ZP binding and ZP penetration tests together with sperm morphology as the most important.

Some of the information provided by these

functional tests can, to a certain degree, already be obtained by the evaluation of sperm morphology according to the strict Tygerberg criteria[18]. Furthermore, Chan and Tucker[24] suggested that the implementation of the strict Tygerberg criteria can reduce drastically the incidence of cases with a diagnosis of idiopathic infertility due to fertilization dysfunction.

It is, therefore, clear that valuable information can be obtained from a sperm morphology evaluation, provided that the evaluation is done correctly, skillfully and accurately. The basic morphology evaluation will, then, always play an important role as a cornerstone in the initial evaluation of a male's fertility status and diagnosis, and even in the prognosis of expected *in vivo* and *in vitro* fertilization.

SPERM MORPHOLOGY EVALUATION PROCEDURES

General aspects

Sperm morphology evaluation can be divided into two categories, i.e. the morphological evaluation of spermatozoa and the evaluation of semen cytology. Both must be regarded as important aspects. Therefore, two types of slides must be prepared, one thicker smear for cytology and one thin smear for the morphology evaluation.

Accurate evaluations of sperm morphology cannot be done if the following, although very basic, principles and steps are not followed:

(1) The correct preparation of slides and smears;

(2) Correct fixation;

(3) Correct staining of the smears;

(4) The number of areas used to evaluate the spermatozoa;

(5) The number of spermatozoa evaluated; and

(6) The magnification used.

Preparation of slides and smears

The slides must be thoroughly cleaned before use, first by washing in a detergent, then rinsed in clean water and then rinsed in alcohol and dried[25]. Coverslips must also be washed with alcohol.

For the morphology evaluation, a small drop of semen should be used so that a very thin smear is prepared with no more than 5–10 spermatozoa present per visual field, at oil immersion magnification (1000–1250×). Thin smears are essential, as this will ensure that each sperm can be visualized separately and all spermatozoa will be on the same focal plane so that the true form and not artefacts will be observed.

The thickness of the smear, and thus the number of sperm per visual field, can be controlled by altering the size of the semen drop and by adjusting the angle and speed of the slide used to make the smear[26,27]. With a lower sperm concentration, the size of the drop is increased, as well as the angle between the base slide and the slide used to make the smear. The slide is also moved more quickly over the sample slide. It is important that the semen drop should be pulled over the sample slide. Pushing the drop may cause artefacts such as loose heads and broken or bent tails.

If the sperm concentration is low ($<5\times10^6$/mL) an aliquot of the semen sample can be spun down and the pellet used to make the morphology smear.

Slides should always be prepared in duplicate. The purpose of this is that one can be stored for later reference purposes or other studies, or is available in cases where the first staining was not successful.

Fixation of smears

Most articles state that the slides must be left to air-dry and fixed in alcohol before staining. Unfortunately this leaves space for different interpretations, as it is not clear at what stage the fixation must take place, i.e. directly after the slides are air-dried, or after being stored and just before staining is to take place. Therefore, many different fixation procedures do exist[28].

These methods differ in the type of fixative used, for example formalin[29], cytology spray fixatives[26] and combinations of alcohol and ether[28,30]. According to Hellinga[31], formalin and sprays should be avoided as this leads to an increased percentage of morphological abnormal spermatozoa, while fixation in 96% alcohol produces the lowest number of abnormal spermatozoa.

A good method to follow is as described by

Mortimer[30]. The smears are left to air-dry and are then fixed for 30 min in a freshly prepared solution of equal parts of analytical grade absolute ethanol and diethyl ether. The slides are again left to air-dry and can then be stained or stored.

Staining of smears

For routine work, a staining method such as the Papanicolaou procedure is preferred[32,33]. The method gives good staining of both spermatozoa and other cells, such as the precursors or germinal epithelium cells and white blood cells[34]. As the Papanicolaou is a basophilic/acidophilic stain, the nucleus of spermatozoa and other cells stain intense blue while the sperm acrosomes appears light blue. The sperm tails stain blue or, if staining conditions are very good, even red, while the midpiece can also stain red but mostly blue–green. Cytoplasmic droplets at the head–neck junction will usually stain blue–green.

The 1992 *WHO Manual*[22] also recommends the use of other staining methods in addition to the Papanicolaou method, such as the Giemsa and Bryan–Leishman stains, as well as the Shorr stain which has been in use in several European countries for many years[35–38].

The Giemsa and Bryan–Leishman stains are not used extensively. With the Giemsa stain spermatozoa without acrosomes may appear normal[39], while Hellinga[31] found that Giemsa often also left the sperm tails unstained and could be associated with an increased percentage of head abnormalities. The advantage of the Shorr stain is the intense staining of the sperm tails compared to the Papanicolaou method. It also has the differentiation ability to stain the sperm tails red (normal) or green which indicates that the tail is non-viable[37]. Meschede *et al.*[40] found the same mean percentages (31.1%) of morphological normal spermatozoa for the same samples stained with the Papanicolaou and Shorr methods, respectively. The 1992 *WHO Manual*[22] also suggests that morphology evaluations could be carried out on wet preparations with the aid of phase contrast optics at a magnification of 600×. However, there are many practical difficulties involved in this method[40], and a significantly lower mean percentage of 12.3% morphological normal spermatozoa was obtained compared to the 31.3% with the Papanicolaou and Shorr methods. The method is also contradictory to the basic principle that the highest magnification possible should be used. If this principle is not followed, only the more gross abnormalities will be identified[18].

For special procedures, rapid staining methods such as the Diff-Quik[41], Testsimplets®[42] and Toluidine blue–pyronine[43] methods can be used. Kruger *et al.*[41] found that the Diff-Quik staining method provided similar results with regard to the percentage of morphological normal spermatozoa (11.3% versus 11.4%, and 13.3% versus 12.7% for the Papanicolaou and Diff-Quik methods, respectively) as evaluated by two technicians. Overstaining with Diff-Quik and intense background staining of the seminal plasma are negative aspects of this method. These negative effects can be overcome by washing of the semen samples before the smears are made.

Spermac®[44] has the advantage of a short staining procedure, while it also provides detailed differentiation staining of the acrosome, postacrosomal region and tail. Due to its intense staining, it also allows for suitable photography. Spermac stains tails and intact acrosomes green and the head nucleus red[45]. (See Section 4 for different staining [Papanicolaou, Diff-Quik, Shorr and Spermac] methods.)

Evaluation of spermatozoa

Number of areas to be used for evaluation

All the spermatozoa should be evaluated in not one, but several areas. This will increase the accuracy of the evaluation as experience has shown that unrepresentative evaluations can be obtained if this is not done. It is, therefore, important that about the same number of spermatozoa should be counted in different areas: 20 spermatozoa per area if 100 spermatozoa are evaluated; and 40 if 200 spermatozoa are evaluated in five different areas. These areas can, for example, be the four corner areas and an area in the middle of the slide. The ability to do this will largely depend on the quality of the smear.

Number of spermatozoa to be evaluated

The number of spermatozoa that are evaluated will largely depend on the time available for the evaluation and the degree of reliability desired. MacLeod[46] has demonstrated that, in most cases, the evaluation of 100 spermatozoa will be sufficient. Eliasson[26] advocated the evaluation of 200 spermatozoa, while Harvey and Jackson[47] also suggested 200 spermatozoa. The WHO (1980)[25] suggested that 100 should be evaluated and the 1992 *Manual*[22] recommended 100 or 200. The consensus is, therefore, that at least 100, but preferably 200, spermatozoa should be evaluated.

Magnification to be used

For the evaluation of sperm morphology a microscope with very good optics should be used, equipped with brightfield illumination and a 100× oil immersion objective with a total magnification of at least 1000×, but preferably 1250×. The use of the highest possible magnification is important. If this is not done, only the grossest abnormalities will be observed. It has been demonstrated that the higher the magnification, the more information and thus better evaluation can be obtained. Singer *et al.*[48] found an average of 5 percentage points more abnormalities at a 1000× magnification compared with the results of evaluations done at a magnification of 400×. They also found 15 percentage points more acrosome abnormalities with the 1000× magnification compared to the 400× magnification.

The use of a micrometer to measure the size of the spermatozoa is also of great importance, especially in the classification of spermatozoa according to size, as too small, too large, as well as to decide whether or not the spermatozoa are possibly elongated. Therefore, inexperienced workers should make use of a built-in micrometer when they begin with sperm morphology evaluations and even experienced workers should make use of sperm measurements from time to time, as normal dimensions may differ depending on the staining method used[18].

Evaluation of semen cytology

For the evaluation of semen cytology, by which is meant the investigation of the sample for the presence of different cells, such as leukocytes and histiocytes, as well as organisms, a thicker smear is prepared. A small drop of egg albumen is added to the semen drop to assure a better adherence of the cellular matter to the slides. The slides are fixed immediately in a 1:1 solution of ether:alcohol and stained together with the slides for morphology evaluations. The slides are screened at a low magnification (15×) and if any cells or organisms are observed a 40× objective is used to make a better diagnosis. Cells looked for are especially white blood cells (polymorphs), epithelial cells, histiocytes and ghost cells. The presence of these cells are recorded separately as: – = no cells; ± = occasional; + = 1–5/HPF; ++ = 5–10/HPF; and +++ = >10/HPF.

SPERM MORPHOLOGY EVALUATION SYSTEMS

Historical background

As mentioned in the Introduction, it has only been since earlier in this century that the morphological appearance of spermatozoa has become a focus of interest, and that it has become accepted that normal and pathological forms could appear simultaneously in a semen sample[1,2].

In 1916, Cary[49] summarized the existing literature and included drawings of atypical spermatozoa. He also stated that the fertilization potential was lowered through the presence of abnormal sperm and thereby was the first person to associate abnormal morphology with the fertility potential of a certain male. In 1931, Moench and Holt[50] supported the statement made by Williams and Savage[51] that the head of the spermatozoa was the biggest single source of information on the reproductive potential of the spermatozoa and that, for the average male, the percentage of head abnormalities will be a good indicator of the reproductive capacity of an individual.

Further advances in the process of sperm morphology evaluation was made possible through the development of new staining techniques[51–54] and the introduction of systems to classify spermatozoa into groups according to the type of abnormality observed[4,50,55]. For example, a new differential staining method was described by Cary and Hotchkiss[4], whereby a better evaluation under oil immersion was possible. This enabled them to more easily classify the sperm in certain groups of abnormalities and to calculate the percentage of abnormal spermatozoa as an extra index of a male's fertility potential.

In 1934, Williams *et al.*[52] divided the spermatozoon into four parts: the head, neck, midpiece and tail, and also described the acrosome for the first time. Williams[54] also made the first major contribution to the classification of spermatozoa, dividing the spermatozoa into six morphological classes. This was possible through the use of a good staining technique which made detailed observations at a 1000× magnification possible. Williams[54] also pointed out that, since evaluation of sperm morphology depends largely on objective findings, repeatable evaluations between different observers were possible if uniform methods were used by all the observers, this would be possible by classifying the abnormal spermatozoa into a limited number of six groups. He further subdivided the normal spermatozoa into three groups:

(1) Perfect oval forms;

(2) Ovals forms with a slightly flat base; and

(3) Those with a slightly tapering base so that the postacrosomal base formed a triangle[54].

Williams' statement[54] was supported by Moench[56], whose statement still holds true today: 'The difficulty in evaluating any semen specimen as to its fertilizing powers lies not in picking out definitely narrow, large, small cells, etc., but in knowing where to draw the line between normal and abnormal.' Hotchkiss *et al.*[55] and Gary and Hotchkiss[4], like Williams[54], also used a similar system of only six classes. Their systems subdivided tapering into three classes: types I, II and III. Their type I could be compared to the third type of normal as described by Williams[54]. After studying 200 patients, Hotchkiss *et al.*[55] decided to classify their type I tapering as normal.

Moench[56] stressed the importance of other cells, such as the germinal epithelium, spermiophages, leukocytes and unknown cells, that could be associated with infertility. Contributions in this regard were also made by Frank *et al.*[57], Hartmann *et al.*[58] and MacLeod[46]. These different systems were later improved by Hotchkiss *et al.*[55], MacLeod and Gold[29], MacLeod[46,59], Freund[19], Eliasson[26], Menkveld[60] and Menkveld *et al.*[18], as will be discussed later.

MacLeod

In 1952, MacLeod and Gold[29] published their well known classification system where the spermatozoa were classified into six groups: (1) oval (normal); (2) megalo (large); (3) small; (4) tapering; (5) amorphous; and (6) duplications. At that stage, MacLeod made the statement that he was not prepared to classify any spermatozoa but the most divergent/bizarre forms as abnormal[29]. In later articles, MacLeod[46,59] included precursors as a seventh group into his classification, which he expressed as a percentage of the total number of cells of germinal origin seen in the semen smear[46].

MacLeod also stressed the important role played by cells other than the spermatozoa in the ejaculate. The temporary appearance of these sperm precursors or 'immature' cells is due to exfoliation of the germinal epithelium cells by the testes and is an indication of a pathological process. This can be caused by exposure of the testes to one or other form of stress caused by a virus infection, mental stress, or even a heavy bout of alcohol drinking. MacLeod came to the conclusion that the presence, or not, of germinal epithelial cells in the semen may serve as a very sensitive indicator of germinal activity and can, as such, be a very important tool in basic research, as semen cytology will reflect sensitively and quickly the response of the testis to environmental influences[46].

Freund

In his introduction and discussion on the results of a sperm morphology evaluation rating project of photomicrographs of 500 spermatozoa by 47 participants, Freund[19] remarked: 'A review of the methods described for the evaluation of sperm morphology reveals a chaotic situation'. There was no definitive consensus on how sperm were to be evaluated for morphology, nor was there agreement on what constituted a 'normal' or 'standard' sperm cell. Most investigators published composite drawings of their concept of an 'ideal type' of a normal spermatozoon, together with several drawings of typical abnormal spermatozoa. According to Freund[19], there was also no standardization in the method of preparing the morphology slides and for the staining methods used. There was also no consensus on the magnification to be used, the number of sperm to be counted and the number of areas where the sperm should be evaluated[19]. In his discussion, Freund[19] also pointed out the many synonymous terms used to describe different abnormal forms. Freund[19] collated these to 12 categories.

Based on the results of the collaborative study, Freund[7] put forward several criteria in order to promote standardization of human sperm morphology evaluation. These points concern the classification of sperm heads into six classes and also addresses tail defects, classification of immature spermatozoa and sperm precursors, as well as primary and secondary criteria for classification of spermatozoa. This will be discussed in detail under general principles of morphology classification.

Eliasson

Eliasson[26] also used the basic six classes of MacLeod[29], but he modified the classification of MacLeod by incorporating neck, midpiece, and tail abnormalities, as well as the presence of cytoplasmic droplets into his classification. As far as could be established, Eliasson[26] introduced the basic principle that the whole spermatozoon must be assessed and a spermatozoon with a 'normal' configuration should have a normal head, midpiece and tail. The other very important contribution made by Eliasson[26] was the introduction of actual measurements for the classification of spermatozoa as too small, too large, or elongated and thus also the normal dimensions of a spermatozoon.

In 1981, Eliasson[61] also pointed out that an abnormal spermatozoon can have several combined defects of the head, neck and tail, and that each of these defects must be counted separately and expressed as a percentage of the total number (100) of spermatozoa counted. With this system, the total sum for normal and abnormal will be more than 100. The true percentage of total abnormal spermatozoa (with one or more abnormalities) is obtained by subtracting the percentage of normal spermatozoa from 100. Eliasson[61], therefore, strongly rejected the counting of only one defect. He also used the principle that borderline normal spermatozoa should be regarded as normal.

David

A whole new concept in sperm morphology evaluation was the multiple entry system introduced by David *et al.*[62] in 1975. The basic classification distinguishes between the following.

(1) *Normal* (the whole spermatozoon).

(2) *Head abnormalities:* seven classes (tapered, thin, small, large, double, amorphous and lysis).

(3) *Flagellum abnormalities:* subdivided into

  (a) Midpiece abnormalities (cytoplasmic droplets, bent tails); and

  (b) tail abnormalities (absent, i.e. loose heads, short tails, coiled tails, and double tails).

In this way, all abnormalities and their combinations are taken into consideration and no abnormality is underestimated in relation to the other. The system allows registration from one single entry for example normal to a combination of four abnormalities and the average number of abnormalities per abnormal spermatozoon can be calculated[63].

This method is not widely used due to its complexity, but its importance lies in the fact that this was the forerunner of the teratozoospermia index (TZI) currently recommended by the WHO[22].

World Health Organization (WHO)

The first *WHO Manual* appeared in 1980[25] with a very basic description of sperm morphology evaluation. The morphology classification recommended was based on the classification system of MacLeod[64]. However, greater emphasis was placed on immature germinal cells (precursors). The categories of pyriform heads, midpiece defects, cytoplasmic droplets and tail defects were added, giving a total of 10 classes, compared to the six[29] and later seven[46,59] of MacLeod. The total of the 10 classes in the WHO[25] system made 100%.

Additional to the classification of spermatozoa, the *WHO Manual*[25] also distinguishes between:

(1) *Immature germinal epithelium cells:* described as germinal cells without tails (precursors) in four categories (spermatogonial cells, primary and secondary spermatocytes, Scb spermatids, and Scd spermatids);

(2) *Leukocytes:* divided into lymphocytes and polymorphonuclear leukocytes. Both are counted

per 100 spermatozoa and converted to 10^6 cells/mL semen.

(3) The presence of epithelium cells is also noted.

The importance of this classification was that the terminology used for immature spermatozoa was not the same as proposed by Freund[19]. Furthermore, head, tail and cytoplasmic droplets are all part of the 100 spermatozoa counted and were not in accordance with the guidelines of Eliasson[61] that multiple defects should be recorded. It is, therefore, clear that this was a single entry system with regard to head and tail abnormalities together totaling up to 100% and no priority was given to one specific abnormality over another.

In the second *WHO Manual*[27] of 1987, even less attention was given to the evaluation of sperm morphology. However, this *WHO Manual*[27] made some important changes to their morphology evaluation guidelines. The first was that the classification changed from a single entry system to a multiple entry system. This was done by removing three categories from the primary classification system, i.e. tail defects, midpiece defects and cytoplasmic droplets. Two new classes were added to the primary system, i.e. round heads and pin heads, thus including nine classes all describing the sperm head and totaling 100%. In addition, two secondary categories were created. The first concerned the midpiece and allowed for three classes, i.e. normal, abnormal and cytoplasmic droplets. The second concerned the tails and allowed two classes, i.e. normal and abnormal. It can be interpreted that the classes in both midpiece and tail categories add up to 100% separately. Although not providing an index of combined head, neck/midpiece and/or tail abnormalities, the incidence of these respective abnormalities could be recorded and expressed as a percentage totaling 100% each.

There is no suggestion that so-called 'main' defects, i.e. head abnormalities, are recorded first in favor of midpiece abnormalities which are of more importance than tail defects, as suggested in recent publications[22,30,40]. The only exception is that the presence of multiple heads takes precedence over any other head defect[25,27], if present, based on the guidelines of Freund[19].

In the 1992 *WHO Manual*[22] much more attention is given to sperm morphology. New guidelines are recommended essentially based on the strict Tygerberg criteria[18,60] as reference is made to the role of spermatozoa obtained from postcoital endocervical mucus in critically defining morphological normal spermatozoa on the basis of natural selection as suggested by Menkveld[60] and Menkveld *et al.*[18,45,65] The previous concept that slightly abnormal spermatozoa should be regarded as normal has also to be changed to the most important concept of the strict Tygerberg criteria, i.e. that slightly abnormal spermatozoa must be regarded as abnormal[18,45,60,65].

The normal sperm measurements are slightly larger than those given in the previous manuals[25,27], i.e. 4.0–5.5 μm versus 3.0–5.0 μm for head length, and 2.5–3.5 μm versus 2.0–3.0 μm for the head width, respectively. The size of the cytoplasmic droplet has been brought down to one-third from the previous, more than half the size of a normal sperm head[25].

The new *WHO Manual*[22] classification now only distinguishes between five classes:

(1) *Normal*: the whole spermatozoon.

(2) *Head size/shape defects*: large, small, tapering, pyriform, amorphous, vacuolated (>20% of head area occupied by unstained vacuolar areas) and double heads or any combination.

(3) *Neck and midpiece defects*: absent tails (i.e. loose heads), non-inserted or bent tails (>90%), distended/irregular/bent midpieces, thin midpieces (i.e. no mitochondrial sheath), or any combination.

(4) *Tail defects*: including short, multiple, hairpin, broken, irregular or coiled tails or tails with terminal droplets, or combinations.

(5) *Cytoplasmic droplets*.

At least 100, but preferably 200 spermatozoa are evaluated and placed in one of the five categories to a total of 100%. If more than one abnormality per spermatozoon is present, all of these abnormalities must be scored separately under each category and a teratozoospermia index (TZI) is calculated. Exactly how this must be done is neither explained nor clear.

Other important aspects referred to in the 1992 *WHO Manual*[22] is the fact that if >20% of a special abnormality is present it must be reported separately. Also of importance is the mention of the fact that specific sterilizing defects do exist, of which the best known is probably the round head sperm defect or globozoospermia syndrome.

Teratozoospermia Index (TZI)

The 1992 *WHO Manual*[22] suggests a 'new' multiparametric scoring system, additional to the evaluation of sperm morphology, based on the fact that many morphological abnormal spermatozoa have multiple defects. According to the 1992 *WHO Manual*[22], and quoted by others[30,40], when multiple defects were present only one was recorded with priority given to the defects of the sperm head over those of the midpiece and to defects of the midpiece over those of the tail. No references are given to substantiate this statement by any of the three sources and no other references could be found in the literature in this regard.

However, according to most morphology evaluating systems published after MacLeod's classification[29], where only sperm heads were considered, abnormalities of the whole spermatozoon is taken into consideration with the evaluation and classification of sperm abnormalities. One of the first to incorporate this system was Eliasson in 1971[26] and 1981[61], as mentioned earlier.

This was followed by the work of David[62] in 1975. The term multiple anomalies index (MAI) was used by Jouannet *et al.*[63] in 1988, who demonstrated that a MAI of 1.56 was found when no pregnancies occurred, versus 1.50 when pregnancies *in vivo* occurred. Jouannet *et al.*[63], therefore, suggested a threshold MAI value of 1.6. This MAI, together with the percentage of motile sperm, was found by them to be the best prognostic indicator of fertility as indicated by multivariate analysis. It must, however, be kept in mind that, in their study, they also found that there was a highly significant correlation ($r = 0.63$, $P < 0.001$) between the MAI and percentage of abnormal spermatozoa present. A multiple scoring system was used by Mortimer[34] and referred to as a TZI[66]. They found a negative correlation with the results of the hyaluronate migration test[66].

The strict Tygerberg criteria method[18] also uses a multiple scoring system, where tail, neck/midpiece and cytoplasmic droplet abnormalities are counted on a separate tally and expressed per 100 spermatozoa counted. This is perhaps the easiest way to calculate a multiple scoring index.

For the calculation of a multiple scoring index, i.e. MAI or preferably the TZI, to keep within the WHO recommendations, it is necessary to primarily record the number of normal and abnormal spermatozoa separately until 100 or 200 spermatozoa have been counted. For each abnormal spermatozoon, the type or combination of abnormalities, i.e. head (size/shape), neck/midpiece and tail defects and cytoplasmic droplets, are each separately and respectively recorded, preferably on a separate counter. An abnormal spermatozoon can, therefore, have a maximal total of four abnormalities[22]. The total number of all separate abnormalities is then divided by the total number of abnormal spermatozoa counted, i.e. 100 minus the percentage of morphological normal spermatozoa[30,34,61].

Düsseldorf classification

The Düsseldorf classification[36,38,67] is unique in so far that it is a more clinically founded classification with more emphasis being placed on elongation of spermatozoa and acrosomes defects, as well as a combination thereof, as an indicator of underlying pathology[67]. The Düsseldorf classification first distinguishes between a normal head and three degrees (types) of elongation of the postacrosomal region: HI°, HII° and HIII°.

Type HI° = slightly elongated with an even distribution between acrosomal and postacrosomal areas.

Type HII° = spermatozoa with a cone- or stalk-like elongation of the postacrosomal segment.

Type HIII° = severe disorder, where spermatozoa show extensive elongation of the postacrosomal region ending in a button-like deformation.

These aberrations are due to functional disorders of the Sertoli cells, due to environmental influences and are reversible up to the HII° stage. Once the severity of the HIII° type is reached the disorder is no longer reversible.

The second defect addressed by the Düsseldorf classification is aberration of the acrosomes. Acrosomes develop from the Golgi complex. Disruption of the acrosome formation are, therefore, of genetic origin, are not reversible, and are correlated with disorders of chromatin condensation. Two degrees (types) of acrosome disorders are distinguished: AI° and AII°.

Type AI° = slight disorders where small or missing acrosomes are present. The outline (form) of the spermatozoa is normal or slightly narrowed.

Type AII° = spermatozoa show the same acrosome defects, but the sperm heads are round with a compact condensation of the chromatin.

A combination of these two disorders is also possible. Furthermore, three degrees of tail defects are also distinguished.

Type I° = broken tails.

Type II° = broken tails at neck or midpiece area with coiling of the tails.

Type III° = short rudimentary (tadpole-like) tails.

Attention is now also paid to the staining behavior and structural shaft disturbances of the tail, as seen with the Shorr staining technique[37].

In total, the Düsseldorf classification[67] distinguishes eight classes:

(1) Normal spermatozoa;

(2) Size defects, too small or too large;

(3) Different degrees of hyperelongation;

(4) Hyperelongation with acrosome defects;

(5) Different degrees of acrosome disorders;

(6) Duplicated forms;

(7) Midpiece and/or tail defects; and

(8) A combination of head and tail defects.

The strength of the Düsseldorf classification, however, lies in the differentiation of elongation and acrosome defects and its bearing on fertilization as will be discussed under the heading of Acrosome Index.

Strict Tygerberg criteria

All classification systems discussed in this chapter were based on what was thought to be a 'normal' spermatozoon. This was derived by consensus of several opinions[19] or based on the description of the modal spermatozoon form seen in ejaculated semen samples[34]. The introduction of the strict Tygerberg criteria[60] brought a new concept into the field of morphology evaluation.

For the first time, the description of a so-called 'normal' spermatozoon was based on biological evidence for normality of spermatozoal forms selected for by natural physiological processes[60]. Based on these criteria, stricter guidelines were outlined for evaluation and classification of spermatozoa. In contrast to other authors[19,25,26,29,34], so-called 'borderline normal' spermatozoa are classified as abnormal. The strict Tygerberg criteria were originally developed in a laboratory and *in vivo* situation[10,60,68] and has thereafter been applied to *in vitro* studies[69], and is thus applicable to *in vivo* and *in vitro* situations and not only to the *in vitro* situation, as has been suggested[37]. Furthermore, the word 'strict' does not refer to actual measurements, as has also been suggested[30], but to the stricter application of the range allowed for normal variations with regard to what can still be regarded as normal, and stricter with regard to the interpretation that slightly abnormal or borderline normal forms must be considered as abnormal.

Establishment of a normal reference population

Rationale Evaluation of sperm morphology of most normal domestic animals reveals a generally homogeneous sperm population in individual species. Man, however, is in a small group of species generating semen specimens that exhibit extreme heterogeneity or pleomorphism of sperm morphology between[18,30,45] and even within specific individuals[58,64]. The homogeneity seen in animals simplifies determining and defining normality for that specific species on account of the appearance of the modal spermatozoon, and is confirmed by proven fertility of the individual animals.

This concept has been applied unsuccessfully to human populations of so-called 'fertile' groups and individual men, with the resultant large differences found between, and even within, laboratories for the evaluation of sperm morphology[19,21].

It has been shown by Mortimer *et al.*[70] and Fredricsson and Björk[71] that strong selection of certain morphological types of spermatozoa occur with migration of spermatozoa through cervical mucus, and that the morphological normality of these populations is significantly increased and of strong prognostic significance[71]. However, the concept[60] of using the appearance of these spermatozoa as a reference population to describe the ideal 'normal' spermatozoon has not been used before.

The strict Tygerberg criteria for an ideal normal spermatozoon, as originally described by Menkveld[60] are, therefore, based on the morphology of post-coital spermatozoa found at the level of the internal cervical os, mostly consisting of an apparently homogeneous sperm population (Figure 1), in contrast to the sperm populations found in the first or lower part of the endocervical canal, as indicated by the presence of epithelial cells[18,62]. The morphology of these spermatozoa at the internal os formed the basis of the strict Tygerberg criteria for the ideal morphologically normal spermatozoon, taking into account the small range of normal biological variations within these populations, but excluding the obvious abnormal forms such as small and elongated[60].

Probably the most important aspect of the evaluation criteria, and therefore the inclusion of the term 'strict'[18], is that the range allowed for the above-mentioned normal variations should be kept as small as possible to ensure repeatable evaluations. This is why the strict Tygerberg criteria[18], in contrast with other evaluating systems[19,25–27,34], regarded spermatozoa with so-called borderline or slightly abnormal head forms as abnormal.

The guidelines of the strict Tygerberg criteria[18] are supported by the morphological appearance of spermatozoa found tightly bound to the human zona pellucida, as seen under hemizona assay conditions[72] and *in vitro*[73]. The morphology of the tightly bound spermatozoa closely resembles that of spermatozoa found in good post-coital cervical mucus and is a further indication for natural selection of spermatozoa defined as morphological normal by the strict Tygerberg criteria.

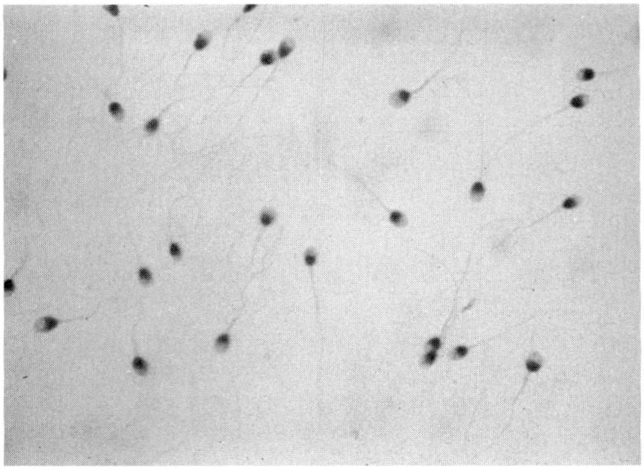

Figure 1 Population of morphologically normal spermatozoa as found in the upper endocervical canal mucus after intercourse and representing a 'normal' reference population for the evaluation of sperm morphology

Description The criteria for a normal spermatozoon are as follows: the head must have a smooth oval configuration with a well-defined acrosome comprising 40–70% of the anterior sperm head. A second, slightly differing type of normal head form is also recognized, i.e. an oval form still having a smooth regular contour, but slightly tapered at the postacrosomal end, as has been described previously[54,55].

Head dimensions are as suggested by Eliasson[26]. The normal length is between 3 and 5 μm, and width between 2 and 3 μm. The head width must be between three-fifths and two-thirds the head lengths.

No neck/midpiece and/or tail defects may be present. The midpiece must be slender, axially attached, ≤1 μm in width and approximately one and one-half times the head length. Cytoplasmic droplets (remnants) which comprise more than half the size of a normal sperm head are regarded as abnormal. Tails must be straight, uniform, slightly thinner than the midpiece, uncoiled and approximately 45 μm long.

The basic morphology classification used for the strict Tygerberg criteria[18] is based on the modification of the methods of MacLeod[29], Eliasson[26] and Freund[19]. The whole spermatozoon (head, neck/midpiece and tail) is taken into consideration for classification, as well as the presence of cytoplasmic droplets, and germinal epithelium and other cells[18].

Spermatozoa heads are classified into seven groups and tallied on an seven-tally laboratory counter as follows:

(1) Normal sperm;

(2) Large heads;

(3) Small heads;

(4) Elongated/tapering heads;

(5) Duplicated heads;

(6) Amorphous heads;

(7) Normal sperm heads with neck/midpiece and/or tail and/or cytoplasmic droplet defects.

All borderline normal forms are regarded as abnormal.

On a separate five-tally laboratory counter, each separate or combination of the following abnormalities or non-spermatozoal cells is counted:

(1) Precursors;

(2) Tail abnormalities;

(3) Neck/midpiece abnormalities;

(4) Cytoplasmic droplets;

(5) Loose heads.

Each of these is recorded separately, i.e. up to three abnormalities per spermatozoon. Precursors (germinal epithelial cells) and loose heads are not regarded as sperm abnormalities. All these abnormalities are, however, expressed as per 100 spermatozoa[18].

A teratozoospermia index (TZI) as suggested by the 1992 *WHO Manual*[22] can thus be easily calculated. This is done by totaling the number of tail and neck/midpiece defects as well as cytoplasmic droplets together and dividing this by 100 minus the percentage of normal spermatozoa.

The value of the strict Tygerberg criteria method as a prognostic tool has been shown in an analysis of the Tygerberg Hospital's IVF results[69]. With ≥15% morphological normal spermatozoa, the fertilization rate was 82.5% with a pregnancy incidence of 25.8% (≥3 ova transferred). When the percentage of normal spermatozoa was ≤14%, there was a drastic drop in the fertilization rate to only 37%, and no pregnancies were recorded. A further modification was introduced by Kruger *et al.*[74] who found that in the group of men with ≤14% normal spermatozoa, two subgroups could be distinguished: those with a good prognosis (G pattern) with between 14 and 5% normal spermatozoa; and those with a poor prognosis (P pattern) with ≤4% morphological normal spermatozoa. Kruger *et al.*[74] included an extra class, comprising of slightly amorphous forms, in their classification. Men with a combination of ≥30% slightly amorphous and normal forms were those with a good prognosis. For *in vivo* fertilization, the same lower cut-off values of ≤4% morphological normal spermatozoa could be established[10].

Acrosome index

From the above data[69] it is clear that although a drastic drop in the fertilization rate occurred when the sperm morphology was ≤4%, normal fertilization in some cases still occurred. With a preliminary investigation[75], it was observed that two distinct morphological patterns could be observed in the cases where fertilization did and did not occur.

In the few men with good fertilization, it was striking to observe a pattern of slightly and moderately elongated spermatozoa, but with morphological normal (size and form) acrosomes (Figure 2). The spermatozoa could be classified as Type HI° and HII° according to the Düsseldorf classification[67]. A typical case is illustrated in Table 1. Although there were only 2% morphological normal spermatozoa, a total of 17% had normal acrosomes. In the group with very poor or no fertilization *in vitro*, it was observed that, in the majority of cases, small and/or abnormal acrosomes were the dominant abnormalities which could be classified predominantly as acrosome defects of AI° or the combination defects A/HI° and A/HII° according to the Düsseldorf classification as illustrated in Figure 3. A typical case is presented in Table 2. This man presented with only 1% morphological normal spermatozoa with a total of only 4% normal acrosomes. In a further study[76], it was found that when the acrosome status was classified into different groups, i.e. normal, small, staining defects and amorphous, and

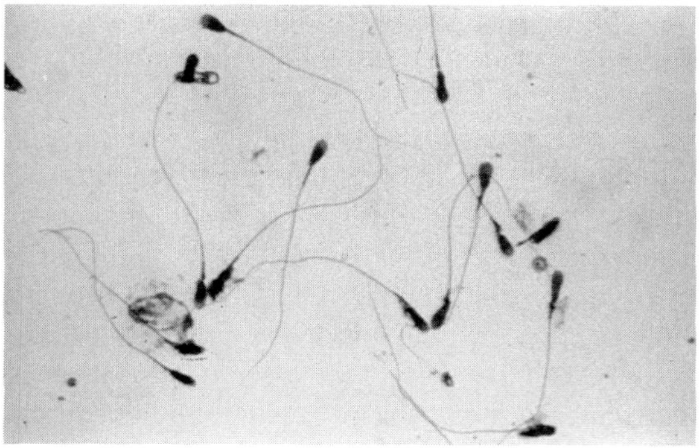

Figure 2 Spermatozoa population of patient K, with only 2% morphologically normal spermatozoa. The spermatozoa show slightly to moderately elongated forms, of which several have morphological normal acrosomes

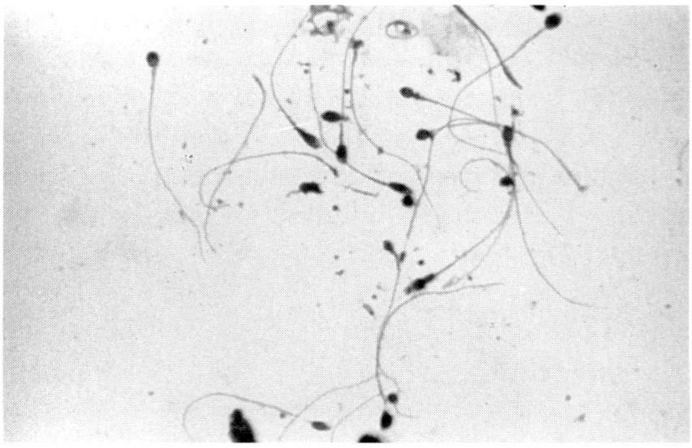

Figure 3 Spermatozoa population of patient T with only 1% morphologically normal spermatozoa. The spermatozoa show a tendency to be smaller than normal and have mostly very small acrosomes

Table 1 Morphology patterns, patient K with 2% morphologically normal spermatozoa; most of the spermatozoa were elongated, some of which had normal acrosomes; after 36 h in CO_2 incubation, 6/6 ova were fertilized

Morphology class	*Percentage*	
	Semen	*Wash/swim-up*
Normal	2	2
Slightly abnormal	2	9
Elongated	41	47
Elongated/abnormal acrosomes	46	26
Small acrosomes	3	0
Amorphous	6	16
Acrosome index (% normal)	17	36

Table 2 Morphology patterns; patient T with only 1% morphologically normal spermatozoa, most spermatozoa were smaller than normal with small acrosomes. After 36 h in CO_2 incubation, 0/4 ova were fertilized

Morphology class	*Percentage*	
	Semen	*Wash/swim-up*
Normal	1	1
Slightly abnormal	0	2
Elongated	0	0
Elongated/abnormal acrosomes	0	0
Small acrosomes	74	70
Amorphous	23	27
Acrosome index (% normal)	4	3

expressed as an acrosome index (% normal acrosomes) no fertilization occurred when the acrosome index was ≤15%. These results are in agreement with previous reports on the role of acrosomal status[77], where it was found that in cases with <30% morphological normal spermatozoa the acrosome status (% normal) was an important prognostic indicator of expected fertilization *in vitro*. Jouannet *et al.*[63] found that the presence of a high frequency of microcephalic sperm was the most statistically significant single sperm abnormality when a pregnancy *in vivo* did not occur. In contrast, it has been noted that elongated spermatozoa of the HI° and HII° are capable of penetrating and migrate through cervical mucus[70,71] and are not associated with a reduced fertilization potential[71,73], as they are capable of binding to the zona pellucida[72,73].

The calculation of the percentage of spermatozoa with normal acrosomes and expressed as the Acrosome Index (% spermatozoa with normal acrosomes and no neck/midpiece, tail, or cytoplasmic droplet abnormalities) can be a valuable additional prognostic morphological parameter in the evaluation of a male's fertility potential, especially in the poor prognosis group with ≤4% morphological normal spermatozoa.

World Health Organization criteria versus strict Tygerberg criteria

After the article of Kruger *et al.*[69] reporting on the good prognostic value of the strict Tygerberg criteria for expected *in vitro* fertilization rates, several papers have been published investigating the usefulness of the strict Tygerberg criteria[18] in this regard[74,78–82]. Reports on comparative studies between the strict Tygerberg criteria and the 1987 WHO criteria[27] have also been published[79,80,82], with most studies finding that the strict Tygerberg criteria were better prognostic indicator of expected fertilization *in vitro* than the WHO criteria[79,80,82]. Although some contradictory results were published on the role of strict Tygerberg criteria versus the WHO criteria[82], it seems that the strict Tygerberg criteria are superior in predicting expected fertilization *in vitro*[79,80] compared to the WHO criteria.

IDENTIFICATION OF MORPHOLOGICAL ABNORMAL SPERMATOZOA

The description and identification of normal spermatozoa has been discussed in detail in a previous section of this chapter. However, in order to achieve the desired standardization in morphology evaluation, it is also very important that clear guidelines be given on the classification of abnormal spermatozoa into specific groups, as has been done by Freund[19] and Eliasson[26].

General principles

Abnormal spermatozoa are those that deviate from the defined criteria for normal, due to differences in size and/or structure or form. Included in these groups are also immature spermatozoa, sperm precursors and spermatozoa with tail and/or neck/midpiece aberrations or defects.

The following six classes, in addition to normal, are identified based on the size or form of the sperm head[19,26].

(1) *Too small:* the heads are smaller than the lower limits of normality.

(2) *Too large:* the heads are larger than the upper limits of normality. Size is the primary criterion as long as the sperm approximate an oval form.

(3) *Duplications:* sperm cells with two or more heads joined together at any location, e.g. neck, midpiece or tail, or by cytoplasmic material not covering the sperm head (see spermatids).

Duplications takes precedence over any other sperm head abnormality classification.

(4) *Elongated/Tapering:* spermatozoa assuming a narrowed form due to flattening of the sides. The term tapering was used by MacLeod[29] and Eliasson[26], but was not included in the classification of Freund[19]. The term 'tapering' may lead to confusion, because it is visualized by many investigators as a spearpoint-like sperm. This is only one of the forms that can be included under the category of tapered. A more appropriate term would be 'elongated' spermatozoa, as those forms termed 'pear-shaped' and 'pyriform' could also be included in this category.

Thus, three basic types of elongated spermatozoa can be identified. Two are the basic elongated forms based on the measurements proposed by Eliasson[26] with the more classic tapering forms. The first is the more general type, which is longer than the upper limits for normality and thinner than the upper limits for normal width, while the second and less common type is shorter than the upper limits for length and thinner than the lower limits for normal width. The third class is the pear-shaped or pyriform sperm. This class can be identified due to the sharp pointed elongated postacrosomal base region of the sperm head. This class may cause confusion because the width is often more than 3 μm, which is the upper normal limit for width, and could potentially also be classified as too large. However, if the principle put forward by Freund[19] that 'the size of the sperm is to be used as *primary criteria* for rating, provided that the shape approximates an oval form', and taking into consideration that this type of abnormality is a specific entity, preference should be given to placing these forms under 'elongated'.

(5) *Amorphous:* all abnormal spermatozoa which do not fall into any of the previous four groups.

(6) *Normal heads with other abnormalities:* the strict Tygerberg criteria[18] include an extra group, i.e. normal heads with other abnormalities, such as a single or combination of neck/midpiece, tail and cytoplasmic droplet defect.

Secondary classification criteria

Immature spermatozoa

Immature spermatozoa are those with a cytoplasmic droplet behind the sperm head or around the midpiece or tail. According to the strict Tygerberg criteria, these sperm are classified first according to the head form, i.e. normal with other defects or one off the abnormal head classes, and then also recorded under cytoplasmic droplets.

A cytoplasmic droplet is deemed to be present when it is larger than one-half the size of a normal sperm head[18,26] or, according to the 1992 *WHO Manual*[22], more than one-third of the normal head.

Sperm precursors

Mature spermatozoa surrounded completely by cytoplasm[18], or all cells from the Scd spermatid stage and earlier, are regarded as precursors, as they have not yet completed their development process[22].

Loose heads

According to the 1992 *WHO Manual*[22], loose heads are counted under neck/midpiece abnormalities. With the strict Tygerberg criteria, these cells are counted separately (like cytoplasmic droplets), under secondary criteria, the rationale being that, in addition to neck abnormalities, the sperm head itself may also be abnormal, which will then not be recorded as such and thus will not add to a representative head evaluation.

Neck/midpiece defects

This category includes bent necks, i.e. the neck and tail forms an angle of ⩾90° with the sperm head. Thickened neck and midpieces are also included, as well as irregular or bent midpieces or abnormally thin midpieces[22].

Tail defects

This category includes bent tails of ⩾90° over any part of the tail except the neck/midpiece region: short tails, coiled tails, or irregular tails, or combinations of these[22].

Loose tails or 'pinheads' are not included in the evaluation. However, if a high incidence (>20%) is present, relative to spermatozoa, this should be noted separately as pinheads and not considered spermatozoa[22].

Unknown cells

The strict Tygerberg criteria[18], in addition to the above-mentioned classes, further provide for an additional group of unknown cells. All cells that cannot be identified positively as either precursors or inflammatory cells are placed in this group.

All the spermatozoa and cells classified under the secondary criteria are expressed as per 100 spermatozoa.

Measurements of spermatozoa

Different dimensions of human spermatozoa are given in the literature[83]. It would seem that the dimensions are influenced by the type of microscopy used, for example light or electron microscopy[83], as well as the staining method used[33,41] According to the 1992 *WHO Manual*[22], dimensions for stained spermatozoa are smaller than for unstained spermatozoa due to slight shrinkage introduced by fixation and staining.

The following normal dimensions, as well as dimensions for the classification of spermatozoa as too large, too small and tapering/elongated, have been published by Eliasson[26] in 1971 and are presented in Table 3. These dimensions are also used for the strict Tygerberg criteria[18] However, experience has shown that the lower limits for normal length are probably too low and should be set at about 4 μm. The normal dimensions proposed by the 1992 *WHO Manual*[22] are also larger than those published by Eliasson[26], i.e. 4.0–5.5 μm and 2.5–3.5 μm. According to the *WHO Manual*, the length:width ratio should be 1.50:1.75 based on the Papanicolaou method[22].

The influences of staining methods are illustrated by the measurements given by Kruger *et al.*[41] for the Diff-Quik method with a length of 5–6 μm and width of 2.5–3.5 μm, in comparison to those of Eliasson[26] based on the Papanicolaou method.

Table 3 Dimensions for the classification of normal and abnormal spermatozoa according to size*

	Dimensions		
Description	*Length (μm)*	*Width (μm)*	
Normal head	3.0–5.0	2.0–3.0	
Normal midpiece	5.0–7.0	1.0	
Normal tail	45.0		
Megalo	>5.0	>3.0	
Small	<3.0	<2.0	
Elongated	>5.0	3.0	Type I
	<5.0	<2.0	Type II

*Adapted from Eliasson 1971[26]

RELIABILITY OF SPERM MORPHOLOGY EVALUATION

The opinion of many workers involved in sperm morphology evaluation is that sperm morphology is a stable semen parameter, when different samples of the same person are compared from time to time, and that the seminal picture is characteristic of a specific person[58,84]. However, Freund[19] found substantial variability in the ratings of percentage of normal sperm morphology among repeated specimens of the same donor. The variability observed was obtained between and within technicians. Freund suggested that, to a great extent, as in the case of sperm counts, this could be due to within and between technician observer variation due to the lack of consensus on normal sperm morphology and general standardization.

The strict Tygerberg criteria[18] created the opportunity to reduce some of the variability obtained with previous methods[21,85] on condition that the basic principles outlined previously, i.e. preparation of smears, number of sperm counted, areas evaluated and stricter adherence to criteria, are carefully followed. The aim, therefore, should be to keep the source of variation as small as possible. Sources of variation are: (1) the number of spermatozoa evaluated; (2) criteria for normality and experience of observers; and (3) additional cell types included under normal.

Number of sperm to be evaluated

The number of spermatozoa that should be evaluated will, to a large degree, depend on the time available and the accuracy desired. MacLeod[29] demonstrated that if 300 spermatozoa were evaluated, the average standard deviation was about 3% and 6% if 100 spermatozoa were evaluated. These deviations were found for mean percentages of 79% and 73% morphologically normal spermatozoa in a group of 'fertile' and 'infertile' males, respectively.

Harvey and Jackson[47] advised that, for maximum accuracy, 400–600 spermatozoa should be evaluated but that for routine practice 200 spermatozoa are sufficient, as this will give values within 3% of those obtained with evaluating more spermatozoa.

However, much lower mean percentages of morphological normal spermatozoa are obtained today, especially with the strict Tygerberg criteria. For example Haidl and Schill[37] found a mean of 29.5% normal spermatozoa in a fertile population with the Düsseldorf classification, and Menkveld *et al.*[18] 16.7% in an infertile population with the strict Tygerberg criteria. Therefore, the deviations obtained in terms of actual percentages will be much smaller.

It is clear, therefore, that the degree of variability can be reduced by evaluating more spermatozoa, but time is also an important factor. Based on the information given earlier in this chapter, evaluating 200 spermatozoa seems to be the golden midway, especially if morphology evaluations are not to be used only for routine purposes.

Evaluation of normal sperm morphology (alone)

The effect of lack of standardization on the evaluation of sperm morphology has been clearly shown by the work of Jequier and Ukombe[21]. The results for morphology evaluations of one semen sample by 27 observers ranged between 15% and 95% normal with a mean (±SD) of 67.3±21.3% morphologically normal spermatozoa.

When evaluations of observers within the same laboratory are compared, the situation is much better. Zaini *et al.*[9] found that, although highly significant correlation coefficients of 0.604, 0.723 and 0.770 were obtained between three technicians, for the percentage of morphological normal spermatozoa, a considerable degree of variation existed between the three technicians' assessments of the same samples, with errors in the region of 40%–60%. In a subsequent article[85], an even larger between-observer variation was found with correlation coefficients of 0.633, 0.534 and 0.389. The role of stricter criteria is demonstrated with the results obtained by the Tygerberg group[18]. The between-observer correlation coefficients were between 0.8675 and 0.6537 ($P<0.0003$) for the results of four observers.

Ayodeji and Baker[85] found within-observer correlation coefficients of 0.611 and 0.791 for two observers, against the 0.9650 ($P<0.0001$) by Menkveld *et al.*[18] for one observer using the strict Tygerberg criteria.

In terms of the coefficient of variation (CV) obtained by repeated counts of sperm morphology on the same slides, the results obtained with the strict Tygerberg criteria[18] were also better than those obtained by MacLeod[59]. MacLeod evaluated 14 series of 100 spermatozoa each on one morphology slide. A CV of 12.3% could be calculated from his results. In the Tygerberg study[18], the CV ranged between 5.21 and 11.62 for 10 repeated morphology evaluations carried out on three different samples, and 27.76 on one sample with an average of only 3.5±0.97% morphologically normal spermatozoa.

From the above it can be concluded that the morphology evaluation results according to the stricter Tygerberg criteria compare favorably with or better than those cited from the literature above. The stricter criteria are thought to play an important role in these results.

Ayodeji and Baker[85] also found that, although the within-observer assessments were more reliable the results still lacked accuracy, and that the assessments by more experienced technicians were generally more reliable. This was also found for the strict Tygerberg criteria[18]. It was found that the error variance (EV), an indication of the relative accuracy between different methods or observers, calculated according to the method of Barnett[86], increased with a decrease in the years of experience of an observer. The smallest (most accurate) EV of 2.89 was obtained for the observer with the longest period of experience and the largest, although still very small, EV of 19.68 was seen for the observer with the shortest period of experience. The same tendency was obtained when the correlation coefficients between observers were compared. The highest correlation coefficient ($r=0.8675$, $P<0.0003$) was obtained between the two observers with the longest period of experience and the lowest correlation coefficient ($r=0.635$, $P<0.0001$) obtained between the observer with the longest and the observer with the shortest periods of experience.

Table 4 Comparison of morphology evaluations between four observers with regard to percentage of morphologically normal and borderline normal spermatozoa; effect of experience on morphology evaluation is also illustrated. Observer 1 has the longest period of experience followed by observer 2, then 3, while observer 4 had the shortest period of experience

Type of spermatozoa	*Observers*					
	4@1		*3@1*		*2@1*	
Normal (%)	12.9	12.4	11.2	11.7	10.2	10.0
Borderline normal (%)	18.6	11.7	13.1	11.7	9.3	9.5
	31.8	24.0	24.2	21.9	19.5	19.2
Number of samples	(*n*=33)		(*n*=39)		(*n*=40)	

Evaluation of normal plus slightly abnormal forms

As soon as another factor is brought into consideration with the basic morphology evaluation, for example incorporating a morphology index, i.e. summation of normal and slightly amorphous forms, as suggested by Kruger *et al.*[74], the variability of the morphology evaluation increases, as shown in Table 4. These increasing differences are due to each observer's interpretation of what can be regarded as a slightly abnormal or borderline spermatozoon. From Table 4 it can be seen that the averages for percentage of morphologically normal spermatozoa between observer 1, with the longest period of experience, and the other three observers are very similar. When the percentage of borderline normals is also taken into consideration, the differences between observer 1 and the other observers once again increases with a decrease in experience. The biggest difference of 6.9 percentage points (18.6% versus 11.7% borderline normal forms) was found between observer 1 with the longest and observer 4 with the shortest experience. A difference of only 0.3 percentage points (19.5% versus 19.2% borderline normal forms) was found between observers 1 and 2 with the longest experience between them. This demonstrates the important role that strict criteria can play in the more accurate evaluation of sperm morphology.

References

1. Joël, C. A. (1971). Historical survey of research on spermatozoa from antiquity to the present. In Joël, C. A. (ed.) *Fertility Disturbances in Men and Women*, pp. 3–47. (Basel: Kager)
2. Hotchkiss, R. S. (1945). *Fertility in Men*. (London: William Heinemann Medical Books)
3. Cary, W. H. (1930). Sterility diagnosis: The study of sperm cell migration in female secretion and interpretation of findings. *N.Y. State J. Med.*, **30**, 131–6
4. Cary, W. H. and Hotchkiss, R. S. (1934). Semen appraisal. A differential stain that advances the study of cell morphology. *J. Am. Med. Assoc.*, **102**, 587–90
5. Moench, G. L. and Holt, H. (1932). Biometrical studies of head lengths of human spermatozoa. *J. Lab. Clin. Med.*, **17**, 297–316
6. Huhner, M. (1921). Methods of examining for spermatozoa in the diagnosis and treatment of sterility. *Int. J. Surg.*, **34**, 91–100
7. Aitken, R. J., Best, F. S. M., Richardson, D. W., Djahanbakhen, O., Mortimer, D., Templeton, A. A. and Lees, M. (1982). Analysis of sperm function in cases of unexplained infertility: conventional criteria, movement characteristics and fertilizing capacity. *Fertil. Steril.*, **38**, 212–21
8. Singer, R., Sagiv, M., Barnet, M., Segenreich, E., Allalouf, D., Landau, B. and Servadio, C. (1980). Motility, vitality and percentage of morphologically abnormal forms of human spermatozoa in relation to sperm counts. *Andrologia*, **12**, 92–6
9. Zaini, A., Jennings, M. G. and Baker, H. W. G. (1985). Are conventional sperm morphology and motility assessments of predictive value in subfertile men? *Int. J. Androl.*, **8**, 427–35
10. Van Zyl, J. A., Kotze, T. J. vW. and Menkveld, R. (1990). Predictive value of spermatozoa morphology in natural fertilization. In Acosta, A. A., Swanson, R. J., Ackerman, S. B., Kruger, T. F., van Zyl, J. A. and Menkveld, R. (eds.) *Human Spermatozoa in Assisted Reproduction*, pp. 319–24. (Baltimore: Williams and Wilkins)
11. Belding, D. L. (1934). Fertility in the male. II. Technique of the spermatozoa count. *Am. J. Obstet. Gynecol.*, **27**, 25–31
12. Freund, M. (1968). Performance and interpretation of the semen analysis. In Rolands, M. (ed.) *Management of the Infertile Couple*, p. 48. (Springfield: Charles C. Thomas Publisher)
13. Farris, E. J. (1949). The number of motile spermatozoa as an index of fertility in man: A study of 406 semen specimens. *J. Urol.*, **61**, 1099–104
14. Rogers, B. J., Bentwood, B. J., Van Campen, H., Helmbrecht, G., Soderdahl, D. and Hale, R. W. (1983). Sperm morphology assessment as an indicator of human fertilizing capacity. *J. Androl.*, **4**, 119–25
15. De Kretser, D. M., Yates, C. and Kovacs, G. T. (1985). The use of IVF in the management of male infertility. *Clin. Obstet. Gyn.*, **12**, 767–73
16. Mahadevan, M. M. and Trounson, A. O. (1984). The influence of seminal characteristics on the success rate of human *in vitro* fertilization. *Fertil. Steril.*, **42**, 400–5
17. Yovich, J. L. and Stanger, J. D. (1984). The limitations of *in vitro* fertilization from males with severe oligospermia and abnormal sperm morphology. *J.* In Vitro *Fertil. Embryo Transf.*, **1**, 172–9
18. Menkveld, R., Stander, F. S. H., Kotze, T. J. vW., Kruger, T. F. and van Zyl, J. A. (1990). The evaluation of morphological characteristics of human spermatozoa according to stricter criteria. *Hum. Reprod.*, **5**, 586–92
19. Freund, M. (1966). Standards for the rating of human sperm morphology. A cooperative study. *Int. J. Fertil.*, **11**, 97–118
20. Fredricsson, B. (1979). Morphologic evaluation of spermatozoa in different laboratories. *Andrologia*, **11**, 57–61
21. Jequier, A. M. and Ukombe, E. B. (1983). Errors inherent in the performance of a routine semen analysis. *Br. J. Urol.*, **55**, 434–6
22. World Health Organization. (1992). *WHO Laboratory Manual for the Examination of Human Semen and Sperm–Cervical Mucus Interaction*, 3rd edn. (Cambridge: Cambridge University Press)
23. Liu, D. Y. and Baker, W. G. (1992). Test of human sperm function and fertilization *in vitro*. *Fertil. Steril.*, **58**, 465–83
24. Chan, S. Y. W. and Tucker, M. J. (1991). Fertilization failure and dysfunctions as possible causes for human idiopathic infertility. *Andrologia*, **23**, 399–414
25. World Health Organization. (1980). *WHO Laboratory Manual for the Examination of Human Semen and Semen–Cervical Mucus Interaction*. (Singapore: Press Concern)
26. Eliasson, R. (1971). Standards for investigation of human semen. *Andrologie*, **3**, 49–64
27. World Health Organization. (1987). *WHO Laboratory Manual for the Examination of Human Semen and*

Semen–Cervical Mucus Interaction, 2nd edn. (Cambridge: Cambridge University Press)
28. Sigg, Ch. and Hornstein, O. P. (1987). *Das Spermiozytogramm. Grundlagen und Diagnostische Anwendung in der Andrologie*. (Erlangen: perimed Fachbuch-Verlagsgesell-Schaft mbH)
29. MacLeod, J. and Gold, R. Z. (1952). The male factor in fertility and infertility. IV. Sperm morphology in fertile and infertile marriage. *Fertil. Steril.*, **2**, 394–414
30. Mortimer, D. (1994). *Practical Laboratory Andrology*. (Oxford: Oxford University Press)
31. Hellinga, G. (1976). *Clinical Andrology*, pp. 15–29. (London: William Heinemann Medical Books)
32. Papanicolaou, G. N. (1942). A new procedure for staining vaginal smears. *Science*, **95**, 438–9
33. Menkveld, R. (1991). Appendices. In Menkveld, R., Oettlé, E. E., Kruger, T. F., Swanson, R. J. and Oehninger, S. (eds.) *Atlas of Human Sperm Morphology*, pp. 115–18. (Baltimore: Williams and Wilkins)
34. Mortimer, D. (1985). The male factor in infertility. Part I: Semen analysis. *Curr. Probl. Obstet. Gynecol. Fertil.*, **8**, 4–87
35. Jeulin, C., Feneux, D., Serres, C., Jouannet, P., Guillet-Rosso, F., Belaisch-Allart, J., Frydman, R. and Testart, J. (1986). Sperm factors related to failure of human *in vitro* fertilization. *J. Reprod. Fertil.*, **76**, 735–44
36. Hofmann, N. and Haider, S. G. (1985). Neue Ergebnisse morphologischer Diagnostik der Spermatogenesestörungen. *Gynäkologe*, **18**, 70–80
37. Haidl, G. and Schill, W.-B. (1993). Sperm morphology in fertile men. *Arch. Androl.*, **31**, 153–7
38. Hofmann, N. (1987). *Wege Zur Andrologie. Einführung in die Praxis*. Erster Teil. (Bremerhaven: Ditzen Druck und Verlags-GmbH)
39. Zaneveld, L. J. D. and Jeyendran, R. S. (1988). Modern assessment of semen for diagnostic purposes. *Semin. Reprod. Endocrinol.*, **6**, 323–37
40. Meschede, D., Keck, C., Zander, M., Cooper, T. G., Yeung, C.-H. and Nieschlag, E. (1993). Influence of three different preparation techniques on the results of human sperm morphology analysis. *Int. J. Androl.*, **16**, 362–9
41. Kruger, T. F., Ackerman, S. B., Simmons, K. F., Swanson, R. J., Brugo, S. S. and Acosta, A. A. (1987). A quick, reliable staining technique for human sperm morphology. *Arch. Androl.*, **18**, 275–7
42. Schirren, C., Eckhardt, U., Jachczik, R. and Carstensen, C. A. (1977). Morphological differentiation of human spermatozoa with Testsimplets[R] slides. *Andrologia*, **9**, 191–2
43. Schütte, B. (1986). Human spermatozoa stained with Toluidine blue-Pyronine. A rapid method for differentiation. *Andrologia*, **18**, 567–96
44. Oettlé, E. E. (1986). Using a new acrosome stain to evaluate sperm morphology. *Vet. Med.*, **81**, 263–6
45. Menkveld, R., Kruger, T. F., Oettlé, E. E., Swanson, R. J., Oehninger, S. and Acosta, A. A. (1991). Basic principles and practical aspects. In: Menkveld, R., Oettlé, E. E., Kruger, T. F., Swanson, R. J. and Oehninger, S. (eds.) *Atlas of Human Sperm Morphology*, pp. 1–6. (Baltimore: Williams and Wilkins)
46. MacLeod, J. (1964). Human seminal cytology as a sensitive indicator of the germinal epithelium. *Int. J. Fertil.*, **9**, 281–95
47. Harvey, C. and Jackson, M. H. (1945). Assessment of male fertility by semen analysis. An attempt to standardize methods. *Lancet*, **ii**, 99–104, 134–7
48. Singer, R., Sagiv, M., Barnet, M., Allalouf, B., Segenreich, E. and Servadio, C. (1981). Head abnormalities assessment of sperm in the routine laboratory. *Andrologia*, **13**, 236–41
49. Cary, H. W. (1916). Examination of semen with reference to gynecological aspects. *Am. J. Obstet. Dis. Women Child.*, **74**, 615–38
50. Moench, G. L. and Holt, H. (1931). Sperm morphology in relation to fertility. *Am. J. Obstet. Gynecol.*, **22**, 199–210
51. Williams, W. A. and Savage, A. (1925). Observations on the seminal micropathology of bulls. *Cornell Vet.*, **15**, 353–75
52. Williams, W. W., McGuigan, A. and Carpenter, H. D. (1934). The staining and morphology of the human spermatozoon. *J. Urol.*, **32**, 201–12
53. Amelar, R. D., Dubin, L. and Schoenfeld, C. (1973). Semen analysis: An office technique. *Urology*, **2**, 605–11
54. Williams, W. W. (1937). Spermatic abnormalities. *N. Engl. J. Med.*, **217**, 946–51
55. Hotchkiss, R. S., Brunner, E. K. and Grenley, P. (1938). Semen analysis of two hundred fertile men. *Am. J. Med. Sci.*, **196**, 362–84
56. Moench, G. L. (1940). Relation of certain seminal findings to fertility with special reference to sperm concentration and the significance of testicular epithelium cells in semen. *Am. J. Surg.*, **47**, 586–96
57. Frank, I. N., Benjamin, J. A. and Segerson, J. E. (1954). Cytologic examination of semen. *Fertil. Steril.*, **5**, 217–26
58. Hartmann, G. G., Schoenfeld, C. and Copeland, E. (1964). Individualism in the seminal picture of infertile men. *Fertil. Steril.*, **15**, 231–53
59. MacLeod, J. (1966). The clinical implications of deviations in human spermatogenesis as evidenced in seminal cytology and experimental production of these deviations. *Ex. Med. Int. Cong. Ser. No. 133.*, pp. 563–74, *Proceedings of the Fifth Congress on Fertility and Sterility*, Stockholm, 16–22 June
60. Menkveld, R. (1987). An investigation of environmental influences on spermatogenesis and semen parameters. *Ph.D. Dissertation, Faculty of Medicine, University of Stellenbosch, South Africa*
61. Eliasson, R. (1981). Analysis of semen. In Burger, H. and De Kretser, D. (eds.) *The Testis*, pp. 381–99. (New York: Raven Press)

62. David, G., Bisson, J. P., Czyglik, F., Juannet, P. and Gernigon, C. (1975). Anomalies morphologiques du spermatozoïde humain. (1) Propositions pour un système de classification. *J. Gynecol. Obstet. Biol. Reprod.*, **4**, Suppl. 1, 17–36
63. Jouannet, P., Ducot, B., Feneux, D. and Spira, A. (1988). Male factors and the likelihood of pregnancy in infertile couples. 1. Study of sperm characteristics. *Int. J. Androl.*, **11**, 379–94
64. MacLeod, J. (1970). The significance of deviations in human sperm morphology. In Rosemberg, E. and Paulsen, C. A. (eds.) *The Human Testis*, pp. 481–94. (New York, London: Plenum Press)
65. Menkveld, R. and Kruger, T. F. (1990). Basic semen analysis. In Acosta, A. A., Swanson, R. J., Ackerman, S. B., Kruger, T. F., van Zyl, J. A. and Menkveld, R. (eds.) *Human Spermatozoa in Assisted Reproduction*, pp. 68–84. (Baltimore: Williams and Wilkins)
66. Mortimer, D., Mortimer, S. T., Shu, M. A. and Swart, R. (1990). A simplified approach to sperm–cervical mucus interaction testing using a hyaluronate migration test. *Hum. Reprod.*, **5**, 835–41
67. Hofmann, N., Freundl, G. and Florack, M. (1985). Die Formstörungen der Spermatozoen im Sperma und Zervikalschleim als spiegel testikulärer Erkrankungen. *Gynäkologe*, **18**, 189–92
68. Van Zyl, J. A., Menkveld, R., Kotze, T. J. vW. and van Niekerk, W. A. (1976). The importance of spermiograms that meet the requirements of international standards and the most important factors that influence semen parameters. *Proceedings of the 17th Congress of the International Urological Society*, Vol. 2, pp. 263–71. (Paris: Diffusion Dion Editeurs)
69. Kruger, T. F., Menkveld, R., Stander, F. S. H., Lombard, C. J., van der Merwe, J. P., van Zyl, J. A. and Smith, K. (1986). Sperm morphologic features as a prognostic factor in *in vitro* fertilization. *Fertil. Steril.*, **46**, 1118–23
70. Mortimer, D., Leslie, E. E., Kelley, R. W. and Templeton, A. A. (1982). Morphological selection of human spermatozoa *in vivo* and *in vitro*. *J. Reprod. Fertil.*, **64**, 391–9
71. Fredricsson, B. and Björk, R. (1977). Morphology of postcoital spermatozoa in the cervical secretion and its clinical significance. *Fertil. Steril.*, **28**, 841–5
72. Menkveld, R., Franken, D. R., Kruger, T. F. and Oehninger, S. (1991). Sperm selection capacity of the human zona pellucida. *Mol. Reprod. Dev.*, **30**, 346–52
73. Liu, D. Y. and Baker, H. W. G. (1992). Morphology of spermatozoa bound to the zona pellucida of human oocytes that failed to fertilize *in vitro*. *J. Reprod. Fertil.*, **94**, 71–84
74. Kruger, T. F., Acosta, A. A., Simmons, K. F., Swanson, R. J., Matta, J. F. and Oehninger, S. (1988). Predictive value of abnormal sperm morphology in *in vitro* fertilization. *Fertil. Steril.*, **49**, 112–17
75. Menkveld, R. (1991). In Menkveld, R., Oettlé, E. E., Kruger, T. F., Swanson, R. J. and Oehninger, S. (eds.). *Atlas of Human Sperm Morphology*. (Baltimore: Williams and Wilkins)
76. Menkveld, R., Rhemrev, J. P. T., Franken, D. R., Vermeiden, J. P. W. and Kruger, T. F. (1995). Acrosomal morphology as a novel criterion for male fertility diagnosis: relation with acrosin activity, morphology (strict criteria) and fertilization *in vitro*. *Fertil. Steril.* (in press)
77. Liu, D. Y. and Baker, H. W. G. (1988). The proportion of human sperm with poor morphology but normal intact acrosomes detected with pisum sativum agglutinin correlates with fertilization *in vitro*. *Fertil. Steril.*, **50**, 288–93
78. Jinno, M., Kobayashi, T., Sugimura, K., Nozawa, S., Katayama, E. and Lida, E. (1990). IVF and sperm morphology. *Mol. Androl.*, **2**, 161–8
79. Oehninger, S., Acosta, A. A., Kruger, T. F., Veeck, L. L., Flood, J. and Jones, H. W. (1988). Failure of fertilization in *in vitro* fertilization: The 'occult' male factor. *J.* In Vitro *Fertil. Embryo Transf.*, **5**, 181–7
80. Enginsu, M. E., Dumoulin, C. J. M., Pieters, M. H. E. C., Bras, M., Evers, J. L. H. and Geraedts, J. P. M. (1991). Evaluation of human sperm morphology using strict criteria after Diff-Quik staining: correlation of morphology with fertilization *in vitro*. *Hum. Reprod.*, **6**, 854–8
81. Kobayashi, T., Jinno, M., Sugimura, K. and Nozawa, S. (1991). Sperm morphological assessment based on strict criteria and *in-vitro* fertilization outcome. *Hum. Reprod.*, **6**, 983–6
82. Morgentaler, A., Harris, D. H., Fung, M. Y. and Powers, R. D. (1993). Sperm morphology as a predictor of IVF results: A comparison of World Health Organization and Tygerberg Methodologies. *Endocr. Fertil. Forum.*, **16**, 2–3
83. Holstein, A. F. and Roosen-Runge, E. C. (1981). *Atlas of Human Spermatogenesis*, p. 204. (Berlin: Grosse Verlag)
84. MacLeod, J. (1965). Seminal cytology in the presence of varicocele. *Fertil. Steril.*, **16**, 735–57
85. Ayodeji, O. and Baker, H. W. G. (1986). Is there a specific abnormality of sperm morphology in men with varicoceles? *Fertil. Steril.*, **45**, 839–42
86. Barnett, V. D. (1969). Simultaneous pairwise linear relationships. *Biometrics*, **25**, 129–42

Evaluation of sperm morphology by computer analysis

9

T. F. Kruger and T. C. du Toit

INTRODUCTION

Historically, sperm morphology assessment has been plagued by subjectivity and by lack of agreement among investigators[1]. However, its reliability and reproducibility have been demonstrated in studies involving experienced scorers who have used standardized criteria[2,3]. Several attempts have been made to use morphometry to quantify sperm morphology[4–9]. It was stated by Jagoe *et al.*[8] that there is potential in computed image processing to be used in routine semen analysis as well as in the study of male infertility. On the other hand, Schrader *et al.*[10] feel that each morphometric parameter may provide important information about different aspects of spermatogenesis. This, however, must be evaluated in clinical practice (assisted reproduction). The previously mentioned research in this field[2] and the work of others[11–14] indicating the value of morphology in predicting results of assisted reproduction lead to a renewed interest in this field of diagnostic andrology and to the development of computerized equipment to be used in clinical practice.

HOW COMPUTER MORPHOLOGY ANALYZERS WORK

Automated sperm morphology analysis (ASMA)[15] instruments work much like current versions of computer-aided sperm analysis instruments for motion, except that no movement information is required. The system consists of a microscope, a video camera, a computer frame grabber and morphology software. The video camera delivers the images to the computer's frame grabber which stores it for analysis[15]. The image is evaluated by the morphology software to determine whether sperm are present. Sperm recognition is based on software specifications for size, shape, color intensity and other characteristics. Once sperm have been recognized and segregated from debris and other objects, metric measurements are performed on the head, midpiece, acrosome and other cytological features. These measurements are the basis for sperm morphological classification. The accuracy and precision of ASMA instruments depend on: (1) the microscope optics, magnification and focusing capabilities; (2) video camera quality; (3) array size of the frame grabber; (4) image processing techniques; (5) definitions of metric measurements[15]; and (6) staining methods used[16].

TECHNICAL DETAIL ON TWO DIFFERENT MORPHOLOGY ANALYZERS

The CellForm–Human (CFH) instrument[17]

The CellForm–Human (CFH) instrument consists of a 386 or 486 IBM-compatible personal computer, an Olympus BH-T or -S microscope equipped with an MTV-3 camera adapter, a 6.7× photo ocular lens, and 40× and 60× dry, brightfield objectives (Olympus Corporation, New York, NY, USA); an automatic microscope stage and autofocus (Robins Scientific, Sunnyvale, CA, USA); a Cohu 4800- or 6400-series video camera (Cohu Electronics, San Diego, CA, USA); and CFH software. CFH runs under the MSDOS operating system in the Windows program environment (Microsoft Corporation, Bellview, WA, USA). The technician selects the microscope objective, loads a stained slide onto the automatic stage, provides information about the specimen to the CFH program, adjusts the microscope's brightness following CFH directions, defines the auto-focus area and initiates the analysis. The instrument automatically locates fields of sperm, recognizes sperm heads separating them from debris and other objects, detects the edge boundary of sperm heads, and performs morphometric measurements on each head. No commercially available, automated morphometry instrument at present analyzes the midpiece or flagellum[17]. Measurements made on the sperm head include: length, width, area, perimeter and width/length. Many other measurements are possible, but this set is sufficient to differentiate normal from abnormal sperm 95% of the time[17].

CFH analysis may be done in an automatic or a manual mode. A typical automatic analysis of 100 sperm takes 3–4 min. In the manual mode, the instrument pauses on each microscopic field to allow the technician to accept or reject individual sperm recognized by the instrument and to make notes or manual measurements on each sperm, if desired. In either mode, images of all sperm are retained by the instrument and can be displayed on the video monitor or printed for inclusion in the patient's chart. Individual sperm heads are classified as normal or abnormal by the instrument using the WHO criteria. Summary statistics and histograms are reported for normal and abnormal sperm on the video monitor and in a printed report. Data files containing individual sperm measurements and the instruments' classification of individual sperm are accessible by the user for further statistical analysis.

Sperm morphology analyzer (IVOS)[16] (Hamilton–Thorne Research®)

The IVOS cell analyzer combines an internal optical system with an internal computer and image-digitizing and analyzing systems. A computer-controlled stage moves the specimen slide between fields. The system may be used for movement analysis of sperm as well as static cell morphology determination. In the sperm morphology application, the optical system uses a narrow-band 662 nm wavelength illumination in conjunction with a 100× oil-immersion objective. Images are produced on a charge-coupled detector and transferred to the digitizer. Clear, high-contrast images of Papanicolaou and Diff-Quik stained cells are produced.

Operation of IVOS

On inserting a slide into the microscope stage, the computer verifies that the illumination is correct and allows the user to electronically manoeuver the slide to select an image containing sperm cells and to adjust the focus. The computer then captures the image, processes it and allows the user to select the next image. Processing can be either in interactive mode or in batch mode.

In interactive mode, an image is captured and processed immediately. The user can select to display the processing of every cell on the screen. The outline of the cell is superimposed with a color line on the microscope image and the classification result is shown in a color-coded table, also superimposed on the image.

Every object located in the image is either accepted as a valid sperm cell for further evaluation, or rejected if it is not in focus, or if it is considered as clutter. A cell is analyzed and classified into one of three categories: normal, subnormal or abnormal[14] with a breakdown of the classification: size: normal, small or large; shape: normal, slightly amorphous, thin, tapered, elongated, round, midpiece or severely amorphous[18]. If the acrosome is smaller than 40% of the sperm head, the cell is abnormal[14,16,18] (Figure 1).

In addition, numerical values are given for the focal quality of the cell, a shape acceptance factor and the area of the cell in pixels. For a cell to be classified as normal, all three parameters of size, shape and acrosome must pass as normal. If both the size and acrosome are normal but the shape is slightly amorphous, then the cell is classified into the subnormal category. In any other case, the cell is classified as abnormal.

In batch mode, the captured images are first stored to disk and processed later to minimize user operation time.

At any stage, the resulting statistics per slide can be viewed by the user, such as the percentage of normal cells.

Hardware

The FERTECH SMA software code is implemented in the IVOS instrument. The IVOS (Hamilton–Thorne Research) is a PC-based imaging computer

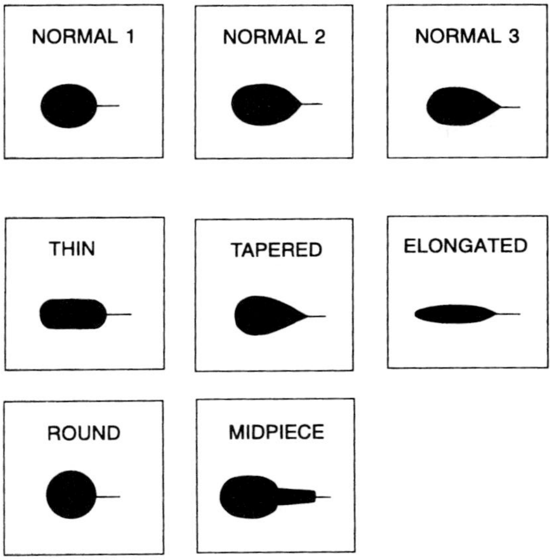

Figure 1 Examples of some normal and abnormal forms. Reproduced from Kruger *et al.* (1995)[16] with permission of the American Society for Reproductive Medicine

consisting of the processing unit, a high-quality Sony Super-VGA color monitor, standard PC keyboard and mouse.

The processing unit contains a 50 MHz 486DX motherboard with 8MB RAM, a DATA Translation DT3851 frame grabber with Super-VGA output, an optical unit, a 80 MB hard disk and a 3.5″ floppy drive. The optical unit consists of a Nikon based microscope developed by HTR with an effective magnification of 1000×, a red illumination lamp, a Sony XC-75 CCD video camera and an electronically controlled mechanical stage to hold a slide. Three push buttons are available to maneuver the stage: the Load button ejects the stage to enable the user to insert a slide into the stage, and then retracts the stage to position the slide under the built-in microscope; the Jog In and Jog Out buttons move the slide under the microscope to allow panning. A Focus knob enables the user to adjust the focusing.

An image is digitized into 256 gray levels and a spatial resolution of 640 columns and 480 rows with aspect ratio of 1.0. The single Super-VGA monitor is used to screen both the PC functions and the real-time video images.

Software

The image processing SMA software is written in Microsoft C++ using the version 7 compiler. The feature extraction and classification are described in more detail below.

Detection

First the intensity range of the input image is normalized. If the lighting is unacceptably low, the image is rejected. Object detection is done by adaptive thresholding the spatial subsampled input image. Template matching is performed on the resulting binary low-resolution image to isolate objects.

Segmentation

Once an object is located, high pass filtering on the original resolution subimage reveals the amount of high-frequency information in the subimage, indicating the focal quality. If this is too low, the object is not properly in focus. In addition, if the size of the object is too large to be a cell, it is regarded as clutter. Objects not in focus or cluttered are completely ignored and not taken into statistical consideration.

To separate the cell from its background a Bayesian-based segmentation technique is implemented operating on both spatial and statistical probabilities. The spatial probability distribution function (pdf) is obtained by fitting a smooth 'bubble' surface over the cell region, with maximum amplitude at the center and decreasing to zero away from the center. The statistical pdf is obtained by dividing the subimage into three regions (entirely cell, entirely background, and unknown) and generating histograms for two of the regions (entirely cell and entirely background). The classical Bayesian classifier separates the two classes, cell and background. A median filter removes spot noise.

A template-based adaptive filter is used to determine the location of the junction of the cell's tail to its head. The head is thus separated from the tail and the orientation of the cell can be normalized.

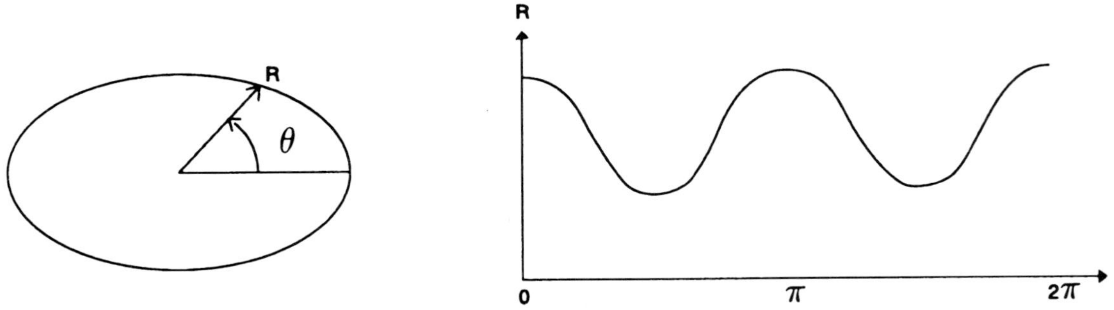

Figure 2 Normal shape signature (to identify normal cells). Reproduced from Kruger *et al.* (1995)[16] with permission of the American Society for Reproductive Medicine

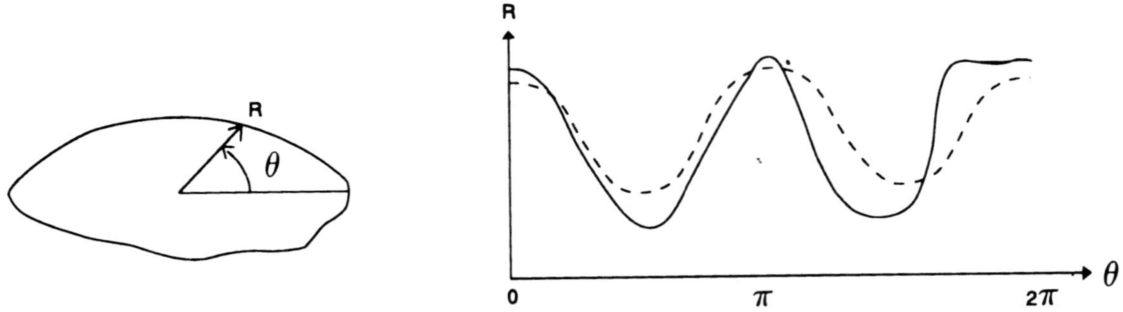

Figure 3 Abnormal shape signature (to distinguish between normal and abnormal cells). Reproduced from Kruger *et al.* (1995)[16] with permission of the American Society for Reproductive Medicine

Classification

The size of the cell head is calculated. If it is too small or too large the cell is considered as abnormal[14,18]. The acrosome is evaluated by measuring the shift of the true gray level centroid of the cell head from its binary centroid. In contrast to the binary centroid, which is at the geometrical center of the head, the true centroid is influenced by the size of the acrosome. Thus, if the acrosome is too small or absent, the true centroid tends to coincide with the geometrical centroid, indicating an abnormal acrosome.

The shape is extracted with a polar transformation using the cell head's centroid as the distance origin and the tail junction as the angular origin. As the cell size has already been extracted and classified at this stage, the polar transformation is normalized with respect to its integral to reveal the 'shape signature' (Figure 2)[16]. The principle behind the shape classification is the isolation of the normal shape[14,18].

For this reason the shape is classified by comparing the cell's signature with the normal signature using a least mean squared-based classifier. Figure 3 shows the principle, with the area between the actual and the normal curve indicating the fit error.

If the error is acceptably small then the shape is considered as normal, otherwise not. If the signature only slightly deviates from the normal form (and the size and acrosome are correct), then the cell is classified into the subnormal (intermediate) class.

The evident advantage of the signature method over the traditional approach to approximate the cell head with an ellipse is that the signature will show out shape errors other than purely the ratio of the major axis to the minor axis. If a cell head has the correct aspect ratio but is distorted, skewed or has a pertubated outline, then the signature method will still throw it out into the abnormal class.

As the above method is very selective of the normal shape, and there are about three variations on the normal or ideal shape, each of three normal signatures is fitted to the cell's signature and the best fit is classified. Similarly, an abnormal shape is subclassified into several other categories being thin, tapered, elongated, round and midpiece (Figure 1). If an abnormal shape does not fall into any of these subclasses, then it is categorized as severely amorphous[14,18].

Processing time

In interactive mode the SMA (program V1.04) captures and processes a single image with one cell in 5.6 s, an image with three cells in 8.9 s and an image with nine cells in 19.2 s. In batch mode, the system captures and stores a single image in 1.7 s.

NEW DEVELOPMENTS IN THE FIELD OF SPERM MORPHOLOGY

In recent studies, sperm morphology was evaluated using computerized sperm analyzers. Four recent studies looked at the value of the computerized system[17,19–21]. Wang *et al.*[20] reported large pairwise differences between a visual classification method and the Cell Soft Morphologizer (CSM). The coefficient of variation (CV) was comparable for the visual and automated methods for normal sperm (~6%), but was not comparable for abnormal sperm. The CVs of morphometric variables (e.g. length, width, etc.) were small, indicating relatively high precision for the analysis. Because 60 min were required to analyze 100 sperm and the cost of the technology was high, Wang concluded that no benefit could be found in the system she had tested above the manual method. Davis *et al.*[17] found good agreement (91%) between a visual type classification method and the Motion Analysis CellForm instrument. The CV for repeated metric measures of the same sperm was 1%. The CV of metric measures from normal sperm ranged from 7.4% to 12.8%, depending on the variable. Metric measures of normal sperm from normal samples were not different from normal sperm from highly abnormal samples. Analysis of 100 sperm took approximately 4 min. Davis[17], however, found the evaluation of the Motion Analysis CellForm system valuable. Both the studies by Wang[20] and Davis[17] looked at comparative analysis between manual and computerized systems on a cell by cell basis.

In a recent study by our own group, we looked at the correlation between sperm morphology (normal forms by strict criteria) comparing the slide by slide evaluation both manually and using the computerized system (IVOS)[21]. A good correlation was observed between the two methods. The computer evaluation of normal and abnormal forms was also compared with the manual evaluation in a clinical study using fertilization as an endpoint. The computerized system identified the percentage normal forms <14% very well and showed a significant difference in fertilization rate at the threshold of <14% normal forms and >14% (Figures 4, 5). This difference was even more pronounced when 10% normal forms was used as a threshold (Figures 4, 5). It was concluded that this new development holds promise for clinical practice.

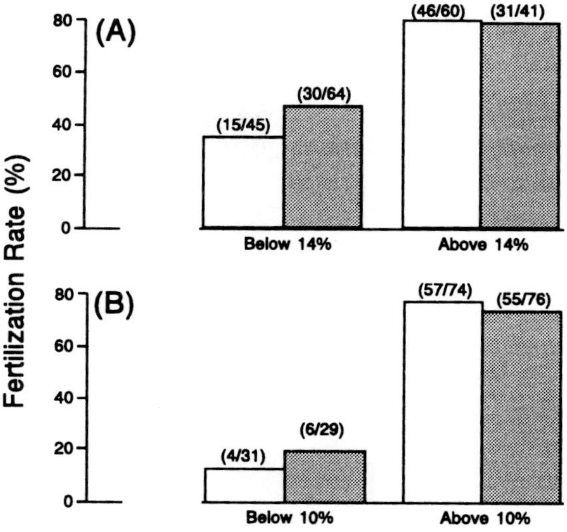

Figure 4 Tygerberg study. (A) Comparison of the ability of the manually recorded method and FERTECH to predict IVF results. A threshold of 14% normal sperm forms was used to divide the two groups of patients. Number of oocytes fertilized/inseminated are provided in parenthesis. (B) Comparison of the ability of the manually recorded method and FERTECH to predict IVF results. A threshold of 10% normal sperm forms was used to divide the two groups of patients. □, manual; ■, FERTECH. Reproduced from Kruger *et al.* (1993)[21] with permission of the American Society for Reproductive Medicine

In a recent study[16] we evaluated the IVOS system against the human reading in a slide by slide evaluation. Thirty slides were compared in each group. The Kappa statistical evaluation was used and man versus man was in the same category as man versus computer (IVOS) looking at percentage normal morphology per slide (Kappa 0.58 and

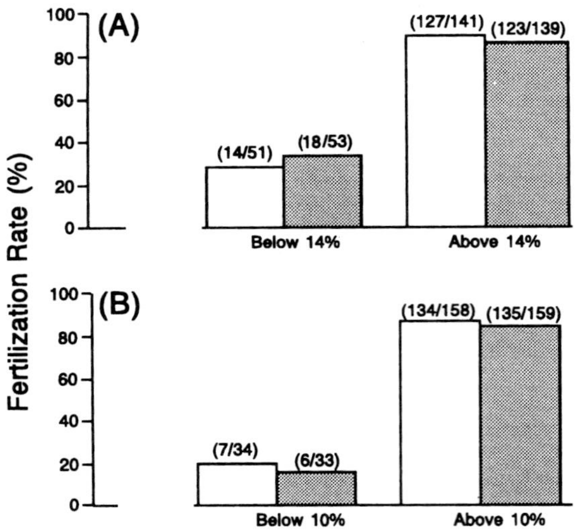

Figure 5 Norfolk study. (A) Comparison of the ability of the manually recorded method and FERTECH to predict IVF results. A threshold of 14% normal sperm forms was used to divide the two groups of patients. (B) Comparison of the ability of the manually recorded method and FERTECH to predict IVF results. A threshold of 10% normal sperm forms was used to divide the two groups of patients. □, manual; ■, FERTECH. Reproduced from Kruger *et al.* (1993)[21] with permission of the American Society for Reproductive Medicine

0.73, respectively; both were in the good agreement group).

When applying the Spearman correlation coefficient in the same experiments it was 0.88 in the man versus man experiment, and 0.85 in the man versus IVOS. The repeatability per cell for the IVOS system was Kappa 0.83 (excellent category).

An accurate length–width ratio is one of the principles to identify normal cells and is used by the different systems available[17,20,21]. This approach, however, is not accurate enough because often a totally amorphous cell can have a normal length–width ratio. Literature has shown that the shape of normal cells is very important in clinical practice[14]. The evident advantage of the signature method used by the IVOS system is to approximate the cell head with an ellipse. The signature will show abnormally shaped cells other than purely the ratio of the major axis to the minor axis. If the cell head has the correct aspect ratio, but is distorted, skewed or has a perturbed outline, the cell will be classified as abnormal with this approach[2,21]. On the other hand, a small acrosome will also be taken into consideration and a cell be classified as abnormal even if the shape is normal[14,16]. This approach simulates the manual strict criteria very well[14,18].

Other factors that could affect accuracy are background on the morphology slide and staining methods[16]. It is of the utmost importance to standardize staining techniques for a given system, otherwise unreliable results will follow. Measurements of spermatozoa stained with different stains, e.g. Papanicolaou[18,22] and Quick Stain[14], differ and this must be taken into consideration when using a computer or manual evaluation. One advantage of the IVOS system is that two options are available taking into account the above-mentioned factors.

Recently we have also compared different staining methods on semen to prepare morphology slides for computer use. Washing of semen samples can reduce background problems and thus gives much more reliable results when using a computerized program to evaluate spermatozoa morphology.

CONCLUSION

The development of the computer has brought an exciting dimension to the basic semen analysis. It can be more objective and holds promise for clinical practice on a day to day basis in assisted reproduction laboratories as well as in andrology laboratories[7,8] and can standardize the evaluation of sperm morphology worldwide[16,22].

References

1. Freund, M. (1966). Standards of the rating of human sperm morphology. *Int. J. Fertil.*, **11**, 97–118
2. Menkveld, R., Stander, F. S. H., Kotze, T. J. vW., Kruger, T. F. and Van Zyl, J. A. (1990). The evaluation of morphological characteristics of human spermatozoa according to stricter criteria. *Hum. Reprod.*, **5**, 586–92
3. Bosmans, E., Janssen, M., Vandeput, H. and

Omberlet, W. (1991). Morphological characterization of human spermatozoa according to strict criteria: a laboratory evaluation. *Hum. Reprod.* (abstr. from the 7th meeting of ESHRE and the 7th World Congress on IVF and assisted procreation), 289–290.
4. Katz, D. F., Overstreet, J. W., Samuels, S. J., Niswander, P. W., Bloom, T. D. and Lewis, E. L. (1986). Morphometric analysis of spermatozoa in the assessment of human male fertility. *J. Androl.*, **7**, 203
5. Schmassmann, A., Mikuz, G., Bartsch, G. and Rohr, H. P. (1982). Spermiometrics: Objective and reproducible methods for evaluating sperm morphology. *Eur. Urol.*, **8**, 274
6. Schmassmann, A., Mikuz, G., Bartsch, G. and Rohr, H. P. (1979). Quantification of human sperm morphology and motility by means of semi-automated image analyses systems. *Microsc. Acta.*, **82**, 163
7. Jagoe, J. R., Washbrook, N. P. and Hudson, E. A. (1986). Morphometry of spermatozoa using semi-automatic image analysis. *J. Clin. Pathol.*, **39**, 1347–52
8. Jagoe, J. R., Washbrook, N. P., Pratsis, L. and Hudson, E. A. (1987). Sperm morphology by image analysis compared with subjective assessment. *Br. J. Urol.*, **60**, 457–62
9. Moruzzi, J. F., Wyrobek, A. J., Mayall, B. H. and Gledhill, B. L. (1988). Quantification and classification of human sperm morphology by computer-assisted image analysis. *Fertil. Steril.*, **50**, 142–52
10. Schrader, S. M., Turner, T. W. and Simon, S. D. (1990). Longitudinal study of semen quality of unexposed workers: sperm head morphometry. *J. Androl.*, **11**, 32–7
11. Enginsu, M. E., Dumoulin, J. C. M., Pieters, M. H. E. C., Evers, J. L. H. and Geraedts, J. P. M. (1993). Predictive value of morphologically normal sperm concentration in the medium for *in-vitro* fertilization. *Int. J. Androl.*, **16**, 113–20
12. Enginsu, M. E., Dumoulin, J. C. M., Pieters, M. H. E. C., Bras, J., Evers, J. L. H. and Geraedts, J. P. M. (1991). Evaluation of human sperm morphology using strict criteria after Diff-Quik staining: correlation of morphology with fertilization *in vitro*. *Hum. Reprod.*, **6**, 854–8
13. Enginsu, M. E., Pieters, M. H. E. C., Dumoulin, J. C. M., Evers, J. L. H. and Geraedts, J. P. M. (1992). Male factor as determinant of *in-vitro* fertilization. *Hum. Reprod.*, **7**, 1136–40
14. Kruger, T. F., Acosta, A. A., Simmons, K. F., Swanson, R. J., Matta, J. F. and Oehninger, S. (1988). Predictive value of abnormal sperm morphology in *in vitro* fertilization. *Fertil. Steril.*, **49**, 112–17
15. Davis, R. O. (1993). Automated sperm morphometry and morphology. In *Course XI Contemporary Methods of Sperm, Oocyte and Embryo Morphology Assessment*, pp. 61–7 (Montreal, Canada: 26th Annual Postgraduate Course of the AFS)
16. Kruger, T. F., Du Toit, T. C., Franken, D. R., Menkveld, R. and Lombard, C. J. (1995). Sperm morphology: assessing the agreement between the manual method (strict criteria) and the sperm morphology analyzer IVOS*. *Fertil. Steril.*, **63**, 134–41
17. Davis, R. O., Bain, D. E., Siemers, R. J., Thal, D. M., Andrew, J. B. and Gravance, C. G. (1992). Accuracy and precision of the CellForm-Human* automated sperm morphometry instrument. *Fertil. Steril.*, **58**, 763–9
18. Menkveld, R., Stander, F. S. H., Kotze, T. J. vW., Kruger, T. F. and Van Zyl, J. A. (1990). The evaluation of morphological characteristics of human spermatozoa according to stricter criteria. *Hum. Reprod.*, **5**, 586–92
19. Wang, C., Leung, A., Tsoi, W., Leung, J., Ng, V. and Lee, V. (1991). Computer-assisted assessment of human sperm morphology: comparison with visual assessment. *Fertil. Steril.*, **55**, 983–8
20. Wang, C., Leung, A., Tsoi, W-L., Leung, J., Ng, V. and Lee, K-F. (1991). Computer-assisted assessment of human sperm morphology: usefulness in predicting fertilizing capacity of human spermatozoa. *Fertil. Steril.*, **55**, 989–93
21. Kruger, T. F., Du Toit, T. C., Franken, D. R., Acosta, A. A., Oehninger, S. C., Menkveld, R. and Lombard, C. J. (1993). A new computerized method of reading sperm morphology (strict criteria) is as efficient as technician reading. *Fertil. Steril.*, **59**, 202–9
22. World Health Organization. (1992). *World Health Organization Manual for the Examination of Human Semen and Sperm–Cervical Mucus Interaction*, 3rd edn. (Cambridge: Cambridge University Press)

Efficiency and predictive value of different methods of morphological evaluation

10

M. E. Enginsu and J. L. H. Evers

INTRODUCTION

The terms *fertility* and *infertility* suggest a binomial partition of patients into disease and health categories which in reality do not exist. Infertility, defined as the inability of a couple to establish a pregnancy, is rare. In the Netherlands, it occurs in about 3% of couples (primary infertility), whereas an estimated 6% do not succeed in obtaining the number of children desired (secondary infertility)[1]. This may be caused by absolute infertility (i.e. sterility) of the man (e.g. due to azoospermia), or of the woman (e.g. premature ovarian failure). However, most of the couples attending infertility clinics are suffering from impaired fertility. For these cases of decreased fecundity the term subfertility is to be preferred.

Traditionally, the woman has been the focal point of the fertility investigation, hence the relegation of this field of clinical medicine to the specialty of gynecology. There exists growing concern about (declining?) fertility, and potential male causes of decreased fertility have been receiving much attention recently. Andrology is emerging as a subspecialty of its own. Evidence is accumulating that at least half of the couples seeking reproductive assistance are suffering from a male problem[2].

SPERM PROCESSING

In vitro fertilization (IVF) has opened a new era in the treatment of the infertile couple. Also, IVF has enabled the scientist to gain more insight in gamete interaction. Since the spermatozoa have to be separated from the seminal plasma before they can capacitate and undergo acrosome reaction (which are prerequisites for fertilization), sperm processing has become an integral part of the routine IVF laboratory procedure. After sperm processing, either the density alone or the density of the motile fraction of the spermatozoa of the final suspension is adjusted prior to insemination. This means that, at most, two of the major sperm parameters, density and motility, are adjusted. The role of the third, morphology, will be considered in more detail in this chapter.

MORPHOLOGY OF HUMAN SPERMATOZOA

When human spermatozoa in the semen come into contact with cervical mucus only a small fraction succeeds in penetration[3]. When the morphology of this portion was evaluated, both after *in vivo*[4] and *in vitro* penetration[5], it was found that the morphologically abnormal spermatozoa were less able to penetrate the mucus than their morphologically normal counterparts.

Morales and coworkers[6] have found that morphologically normal spermatozoa swim faster than abnormal spermatozoa. Normal spermatozoa also have higher rolling and flagellar beat frequencies and flagellar amplitude[6].

Sperm penetration assay (SPA) and hemizona assay (HZA) are two diagnostic tests used for the detection of abnormalities of male origin. The results of these tests have shown that normal morphology correlates highly with positive test results, suggesting that morphologically normal spermatozoa have a better chance of binding to the human zona pellucida and of forming a male pronucleus in a hamster oocyte[7,8].

These results support the notion that the motility of the spermatozoa is highly related to their morphology. Therefore, in assisted reproductive technologies (ART), morphology evaluation may become the cornerstone of semen analysis.

Morphology evaluation techniques

A reliable morphology evaluation technique begins with well prepared slides and a suitable staining technique[9]. Papanicolaou staining is widely used for this purpose. However, the time spent for this procedure (approximately 1 h) causes a shrinkage of the sperm head due to its exposure to the fixative and staining solutions. When living sperm heads of native samples were compared with Papanicolaou stained ones, the measurements of the stained sperm heads were within the 95% confidence intervals of the native sperm[10]. In the Diff-Quik staining technique, spermatozoa are exposed to the fixative and to two staining solutions for not more than 30 s. Since the shrinkage problem is eliminated with this technique, the morphology of the sperm head can be evaluated more reliably. Furthermore, the latter technique is time saving and the background of the slides gives better contrast.

The percentage of morphologically normal spermatozoa, evaluated with conventional WHO criteria, has been reported to correlate positively with fertilization results[11–13]. However, a positive correlation between IVF results and the percentage of normal morphology does not offer the clinician a decisive cut-off point to include (or to exclude) the patients from an IVF program.

After the introduction of new, more strict, evaluation criteria by Kruger and co-workers[14], based on the morphology of the spermatozoa that have eventually penetrated cervical mucus and that can bind to the zona pellucida, morphology evaluation has been the focal point of much debate. We have compared the predictive value of both the conventional WHO criteria and the new morphology evaluation using strict criteria (MEUSC) simultaneously on IVF patients with normal sperm density and motility parameters[15]. The main differences between the MEUSC and the WHO criteria are that in MEUSC all borderline forms are considered abnormal and the sperm head should have a smooth oval shape.

Since individual parameters may not offer the ultimate answer for diagnosing male factor subfertility, it has been suggested to combine them and study the predictive value of these combined semen parameters[16,17]. In addition to the conventional WHO parameters (sperm density and motility characteristics), we have evaluated progressive motile sperm density (PMSD; by multiplying the percentage of progressive motile spermatozoa with sperm density), post swim-up MEUSC scores (MEUSCi) and the number of morphologically normal spermatozoa in the insemination medium (IMNS; by multiplying the sperm density of the swim-up fraction, MEUSCi and the volume used for insemination)[18,19]. This chapter will give an overview of our results.

Although the highest correlations between the fertilization outcome and the semen parameters were in favor of morphology scores, a positive correlation between the fertilization outcome and all other semen parameters was also detected (Table 1).

Therefore, to evaluate the predictive value of each parameter, in addition to the correlation coefficiencies, we have used the receiver operating characteristics (ROC) curves as detailed by Metz[20]. Cohen's kappa statistics were calculated to decide on the most appropriate clinical cutoff point[21].

Of the conventional semen parameters evaluated in practice, the best cutoff points to predict fertilization outcome according to their kappa values were found to be: sperm density 20 million/mL, motility 30%, progressive motility 30%, progressive motile sperm density 3 million/mL, morphology WHO criteria 14% normal forms, morphology with strict criteria 5% normal forms, morphology with strict criteria in the insemination medium 8% normal forms, number of sperm in the insemination medium 5800/mL. These cutoff points indicate fertilization failure is to be expected if semen analysis results fall below these values for *in vitro* conditions (Table 1).

Morphology evaluation using strict criteria enclosed a larger area (below and to the right of the curve) than any of the other parameters (Figure 1).

Predictive values of test results

In clinical practice, the predictive value of a test result is more important than its distribution among diseased (infertile) and non-diseased (fertile) couples[22]. Likelihood ratios, in contrast to the more

Table 1 Comparison of different parameters of semen samples on the basis of correlation with fertilization *in vitro* (Cohen's Kappa, Pearson correlation coefficient)

Parameter	*Cut-off*	*Kappa*	*r*	*P*
Morphology evaluation using strict criteria (MEUSC)	5	0.55	0.57	0.001
Morphology (WHO)	14	0.31	0.38	0.001
Motility (WHO)	30	0.22	0.25	0.001
Progressive motility (WHO)	30	0.18	0.19	0.010
Sperm density (WHO)	20	0.27	0.23	0.001
Progressive motile sperm density (PMSD)	3	0.37	0.33	0.001
MEUSC in insemination medium (MEUSCi)	8	0.47	0.62	0.001
Inseminated morphologically normal spermatozoa (IMNS)	5800	0.25	0.34	0.001

r and *P* = Pearson's correlation coefficient and probability; Kappa = Cohen's kappa (<0.4 = poor agreement; 0.4–0.75 = good agreement)

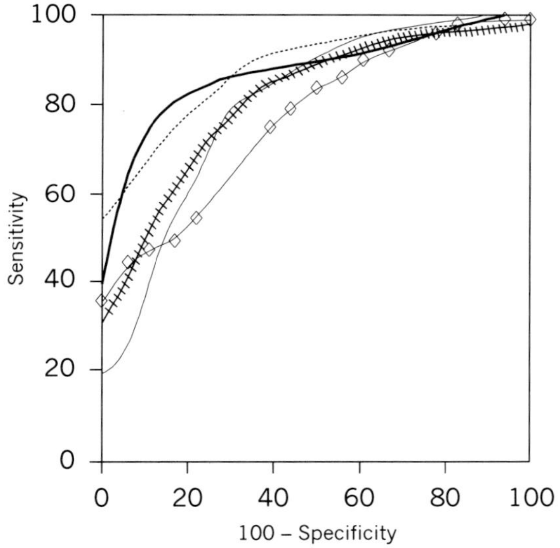

Figure 1 Receiver operating characteristic (ROC) curves of semen parameters; only the five best parameters were included in the figure. ___, MEUSC; ___, PMSD; ++++, morphology (WHO); - - -, MEUSCi; ◇, IMNS

conventionally used positive and negative predictive values, are not affected by the prevalence of disease in the population studied. Therefore, they can be used to compare the outcome of the same test in different populations and to compare different tests of the same disease entity in the same population. The positive likelihood ratio (LR+) indicates the likelihood of a positive test (abnormal) result in a patient with the disease over the likelihood of a positive test result in a patient without the disease. The negative likelihood ratio (LR–) indicates the likelihood of a negative (normal) test result in a patient with the disease over the likelihood of a negative test result in a patient without the disease. Calculation of the LR yields a score that allows categorization of test results. Comparison of different methods can also be detected by calculating the confidence intervals (CI) of the likelihood ratios[23]. Since subfertility is defined as the *absence of conception*, one may use the likelihood ratios to estimate the properties of a given test to predict conception (or for that matter fertilization in case of IVF), or to predict disease (i.e. absence of conception; fertilization failure at IVF) which constitutes the reciprocal value of the LRs. For the sake of clarity an overview of the results of both estimations for all parameters is offered in Table 2.

The likelihood of finding an abnormal MEUSC result (<5% normal forms) in a patient whose oocytes were subsequently not fertilized was 8.6 times the likelihood of an abnormal test in a patient without fertilization failure (95% CI 6.8–11.1). For the best WHO parameter, the percentage of progressive motility, this likelihood ratio was only 5.2 (95% CI 3.9–6.6), which is significantly worse.

The likelihood ratios for PMSD and for IMNS were 4.4 (95% CI 3.6–5.6) and 3.9 (95% CI 2.7–5.3), respectively, both of which indicate a significantly worse performance than MEUSC. The only parameter which did not show a significant difference was MEUSCi with a likelihood ratio of 7.4 (95% CI 5.5–10.7), which was not significantly different from PMSD but was significantly better than IMNS (Figure 2).

The likelihood of finding normal MEUSC results (⩾5% normal forms) in a patient whose oocytes were fertilized was four times that in a

Table 2 The likelihood ratios of semen parameters with the 95% confidence intervals

Test	*Diagnosing infertility*				*Diagnosing fertility*			
	LR+	*95% CI*	*LR–*	*95% CI*	*LR+*	*95%CI*	*LR–*	*95% CI*
Morphology evaluation using strict criteria (MEUSC)	8.6	6.8–11.1	0.25	0.00–0.44	4.0	2.4–11.7	0.12	0.09–0.15
Morphology (WHO)	4.6	3.2–6.7	0.60	0.20–0.87	1.7	0.9–5.0	0.22	0.16–0.32
Motility (WHO)	4.6	3.7–5.8	0.81	0.53–1.14	1.2	0.9–1.8	0.22	0.18–0.28
Progressive motility (WHO)	5.2	3.9–6.6	0.78	0.53–1.14	1.3	0.9–2.2	0.19	0.16–0.24
Sperm density (WHO)	3.3	2.5–4.1	0.83	0.53–1.14	1.2	0.8–2.2	0.30	0.24–0.39
Progressive motile sperm density (PMSD)	4.4	3.6–5.6	0.71	0.44–1.02	1.4	0.9–2.2	0.23	0.18–0.29
MEUSC in insemination medium (MEUSCi)	7.4	5.5–10.7	0.36	0.09–0.68	2.8	1.4–10.7	0.13	0.10–0.17
Inseminated morphologically normal spermatozoa (IMNS)	3.9	2.7–5.3	0.68	0.28–1.12	1.5	0.9–3.5	0.26	0.20–0.36

Table 3 Combined results of morphology evaluation using strict criteria (MEUSC) and progressive motile sperm density (PMSD) in prediction of fertilization *in vitro*

Category	*n*	*Fertilization**	*Pregnancy**
I MEUSC <5% and PMSD <3×10⁶/mL	11	17%[a]	0%[d]
II MEUSC <5% or PMSD <3×10⁶/mL	47	27%[b]	7%[e]
III MEUSC >5% and PMSD >3×10⁶/mL	235	72%[c]	25%[f]

*Fertilization rates were calculated per oocyte and pregnancy rates were calculated per embryo transfer. [a–f]indicate significant differences between $P<0.03$ and $P<0.00001$

patient with a fertilization failure (95% CI 2.3–11.7). For the best WHO parameter, the percentage of normal morphology, this likelihood was 1.7 (95% CI 0.9–5.0). Although the difference between these figures, for MEUSC and WHO morphology, respectively, is not significant, MEUSC was significantly better than all other WHO parameters. The likelihood ratio for PMSD was 1.4 (95% CI 0.9–2.2), significantly worse than MEUSC, whereas the differences between MEUSC, IMNS and MEUSCi were not significant (Figure 3).

Since PMSD was the second best parameter of the native semen analysis, the patients were categorized according to their MEUSC and PMSD results (Table 3). When both parameters were below their respective cutoff points, the fertilization rate was significantly reduced (17%) and no pregnancies were achieved ($P<0.00001$). When only one of these parameters was above the cutoff point, the fertilization rate was increased to 27% and the pregnancy rate was 7%. The best fertilization and pregnancy rates were obtained if both parameters were above their respective cutoff points, with 73% fertilization and 25% pregnancy rates.

Measuring outcomes in assisted reproductive technologies

Assisted reproductive technologies (ART) such as IVF are expensive for the health care system and demanding on the patient. Therefore, a need exists for a reliable parameter to estimate the outcome of applying these techniques in terms of pregnancies, conceptions or fertilizations obtained. The occurrence of fertilization is difficult to predict from sperm tests alone, since multiple, also female, factors are known to influence it. This is reflected in Table 2, regarding the likelihood of a normal test result in patients fertilizing their oocytes. Deficient sperm quality, however, may be the sole determinant of failure of fertilization at IVF. Therefore, the likelihood of an abnormal test in patients failing fertilization seems to be the most important factor to take into account when counseling a couple regarding the male determinant of their pregnancy chances with ART. Although the prediction of a fertilization failure by semen analysis result should evoke substantial concern regarding the question of whether or not to start IVF, the prediction of successful

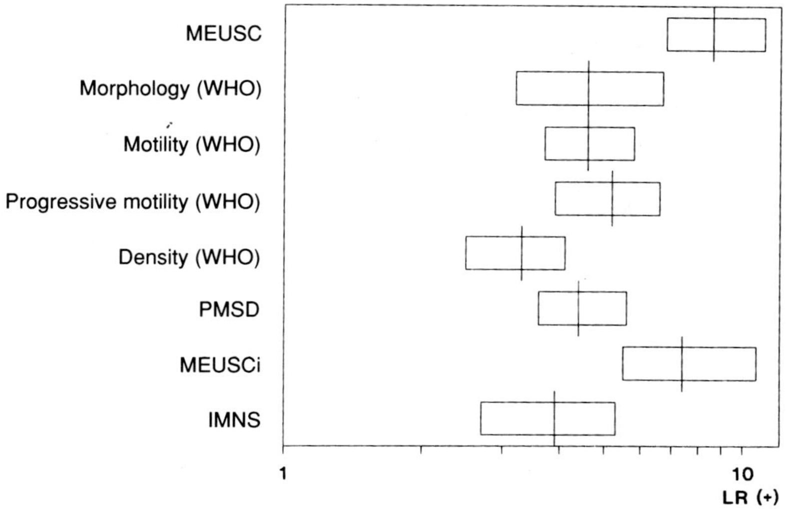

Figure 2 Positive likelihood ratios (LR+), within their 95% confidence intervals, for MEUSC and conventional WHO parameters. Positive likelihood ratios (LR+) for an abnormal test: the likelihood of having an abnormal test result, in a patient with fertilization failure (0% fertilization), divided by the likelihood of having an abnormal test result in a patient with fertilization

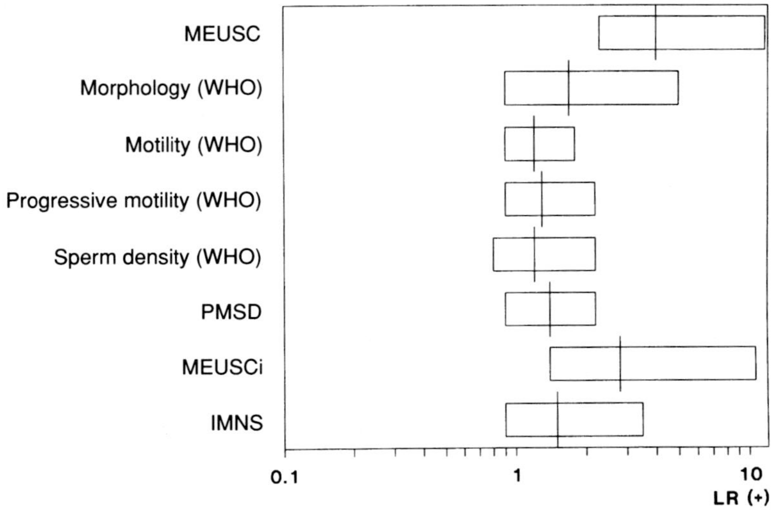

Figure 3 Positive likelihood ratios (LR+), within their 95% confidence intervals, for MEUSC and conventional WHO parameters. Positive likelihood ratios (LR+) for a normal test: the likelihood of having a normal test result in a patient with fertilization, divided by the likelihood of having a normal test result in a patient with fertilization failure

fertilization on the basis of semen analysis results should always be considered with reserve. MEUSC is superior to semen analysis according to WHO criteria in detecting couples with an inadequate male factor. Additional parameters, such as PMSD and MEUSCi, give a better insight into a couple's IVF potential than the individual conventional parameters, allowing the clinicians to tailor their treatment. However, for the evaluation of the morphology score in the insemination medium, one should add the swim-up (or the respective alternative routine sperm processing) procedure into the routine protocol. Although MEUSCi predicts both the fertile and the infertile patient better than the PMSD (Table 2), this is not significant. Evaluation of PMSD, on the other hand, is a part of the routine procedure which is done on the native semen sample. In a previous study from our group, it was shown that when both MEUSC scores in the native sample and in the insemination medium fall below their respective cutoff point, no pregnancies may be expected[19]. Since this information can also be obtained with the use of PMSD (Table 3) instead of MEUSCi, the latter does not offer additional clinical value.

Differences in cutoff points

Differences in cutoff points for strict criteria between our studies and others originate from differences in the interpretation of the IVF results. The suggested 5% cutoff points in our studies[15,18,19] is based on the occurrence of fertilization. The original articles describing strict criteria[24,25] have suggested that the cutoff points should be set at 14%, since there was a significant difference between the fertilization rates below (49.5% fertilization rate) and above (88.3% fertilization rate) 14% normal morphology. The drawback of this approach is that it only predicts optimal fertilization rates. As discussed above, identifying patients with an optimal chance of fertilization is of only secondary importance. The identification of patients that do not stand a fair chance at fertilization by ART is pivotal.

In search of a standard for morphology evaluation, the WHO has changed both the definition and the cutoff point for normal morphology in its most recent laboratory manual in 1992[10]. It is stated that morphology should be evaluated strictly. Normal sperm should have an oval shape and all borderline forms should be considered abnormal. This definition fits perfectly with the strict criteria. The cutoff point was also lowered from 50% to 30% morphologically normal spermatozoa. However, 30% normal morphology is still higher than the 14% normal forms (for WHO criteria) suggested in the present study, based on ROC curves. A possible explanation to this rather high cutoff point can be that the studies of WHO are aimed at *in vivo* conditions, whereas all our studies were performed in an IVF population.

Besides the descriptive basic semen analysis, additional diagnostic tests have been developed to detect disorders of sperm function. However, many of the additional tests are too time consuming, cumbersome and sometimes too expensive to include them into the routine male factor evaluation. At this point the World Health Organization plays a crucial role, since its manual for human semen examination is widely used as a reference guide in fertility centers. In their latest manual, besides the conventional parameters (density, motility and morphology), computer-assisted sperm analysis (CASA), hypo-osmotic swelling test (HOST), sperm penetration assay (SPA), hemizona assay (HZA) and acrosome reaction tests are recognized as additional tests that can be used routinely. Since the methodology and the diagnostic value of these additional tests are the subjects of other chapters of this book, we did not include our observations. However, we strongly believe that, prior to including any additional test into routine, the diagnostic value of the basic semen analysis should be estimated for one's own laboratory. Because of their financial disadvantages and technical difficulties, the application of these tests should be restricted to cases of persisting unexplained subfertility.

CONCLUSION

In conclusion, MEUSC, when falling below its cutoff point of 5% normal forms, predicts a subsequent fertilization failure at IVF. It is significantly better than the conventional WHO parameters. In view of the need for identifying poor prognosis patients, given the results of the series of experiments described in this chapter, and taking into account the laborious detail and financial burden of the additional tests, MEUSC in the native sample constitutes a suitable and reliable first-line screening tool for couples seeking IVF treatment.

References

1. Evers, J. L. H., te Velde E. R. (1993). Vruchtbaarheidsstoornissen. In Treffers, P. E. (ed.) *Obstetrie en Gynaecologie: De Voortplanting van de Mens*, p. 463. (Utrecht: Wetenschappelijke uitgeverij Bunbe)
2. World Health Organization. (1993). Rowe, P. J., Hargreave, T. B., Mellows, H. J. and Comhaire, F. H. (eds.) *WHO Manual for the Standardized Investigation and Diagnosis of the Infertile Couple*. (Cambridge, Cambridge University Press)
3. Settlage, D. S. F., Motoshima, M. and Tredway, D. R. (1973). Sperm transport from the external os to the Fallopian tubes in women: a time and quantitation study. *Fertil. Steril.*, **24**, 655
4. Hanson, F. W. and Overstreet, J. W. (1981). The interaction of human spermatozoa with cervical mucus *in vivo*. *Am. J. Obstet. Gynecol.*, **140**, 173
5. Fredricsson, B. and Bjork, G. (1977). Morphology of post-coital spermatozoa in the cervical secretion and its clinical significance. *Fertil. Steril.*, **28**, 8415
6. Moralles, P., Overstreet, J. W. and Katz, D. F. (1988). Changes in human sperm motion during capacitation *in vitro*. *J. Reprod. Fertil.*, **83**, 119–28
7. Kruger, T. F., Swanson, R. J., Hamilton, M., Simmons, K. F., Acosta, A. A., Matta, J. F., Oehninger, S. and Morshedi, M. (1988). Abnormal sperm morphology and other semen parameters related to the outcome of the hamster oocyte human sperm penetration assay. *Int. J. Androl.*, **11**, 107
8. Oehninger, S., Coddington, C. C., Scott, R., Franken, D. R., Burkman, L. J., Acosta, A. A. and Hodgen, G. D. (1989). Hemizona assay: assessment of sperm dysfunction and prediction of IVF outcome. *Fertil. Steril.*, **51**, 665
9. World Health Organization. (1987). *Laboratory Manual for the Examination of Human Semen and Sperm–Cervical Mucus Interactions* 2nd edn, pp. 9–11. (Cambridge: Cambridge University Press)
10. World Health Organization. (1992). *Laboratory Manual for the Examination of Human Semen and Sperm–Cervical Mucus Interactions*, 3rd edn, p. 14. (Cambridge: Cambridge University Press)
11. Rogers, B. J., Bentwood, B. J., Van Campen, H., Helmbrecht, G., Sodendahl, D. and Hale, R. W. (1983). Sperm morphology assessment as an indicator of human fertilizing capacity. *J. Androl.*, **4**, 119–25
12. Chan, S. Y. W., Wang, C., Chan, S. T. H., Ho, P. C., So, W. W. K., Chan, Y. F. and Ma, H. K. (1988). Predictive value of sperm morphology and movement characteristics in the outcome of *in vitro* fertilization of human oocytes. *J.* In Vitro *Fertil. Embryo Transf.*, **6**, 142–8
13. Liu, D. Y., Lopata, A., Johnston, W. I. H. and Baker, H. W. G. (1989). Human sperm–zona-pellucida binding, sperm characteristics and *in vitro* fertilization. *Hum. Reprod.*, **4**, 696–701
14. Kruger, T. F., Acosta, A. A., Simmons, K. F., Swanson, R. J., Matta, J. F., Veeck, L. L., Morshedi, M. and Brugo, S. (1987). New method of evaluating sperm morphology with predictive value for human *in vitro* fertilization. *Urology*, **30**, 248–51
15. Enginsu, M. E., Dumoulin, J. C. M., Pieters, M. H. E. C., Bras, M., Evers, J. L. H. and Geraedts, J. P. M. (1991). Evaluation of human sperm morphology using strict criteria after Diff-Quik staining: correlation of morphology with fertilization *in vitro*. *Hum. Reprod.*, **6**, 854–8
16. Francavilla, F., Romano, R., Santucci, R. and Poccia, G. (1990). Effect of sperm morphology and motile sperm count on outcome of intrauterine insemination in oligospermia and/or asthenozoospermia. *Fertil. Steril.*, **53**, 892–7
17. Glazener, C. M. A., Kelly, N. J., Weir, M. J. A., Davis, J. S. E., Cornes, J. S. and Hull, M. G. R. (1987). The diagnosis of male infertility – prospective time specific study of conception rates related to seminal analysis and postcoital sperm–mucus penetration and survival in otherwise unexplained infertility. *Hum. Reprod.*, **2**, 665–71
18. Enginsu, M. E., Dumoulin, J. C. M., Land, J. A., Evers, J. L. H. and Geraedts, J. P. M. (1992). Male factor as determinant of *in vitro* fertilization outcome. *Hum. Reprod.*, **7**, 1136–40
19. Enginsu, M. E., Dumoulin, J. C. M., Pieters, M. H. E. C., Evers, J. L. H. and Geraedts, J. P. M. (1993). Predictive value of morphologically normal sperm concentration in the medium for *in vitro* fertilization. *Int. J. Androl.*, **16**, 113–20
20. Metz, C. (1978). Basic principles of ROC analysis. *Semin. Nucl. Med.*, **8**, 283–98
21. Fleis, J. L. (1981). *Statistical Methods for Rates and Proportions*, p. 56. (Toronto: John Wiley)
22. Overstreet, J. W. and Katz, D. F. (1981). Sperm transport and capacitation. In Sciarra, J. J. (ed.) *Gynecology and Obstetrics*, Vol. 5, ch. 45, pp. 1–10. (New York: Harper & Row)
23. Sacket, D. L., Haynes, R. B. and Tugwell, P. (1985). *Clinical Epidemiology: A Basic Science for Clinical Medicine*, pp. 108–124. (Boston: Little, Brown and Company)
24. Acosta, A. A., Oehninger, S., Morshedi, M., Swanson, R. J., Scott, R. and Irianni, F. (1988). Assisted reproduction in the diagnosis and treatment of the male factor. *Obstet. Gynecol. Surv.*, **44**, 1–18
25. Kruger, T. F., Acosta, A. A., Simmons, K. F., Swanson, J. R., Matta, J. F. and Oehninger, S. (1988). Predictive value of abnormal sperm morphology in *in vitro* fertilization *Fertil. Steril.*, **49**, 112–17

Male genital tract infections 11

F. H. Comhaire

INTRODUCTION

Infection and/or inflammation of the male accessory sex glands (MAGI) is recorded in variable frequency among subfertile men with impaired semen quality, and in patients with sexual or ejaculatory dysfunction[1]. The large differences in occurrence are related to regional differences in frequency of sexually transmitted diseases, sexual habits and general health condition of the population[2]. Other factors which influence the occurrence of MAGI are smoking and the presence of varicocele, both of which seem to promote infection.

EPIDEMIOLOGICAL DATA

In a large study by the World Health Organization[3], male accessory gland infection was found in 6.9% of men with impaired semen quality. However, MAGI is rarely the only demonstrable cause of couple infertility since it is commonly associated with other factors in the male, such as varicocele or immunological factors, or in the female partner, including ovulatory disturbances or tubal pathology[4]. MAGI is associated with sexual dysfunction, namely inadequate coital erection, and ejaculatory disturbances such as painful or abnormal ejaculation[1].

PATHOGENESIS

Neisseria gonorrhoea has recently become more frequent. When treated inadequately, infection with this pathogen may cause severe damage to the epididymis resulting in progressive obstruction of sperm transport with oligozoospermia or azoospermia, and disruption of the blood–testis barrier with formation of antisperm antibodies.

Chlamydia trachomatis causes minor symptoms of urethritis and may remain untreated as symptoms tend to disappear spontaneously. The infection, however, may spread along the vas deferens to cause chronic epididymitis which is characterized by a chronic and remittent course[5]. Areas of granuloma formation may cause partial or total obstruction, and epididymal dysfunction which is associated with asthenozoospermia. Again, disruption of the blood–testis barrier may initiate production of antisperm antibodies.

Trivial cysto-urethritis is probably the most frequent cause of MAGI in western countries. *Escherichia coli*, *Streptococcus faecalis*, *Klebsiella* species and *Proteus* species are the most commonly identified pathogens[6,7]. It is the inadequate or insufficient treatment of trivial cysto-urethritis which will result in chronic bacterial infection of the accessory sex glands, mostly the prostate. Infection descending along the genital tract will cause chronic swelling and inflammation of the epididymis, typically at its caudal part and the transition to the vas deferens.

Chronic and excessive tobacco use significantly increases the prevalence of cysto-urethritis and MAGI, probably by causing chemical irritation of the bladder and urethral mucosa, which become more susceptible to bacterial invasion. It has also been suggested that the increased venous flow of testicular blood through the plexus of Santorini, which surrounds the prostate and seminal vesicles, occurring in patients with varicocele may increase the susceptibility of these glands to infection[8].

EFFECTS OF MAGI ON ACCESSORY GLAND FUNCTION AND SPERMATOGENESIS

Both chronic and acute infection of the accessory sex glands result in diminished secretory function. This manifests itself by a lowered concentration and output-per-ejaculate of secretory products (Table 1)[9].

In the case of prostatitis, semen liquefaction may be abnormal (Table 2) due to impaired secretion of prostate specific antigen, which is the major enzyme responsible for this phenomenon[10]. Decreased secre-

Table 1 Secretory products of the accessory sex glands

Epididymis	Neutral alpha-glucosidase
	Free L-carnitine
	Glyceryl-phosphoryl-choline
Seminal vesicles	Fructose
	Fluid volume
	Prostaglandins
Prostate	Citric acid
	Acid phosphatase
	Gamma glutamyltranspeptidase
	Zinc, calcium
	Semen liquefaction

Table 2 Relation between semen consistency, abnormal sperm quality and male accessory gland infection (MAGI). Reproduced with permission of Blackwell Science Ltd from Comhaire *et al.* (1987)[3]

	N	%*
No MAGI + normal spermatozoa	3117	2.3
No MAGI + abnormal spermatozoa	2807	12.9
MAGI + abnormal spermatozoa	440	33.9 ($P<0.001$)

*Percentage of cases with abnormal consistency or impaired liquefaction of semen

Table 3 Male accessory gland infection is diagnosed if the patient has oligo- or astheno- or teratozoospermia and fulfills the following criteria. Reproduced with permission of Blackwell Science Ltd from Comhaire *et al.* (1980)[15]

History and physical signs
- history of urinary infection
- and/or epididymitis
- and/or sexually transmitted disease
- and/or thickened or tender epididymis
- and/or thickened vas deferens
- and/or abnormal rectal examination

Prostatic fluid
- abnormal prostatic expression fluid
- and/or abnormal urine after prostatic massage

Ejaculate signs
- more than 1 million/mL white blood cells
- culture with significant growth of pathogenic bacteria
- abnormal appearance and/or viscosity and/or pH and/or abnormal biochemistry of the seminal plasma

Any of the following combinations should be present
- a history or physical sign with a prostatic sperm
- or a history or physical sign with an ejaculate sign
- or a prostatic sign with an ejaculate sperm
- or at least two ejaculate signs in each ejaculate
- one of A and one of B
- or one of A and one of C
- or one of B and one of C
- or two of C in each ejaculate

tion of acidic products by the prostate, particularly of citric acid, will also result in a more alkaline pH of the ejaculate[11,12]. On the other hand, decreased secretion by the seminal vesicles reduces the ejaculate volume. There is still some controversy over the effects of infection on sperm characteristics[13].

DIAGNOSIS OF MALE ACCESSORY GLAND INFECTION

In its clinical manual, the World Health Organization suggests a system of complementary criteria for the diagnosis of MAGI[14] as developed by Comhaire *et al.*[15]. This rather complex system (Table 3) includes elements from history-taking, physical examination and analysis of urine, prostate expression fluid and semen. In addition, echographic findings may contribute to the diagnosis (Figure 1)[16]. Other authors recommend the measurement of polymorphonuclear-elastase activity in seminal plasma[17–19].

Several problems may arise from the implementation of these criteria. For example, the cytological examination of prostate expression fluid may not give an abnormal result in cases where infection is restricted to the epididymides. Also, sperm culture may be positive with a significant number of colony forming units (CFU) due to urethral or skin contamination[20], and bacterial culture will fail to detect infection by, for example, *Chlamydia*. Problems may also occur with sperm culture, in so far that bacteriostatic substances secreted by the prostate, such as muramidase[21–23], may inhibit bacterial growth. In order to overcome the bacterial growth, it is recommended to perform a dilution of at least 1:1 semen with sterile physiological salt solution before plating[15].

The identification of polymorphonuclear white blood cells may be difficult as these cells are commonly confused with other 'round cells', namely spermatogenic cells. Peroxidase staining (LeucoScreen, FertiPro, Lotenhulle, Belgium) of the fresh ejaculate may help to overcome this problem, since the former will present a positive stain as against the latter remaining unstained (Figure 2)[24]. This staining method, orig-

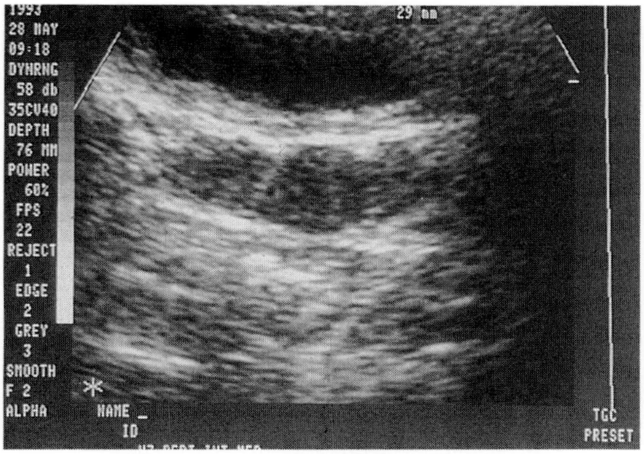

Figure 1 Transabdominal echogram of the seminal vesicles in a patient with acquired severe oligozoospermia and chronic vesiculitis. The seminal vesicles are distended and their wall is thickened

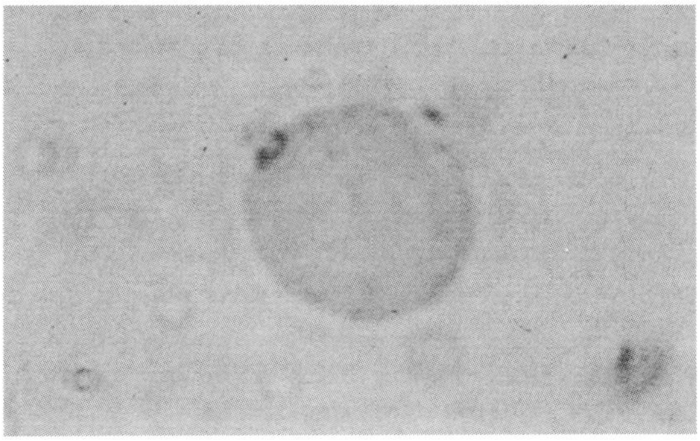

(A)

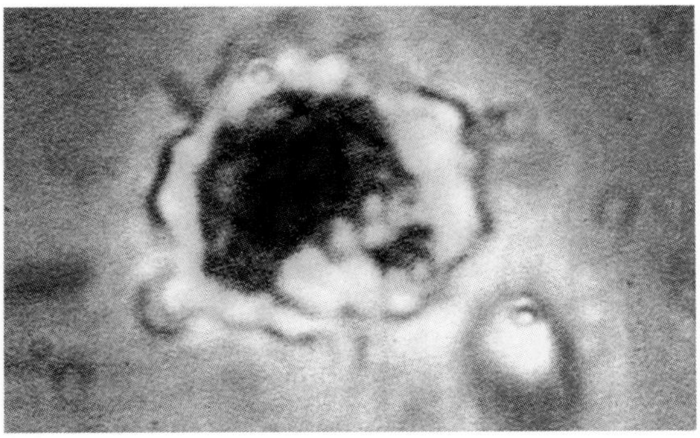

(B)

Figure 2 Peroxidase-positive and peroxidase-negative stained cells. (A) A peroxidase-negative cell, probably an 'immature' germ cell, counterstained with cyanosine; (B) a peroxidase-positive white blood cell. Reproduced with permission of the World Health Organization (1987)[24]

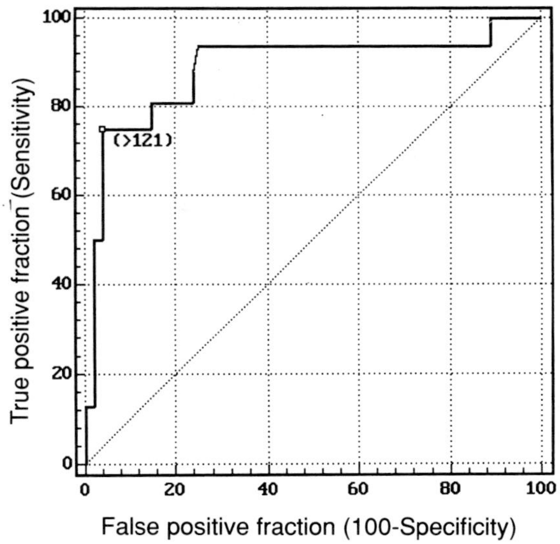

Figure 3 Receiver operating characteristic curve analysis of IL-6 in cases with or without accessory gland inflammation (sensitivity 75%, specificity 96%). Reproduced with permission of Munksgaard International Publishers from Comhaire *et al.* (1994)[27]

inally described by Endtz[25], is a simple and rapid method to differentiate nucleated round cells in the ejaculate. Nonetheless, degenerated and degranulated polymorphonuclear white blood cells may stain negative, and the peroxidase staining technique may therefore underestimate the number of white blood cells. Immunofluorescent identification using monoclonal antibodies against antigens on white blood cells may give more reliable results, but is impractical and too expensive for routine application[26].

Recently, measurement in seminal plasma of the amount of Interleukin-6 (IL-6) (Eurogenetics, Tessenderlo, Belgium) was found to be a sensitive and specific marker of inflammatory reaction (Figure 3). This enzyme-linked immunosorbent assay (ELISA) determination may turn out to be a great help for the diagnosis of accessory gland inflammation in the future[27].

Among the many biochemical markers of accessory sex gland function, citric acid seems to be superior in the detection of secretory deficiency among patients with MAGI (Figure 4)[11]. Patients with oligozoospermia and epididymal inflammation present a decreased concentration of neutral alpha-glucosidase in seminal plasma (EpiScreen, FertiPro, Lotenhulle, Belgium), but

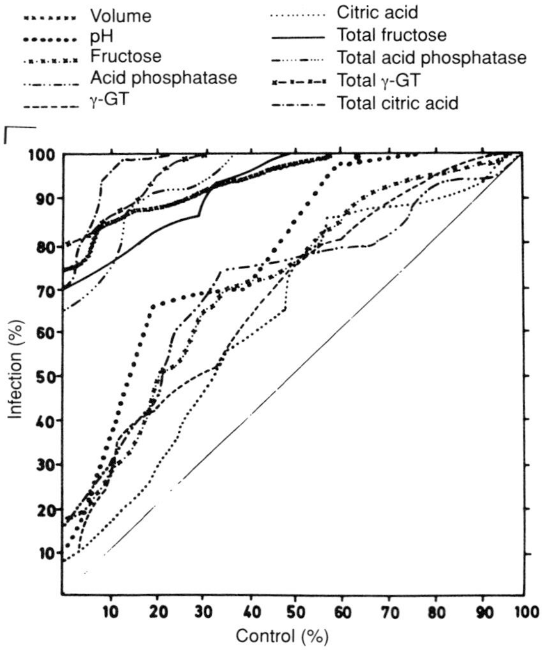

Figure 4 Receiver operating characteristic curves of physical and biochemical markers of semen of infected compared with non-infected infertile men. Reproduced with permission of W. Zuckschwerdt Verlag Comhaire *et al.* (1986)[11]

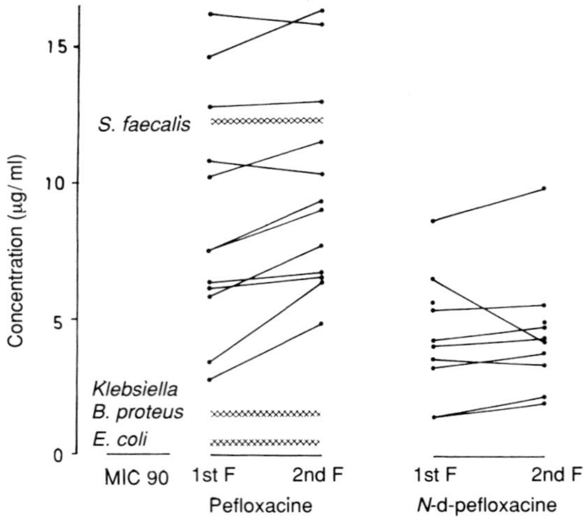

Figure 5 Concentration of pefloxacine and its N demethylated derivative (N-d-pefloxacine) in fractions 1 (1st F) and 2 (2nd F) of split ejaculates of patients with male accessory gland infection. Minimal inhibitory concentrations (MIC 90, crossed lines) of pefloxacine for more common aerobic urinary tract pathogens are also shown. Reproduced with permission of Williams & Wilkins from Comhaire (1987)[29]

the latter is not seen in cases with alleged epididymitis and normal sperm concentration (unpublished observations).

In summary, the diagnosis of MAGI should probably rely mainly on the combination of bacteriological, cytological and biochemical analyses of seminal plasma. This should include the measurement of IL-6, of markers of secretory function such as citric acid and alpha-glucosidase, and peroxidase staining of round cells.

TREATMENT

Treatment of MAGI aims at the eradication of all bacterial pathogens. In cases of infection with *E. coli*, *Proteus* species or *Klebsiella*, fluorinated quinolone derivatives are to be used, such as pefloxacine, ofloxacine, norfloxacine or ciprofloxacine[28]. The concentrations of these antibiotics in the first and second fraction of the ejaculate of men with MAGI are between 30 and 90 times higher than the minimal inhibitory concentration 90 (MIC 90) of these bacteria (Figure 5)[29]. The quinolones are not sufficiently effective against *Streptococcus*, and infection with this requires treatment with semi-synthetic penicillin derivatives such as ampicillin or amoxicillin, or with trimethoprim[30–32]. Initial antibiotic treatment should be given in a sufficiently high dose and for at least 10 days, since it takes about 7 days before a steady-state bactericidal concentration is reached in the diseased glands.

It is also recommended to continue treatment after this initial period, using either doxycycline in a dose of 200 mg day^{-1}, or trimethoprim 300 mg day^{-1} for another 30–90 days. The long-lasting treatment aims at preventing recurrence of infection or, alternatively, reinfection by the same or a different pathogen. In addition, *Chlamydia* infection will also be eradicated by doxycycline treatment[33,34].

In the past it has been suggested that adding a non-steroidal anti-inflammatory drug (e.g. indomethacin, naproxen) to the antibiotic increases the effectiveness of treatment[35]. However, there are no studies available to sustain this suggestion so that the indication for such adjuvant treatment is empirical.

RESULTS OF TREATMENT

In general, antibiotic treatment will not result in a clearcut improvement of sperm characteristics in comparison with that seen after placebo intake[4,36,37]. Sperm motility and morphology usually do improve, white blood cells may disappear and sperm culture will eventually become negative in most cases, but such effects have also been observed in placebo-treated controls. The biochemical make-up of seminal plasma does not usually change, as far as markers of accessory gland function are concerned. Data on IL-6 concentration in seminal plasma are not yet available, but the concentration of this cytokine may well be a good indicator of regression of the inflammatory condition.

Also, it is not clear whether antibiotic treatment results in improvement of the conception rate among couples with infertility due to MAGI-associated sperm deficiency. Several open studies do suggest a beneficial effect[35,36], but the results of double-blind studies[4] are less convincing. It should, however, be mentioned that no double-blind studies using the third-generation quinolones have been performed so far.

With regard to the results of IVF, it has been suggested that fertilization rates are improved after antibiotic treatment and elimination of white blood cells from the ejaculate. This effect has been ascribed to the increase of radical oxygen species (ROS)[38] which is claimed to interfere with the *in vitro* oocyte fertilizing capacity of spermatozoa. However, the use of newer methods of sperm selection and separation by means of discontinuous Percoll gradient (Perwash, FertiPro, Lotenhulle, Belgium) may eliminate such toxic effects of ROS, while rapidly separating white blood cells from spermatozoa[39]. Hence, doubts have risen on the necessity of antibiotic treatment of the male before artificial insemination[40,41] and *in vitro* fertilization[42].

CONCLUSIONS

Male accessory gland infection is a common finding in subfertile men. However, it seldom occurs as an isolated pathology. The diagnosis has become easier thanks to advanced biochemical measurements in seminal plasma, improved techniques of bacterial culture and cytological investigations. Treatment with newer antibiotics is highly effective in terms of eradication of bacterial pathogens. Further studies are needed to evaluate the potential of such treatment to improve the *in vivo* and *in vitro* fertilizing capacity of spermatozoa.

In view of these considerations, it is mandatory to prevent MAGI and subfertility which is associated with it, by means of early and radical treatment of infections of the urethro-genital tract including those caused by sexually transmitted disease and those resulting from trivial pathogens.

References

1. Comhaire, F. H., Farley, T. and Rowe, P. (1988). Sterility and sexuality from the andrologist's standpoint. In Eicher, W. and Kockott, G. (eds.) *Sexology*, pp. 81–102. (Berlin/Heidelberg: Springer Verlag)
2. Rowe, P. J. (1988). WHO's approach to the management of the infertile couple. In Negro-Vilar, A., Isidori, A. Paulson, J., Abdelmassih, R. and De Castro, M. P. P. (eds.) *Andrology and Human Reproduction*, pp. 219–309. (New York: Serono Symposia Publications from Raven Press)
3. Comhaire, F. H., de Kretzer, D. M. I., Farley, T. M. M. and Rowe, P. J. (1987). Towards more objectivity in diagnosis and management of male infertility; results of a World Health Organization multicenter study. *Int. J. Androl.*, **10** (Suppl. 7), 1–53
4. Comhaire, F. H., Rowe, P. J. and Farley, T. M. M. (1986). The effect of doxycycline in infertile couples with male accessory gland infection: a double blind prospective study. *Int. J. Androl.*, **9**, 91–8
5. Gerris, J., Schoysman, R. and Piessens-De Nef., M. (1985). A possible role of *Chlamydia trachomatis* as a causative agent in epididymal infertility. *Acta Eur. Fertil.*, **16**, 179–82
6. Taylor-Robinson, D., Furr, P. M. and Evans, R. T. (1986). The antibiotic susceptibility of possible aetiologic agents in prostatitis with views on rational therapy. In Weidner, W., Brunner, H., Krause, W. and Rothauge, C. F. (eds.) *Therapy of Prostatitis*, pp. 3–13. (München: W. Zuckschwerdt Verlag)
7. Ghormley, K. O., Cook, E. N. and Needham, G. M. (1954). Bacterial flora in chronic prostatitis. *Am. J. Clin. Pathol.*, **24**, 186–93

8. Comhaire, F. (1986). Varicocele and its role in male infertility. *Oxford Rev. Reprod. Biol.*, **8**, 165–213
9. Wolff, H., Bezold, G., Zebhauser, M. and Mewrer, M. (1991). Impact of clinically silent inflammation on male genital tract organs as reflected by biochemical markers in semen. *J. Androl.*, **12**, 331–4
10. McGee, R. S. and Herr, J. C. (1988). Human seminal vesicle-specific antigen is a substrate for prostate specific antigen. *Biol. Reprod.*, **39**, 499–510
11. Comhaire, F., Pieters, O., Debrock, M., Vermeulen, L., Rowe, P. and Farley, T. (1986). Importance of male accessory gland infection in fertility disorders. In Weidner, W., Brunner, H., Krause, W. and Rothaugel, C. F. (eds.) *Therapy of Prostatitis*, pp. 223–9. (München: W. Zuckschwerdt Verlag)
12. Anderson, R. and Fair, W. (1976). Physical and chemical determinations of prostatic secretion in benign hyperplasia, prostatitis and adenocarcinoma. *Invest. Urol.*, **14**, 137–40
13. Teague, N. S., Boyersky, S. and Glenn, J. F. (1971). Interference of human spermatozoa motility by *Escherichia Coli. Fertil. Steril.*, **22**, 281–5
14. Rowe, P. J., Comhaire, F. H., Hargreave, T. B. and Mellows, H. (1993). *WHO Manual for the Standardized Investigation and Diagnosis of the Infertile Couple.* (Cambridge: Cambridge University Press)
15. Comhaire, F., Verschraegen, G. and Vermeulen, L. (1980). Diagnosis of accessory gland infection and its possible role in male fertility. *Int. J. Androl.*, **3**, 32–45
16. Purvis, K. and Christiansen, E. (1993). Infection in the male reproductive tract. Impact, diagnosis and treatment in relation to male infertility. *Int. J. Androl.*, **16**, 1–13
17. Wolff, H. and Anderson, D. J. (1988). Evaluation of granulocyte elastase as a seminal marker for leukocytospermia. *Fertil. Steril.*, **50**, 129–32
18. Micic, S., Macura, M., Lalic, N. and Dotlic, R. (1989). Elastase as an indicator of silent genital tract infection in infertile men. *Int. J. Androl.*, **12**, 423–9
19. Cumming, J. A., Dawes, J. and Hargreave, T. B. (1990). Granulocyte elastase levels do not correlate with anaerobic and aerobic bacterial growth in seminal plasma from infertile men. *Int. J. Androl.*, **13**, 273–7
20. Bowie, W., Pollock, H. M., Forsyth, P. S., Floyd, J. F., Alexander, E. R., Wang, S.-P. and Holmes, K. K. (1977). Bacteriology of the urethra in normal men and in men with nongonococcal urethritis. *J. Clin. Microbiol.*, **6**, 482–8
21. Comhaire, F. H., Vermeulen, L. and Verschraegen, G. (1980). Relation between bactericidal capacity, concentration of muramidase and other biochemical substances in semen plasma. In Salvadori, S., Semm, K. and Vadora, E. (eds.) *Fertil. Steril.*, pp. 477–9. (Edizione Internationali Gruppo Editoriale Medico)
22. Rozansky, R., Gurevitch, J., Brzezinsky, A. and Eckerling, B. (1949). Inhibition of the growth of *Staphylococcus aureus* by human semen. *J. Lab. Clin. Med.*, **34**, 1526–9
23. Rusk, J., Tallgren, L. G., Alfthan, O. S. and Johansson, C.-J. (1973). The antibacterial activity of semen and its relation to semen proteins. *Scand. J. Urol. Nephrol.*, **7**, 23–9
24. World Health Organisation (1987) *WHO Laboratory Manual.* (Cambridge: Cambridge University Press)
25. Endtz. (1972). Een methode om het vochtige urinesediment en het vochtige menselijk sperma rechtstreeks te kleuren. *Ned. T. Geneesk.*, **117**, 681–9
26. Eggert-Kruse, W., Tilgen, W., Bellmann, A., Runnebaum, B. and Rohr, G. (1992). Differentiation of round cells in semen by means of monoclonal antibodies and relationship with male infertility. *Fertil. Steril.*, **58**, 1046–55
27. Comhaire, F., Bosmans, E., Ombelet, W., Punjabi, U. and Schoonjans, F. (1994). Cytokines in semen of normal men and of patients with andrological diseases. *Am. J. Reprod. Immun.*, **31**, 99–103
28. Naber, K. E., Adam, D. and Kees, F. (1987). *In vitro* activity and concentration in serum, urine, prostate secretion and adenoma tissue of Ofloxacin in urological patients. *Drugs*, **34** (S1), 44–50
29. Comhaire, F. H. (1987). Concentration of Pefloxacine in split ejaculates of patients with chronic male accessory gland infection. *J. Urol.*, **138**, 828–30
30. Fortune, A. (1980). Co-trimoxazole in the treatment of prostato-vesiculitis associated with a diagnosis of male infertility. *Br. J. Sexual Med.*, **7**, 16–18
31. Drach, G. W. (1974). Trimethoprim/Sulfamethoxazole therapy of chronic bacterial prostatitis. *J. Urol.*, **111**, 637–9
32. Nielsen, M. L. and Hansen, I. (1972). Trimethoprim in human prostatic tissue and prostatic fluid. *Scand. J. Urol. Nephrol.*, **6**, 244–8
33. Oosterlinck, W., Wallijn, E. and Wyndaele, J. J. (1976). The concentration of Doxycycline in human prostate gland and its role in the treatment of prostatitis. *Scand. J. Infect. Dis.*, Suppl. **9**, 85–8
34. Harrison, R. F., de Louvois, J., Blades, M. and Hurley, R. (1975). Doxycycline treatment and human infertility. *Lancet*, **i**, 605–7
35. Hommonai, T. Z., Sasson, S., Paz, G. and Kraicer, P. F. (1975). Improvement of fertility and semen quality in men treated with a combination of anticongestive and antibiotic drugs. *Int. J. Fertil.*, **20**, 45–9
36. Baker, H. W. G., Straffon, W. G. E., Murphy, G., Davidson, A., Burger, H. G. and de Kretser, D. M. (1979). Prostatitis and male infertility: a pilot study. Possible increase in sperm motility with antibacterial chemotherapy. *Int. J. Androl.*, **2**, 193–201
37. Baker, H. W. G., Straffon, W. G. E., McGowan, M. P., Burgers, H. G., de Kretser, D. M. and Hudson, B. (1984). A controlled trial of the use of erythromycin for men with asthenospermia. *Int. J. Androl.*, **7**, 383–8
38. Aitken, R. J. and West, K. M. (1990). Analysis of the

relationship between reactive oxygen species production and leucocyte infiltration in fractions of human semen separated on Percoll gradients. *Int. J. Androl.*, **130**, 433–9
39. Wang, P. C., Balmaceda, J. R., Blanco, J. D., Gibbs, R. S. and Asch, R. (1986). Sperm washing and swim-up technique using antibiotics removes microbes from human semen. *Fertil. Steril.*, **45**, 97–100
40. Lumpkin, M. M., Smith, T. E., Coulam, C. B. and O'Brien, P. C. (1987). *Ureaplasma urealyticum* in semen for artificial insemination: its effect on conception and semen analysis parameters. *Int. J. Fertil.*, **32**, 122–30
41. Eggert-Kruse, W., Hofmann, H., Gerhard, I., Bilke, A., Runnebaum, R. and Petzoldt, D. (1988). Effects of antimicrobial therapy on sperm–mucus interaction. *Hum. Reprod.*, **3**, 861–9
42. Stoval, D. W., Bailey, L. E. and Talbert, L. M. (1993). The role of aerobic and anaerobic semen cultures in asymptomatic couples undergoing *in vitro* fertilization: effects of fertilization and pregnancy rates. *Fertil. Steril.*, **59**, 197–201

Antisperm antibodies 1: laboratory techniques

12

M.-L. Windt and G. F. Doncel

INTRODUCTION

Although antigenicity of spermatozoa was first described by Landsteiner[1] in 1899, the possible role of antisperm antibodies (ASAs) as a factor of male infertility was not noticed until the middle of this century[2]. The blood–testis barrier formed by the tight junctions of the Sertoli cell provides immunological protection for sperm antigens[3]. Disruption of this barrier by various pathogenetic mechanisms, such as vasectomy[4], testicular trauma, testicular torsion[5], infection[6] and testicular surgery[7] has been associated with the formation of ASAs. However, there are some regions of the male genital tract, such as rete testis and ductus efferentes, where a strict sequestration of sperm does not occur[8]. Therefore men, as well as women, through sexual intercourse are regularly exposed to considerable doses of highly antigenic cells.

Since auto- (male) or isoimmune (female) pathogenetic ASAs are not a common finding in the general population[9], an important suppression of such response must be in place. Systemic and local (genital) immunoregulatory mechanisms control the development of antispermatic immunity. However, genetic predispositions, non-physiological routes of inoculations[10,11] and adjuvant-like conditions, such as genital tract infections[12] may impair or override those mechanisms, favoring a type of immune response that can lead to sperm dysfunction.

The immunological response to sperm is polyclonal and a heterogeneous population of ASAs directed against different domains of sperm surface antigens occurs in different individuals[13]. Different ASA isotypes can be stimulated, either singly or concomitantly, by the same population of sperm[9]. As a result, a wide spectrum of ASA-mediated effects on sperm function and sperm–egg interactions has been documented *in vitro*[14,15]. How such effects occur, however, remains elusive.

In spite of the knowledge that the surface of mammalian sperm is regionally organized[16], the identity of only a limited number of membrane proteins is known.

Furthermore, if the antigenic character of the freshly ejaculated human sperm is poorly known, that of spermatozoa after incubation under capacitating conditions is much less so. Several authors have pointed out that there is greater binding of serum immunoglobulins to capacitated sperm than those isolated soon after ejaculation[17,18]. Certain ASAs have a cytotoxic effect on spermatozoa and can cause cell death and immobilization of sperm cells. Immobilization and agglutination of spermatozoa caused by ASA in seminal plasma, the cervical mucus and on the sperm cells themselves can prevent spermatozoa reaching the ovum[19–24]. *In vivo*, antibody binding to sperm with subsequent complement fixation is thought to be of major pathogenetic importance in sperm dysfunction[25,26]. In fertilization *in vitro*, several modes of action have been postulated: (1) direct binding to sperm receptors for zona ligands; (2) adjacent cross-linking which blocks zona receptors by steric hindrance; and (3) interference with sperm capacitation.

Benoff *et al.*[27] recently published data which support the hypothesis that ASAs inhibit capacitation-associated increases in both surface sperm receptors and spontaneous acrosome loss, stabilizing plasma membrane structure by antibody cross-linkages. Such stabilization would both slow the normal lateral diffusion and aggregation of sperm membrane proteins associated with the instruction of acrosome exocytosis, as well as inhibit sterol-acceptor-induced cholesterol loss. Ultimately, cumulus dispersion, zona pellucida binding and penetration and oolemma fusion can be impeded[28–31].

Antisperm antibodies can be detected in serum, seminal plasma, cervical mucus, other reproductive tract fluids (tubal fluid, follicular fluid, uterine fluid) and on the surface of spermatozoa. IgA and IgG are the two major immunoglobulin classes of ASA detected in both males and females[32–35]. The IgM class is sometimes detected in the serum of antibody-positive females[36–39], but seldom in seminal fluid or on the sperm surface. This finding, however, can be of pathogenetic significance[40].

METHODOLOGY

Detection of ASAs in the various biological fluids where they can be found plays an important role in the clinical evaluation and in estimating the prognosis of the couple's immunological infertility.

Serum titers of ASA have been used as an indication of possible infertility. However, ASAs in serum, although very useful in the screening process, do not necessarily impair fertility unless these circulating antibodies are also present within the reproductive tract or are detectable on living spermatozoa[20]. Detection of ASA in cervical mucus, seminal plasma and on the sperm surface is mandatory[41].

Besides the traditional methods for detection of agglutinating and immobilizing ASA, newer procedures have been developed. These tests allow identification of antibody class and localization and can be applied directly to the sperm cell or indirectly to blood serum, seminal plasma and cervical mucus. These tests include the mixed antiglobulin reaction (MAR) test, the direct and indirect immunobead test (IBT) and an enzyme-linked immunosorbent assay (ELISA).

The sperm–cervical mucus contact (SCMC) test is also a valuable screening test to ascertain the *in vivo* effect of sperm antibodies in cervical mucus and on the sperm membrane.

Some methods are of use as screening tests, while others are of importance in prognosis and research. To help patients with a sperm antibody-related infertility problem, the whole battery of tests should be performed in order to obtain the exact profile of the problem.

Agglutination

Kibrick: gelatin agglutination test (GAT)

This macroscopic method[42–51] for the detection of agglutinating antibodies was described by Kibrick in 1952. It has since been replaced by more accurate microagglutination methods.

Franklin and Dukes: tube slide agglutination test (TSAT)

This microscopic method was introduced by Franklin and Dukes in 1964 and has been employed extensively[52]. It also has been replaced in many laboratories by the simpler tray agglutination text (TAT) introduced by Friberg in 1974[53].

Friberg: tray agglutination test (TAT)

A mixture of test sample and donor spermatozoa is made with a microsyringe on tissue typing plates and then examined under an inverted microscope to ascertain the titer, type and degree of sperm agglutination.

Method

A semen sample of a fertile donor is layered with Baker's medium containing 1% bovine serum albumin (BSA) for 1 h to obtain motile spermatozoa. A sperm concentration of 30×10^6/mL is used.

Thawed test samples (serum, seminal plasma, cervical mucus) are diluted serially in tissue culture plates (Sterilin Titertrek, Feltham Middlesex, UK) with Baker's medium with added 1% bovine serum albumin (BSA). Screening is done at a 1:4 dilution. All positive samples are then serially diluted to 1:1024. Five μL of diluted test sample is transferred to a disposable microchamber (Design AB, Moss, Norway) containing 3 mL of liquid paraffin and incubated for 1 h at 37°C in a moist Petri dish. Known positive and negative control samples are included in the test procedure. After 1 h incubation, the samples are examined for agglutination under an inverted light microscope. The examination is repeated after 2 h of incubation. A 100× magnification is used for the detection of agglutination and 400× for the identification of the type of agglutination. The test is regarded as positive when an obvious agglutination of spermatozoa is noted:

3+ all spermatozoa agglutinated

2+ large agglutinates together with free spermatozoa

1+ scattered and small agglutinates

All positive test samples are tested a second time to ascertain positivity and only titers ≥1:32 are considered of clinical importance. Titer values represent the highest dilution where a 1+ agglutination of donor sperm is observed.

The TAT has several advantages: it is easy to perform and read, it is simple and sensitive, the type of agglutination (head/head, tail/tail or mixed) is revealed in each test and a large number of tests can be done at one time with a single donor sperm sample[53]. The method, however, requires fresh donor sperm of excellent quality.

The TAT is the most used screening test for ASA in serum and seminal plasma[47,50,54–62] and correlates well with most other ASA tests[44,49,63,64].

Immobilization

Tests for sperm-immobilizing antibodies depend on the complement system and the presence of sperm antibodies. Interaction of antibody molecules with sperm antigen activates the complement system and disrupts the permeability and integrity of the sperm's cell membrane. The ultimate effect can be detected as a loss of motility followed by cell death[65]. After antibody–antigen binding, complement components bind to the Fc part of the antibody molecule and cause cell lysis by subsequent activation of the lytic complement factors.

The sperm immobilizing test (SIT) as described by Isojima *et al.*[66,67] is the method most often applied[48,59,62,68].

Isojima: sperm immobilizing test (SIT)

The test is usually performed together with the TAT so that the same semen sample and sample dilutions are used. Donor semen preparation and test sample dilutions are exactly as for the TAT. Only a 1:4 dilution of each test sample is screened for immobilization. Guinea pig complement at a dilution of 1:8 in Baker's solution is used. The complement solution is divided into two portions: one is utilized as a positive complement source, and the other as a negative souce after inactivation at 56°C for 1 h[45]. Five µL of a 1:4 test sample dilution is transferred in duplicate to a disposable microchamber containing 3 mL of liquid paraffin (as for TAT). Two µL of motile donor sperm suspension (concentration 30×10^6/mL) is added to each 5 µL sample and mixed thoroughly. The microchambers are then incubated at 37°C in moist Petri dishes for 30 min to allow antibody–antigen binding. After 30 min, 5 µL of fresh complement (positive sample) is added to one sample drop. Five µL of the inactivated complement is added to the duplicate drop (negative control). Microchambers are then incubated for another hour. Results are read under an inverted light microscope (as for TAT) at 100× magnification. The percentage of motile spermatozoa in the duplicate sample drops is estimated. The sperm-immobilization value (*SIV*) is then calculated.

$$SIV = \frac{C}{T}$$

C= % motility in sample incubated with inactivated complement (negative); *T*= % motility in sample incubated with fresh, active complement (positive). A *SIV* of >2 is regarded as positive[66,67].

The SIT method, as the TAT, is easy to perform and a large number of samples can be tested with one donor sample. SIT is usually less sensitive than the TAT. An excellent fresh donor sample is required to obtain sufficient motile spermatozoa for the test. SIT cannot detect antibodies incapable of fixing complement (e.g. IgA).

Mixed agglutination reactions

ASAs in serum and seminal plasma are not necessarily an indication of infertility in males. The impairment of fertility may be more related to the amount of ASA on the sperm cell itself[69,70].

Several assays have been developed which can demonstrate the binding of antibodies directly to the sperm surface. These assays can also be adapted to detect antibodies in serum, seminal plasma and cervical mucus by doing an indirect test.

Antibodies are then first allowed to adsorb to donor spermatozoa before testing.

Mixed antiglobulin reaction test (MAR test)

The MAR test was developed to detect surface ASA[70] and has since been used by numerous laboratories[44,45,54,60,61,71–73]. The test is a modification of the Coombs test described in 1956 by Coombs *et al.*[74]. The MAR test is performed by mixing three ingredients as single drops on a slide and covering it with a cover slip[69,70]:

(1) the semen sample;

(2) a suspension of group O, Rh-positive, human red cells of R_1R_2 type, sensitized with human incomplete anti-D antibody.

(3) rabbit or goat, undiluted, monospecific anti-IgG antiserum.

The reaction is then observed after 10 min of incubation under a light microscope. The red cells are coated with IgG (anti-D) as well as the sperm cells if they have antibodies on them. The added anti-IgG antiserum will then link together the two kinds of cells. Agglutination will be seen as mixed clumps of spermatozoa and red blood cells with a slow 'shaky' movement when observed under a light microscope.

The results are noted as percentages of motile spermatozoa incorporated into the mixed agglutinates. The site of attachment is also noted. No interpretation of the test is given unless agglutination of red blood cells and the presence of sufficient motile spermatozoa are observed. A MAR test is rendered positive when >10% agglutination is seen, but is considered of clinical significance only when >80% agglutination is present[69].

The advantage of the MAR test is that it can be applied directly to fresh, untreated semen samples. The result can be obtained within a few minutes and is therefore quick, simple and repeatable[69,70,75]. The MAR test correlates well with most other sperm antibody tests, e.g. agglutinating titer in serum[69], SCMC tests and immunobead test[39]. It does not correlate well with agglutinating titers in seminal plasma[69].

Although the MAR test is still the ideal method for screening of autosperm antibodies[45,55,76], it has certain limitations:

(1) It cannot be used in patients with oligozoospermia, asthenozoospermia and azoospermia.

(2) It is difficult to quantitate.

(3) The IgG MAR cannot detect IgA and the erythrocyte IgA MAR was shown to be less sensitive than the IgG MAR[76].

(4) Must be performed on a fresh sample.

(5) Can be influenced by debris, mucus, and microbial factors[77].

SpermMar (latex MAR)

Recently, Ortho Diagnostic Systems introduced a SpermMar kit that relies on an antiserum against the Fc component of human IgG to induce mixed agglutination between antibody-coated sperm and latex beads conjugated with human IgG[59,60,68,78,79]. This assay can be used for direct detection on unwashed spermatozoa, but also indirectly on serum and seminal plasma.

Ten microliters of unwashed sperm are mixed with 10 μL of SpermMar latex particles and 10 μL of the antiserum against the Fc component of human IgG on a microslide, covered with a coverslip and incubated for 2–3 min. The reaction is examined by phase contrast microscopy at 400×, and the percentage of motile spermatozoa incorporated in mixed agglutinates is recorded[61,78,80]. Different laboratories have different values for positivity, including >40%[59–61] and >10%[60,78–80].

The SpermMar was shown to correlate relatively well with most other sperm antibody detection methods including flow cytometry[80], IBT[68,78,82] TAT[61], GAT[68] and SIT[68].

The main advantage of the SpermMar compared to the erythrocyte MAR is the convenience of the kit, since the preparation of IgG-sensitized erythrocytes is not always available[79] and also unwashed spermatozoa can be used[78,81]. The SpermMar circumvents the use of erythrocytes and is also time- and cost-efficient[68,82]. It should be used as a screening test for identifying sperm with antibodies of the IgG class on their surface and should be confirmed with the IBT[68,78].

The disadvantage of the SpermMar (IgG labeled), is that it cannot detect IgA and this should then be carried out using the IBT[68,78]. It also seems that an indirect SpermMar is difficult to interpret and antibodies in serum should rather be detected with the TAT and SIT.

Immunobead test (IBT)

Traditionally, the identification of patients with sperm antibodies has depended on tests on blood serum[37,39]. This has been criticized, since serum antibodies are not necessarily an indication of the antibody activity in the seminal plasma and on the sperm membrane[37,38]. It is possible that, in some patients, sperm antibodies can be detected in seminal plasma and on the sperm membrane, but not in serum[39]. Therefore, there is a growing emphasis on the investigation of local rather than systemic immunity to spermatozoa and it has become essential to develop assays for sperm-bound antibodies[37].

It was further stated by Adeghe *et al.*[39] that it is no longer sufficient to merely demonstrate sperm antibodies without also determining their isotype, surface specificity and concentration.

The IBT was developed by Clarke *et al.*[35,39] and permits a complete characterization (immunoglobulin class, localization of attachment) of sperm-bound antibodies as well as antibodies in seminal plasma and serum. The test can, therefore, be done directly on spermatozoa or indirectly on serum and fluids of the reproductive tract, e.g. seminal plasma, cervical mucus and follicular fluid[37].

Direct IBT

The immunobead reagent consits of polyacrylamide beads, 5–10 μm in diameter and covalently bound to rabbit anti-human immunoglobulins of either the IgA, IgG or IgM class. The reagent can be purchased in lyophilized form (50 mg) and is reconstituted by adding 10 mL of sterile Tyrode's solution. The reconstituted reagent is stable for 4–6 weeks at 4°C[35–37]. Before use, an aliquot of the reagent is washed once with Tyrode's solution containing 0.3% BSA (Cohn fraction V) (TBSA) and then resuspended to 5 mg/mL in Tyrode's solution containing 5% BSA (TBSA-5).

Semen samples to be tested are washed three times in TBSA (600 g, 5 min., room temperature) and resuspended to a sperm concentration of $10–25\times10^6$/mL motile spermatozoa in TBSA-5. A drop of immunobead reagent is mixed with an equal drop of washed sperm (5 μL), covered with a cover slip and incubated in a moist Petri dish for 10 min at room temperature.

Any antibody attached to the sperm membrane will react with the anti-human immunoglobulin on the immunobead and sperm–immunobead binding can be observed under phase contrast optics at 400× magnification. All motile spermatozoa are noted and the percentage of motile sperm with attaching beads are of importance. The localization and number of attached beads are also noted[35,37]. A motile sperm is scored positive when one or more beads are attached to the sperm surface[35]. The semen sample is scored positive when 20% or more of the motile spermatozoa show positive binding. The localization of bead binding (head, midpiece, neck, tailtip and tail) and the number of beads per spermatozoa are also noted, as this may be of clinical and prognostic value[30,83].

Although there are modifications of this method in the literature regarding the sperm concentration used, washing and resuspension mediums, incubation times and interpretation of the results, the method above is the one most used by researchers[29,30,35,37–39,45,55,57,58,83–95].

Indirect IBT

The indirect IBT can be performed on seminal plasma of semen samples with too few motile spermatozoa for a direct IBT and also on serum, cervical mucus and follicular fluid to obtain information of the antibody status in these fluids[35,37]. Samples for the indirect IBT can be stored frozen until analyzed[35].

Serum, follicular fluid or liquefied cervical mucus (2 mg/mL bromelin in Tyrode's buffer) are incubated at 56°C for 30 min to inactivate complement[37]. Seminal plasma is filtered (0.45 μm) before use[35,37]. Aliquots (200–500 μL) of test samples (possibly containing antibodies) are incubated with donor semen (25–50 μL, negative by direct IBT and of good quality – can use layered samples to obtain good motility) for 1 h[19,39]. Samples can be used diluted or undiluted[29,39,96]. An initial sperm concentration of $40–80\times10^6$/mL should be used to obtain $1–4\times10^6$/25–50 μL motile spermatozoa for the final incubation.

The incubated samples are now washed as for the direct IBT, a drop of immunobead reagent is added and the mixture is observed after 10 min incubation under phase contrast at 400× magnification[35,37]. Any antibody present in the test fluid will bind to antigen on donor sperm cells. Bound antibody will then react with the immunobead reagent. Interpretation of the results is as for the direct IBT.

The indirect IBT is used mainly for the indication of antibody type and localization in serum and seminal plasma. Implementation of the method for the determination of antibody titers is not very practical when the extensive washing procedure is taken into consideration.

When used to determine titers, the endpoint for titer estimation is taken as the highest dilution where 50% or more of the sperm still have beads attached[84]. Again, variation with regard to donor sperm concentration, test sample volume and dilution, incubation times and interpretation of the results exists in the literature[29,35,37,39,51,56,60,62,73,84,88,94,96–100].

The IBT was shown to correlate very well with most other ASA tests, i.e. SCMC[70,82], SIT[38,83,97,102,103], MAR[38,39,44,78], ELISA[104], RIA[105] and immunofluorescence[103].

The IBT is an immunological specific test, indicative of antibodies specifically attached to the sperm membrane[30,35,38]. It has been found to be an excellent screening test for sperm-bound antibodies[35,83,102]. The IBT correlates well with and is more sensitive than other traditional tests[35,38,39,64,103,106,107]. The IBT also has other advantages over most traditional tests: it allows determination of the antibody class attached to spermatozoa, the localization on the spermatozoa and the proportions of spermatozoa coated with antibody[23,35,36,38,83,97,102]. It can also give semi-quantitative information, that is, the number of immunobeads bound to a specific region of the spermatozoon[37]. Detection of immunoglobulin class and localization of antibodies on the spermatozoa can be of clinically diagnostic and prognostic value[30,83]. Sperm antibodies of the IgA class and directed at the sperm head, seems to be of great importance in reproduction[29,83,96,97].

The IBT is also a relatively simple procedure, inexpensive, quick and easy to perform[37,38,97,102]. It is very convenient, utilizing only a bench centrifuge, light microscope, commercially available immunobeads, and takes less than 30 min to perform[37]. The specificity of binding between immunobeads and sperm-bound antibodies was tested with cross-inhibition tests, proving the high specificity of the IBT[35,96,97]. Non-specific binding was also found to be minimal[97].

The IBT can also be done indirectly on reproductive fluids, seminal plasma, follicular fluid, cervical mucus and serum. The immunoglobulin class thus detected can be of clinical importance[108]. The direct and indirect IBT are therefore reliable, valid, specific and reproducible tests for the detection of sperm-bound antibodies and sperm antibodies in reproductive fluids and serum.

The few disadvantages of the IBT include the fact that titer determination is slightly cumbersome due to the several washing steps included. Furthermore, it is not truly quantitative[38,39]. The IBT also requires fresh motile spermatozoa of good quality. Usually spermatozoa from only one donor are used, allowing for individual differences in tests done with different donors. It is very important to wash spermatozoa thoroughly, since free immunoglobulins in the reaction mixture can potentially inhibit the interaction between anti-immunoglobulin on the immunobeads and immunoglobulin bound to the sperm surface[35,38].

Recently, a modification of the IBT has also been used widely in the literature (SpermCheck, Bio-Rad Laboratories, Inc. USA)[61,82,109]. The SpermCheck Assay is based on a modification of the immunobead test[109] and consists of latex beads coated with antihuman IgG, IgA and IgM[61]. The assay is supplied with a wash buffer, controls and a bead reagent which detects all the three major classes of ASA (IgG, IgA and IgM) in a single test[63]. Semen is washed three times with SpermCheck wash buffer. After preparation, 50 μL of latex bead reagent is mixed with 5 μL of sperm suspension. Regional binding of beads to motile spermatozoa is noted and a total binding of 17% is considered positive[61]. SpermCheck can also be used for an indirect ASA test on serum[61]. When compared to the immunobead test (direct and indirect) on semen and serum, SpermCheck was shown to have a slightly greater sensitivity and was easier to perform[82].

Sperm-cervical mucus contact test (SCMC)

The SCMC test was introduced in 1976 by Kremer and Jager, who postulated that the interaction between the antisperm antibody-coated spermatozoa and the long glycoprotein micelles in cervical mucus is the cause of a non-progressive shaking phenomenon of spermatozoa in cervical mucus[110]. The shaking appeared to be complement-independent, since it still occurred after mucus was heated to 56°C for 30 min[110]. The interaction is explained as follows:

(1) Progressively moving spermatozoa, coated with sperm antibody, stick to the network of long glycoprotein micelles in normal cervical mucus[110]. In 1981, Jager *et al.*[111] showed that the Fc part of the IgG ASA plays an important role in the occurrence of the shaking phenomenon.

(2) The same shaking phenomenon appears when ASAs are present in the cervical mucus. Spermatozoa swimming through the positive mucus become sensitized and the reaction is similar to the previous one. It is also possible that the glycoprotein micelles are coated with sperm antibodies and that the shaking phenomeon develops thereby[110].

(3) A positive SCMC test is caused mainly by IgA in cervical mucus and on the sperm surface, although it can also be caused by IgG on the spermatozoal surface[112,113]. Positive SCMC tests were shown to correlate well with reduced penetration into cervical mucus, and sperm agglutination titer in seminal plasma and cervical mucus. The test is performed as follows, according to method I of Kremer *et al.*[110]

Semen samples to be tested (1 mL) are left upright in a tube for 30 min at 37°C to allow agglutinated and dead spermatozoa, as well as debris to settle to the bottom. Freely swimming spermatozoa are obtained by aspirating 0.1 mL of the sample from approximately 0.5 mm under the fluid surface.

Cervical mucus to be used must be of good quality with no epithelial or blood cells, indicating good estrogenic stimulation. The pH must be >7.0.

A drop of the mucus is placed on a glass slide and a drop of semen is added, mixed with the mucus, and covered with a coverslip. A drop of semen alone is also investigated simultaneously to compare the motility in both samples. The slides are then placed in a moist Petri dish for 30 min at room temperature and then examined.

SCMC tests usually include donor semen and donated mucus, as well as that of the husband and wife:

(a) patient sperm and donor mucus;

(b) donor sperm and donor mucus;

(c) donor sperm and patient mucus; and

(d) patient sperm and patient mucus.

By including all these controls (cross-matched test) it is possible to ascertain where the sperm antibodies are present.

The interpretation of the test is conducted as described by Jager *et al.* in 1979[114]. The samples are examined at a magnification of 400× (phase contrast) and the percentage of progressively motile spermatozoa (% PM), as well as the percentage of locally motile spermatozoa with quick shaking movements (% LM) are estimated in order to obtain the shaking percentage (% S).

$$\%S = \frac{\%LM}{\%PM + \%LM} \times 100$$

The whole slide is screened and all percentages are estimated as multiples of 10.

Tests are read after 15–30 min and are considered positive when %S>30%, but are thought to be of clinical importance only when %S>75%[113,114].

SCMC tests are valid only when the cervical mucus is of excellent quality without any foreign cells and debris and when semen samples contain sufficient concentrations of spermatozoa with good motility[114].

The SCMC test is easy and quick to perform, gives a good indication of the *in vivo* situation of the infertile patient with an immunological factor and is still used in many laboratories as a screening test for isoantibodies[47,55,60,71].

Newer tests

Enzyme-linked immunosorbent assay (ELISA)

It has become increasingly clear that antibodies which do not agglutinate or immobilize spermatozoa may nevertheless interfere with fertilization. Traditional assays for ASA detection in serum and seminal plasma, and based on immobilization and agglutination, are not conclusive[115]. Additional assays are, therefore, needed which will detect the full range of immunoglobulin reactivity with spermatozoa.

Enzyme-linked immunosorbent assays (ELISAs) and radioimmunoassays (RIAs) for sperm antibody detection have recently been developed to meet this demand.

The ELISA method consists of a series of additions of reagents separated by washings. In this method, enzymes linked to antibodies or antigens, forming complexes with both immunological and enzymatic activity, are used. Degradation by the enzymes of a chromogenic substrate yields an amplification factor which enables accurate and sensitive detection of the presence of the enzyme-bound antibody[116].

In general, antigen is immobilized by passive adsorption to a solid phase. The test sera are then incubated with the solid phase. Antibody in the serum becomes attached to the antigen. Several washes are performed to remove unreacted serum components. Incubation with the antiglobulin–enzyme conjugate follows. This complex becomes attached to any antibody fixed to antigen. Enzyme substrate is now added and the color change of the substrate is a measure of the amount of conjugate fixed. This again is proportional to the antibody level in the test sample[116].

The solid phase used includes test tubes, beads, disks and microtitration plates made of polyvinyl, polypropylene, glass or silicone rubber. The enzyme conjugate can be either alkaline phosphatase (with substrate *para*-nitrophenylphosphate), horseradish peroxidase (substrate *ortho*-phenyl diamine), glucose oxidase and β-*d*-galactosidase[116]. No generally accepted way of expressing the results is established. All methods rely on optical density readings with a spectrophotometer[116].

In past years, several researchers performed ELISAs to detect ASA in serum and seminal plasma[115–121]. Many different methods were used, differing mainly in the type of antigen used[115,117–119,121]. Most researchers used whole sperm as antigen, while some used a sperm membrane extract[115,117–119,121].

In the whole-cell ELISA fixation of spermatozoa to the solid phase is very problematic, since fixatives can cause high background values[117,118], poor repeatability[118], binding of circulating immunocomplexes[118], denaturation and loss of surface antigens[20,104,119] and breakdown of the sperm plasma membrane – leading to exposure of intracellular antigens not important in reproduction[20,104].

The antigen-extract ELISA eliminates some of the problems of the whole-sperm ELISA (fixation and centrifugation). Alexander *et al.*[118] used a 0.3 M lithium 3,5 diidosalicylate (LIS) sperm membrane extract claiming that it selectively extracts glycoproteins that bind to sperm antibodies. Some authors, however, feel that membrane extracts may contain antigens not associated with the fertilization process and are not of real clinical value[20,104,120]. Other authors find the sperm membrane extract superior to the whole-cell ELISA, with good reproducibility, small interassay variability and very easy to perform[121–123].

When the ELISA was compared to other established methods, the results were conflicting. Many authors found it to be more sensitive than the traditional methods such as the TAT, GAT and SIT and also reported good correlation with these tests[117–119,121,124–127]. Others reported different results. Eggart-Kruse *et al.*[71] implemented a commercially available ELISA kit and compared its results with those of the SCMC and MAR test. Very poor correlations were found and they concluded that the ELISA method cannot be recommended for the detection of ASA during an infertility investigation. They further concluded that circulating ASA, detected with ELISA in infertile couples do not necessarily indicate immunologic infertility or a reduced chance of conception.

A study done by Bronson *et al.*[104] reported that the use of live spermatozoa (such as in the IBT) in the detection of sperm reactive antibodies is very important since their results showed that the IBT was more sensitive than the ELISA they performed.

The usefulness and superiority of the ELISA for

the detection of ASA when compared to other sperm antibody tests reside mainly in the fact that the ELISA obviates the need for fresh, good quality semen, is non-subjective, is quantitative, and also immunoglobulin-specific[115,116,119,124,125]. Other factors making the ELISA extremely useful are its sensitivity[115,117,119,124,125,128], relative simplicity and rapidity[115,118,121]. The ELISA is also thought to be inexpensive, especially when compared to the RIA and IBT[117,118,128]. The test allows high-volume qualitative screening[117–119] and can easily be automated[118]. In the ELISA test pooled semen is used as antigen. This prevents a factor from one ejaculate being a major influence on the assay[118,119]. Semen used in the ELISA need not be of excellent quality[119] and microtiter plates coated with antigen can be stored for later use[117,118].

The fact that ASAs detected with ELISA include those that cause neither agglutination nor immobilization, but can still influence fertility, makes the assay valuable. The ELISA assay for ASA is, however, not without disadvantages.

In most ELISA assays, glutaraldehyde-fixed spermatozoa are used as antigen. A few authors found that this fixative can change or remove the antigenicity of the spermatozoa, causing false negative or positive results. Glutaraldehyde also causes high background values[20,104,119]. The use of sperm membrane extracts solves this problem. A new assay employing a soluble extract of sperm surface antigens fixed to a pin without methanol or glutaraldehyde has recently been reported[12]. This assay, named syncheon ELISA (Elias Medizintechnik, Freiburg, Germany) represents a quantitative assay for the determination of ASA (IgG, IgA, IgM) in serum and seminal plasma. However, some authors pointed out that extracts will expose intracellular antigens that play no role in reproduction[20,104]. Mathur *et al.*[120] stated that the ELISA assays are reliable only when purified antigen is used, as the presence of Fc receptors on the sperm or binding of adsorbed microbial antigens may lead to non-specific binding of immunoglobulins to sperm cells[107].

A recent study by Menge and Naz[62] utilized the sperm antibody fertilization antigen-1 (FA-1) as the solid phase in an ELISA assay. This antigen has been shown to be involved in human immunological infertility[129–131] and the authors suggested that an ELISA assay using this sperm-specific antigen (FA-1) should aid in elucidating the role of sperm antibodies in human infertility.

In conclusion ELISA, a quantitative ASA test, is potentially useful clinically or in research and may provide convenience and accuracy not possible with other assays[132]. The most recent data on the ELISA test for ASA, however, show disappointing results[71].

Other methods

Some sperm antibody detection tests which are not used in a routine, screening manner have also been described in the literature. These include the use of flow cytometry (FacScan) and RIA techniques and were mainly used for specific research protocols.

Flow cytometry / immunofluorescence

The use of flow cytometry and immunofluorescent staining of spermatozoa for the detection of sperm antibodies is a field that gained some attention in recent years[78,79,97,102,106,132,133]. Although it is not available to all routine laboratories, it is of importance due to its high specificity and sensitivity[79]. The method can utilize either fixed whole sperm or unfixed, intact spermatozoa as antigen[79,102,106,132].

In general, spermatozoa are washed free of seminal plasma (in some cases, fixed) and then incubated with monoclonal mouse anti-human antibodies. After another wash procedure, cells are incubated with fluorescein isothiocyanate (FITC) labeled goat anti-mouse antibody. Samples are then analyzed with a FacScan[79,97,132] or viewed for fluorescence[78,102,106,133].

It seems to be important to use intact sperm cells as antigen in flow cytometry assays (FCA) since plasma membrane integrity can be altered by fixatives, detergents and permeabilizing agents and air-drying[79,132]

When studies were conducted to ascertain the correlation between an immunofluorescent assay and other traditional assays, Daru and Mathur[102] found good correlation between IgG-IBT, cytotoxic assays and an indirect immunofluorescent assay on serum, seminal plasma and cervical mucus[102]. A study reported by Haas *et al.*[106] revealed that the IBT is more sensitive than the FCA, indicating that the FCA may miss low-titered sperm antibodies.

When the same sperm source was used (live spermatozoa) and antibody titers were relatively high, the IBT and the FCA were comparable[106]. The authors also concluded that the use of fixed spermatozoa in sperm antibody assays is inclined to give false positive results due to the disturbance of surface antigens and exposure of internal antigens[106].

Advantages of the FCA are its objectivity and specificity based on the highly specific interaction of monoclonal antibodies with immunoglobulins on the cell surface that does not require microscopic estimations. It may also be feasible in the case of immotile spermatozoa. Another unique feature of the FCA is the possibility to detect cell heterogeneity in terms of different antibodies on the cell surface[79].

The disadvantage is the fact that the procedure involves numerous washings and also requires very complicated and expensive equipment.

Radioimmunoassay (RIA)

The radioimmunoassay has been employed extensively in science to detect cell surface-bound antibodies. It has also been investigated recently as a direct method for the detection of ASAs on the sperm surface as well as indirectly to detect them in sera and seminal plasma[49,104,106].

When used as an indirect assay, several problems have been encountered, since patients' serum contains antibodies to both the sperm surface and internal sperm antigens[106]. This causes false positive results which may be increased by the fact that various fixatives used in the assay can cause abnormal surface morphology and antigen expression[106]. When compared to assays that employ live unfixed spermatozoa (IBT, GAT, TAT)[49,104,106], this assay seems to be less sensitive[106], especially when low titers are observed.

Therefore, although the RIA is a widely used method in the medical science field, currently available RIA methods for sperm antibodies that use extractive antigen preparations from sperm do not give reliable results[49]. The main reason for this is that researchers have not been able to identify one or more sperm antigens that directly and absolutely correlate with infertility[49]; identification of such a particular antigen have failed. The currently used RIA methods could not detect IgA and IgM. Gandini *et al.*[49] conclude that the RIA test cannot, at this stage, compete with other more widely used methods such as the TAT, MAR and IBT[27].

CONCLUDING REMARKS

In a recent review by Adeghe[55], many aspects of immunological infertility are discussed and we agree with him regarding testing for ASA. Patients (male and female) should be routinely tested for ASA as part of a standard semen analysis. Since many tests are available, those with sensitivity, specificity and reproducibility should be favored. Furthermore, these tests should be of clinical and prognostic value. It is, therefore, important to determine the immunoglobulin class, surface specificity and quantity. It is relevant to test for ASAs present on the surface of live sperm since these antibodies are of clinical importance.

An ideal test must, therefore, be able to test sperm-bound antibodies, must be simple and inexpensive, must not require expensive and complicated equipment, and must not be time-consuming. Taking this into consideration, we are using the following protocol in the Reproductive Biology Unit and Andrology Laboratory (Tygerberg Hospital), as follows.

Screen the female serum with the TAT and SIT and use the SCMC for detection of sperm antibodies in cervical mucus (if suitable mucus is available). Positive results can be followed up with the indirect IBT for determination of immunoglobulin class and localization.

Screen the male spermatozoa with the MAR test and follow up positive results with the TAT and SIT for serum and seminal plasma ASA titers. For immunoglobulin class and localization, the direct IBT is performed. In cases of poor sperm motility and suspected ASA, the seminal plasma is tested with either the TAT or SIT. Following this approach there should be enough information about the patient's sperm immunology to implement successful treatment.

Due to the fact that results with the ELISA[134], RIA and FacScan methods are still conflicting, these methods are not incorporated into our sperm antibody testing regimen.

In our own experience, the TAT and SIT are the most valuable ASA tests for screening female serum. All patients visiting the Unit for the first time are screened for ASA (TAT and SIT). During the period January 1993–March 1994, 385 female sera were screened and 19 of them had a TAT titer ≥1:16. No positive SIT titers were encountered for this period. Good cervical mucus is seldom found and, therefore, the SCMC test for screening is infrequently used.

All male patients with adequate semen samples are screened for ASA with the MAR test. We find this an excellent and valid test for ASA. All positive patients (MAR ≥10%) are also tested with the direct IBT and titers in seminal plasma and serum are tested with the TAT and SIT when available. We find that positive MAR tests correlate very well with the positivity for IgA and IgG in the direct IBT. Serum titers also correlate with the MAR test and the direct IBT. We seldom find high TAT titers in seminal plasma of ASA-positive men and seldom find positive SIT titers in either serum or seminal plasma in ASA-positive men. From the period January 1993–March 1994, 952 MAR tests were performed and 49 patients had a positive (≥10%) MAR test (5.1%). Sixty males were tested for ASA with TAT and SIT. Only one positive SIT serum was found (1.67%) and four patients' sera had TAT titers ≥1:16 (6.67%). All seminal plasma titers were negative.

References

1. Landsteiner, K. (1899). Zur Kenntnis der spezifisch auf Blutkorperchen wirkende Sera. *Zentralbl. Bakeriol.*, **25**, 546
2. Rumke, P. and Hellinga, G. (1959). Autoantibodies against spermatozoa in sterile men. *Am. J. Clin. Pathol.*, **32**, 357–63
3. Furuya, S., Kumamoto, Y. and Sugiyama, S. (1978). Fine structure and development of Sertoli junctions in human testis. *Arch. Androl.* **1**, 211–19
4. Sotolongo, J. R. (1982). Immunological effects of vasectomy. *J. Urol.*, **127**, 1063–6
5. Anderson, J. B. and Williams, R. C. N. (1990). Fertility after torsion of the spermatic cord. *Br. J. Urol.*, **65**, 225–30
6. Jarow, J. P., Kirkland, J. A. and Assimos, D. G. (1990). Association of antisperm antibodies and infertility in patients with testicular cancer. *Urology*, **36**, 154–6
7. Hjort, T., Husted, S. and Linnet-Jepsen, P. (1974). The effect of testis biopsy on autosensitization against spermatozoal antigens. *Clin. Exp. Immunol.*, **18**, 201–12
8. Marsh, L. D. and Alexander, N. J. (1982). Effects on the efferent ducts in *Macaca mulatta*. *Am. J. Pathol.*, **107**, 310–15
9. Haas, G. G. Jr., D'Cruz, O. J. and DeBault, L. E. (1990). Assessment by fluorescence-activated cell sorting of whether sperm-associated immunoglobulin IgG and IgA occur on the same sperm population. *Fertil. Steril.*, **54**, 127–32
10. Wolff, H. and Schill, W. B. (1985). A modified enzyme-linked immunosorbent assay (ELISA) for the detection of antisperm antibodies. *Andrologia*, **17**, 426–39
11. Tung, K. S. K., Teuscher, C., Goldberg, E. H. and Wild, G. (1981). Genetic control of antisperm antibody response in vasectomized guinea pigs. *J. Immunol.*, **127**, 835–9
12. Heidenreich, A., Bonfig, R., Wilbert, D. K., Strohmaier, W. L. and Engelmann, U. H. (1994). Risk factors for antisperm antibodies in infertile men. *Am. J. Reprod. Immunol.*, **31**, 69–76
13. Witkin, S. S., Vogel-Roccuzzo, R., David, S. S., Berkeley, A., Goldstein, M. and Graf, M. (1988). Heterogeneity of antigenic determinants on human spermatozoa: relevance to antisperm antibody testing in infertile couples. *Am. J. Obstet. Gynecol.*, **159**, 1228–31
14. Clarke, G. N. (1988). Sperm antibodies and human fertilization. *Am. J. Reprod. Immunol. Microbiol.*, **17**, 65–71
15. Bronson, R. A. (1990). Sperm antibodies and human fertilization. *Immunol. Allergy Clin. North Am.*, **10**, 165–84
16. Friend, D. S. (1982). Plasma-membrane diversity in a highly polarized cell. *J. Cell Biol.*, **93**, 243–9
17. Fusi, F., Bronson, R. A. (1990). Effect of incubation time in serum and capacitation on spermatozoal reactivity with antisperm antibodies. *Fertil. Steril.*, **54**, 887–93
18. Monroe, J. R., Altenbern, D. C., Mathur, S. (1990). Changes in sperm antibody tests results when spermatozoa are subjected to capacitating conditions. *Fertil. Steril.*, **54**, 1114–20
19. Bronson, R., Cooper, G. and Rosenfeld, D. (1984). The role of sperm antibodies in infertility. *Res. Reprod.*, **16**, 1–2
20. Bronson, R., Cooper, G. and Rosenfeld, D. (1984). Sperm antibodies: their role in infertility. *Fertil. Steril.*, **42**, 171–83

21. Menge, A. C. and Behrman, S. J. (1980). Immunologic problems of infertility. In Gold, J. J. and Josimovich, J. B. (eds.) *Gynecologic Endocrinology*, 3rd edn, pp. 690–707. (London: Harper and Row)
22. Alexander, N. J. (1984). Antibodies to human spermatozoa impede sperm penetration of cervical mucus or hamster eggs. *Fertil. Steril.*, **41**, 433–9
23. Brannen-Brock, L. R. and Hall, J. L. (1985). Effect of male antisperm antibodies on sperm fertilizability *in vitro*. *Arch. Androl.*, **15**, 15–19
24. Rumke, P. (1984). Autoimmunity against sperm in infertile men. *Asian Pac. J. Allergy Immunol.*, **2**, 329–35
25. Mathur, S., Williamson, H. O., Derrick, F. C., Madyastha, P. R., Melchers, J. T. III, Holtz, G. L., Baker, E. R., Smith, C. L. and Fudenberg, H. H. (1981). A new microassay for spermocytotoxic antibody: comparison with passive hemagglutination assay for antisperm antibodies in couples with unexplained infertility. *J. Immunol.*, **126**, 905–9
26. Bronson, R. A., Cooper, G. W. and Rosenfeld, D. L. (1983). Complement-mediated effects of sperm head directed human antibodies on the ability of human spermatozoa to penetrate zona-free hamster eggs. *Fertil. Steril.*, **40**, 91–5
27. Benoff, S., Cooper, G. W., Hurley, I., Mandel, F. S. and Rosenfeld, D. L. (1993). Antisperm antibody binding to human sperm inhibits capacitation induced changes in the levels of plasma membrane sterols. *Am. J. Reprod. Immunol.*, **30**, 113–30
28. Yovich, J. L., Kay, D., Stanger, J. D. and Boettcher, B. (1984). *In vitro* fertilization of oocytes from women with serum antisperm antibodies. *Lancet*, **18** (1873), 369–70
29. Bronson, R. A., Cooper, G. W. and Rosenfeld, D. L. (1982). Sperm-specific isoantibodies and autoantibodies inhibit the binding of human sperm to the human zona pellucida. *Fertil. Steril.*, **38**, 724–9
30. Bronson, R., Cooper, G. and Rosenfeld, D. (1981). Ability of antibody-bound human sperm to penetrate zona-free hamster ova *in vitro*. *Fertil. Steril.*, **36**, 778–83
31. Tzartos, S. J. (1979). Inhibition of *in-vitro* fertilization of intact and denuded hamster eggs by univalent anti-sperm antibodies. *J. Reprod. Fertil.*, **55**, 447–55
32. Clarke, G. N., Stojanoff, A., Cauchi, M. N. and Johnston, W. I. (1985). The immunoglobulin class of antispermatozoal antibodies in serum. *Am. J. Reprod. Immunol. Microbiol.*, **7**, 143–7
33. Clarke, G. N. (1984). Detection of antispermatozoal antibodies of IgG, IgA, and IgM immunoglobulin classes in cervical mucus. *Am. J. Reprod. Immunol.*, **6**, 195–7
34. Clarke, G. N., Hsieh, C., Koh, H. and Cauchi, M. N. (1984). Sperm antibodies, immunoglobulins and complement in human follicular fluid. *Am. J. Reprod. Immunol.*, **5**, 179–81
35. Clarke, G. N., Elliot, P. J. and Smaila, C. (1985). Detection of sperm antibodies in semen using the immunobead test: A survey of 813 consecutive patients. *Am. J. Reprod. Immunol. Microbiol.*, **17**, 118–23
36. Ackerman, S. B., Graff, D., Van Uem, J. F. H. M., Swanson, R. J., Veeck, L. L., Acosta, A. A. and Garcia, J. E. (1984). Immunologic infertility and *in vitro* fertilization. *Fertil. Steril.*, **42**, 474–7
37. Clarke, G. N. Protocol for detection of auto-antibodies to sperm cells using the immunobead reagent. *Chemlab/Bio Rad Laboratories Bulletin 1170.*
38. Clarke, G. N., Stojanof, A. and Cauchi, M. N. (1982) Immunoglobulin class of spermbound antibodies in semen. In Branatov, K. (ed.) *Immunology of Reproduction. Proceedings of the Fifth International Symposium on Immunology of Reproduction*, 26–29 May, pp. 482–5. (Sofia, Varna, Bulgaria: Bulgarian Academy of Sciences Press)
39. Adeghe, J.-H. A., Cohen, J. and Sawers, S. R. (1986). Relationship between local and systemic autoantibodies to sperm, and evaluation of immunobead test for sperm surface antibodies. *Acta Eur. Fertil.*, **17**, 99–105
40. Yeh, W.-R., Acosta, A. A., Seltman, H. J. and Doncel, G. (1995). Impact of immunoglobulin isotype and sperm surface location of antisperm antibodies on fertilization *in vitro* in the human. *Fertil. Steril.*, **63**, 1287–92
41. Haas, G. G. Jr, Schreiber, A. D. and Blasco, L. (1983). The incidence of sperm-associated immunoglobulin and C_3, the third component of complement, in infertile men. *Fertil. Steril.*, **39**, 542–7
42. Kibrick, S., Belding, D. L. and Merrill, B. (1952). Methods for the detection of antibodies against mammalian spermatozoa: gelatin agglutination test. *Fertil. Steril.*, **3**, 430–5
43. Rumke, P. (1954). The presence of sperm antibodies in the serum of two patients with oligozoospermia. *Vox Sang. (Basel)*, **4**, 135–9
44. Dondero, F., Lenzi, A., Gandini, L., Lombardo, F. and Culassao, F. (1991). A comparison of the direct immunobead test and other tests for sperm antibodies detection. *J. Endocrinol. Invest.*, **14**, 443–9
45. Shulman, S. (1988). Autoimmune aspects of human infertility. *In Vivo*, **2**, 57–60
46. Shulman, S. and Moskovljevic, P. M. (1991). Antibodies to spermatozoa. XII. The critical performance of the Gelatin Agglutination Tests (GAT). *Acta Eur. Fertil.*, **22**, 69–74
47. Henry, W. F. (1989). Detection and treatment of antispermatozoal antibodies in men. *Reprod. Fertil. Dev.*, **1**, 205–20
48. Mohan, H., Yadav, S., Singh, U., Kadian, A. and Mohan, P. (1990). Circulating iso and autoantibodies to human spermatozoa in infertility. *Indian J. Pathol. Microbiol.*, **33**, 161–5
49. Gandini, L., Lombardo, F., Lenzi, A. and Dondero, F. (1991). Radioimmuno binding test for anti-sperm antibody detection: analysis and critical revision of various methodological steps. *Andrologia*, **23**, 61–8
50. Lenzi, A., Gandini, L., Lombardo, F., Cappa, M., Nandini, P., Ferro, F., Borrelli, P. and Dondero, F.

(1991). Antisperm antibodies in young boys. *Andrologia*, **23**, 233–5

51. Purvis, K. and Egdetveit, I. (1993). Use of particle filters for increased practicability in sperm processing: application to the direct immunobead test. *Fertil. Steril.*, **59**, 1135–7
52. Franklin, R. R. and Dukes, C. D. (1964). Antispermatozoal antibody and unexplained infertility. *Am. J. Obstet. Gynecol.*, **89**, 6–9
53. Friberg, J. (1974). A simple and sensitive micromethod for demonstration of sperm-agglutinating activity in serum from infertile men and women. *Acta Obstet. Gynecol. Scand.*, (Suppl. 36), 21–9
54. Meinertz, H. (1991). Antisperm antibodies in split ejaculates. *Am. J. Reprod. Immunol.*, **26**, 110–13
55. Adeghe, J. H. (1993). Male subfertility due to sperm antibodies: a clinical overview. *Obstet. Gynecol. Surv.*, **48**, 1–8
56. De Almeida, M., Zouari, R., Jouannet, P. and Feneux, D. (1991). *In vitro* effects of anti-sperm antibodies on human sperm movement. *Hum. Reprod.*, **6**, 405–10
57. Janssen, H. J., Bastiaans, B. A., Goverde, H. J., Hollanders, H. M., Wetzels, A. A. and Schellekens, L. A. (1992). Antisperm antibodies and *in vitro* fertilization. *J. Assist. Reprod. Genet.*, **9**, 345–9
58. Kahn, J. A., Sunde, A., von Düring, V., Sørdal, T., Remen, A., Lippe, B., Siegel, J. and Molne, K. (1993) Formation of antisperm antibodies in women treated with fallopian tube perfusion. *Hum. Reprod.*, **8**, 1414–19
59. Hinting, A., Vermeulen, L., Goethals, I., Dhont, M. and Comhaire, F. (1989). Effect of different procedures of semen preparation on antibody-coated spermatozoa and immunological infertility. *Fertil. Steril.*, **52**, 1022–6
60. Kremer, J. and Jager, S. (1992). The significance of antisperm antibodies for sperm-cervical mucus interaction. *Hum. Reprod.*, **7**, 781–4
61. Lähteenmäki, A. (1993). *In vitro* fertilization in the presence of antisperm antibodies detected by the mixed antiglobulin reaction (MAR) and the tray agglutination test (TAT). *Hum. Reprod.*, **8**, 84–8
62. Menge, A. C. and Naz, R. K. (1993). Immunoglobulin (Ig) G, IgA, and IgA subclass antibodies against fertilization antigen-1 in cervical secretions and sera of women of infertile couples. *Fertil. Steril.*, **60**, 658–63
63. Morroll, D. R., Lieberman, B. A. and Matson, P. L. (1993). The detection of antisperm antibodies in serum: a comparison of the tray agglutination test, indirect immunobead test and indirect SpermCheck assay. *Int. J. Androl.*, **16**, 207–13
64. Andolz, P., Bielsa, M. A., Martinez, P., Garcia-Framis, V., Benet-Rubinat, J. M. and Egozcue, J. (1990). Detection of antisperm antibodies in serum, seminal plasma and cervical mucus by the immunobead test. *Hum. Reprod.*, **5**, 685–9
65. Weir, D. M. (1977). The interaction of antibody with antigen. In *Immunology, an Outline for Students of Medicine and Biology*, 4th edn, pp. 172–200. (London, New York: Churchill Livingstone)
66. Isojima, S., Shun, T. and Ashikata, Y. (1968). Immunologic analysis of sperm-immobilizing factor found in sera of women with unexplained sterility. *Am. J. Obstet. Gynecol.*, **101**, 677–83
67. Isojima, S., Tsuchiya, K., Koyama, K., Tanaka, C., Nako and Adachi, H. (1972). Further studies on sperm immobilizing antibody found in sera of unexplained cases of sterility in women. *Am. J. Obstet. Gynecol.*, **112**, 199–207
68. Kay, D. J. and Boettcher, B. (1992). Comparison of the SpermMar test with currently accepted procedures for detecting human sperm antibodies. *Reprod. Fertil. Dev.*, **4**, 175–81
69. Jager, S., Kremer, J. and Van Slochteren-Draaisma, T. (1978). A simple method of screening for antisperm antibodies in the human male. Detection of spermatozoal surface IgG with the direct mixed antiglobulin reaction carried out on untreated fresh human semen. *Int. J. Fertil.*, **23**, 12–21
70. Schulman, S. (1986). Sperm antigens and autoantibodies: Effects on fertility. *Am. J. Reprod. Immunol. Microbiol.*, **10**, 82–9
71. Eggert-Kruse, W., Huber, K., Rohr, G. and Runnebaum, B. (1993). Determination of antisperm antibodies in serum samples by means of enzyme-linked immunosorbent assay – a procedure to be recommended during infertility investigation? *Hum. Reprod.*, **8**, 1405–13
72. Hendry, W. F. (1991). Corticoid therapy – risk/benefit? *Fertil Steril.*, **55**, 652–3
73. Hirsch, I. H., Sedor, J., Callahan, H. J. and Staas, W. E., Jr. (1990). Systemic sperm autoimmunity in spinal-cord injured men. *Arch. Androl.*, **25**, 69–73
74. Coombs, R. R. A., Marks, J. and Bedford, D. (1956). Specific mixed agglutination: Mixed erythrocyte–platetlet anti-globulin reaction for detection of platelet antibodies. *Br. J. Haematol.*, **2**, 84–94
75. Hendry, W. F. and Stedronska, J. (1980). Mixed erythrocyte–spermatozoa antiglobulin reaction (MAR test) for the detection of antibodies against spermatozoa in infertile males. *J. Obstet. Gynecol.*, **1**, 59–62
76. Hendry, W. F., Stredonska, J. and Lake, R. A. (1982). Mixed erythrocyte spermatozoa antiglobulin reaction (MAR-test) for IgA antisperm antibodies in subfertile males. *Fertil. Steril.*, **37**, 108–12
77. Mathur, S., Williamson, H. D., Landgrebe, S. C., Smith, S. L. and Fudenberg, H. H. (1979). Application of passive hemagglutination for evaluation of antisperm antibodies and a modified Coomb's test for detecting male auto-immunity to sperm antigens. *J. Immunol. Method.*, **30**, 381–6
78. Hellstrom, W. J. G., Samuels, S. J., Waits, A. B. and Overstreet, J. W. (1989). A comparison of the usefulness of SpermMar and Immunobead tests for the detection of antisperm antibodies. *Fertil. Steril.*, **52**, 1027–31

79. Foresta, C., Varotto, A. and Caretto, A. (1990). Immunomagnetic method to select human sperm without sperm surface-bound autoantibodies in male autoimmune infertility. *Arch. Androl.*, **24**, 221–5
80. Nikolaeva, M. A., Kulakov, V. I., Ter-Avanesov, G. V., Terekhina, L. N., Pshenichnikova, T. J. and Sukhikh, G. T. (1993). Detection of antisperm antibodies on the surface of living spermatozoa using flow cytometry: preliminary study. *Fertil. Steril.*, **59**, 639–44
81. Sinisi, A. A., Di Finizio, B., Pasquali, D., Scurini, C., D'Apuzzo, A. and Bellastella, A. (1993). Prevalence of antisperm antibodies by Sperm MAR test in subjects undergoing a routine sperm analysis for infertility. *Int. J. Androl.*, **16**, 311–14
82. Khoo, D., Feigenbaum, S. L. and McClure, R. D. (1991). Screening assays for immunologic infertility: a comparative study. *Am. J. Reprod. Immunol.*, **26**, 11–16
83. Wang, C., Baker, H. W. G., Jennings, M. G., Burger, H. G. and Lutjen, P. (1985). Interaction between human cervical mucus and sperm surface antibodies. *Fertil. Steril.*, **44**, 484–8
84. Clarke, G. N., Lopata, A. and Johnston, W. I. H. (1986). Effect of sperm antibodies in females on human *in vitro* fertilization. *Fertil. Steril.*, **46**, 435–41
85. Boettcher, B., Kay, D. J. and Fitchett, S. B. (1982). Successful treatment of male infertility caused by antispermatozoal antibodies. *Med. J. Aust.*, **2**, 471–4
86. Lenzi, A., Gandini, L., Lombardo, F., Micara, G., Culasso, F. and Dondero, F. (1992). *In vitro* sperm capacitation to treat antisperm antibodies bound to the sperm surface. *Am. J. Reprod. Immunol.*, **28**, 51–5
87. Hamilton, F., Gutlay-Yeo, A. L. and Meldrum, D. R. (1989). Normal fertilization in men with high antibody sperm binding by the addition of sufficient unbound sperm *in vitro*. *J.* In Vitro *Fertil. Embryo Transf.*, **6**, 342–4
88. Almagor, M., Margalioth, E. J. and Yaffe, H. (1992). Density differences between spermatozoa with antisperm autoantibodies and spermatozoa covered with antisperm antibodies from serum. *Hum. Reprod.*, **7**, 959–61
89. Liu, D. Y., Clarke, G. N. and Baker, H. W. (1991). Inhibition of human sperm–zona pellucida and sperm–oolemma binding by antisperm antibodies. *Fertil. Steril.*, **55**, 440–2
90. Witkin, S. S. and Chaudhry, A. (1989). Relationship between circulating antisperm antibodies in women and autoantibodies on the ejaculated sperm of their partners. *Am. J. Obstet. Gynecol.*, **161**, 900–3
91. Kortebani, G., Gonzales, G. F., Berrera, C. and Mazzolli, A. B. (1992). Leukcocyte populations in semen and male accessory gland function: Relationship with antisperm antibodies and seminal quality. *Andrologia*, **24**, 197–204
92. Francavilla, F., Romano, R., Santucci, R., Marrone, V. and Corrao, G. (1992). Failure of intrauterine insemination in male immunological infertility in cases in which all spermatozoa are antibody-coated. *Fertil. Steril.*, **58**, 587–92
93. Gonzales, G. F., Kortebani, G. and Mazzolli, A. B. (1992). Effect of isotypes of antisperm antibodies on semen quality. *Int. J. Androl.*, **15**, 220–8
94. Jarow, J. P. and Sanzone, J. J. (1992). Risk factors for male partner antisperm antibodies. *J. Urol.*, **148**, 1805–7
95. Vigano, P., Fusi, F. M., Brigante, C., Busacca, M. and Vignali, M. (1991). Immunomagnetic separation of antibody-labelled from antibody-free human spermatozoa as a treatment for immunologic infertility. A preliminary report. *Andrologia*, **23**, 367–71
96. Clarke, G. N. (1985). Induction of the shaking phenomenon by IgA class antispermatozoal antibodies from serum. *Am. J. Reprod. Immunol. Microbiol.*, **9**, 12–14
97. Clarke, G. N., Stojanoff, A., Cuachi, M. N., McBain, J. C., Speirs, A. L. and Johnston, W. I. H. (1984). Detection of antispermatozoal antibodies of the IgA class in cervical mucus. *Am. J. Reprod. Immunol.*, **5**, 61–5
98. Haas, J. J. Jr and D'Cruz, O. J. (1991). The predominance of IgG1 and IgG3 subclass antisperm antibodies in infertile patients with serum antisperm antibodies. *Am. J. Reprod. Immunol.*, **26**, 104–9
99. Matsuda, T., Muguruma, K., Horii, Y., Ogura, K. and Yoshida, O. (1993). Serum antisperm antibodies in men with vas deferens obstruction caused by childhood inguinal herniorrhaphy. *Fertil. Steril.*, **59**, 1095–7
100. Bronson, R. A., O'Connor, W. J., Wilson, T. A., Bronson, S. K., Chasalow, F. I. and Droesch, K. (1992). Correlation between puberty and the development of autoimmunity to spermatozoa in men with cystic fibrosis. *Fertil. Steril.*, **55**, 1199–204
101. Pretorius, E., Franken, D. R., Shulman, S. and Gloeb, J. (1986). Sperm cervical mucus contact test and immunobead test for sperm antibodies. *Arch. Androl.*, **16**, 199–202
102. Franco, J. G., Schimberni, M. and Stone, S. C. (1987). An immunobead assay for antibodies to spermatozoa in serum. Comparison with traditional agglutination and immobilization tests. *J. Reprod. Med.*, **32**, 188–90
103. Daru, J. and Mathur, S. (1990). A comparison of sperm antibody assays. *Am. J. Obstet. Gynecol.*, **163**, 1622–9
104. Bronson, R., Cooper, G., Rosenfeld, D. and Witkin, S. S. (1984). Detection of spontaneously occurring sperm-directed antibodies in infertile couples by immunobead binding and enzyme-linked immunosorbent assay. *Ann. N.Y. Acad. Sci.*, **438**, 504–7
105. Haas, J. J. Jr, Lambert, H., Stern, J. E. and Manganiello, P. (1990). Comparison of direct radiolabeled antiglobulin assay and the direct immunobead binding test for detection of sperm-associated antibodies. *Am. J. Reprod. Immunol.*, **22**, 130–2
106. Shulman, S. and Hu, C. (1992). A study of the detection of sperm antibody in cervical mucus with

a modified immunobead method. *Fertil. Steril.*, **58**, 387–91
107. Haas, G. G. Jr, D'Cruz, O. J. and DeBault, L. E. (1991). Comparison of the indirect immunobead, radiolabeled and immunofluorescence assays for immunogold G serum antibodies to human sperm. *Fertil. Steril.*, **55**, 377–88
108. Mandelbaum, S. L., Diamond, M. P. and DeCherney, A. H. (1987). The impact of antisperm antibodies on human infertility. *J. Urol.*, **138**, 1–8
109. Sugi, T., Makino, T., Maruyama, T., Nozawa, S. and Iizuka, R. (1993). Influence of immunotherapy on antisperm antibody titer in unexplained recurrent aborters. *Am. J. Reprod. Immunol.*, **29**, 95–9
110. Kremer, J. and Jager, S. (1976). The sperm cervical mucus contact test: A preliminary report. *Fertil. Steril.*, **27**, 335–40
111. Jager, S., Kremer, J., Kuiken, J. and Mulder, I. (1981). The significance of the Fc part of antispermatozoal antibodies for the shaking phenomenon in the sperm cervical–mucus contact test. *Fertil. Steril.*, **36**, 792–7
112. Jager, S., Kremer, J., Kuiken, J. and Van Slochteren-Draaisma, T. (1980). Immunoglobulin class of antispermatozoal antibodies from infertile men and inhibition of *in vitro* sperm penetration into cervical mucus. *Int. J. Androl.*, **3**, 1–14
113. Kremer, J. and Jager, S. (1980). Characteristics of anti-spermatozoal antibodies responsible for the shaking phenomenon with special regard to immunoglobulin class and antigen-reactive sites. *Int. J. Androl.*, **3**, 143–52
114. Jager, S., Kremer, J. and Van Slochteren-Draaisma, T. (1979). Presence of sperm agglutinating antibodies in infertile men and inhibition of *in vitro* sperm penetration into cervical mucus. *Int. J. Androl.*, **2**, 117–30
115. Witkin, S. S. (1983). Enzyme-linked immunosorbent assay (ELISA) for detection of antibodies to spermatozoa. *Res. Reprod.*, **15**, 1–2
116. Voller, A., Bartlett, A. and Bidwell, D. E. (1978). Enzyme immunoassays with special reference to ELISA techniques. *J. Clin. Path.*, **31**, 507–20
117. Ing, R. M. Y., Wang, S. X., Brennecke, A. M. and Jones, W. R. (1985). An improved indirect enzyme-linked immunosorbent assay (ELISA) for the detection of antisperm antibodies. *Am. J. Reprod. Immunol. Microbiol.*, **8**, 15–19
118. Alexander, N. J. and Bearwood, D. (1984). An immunosorption assay for antibodies to spermatozoa: comparison with agglutination and immobilization tests. *Fertil. Steril.*, **41**, 270–6
119. Mathur, S. (1985). Immune and immunogenetic mechanisms in infertility. *Contr. Gynecol. Obstet.*, **14**, 138–50
120. Paul, S., Baukloh, V. and Mettler, L. (1983). Enzyme-linked immunosorbent assays for sperm antibody detection and antigenic analysis. *J. Immunol. Meth.*, **56**, 193–9
121. Marquant-Le Guienne, B. and De Almeida, M. (1986). Role of guinea-pig sperm autoantigens in capacitation and the acrosome reaction. *J. Reprod. Fertil.*, **77**, 337–45
122. Yan, Y. C., Wang, L. F. and Koide, S. S. (1986). Characterization of sperm agglutinating monoclonal antibody and purification of the human sperm antigen. *Int. J. Fertil.*, **31**, 77–85
123. Howe, S. E. and Lynch, D. M. (1986). Quantitation of sperm bindable IgA and IgG in seminal fluid. *Am. J. Reprod. Immunol. Microbiol.*, **11**, 17–23
124. Lynch, D. M., Leali, B. A. and Howe, S. E. (1986). A comparison of sperm agglutination and immobilization assays with a quantitative ELISA for antisperm antibody in serum. *Fertil. Steril.*, **46**, 285–92
125. Smithwick, E. B. and Young, L. G. (1990). Solid-phase indirect immunogold localization of human sperm antigens reacting with antisperm antibodies in human sera. *J. Androl.*, **11**, 246–54
126. Howe, S. E., Grider, S. L., Lynch, D. M. and Fink, L. M. (1991). Antisperm antibody binding to human acrosin: a study of patients with unexplained infertility. *Fertil. Steril.*, **55**, 1176–82
127. Herr, J. C., Flickinger, C. J., Howards, S. S., Yarboro, S., Spell, D. R., Caloras, D. and Gallien, T. N. (1986). An enzyme-linked immunosorbent assay for measuring antisperm autoantibodies following vasectomy in Lewis rats. *Am. J. Reprod. Immunol. Microbiol.*, **11**, 75–81
128. Naz, R. K. (1987). Involvement of fertilization antigen (FA-1) in involuntary immunoinfertility in humans. *J. Clin. Invest.*, **80**, 1375–83
129. Bronson, R. A., Cooper, G. W., Margalioth, E. J., Naz, R. K. and Hamilton, M. S. (1989). The detection in human sera of antisperm antibodies reactive with FA-1, an evolutionary conserved antigen, and with murine spermatozoa. *Fertil. Steril.*, **52**, 457–62
130. Naz, R. K., Chaudhry, A. and Witkin, S. S. (1990). Lymphocyte proliferative response to fertilization antigen in patients with antisperm antibodies. *Am. J. Obstet. Gynecol.*, **163**, 610–13
131. Fichorova, R. N. and Nakov, L. S. (1993). The use of ELISA to evaluate human antibody binding to epididymal sperm from different species. *Am. J. Reprod. Immunol.*, **29**, 109–15
132. Sinton, E. B., Rieman, D. C. and Ashton, M. E. (1991). Antisperm antibody detection using concurrent cytofluorometry and indirect immunofluorescence microscopy. *Am. J. Clin. Pathol.*, **95**, 242–6
133. Naz, R. K. (1992). Effects of antisperm antibodies on early cleavage of fertilized ova. *Biol. Reprod.*, **46**, 130–9
134. Windt, M.-L., Bouic, P. J. D., Menkveld, R. and Kruger, T. F. (1989). Anti-spermatozoa antibody tests: correlation between traditional methods and an enzyme-linked immunosorbent assay (ELISA). *Arch. Androl.*, **23**, 139–45

Antisperm antibodies 2: clinical aspects 13

W.-R. Yeh, A. A. Acosta and J. P. Van der Merwe

INTRODUCTION

The existence of antisperm antibodies (ASA) has long been noted, since the antigenicity of spermatozoa was first demonstrated by Landsteiner and Metchnikoff in 1899. Nevertheless, their presence raised the question of whether such antibodies could cause male infertility. In 1932, Baskin found that temporary infertility in women could be achieved by the injection of human spermatozoa[1]. In 1959, Katsh[2] reported that infertility could be induced in female guinea pigs by intraperitoneal injection of homologous sperm. In the same year, Rümke and Hellinger[3] noted the presence of autoantibodies against spermatozoa in a significant number of men with infertility. McLaren and others also demonstrated reduction of fertility in female mice when iso-immunized with a subcellular sperm fraction[4,5]. In 1981, Yanagimachi reported that the acrosome reaction and sperm– ovum interactions could be impaired by sperm autoantibodies induced in male guinea pigs[6]. Later, Bronson *et al.* developed the immunobead test (IBT) for quantitative detection of antibodies bound to the motile sperm. The correlation between ASA and reproduction results has been extensively investigated in attempts to find out the mechanisms involved in antisperm antibodies impairment of human fertility.

The introduction of assisted reproduction technologies in the therapeutic armamentarium of infertility allowed the use of new endpoints, namely fertilization, implantation and cleavage rates, to evaluate the net impact of the presence of ASA. A wide spectrum of results is present in the literature; however, the majority agreed that fertilization rates are reduced in the presence of ASA.

DIFFERENT TYPES AND DISTRIBUTION OF ASA

The association of antibody activity with the classical r-globulin fraction of serum has long been shown by Kabat[7]. There are three major structural types of antisperm immunoglobulins in humans: immunoglobulin G (IgG), immunoglobulin A (IgA) and immunoglobulin M (IgM). Immunoglobulins are glycoproteins composed of a basic unit made up of four polypeptide chains (Figure 1). The interchain disulfide bonds can be broken by reduction with excess of a sulfydryl reagent. The reduced molecule can be further separated into two different sizes of peptide chains, heavy and light, by lowering the pH.

The primary sequence of amino acids near the amino-terminal portion of the polypeptide possesses a structural complementariness with a specific region of the antigen and is given the name Fab (fragment antigen binding). The carboxyl-terminal portion, constant and obtainable in crystalline form, is termed fragment crystallizable (Fc).

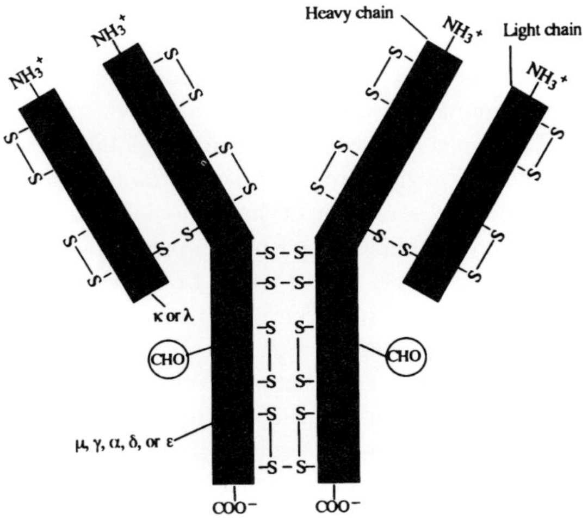

Figure 1 Sequencing studies revealed that immunoglobulin heavy and light chains each contain an amino-terminal variable region that contains 100–110 amino acids and differs from one antibody to the next. The remainder of the molecule contains a small number of constant regions, designated κ or λ in light chains and μ, γ, α, δ or ε in heavy chains

The three classes of sperm immunoglobulins in humans are defined by structural differences in the Fc portion of their heavy chains. The molecular weight can vary from 150 000 for IgG to 900 000 for IgM. IgG and IgA are the two major immunoglobulin classes of antisperm antibodies in the sera of immunologically infertile couples. Whereas IgA is the predominant form of immunoglobulins in local secretions and is commonly composed of two molecules, IgM makes up approximately 10% of normal serum immunoglobulins and exists as a pentamer. IgM antibodies are most prominent in mediating sperm plasma membrane damage and/or sperm immobilization when they interact with immune complements.

In the reproductive tract, IgA is the major immunoglobulin and is produced by plasma cells and epithelial cells. The reproductive tract antibodies differ from circulating antibodies in their relative immunoglobulin concentration and in the structure of immunoglobulins and, consequently, could also differ in antibody affinity and biological activities. Sex steroids influence the immunoglobulin levels in the reproductive tract in an intricate way. An experimental study with ovariectomized rats has shown that estradiol administration would yield a declined level of IgG and IgA in cervical and vaginal content; however, the IgA content in the uterine secretions increased[8]. A different response of each compartment of the female reproductive tract to the hormonal stimulus was demonstrated.

The molecular weight of immunoglobulins and concentration gradient play an important role in the regulation of secretion of immunoglobulins from serum into the different parts of reproductive tract. Within 3–6 h, IgG is transferred from blood to the uterine lumen of ovariectomized rats treated with estradiol[9]. In contrast, IgA takes several days to move into the uterine lumen. While IgG moves down a concentration gradient, IgA accumulation within the uterus is against such a gradient. Evidently, in addition to the leakage of antibodies from systemic serum, some antibodies are being made locally.

It has been well demonstrated that many substances can be readily absorbed through the epithelium of the vagina, cervix and uterus. Moreover, the route of antigen absorption will unavoidably affect local antibodies production. Generally speaking, the immune response was significantly weaker after local vaginal and/or cervical immunization than after systemic immunization. While intraperitoneal and oral immunization with sheep red blood cells (sRBC) produce a significant amount of anti-sRBC antibodies in uterine and vaginal secretions, subcutaneous immunization results in only a weak response. The intragastric immunization of women with polio vaccine results in IgA antibodies in uterine and vaginal secretions[10]. An intriguing study demonstrated that orally ingested sperm reduced fecundity in the rat with production of antisperm antibodies[11].

Several reports have documented that there is a local immune system in the human uterine cervix. The presence of immunoglobulin-producing cells and its local biosynthesis has been demonstrated. The antibody levels in cervical mucus vary markedly during the whole cycle. Concentrations of immunoglobulins in cervical secretions, mainly IgA and IgG, decrease to extremely low levels at midcycle. This decrease is probably due to the preovulatory estradiol rise which will lead to cervical mucus production. Specific antibodies were observed in human cervical mucus against several microorganisms. Lactoferrin and IgG, IgA, and IgM secretory pieces were noted localized in the female reproductive tract by indirect immunofluorescence[12].

By analyzing human Fallopian tubal fluid, the total Fallopian tube immunoglobulin levels are about 10% those of serum and are mainly composed of IgG and IgA. An immunofluorescence study showed that IgG and IgA staining is present along the basement membrane of the Fallopian tubes[13]. Immunological complements are not present in the Fallopian tube fluid to any appreciable extent. Only immunoglobulin A (IgA) antisperm antibody was found significantly more frequently in infertile patients than in fertile controls. This finding suggests that IgA may be a factor that mediates immunologic infertility at the level of the Fallopian tube.

Antibodies in each reproductive compartment are different thoughout the menstrual cycle, and may not be a reflection of antibodies present in serum. Immunoglobulins predominantly of the IgA class directed against specific regions of the sperm surface were present in uterotubal lavages but not in serum, implying their local production. The antisperm antibodies in peritoneal fluid, however, were consistent with those found in serum, indicating their nature as transudates. In that sense, the presence of antisperm antibodies in serum may not precisely reflect the true immunologic status of the female reproductive tract.

ANALYSIS OF ANTISPERM ANTIBODIES

The agglutination technique, commonly used in the past, was first described by Franklin and Dukes in 1964[14]. Subsequently, Kibrick and Friberg modified it and developed the Kibrick's gelatin agglutination test and tray agglutination test, respectively[15]. Unfortunately, since cell agglutination can possibly be caused by serum protein or microorganisms, the agglutination tests would misinterpret the contaminated specimens as positive for antisperm antibodies[16,17].

Evidence has shown that antibodies directed against sperm do not necessarily impair fertility unless these circulating antibodies are also present within the reproductive tract[18,19] and the most direct evidence of autoimmunity to the sperm is the presence of immunoglobulins on sperm surface[20]. Given these considerations, several diagnostic techniques were developed in an attempt to allow the identification of cell bound immunoglobulins on the sperm surface (Table 1). In 1978, Jager developed a simple screening method of mixed agglutination reaction (MAR) to detect IgG on spermatozoal surface[21] (see Chapter 12). The tested semen was mixed with sensitized human Rh-positive red blood cells and rabbit antihuman antiglobulin to see if cell agglutination occur. It is now widely used as a fast screening test for the presence of antisperm antibodies due to its relative sensitivity, useful performance and cost efficiency. However, the IgA-MAR developed later is difficult to read compared with the IgG-MAR and the relatively large size of RBC agglutinates limits its ability to determine the regional binding of antibody to the sperm surface.

Radiolabeled antiglobulin assay

In 1980, the radiolabeled antiglobulin assay used xenogeneic radioiodinated antiglobulins to trace quantitatively the existence of human antisperm antibodies[22]. When utilizing living sperm as antibody targets, they are highly specific and sensitive. However, the regional specificity of antibody binding and the proportion of sperm bound cannot be determined by these techniques. In addition, the procedure requires equipment which is expensive and not readily available in smaller hospitals.

Table 1 Laboratory tests for analysis of ASA

Sperm agglutination test
Franklin–Dukes test
Kibrick's gelatin test
tray agglutination test
Mixed agglutination reaction (MAR)
Radiolabeled antiglobulin assay
Panning procedure
Immunobead test (IBT)
direct IBT
indirect IBT
Complement-dependent immobilization test
Enzyme-linked immunosorbent assay (ELISA)
Immunofluorescent test

Panning procedure

The panning procedure of adding mouse anti-rabbit sperm sera to microtiter wells previously coated with immunoglobulin and allowing anti-immunoglobulin molecules to bind is good for screening[23]. The procedure has the advantage that they are cheap, simple, do not need sperm fixation and may be used with relatively dilute sperm cell suspensions and with sperm of low motility. The drawback is that it does not allow assessment of individual sperm, nor does it provide information regarding regional distribution of immunoglobulins bound on the sperm surface.

Immunobead test (IBT)

The immunobead test (IBT) (see Chapter 12) uses rabbit antihuman immunoglobulin-linked polyacrylamide microspheres as immunobeads (Figure 2). The immunobeads will adhere to the surface of sperm that are antibodies-bound. Quantification can be made by visualization of the number of beads bound to the sperm. Furthermore, the test provides information concerning the regions of sperm surface to which antisperm antibodies are directed and the proportion of sperm which shows antibodies for each

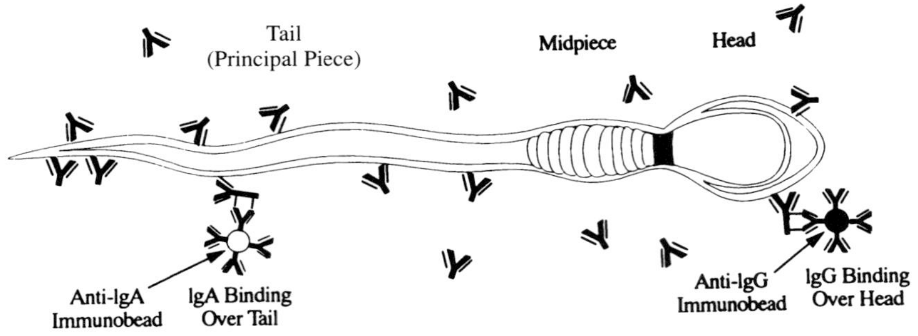

Figure 2 Schematic drawing of the immunobead test. Anti-IgA or anti-IgG covalently linked to polyacrylamide beads binds to IgA or IgG bound to the sperm surface. Quantification of antisperm antibody is by visualization of beads bound to the sperm surface

immunoglobulin class. Compared to agglutination and complement immobilization IBT is specific, sensitive and reproducible[24,25]. ASA can be tested by either the direct or indirect method. Direct IBT is used for the detection of antibodies bound to the surface of motile sperm, and indirect IBT is used for the detection of antisperm antibodies in serum, follicular fluid, cervical mucus and seminal plasma. Since the different types of immunoglobulin will react in different ways it is optimal to determine the immunobead bindings individually (IgG, IgA, IgM) to distinguish the differences. The ultrastructural views under electron microscopy have shown that the beads appeared as electron-dense spheres with a microfibrillar coat on the surface composed of microfilaments radially displaced on the whole bead surface[26,27].

Complement-dependent immobilization test

The complement-dependent immobilization test uses immune complements to interact with IgM or IgG antibodies to form a membrane-attack complex, which is capable of creating damage on the plasma membrane of sperm[28,29]. IgA immunoglobulins do not bind with immune complements and will not result in cell injury. There is a direct correlation between regional specificity of antisperm antibodies to the spermatozoal surface and complement-mediated sperm immobilization[30]. Despite its high specificity for the detection of antisperm antibodies, false-negative results may occur. A recent study has shown the expression of complement inhibitors on human sperm surface, yet their presence does not offer protective effects in restricting antisperm antibodies and complement-mediated injury[31].

Enzyme-linked immunosorbent assay (ELISA)

Enzyme-linked immunosorbent assay (ELISA), first described in 1971, has been widely used in the detection and quantitation of sperm autoimmunity[32–37]. ELISA uses an antiglobulin, conjugated to an enzyme, and a solid phase as a support for one of the immunoreagents. The existence of trace amounts of naturally occurring antisperm antibodies in the majority of men and women, however, reduces the accuracy of the predictive value of ELISA[38]. The method of spermatozoa fixation is important in determining which antigens are presented to the test specimen. Nevertheless, the fixation may damage the sperm surface and cause the loss of some surface antigens and expose the intracellular antigens. In this way, this assay inevitably detects antibodies that interact with either the surface antigens or the subsurface antigens[39]. The relationship between the antibodies' interaction with subsurface antigens and sperm function needs further studies to elucidate it[40]. Another specific shortcoming of the ELISA is that it does not reveal the location of antibody binding on the sperm. In addition, some antibodies remain under-detected by ELISA. A reverse ELISA (antibody capture) has been developed with higher sensitivity and specificity than conventional ELISA in detecting sperm antibodies of different isotypes[38].

Immunofluorescence tests

Immunofluorescence tests utilize fluorescein-conjugated antiglobulins to detect sperm-bound antibodies[41,42]. These procedures can define the binding locus on sperm surface for both IgG and IgA. Unfortunately, a high false-positive result may occur due to the exposure of internal antigens to antiglobulins during the methanol fixation.

POSSIBLE CLINICAL RELEVANCE OF ANTISPERM ANTIBODIES

The potential mechanisms of action concerning how the antisperm antibodies affect human fertility include: (1) interference with sperm production by the testes; (2) restriction of the capability of sperm to penetrate or survive in cervical mucus; (3) reduction of the sperm motility and hindering of its transport; (4) damage of the integrity of sperm plasma membrane if complement mediated; (5) interference with sperm capacitation and/or acrosome reaction; (6) interference with sperm–zona pellucida binding and/or penetration; (7) inhibition of sperm–oolemma fusion; (8) inhibition of the early cleavage of fertilized eggs; (9) suppression of the development of embryo; (10) interference with the implantation process (Table 2).

In the male, spermatogenesis can possibly be impaired as a result of immunologically mediated testicular damage. Locally produced and/or systemically derived sperm autoantibodies may attach to the sperm in the epididymis and suppress spermatozoa maturation, cause resorption or agglutination, or enhance sperm engulfment by activated macrophages[43].

A study investigating the effect of antisperm antibodies on semen quality has demonstrated that semen parameters were altered most frequently when IgM was present in association with IgA and/or IgG[44]. The presence of cytotoxic sperm antibodies in the seminal plasma adversely affects sperm motility as early as 4 h after semen collection[45]. A significant decline in the percentage of motile sperm and a reduced sperm swimming speed were observed in semen from infertile men with antisperm antibodies. Although the real mechanism by which sperm antibodies restrict sperm motion is not completely understood; the Fc region of the immunoglobulin molecule has been implicated in this inhibition process. The binding of Fab fragments to spermatozoa leads to much less impairment of sperm motility than intact immunoglobulins[46].

Table 2 Potential influences of ASA on human fertility

- Interference with sperm production by the testes
- Restriction of the capability of sperm to penetrate or survive in cervical mucus
- Reduction of the sperm motility and hindering of its transport
- Damage of the integrity of sperm plasma membrane
- Interference with sperm capacitation and/or acrosome reaction
- Interference with sperm–zona pellucida binding and/or penetration
- Inhibition of sperm–oolemma fusion
- Inhibition of early cleavage of fertilized eggs
- Suppression of the development of embryo
- Interference with the implantation process

A major site of impaired fertility in men with sperm autoimmunity rests at the level of restricted sperm entry and motility within cervical mucus[47–49]. A correlation has been demonstrated between the immunoglobulin-bound spermatozoa and the number of motile sperm noted within cervical mucus in the postcoital test[50].

Acrosome reaction

In 1980 Tung *et al.* demonstrated that acrosome reaction of guinea pig spermatozoa was completely inhibited in the presence of antisperm antibody molecules *in vitro*[6,51]. Later, through electron microscopy, Tsukui reported that sperm antibodies could interfere with acrosome reaction[52]. Actually, human sperm acrosome reaction is difficult to be accurately assessed by motility pattern or morphological criteria. When acrosome reaction was assessed by using lectin–*Pisum sativum* agglutinin (PSA) labeled with fluorescein isothiocyanate (FITC), antisperm antibodies of any immunoglobulin class did not significantly affect the acrosome reaction rate[53,54]. Meanwhile, quantitative analysis of sperm ultrastructure revealed no significant difference in acrosomal morphology of antibody-coated sperm[55].

When spermatozoa contact the zona pellucida of

the egg they become tightly bound. This species-specific binding suggests that sperm surface has zona-pellucida-binding receptors and the zona has sperm-binding receptors. The presence of antisperm antibodies could interfere with sperm–zona attachment by blocking the receptor site through steric hindrance or epitope specificity. Overwhelming evidence has documented that the existence of antisperm antibodies will inhibit the binding and/or penetration of human sperm to the zona pellucida[52,56–62]. It is believed that there are two kinds of sperm antibodies, one with both activities of sperm immobilization and sperm–zona binding inhibition and another with immobilizing activity only. Most sperm-immobilizing antibodies are capable of blocking sperm–zona interaction even without the presence of immune complement.

By analyzing the result of *in vitro* fertilization, sperm autoantibodies do not seem to hamper embryonal development and implantation[63]. However, a recent study has shown that the antisperm antibodies could lead to abnormally early cleavage of zygotes[64]. Since human gene expression first occurs during the 4–8 cell stages[65], the sperm cell may share antigenic specificity with a developing embryo and provide a cleavage signal to the fertilized ova. The specific sperm surface antigens, if bound to sperm antibodies, will result in late, unequal cleavage and degenerated embryo. Further studies are needed.

Whether antisperm antibodies are directly involved in pregnancy failure is still open to speculation. There is evidence in animal experiments that sperm antibodies could adversely affect post-fertilization events[66]. The mechanism may be partly explained by the fact that sperm share common antigen(s) with lymphocytes and trophoblastic tissues[67,68]. Another plausible explanation is that antisperm antibodies may be a marker for defective immunosuppression, thus exposure of sperm-sensitized pregnant women to sperm may arouse the maternal immune system to respond to paternal antigens on the fetus. Among 109 infertile couples, antisperm antibodies of the IgA and IgG classes were present in nearly 40% of women with a history of miscarriages[69]. Another study detected antisperm antibodies in 36.4% of 44 women with recurrent abortions and 14.6% of 616 female partners of infertile couples which showed a significant association between recurrent miscarriages and IgG tail-directed antisperm antibodies[70]. Different conclusions were reached by Clarke *et al.*[71], who found that only 1.4% of circulating sperm antibodies, either IgG or IgA, could be found in 70 women with a history of recurrent spontaneous abortions. The correlation between sperm autoimmunity and early abortion needs further clarification.

ETIOLOGY

Specific antigens appear on the sperm surface from the beginning of spermatogenesis in puberty. It still remains unclear how these self-antigens can be tolerated and stay unrecognized by the immune system. Meanwhile, although women are inoculated intravaginally with spermatozoa during coitus, it will not usually result in the development of antisperm antibodies. Evidence exists that a population of intraepithelial suppressor T lymphocytes was identified in the epididymis by immunoperoxidase staining with monoclonal antibodies to T-cell surface antigens[72]. Moreover, a decreased number of T-suppressor cells was noted in approximately one-third of men with antisperm antibodies. Therefore, it was suggested that T-suppressor cells may play an important role in preventing the development of autoimmunity to sperm; also, a broad spectrum of immunosuppressive effects on lymphocyte function by seminal plasma has been documented[73,74]. Proliferation of T lymphocytes will be blocked or suppressed by antigen, mitogen and allogenic cells. Complement activity is also inhibited by several protease inhibitors in seminal plasma.

Thus far, the true etiology of the development of antisperm antibodies cannot be positively identified. Certain factors, however, have been proposed to be associated with their development *in vivo* (Table 3). Naturally occurring orchitis leading to immunological infertility occurs in the black mink *Mustela vison* after seasonal regression of the testes[75]. Acute experimental unilateral orchitis was induced in rabbits, causing the production of antisperm antibodies in serum and histological changes in contralateral testicles, therefore impairing fecundity[76].

During genitourinary tract infection, leukocytes and lymphocytes may encounter sperm antigens to which the immune system is not tolerant. Seminal antisperm antibodies activity was significantly

Table 3 Possible factors related to the development of antisperm antibodies

Testicular trauma or orchitis
Genitourinary tract infection
Vasectomy with or without vasovasostomy
Genital tract obstruction
Spinal cord injury
Female sexual practices
Homosexuality
Prostitution
Intrauterine insemination

increased in cases with genital mycoplasmas and *Chlamydia trachomatis*[77,78]. A recent study has shown that *Ureaplasma urealyticum* and *Escherichia coli* appear to be the bacteria most frequently found in cultures from semen of infertile men, and antisperm antibodies are the probable cause of male infertility[79]. Nevertheless, subsequent studies could not confirm these results[80].

Vasectomy

Serum sperm antibodies are present in 50–80% of men who have undergone vasectomy with or without subsequent vasovasostomy[81]. Most show an initial response within 6 weeks–6 months, and titers generally increase over time and may persist for years. Following vasectomy, certain men have abnormalities in seminiferous tubule and Leydig cell functions. Sperm antibodies are most likely to be present in those who demonstrate normal seminiferous tubular activity after vasectomy[82,83]. It has been hypothesized that vasectomy-induced obstruction to sperm transport would cause the development of sperm autoimmunity by allowing entry of sperm antigens into the circulation. Soluble sperm antigens most probably leak from the epididymis after spermatozoa degradation[84]. The immunological status of patients after vasovasostomy has been found to have a high incidence of sperm antibodies associated with significant raised fibronectin levels which may contribute to infertility by its agglutination effect[85–88]. A significantly higher incidence of antisperm antibodies was seen in the men who achieved patency than those who did not[89].

Similar to other men with congenital or acquired obstruction of their genital tract, antisperm antibodies may occur in about one-third of patients with cystic fibrosis[90,91]. The sperm dysfunction may be induced by the presence of sperm antibodies with activated complement-mediated events and interfering with sperm–egg interactions.

The correlation between sperm immunity and spinal cord-injured men remains in dispute. Long-term anejaculation and sperm retention will result in the development of antisperm antibodies in the seminal plasma of spinal cord-injured patients with nearly 80% incidence[92]. This association, however, could not be confirmed by others[93].

The association between female sexual practices and the development of antisperm antibodies also needs further investigation. In a preliminary study with 39 patients, female sexual practices do not appear to be related to the development of sperm autoimmunity[94].

A high incidence of antisperm antibodies was documented in the sera of homosexual men[95,96]. Reportedly, the immunoglobulin isotypes are different in the homosexual and heterosexual infertile male populations. While head-directed antibodies of the IgM class predominate in homosexual men, tail-directed IgG antibodies are more frequently detectable in the sera of heterosexuals. It is most likely that the immune system in colonic submucosa or Peyer's patches is sensitized to the sperm antigen, and then locally stimulated to secrete antisperm antibodies.

A high antisperm antibodies rate was reported among prostitutes[97]. Approximately 40–45% of prostitutes are positive for sperm antibodies, and the incidence further increases to more than 60% in those women who have never used contraceptive methods. These results may be explained by repeated inoculations with multiple different sperm antigens and/or microorganisms.

It has also been hypothesized that intrauterine insemination will cause the formation of antisperm antibodies[98,99]. In a prospective study of 53 enrolled patients, however, there was no difference in serum antisperm antibodies level after intrauterine insemination when the immunobead tests were used[100]. More studies are needed.

PROPOSED TREATMENTS FOR ANTISPERM ANTIBODY

At this point, there is still no unique way to improve the sperm performance and/or promote the fecundity of those who suffer from antisperm antibodies.

Table 4 Proposed therapeutic modalities for ASA

- Use of condoms
- Immunization with partner's lymphocytes or leukocytes
- Systemic administration or local application of corticosteroids
- *In vitro* sperm processing
- Intrauterine insemination (IUI)
- *In vitro* fertilization and embryo transfer (IVF & ET)
- GIFT
- Assisted fertilization

The possible therapeutic methods that have been offered in cases of immunological infertility include: (1) use of condoms; (2) immunization with partner's lymphocytes or leukocytes; (3) systemic administration or local application of corticosteroids; (4) *in vitro* sperm processing; (5) intrauterine insemination; (6) IVF; (7) GIFT; and (8) assisted microfertilization (Table 4).

Traditionally, when sperm-agglutinating antibodies were found in sera and/or in cervical mucus of infertile women, several months of condom therapy was the predominant therapy[14,101]. The results seem to be ineffective in decreasing the antibody titers[102]. Although decreased, there is always a resurgence of sperm antibodies level after cessation of condom therapy.

A recent study has revealed that immunization by intradermally injecting 4×10^7 paternal lymphocytes, collected from 30 mL of heparinized paternal whole blood separated on a Ficoll-Hypaque gradient, into the forearms of each patient four times at intervals of 2–4 weeks could significantly reduce the antisperm antibody titers[103]. The mechanism of action may be partly explained by the increased suppressor T cells and decreased cytotoxic T cells and B cells after immunotherapy. The clinical applications require further elucidation.

In an effort to achieve immunosuppression, either a high-dose short-course regimen (96 mg methylprednisolone orally taken daily for 7 days) or a low-dose long-course regimen (2 mg dexamethasone acetate intramuscularly injected daily for 13 weeks) has been reported to be effective in decreasing the titer of antisperm antibodies[104–106]. The apparent pregnancy success rates were reported to be about 22% where the men were treated and about 14% in treated women[107,108]. The decreased antibody levels were probably due to increased immunoglobulin catabolism and decreased in its synthesis after steroid administration[109]. Such treatment, however, is not without hazard and side-effects were common. Most patients complained of dyspepsia and facial flushing was also commonly reported. To minimize the side-effects derived from steroids, local hydrocortisone was tried in infertile women with antisperm antibodies[110,111]. The initial results of 47 infertile women revealed that this local treatment seemed to be promising in dealing with immunological infertility.

Table 5 Proposed *in vitro* processing of semen to separate or elute antisperm antibodies

Rapid dilution and washing of sperm
Immunobinding on Mage's plate
Immunomagnetic separation
Add albumin to semen collection parts
In vitro sperm capacitation

In vitro processing of semen to remove the antisperm antibodies was advocated on the assumption that spermatozoa become coated with antibodies mostly at the time of ejaculation (Table 5). If sperm are exposed to antibodies in seminal plasma, then a time-dependent transfer of seminal antibodies to the sperm surface must occur after ejaculation. Rapid dilution and washing of semen resulted in a variable decrease in IgG and/or IgA binding[112]. None the less, immunobinding to Mage's plate was reported to be quite effective in increasing the proportion of antibody-free motile spermatozoa[113,114]. An efficient selection of antibody-free spermatozoa can be achieved prior to swim-up migration by immunobinding to polystyrene Petri dishes coated with purified antihuman immunoglobulin antibodies (Mage's plate). The obtained non-adherent sperm populations were depleted of 27–100% of IgG and IgA antibodies. Another *in vitro* technique of immunomagnetic separation by incubation of semen with immunoglobulin-linked magnetic microspheres (Magnetic protAspheres, Boehringer) was also undertaken to separate antibody-free sperm from antibody-coated sperm[115]. The preliminary report demonstrated that it only partially worked in the separation of IgA-bound spermatozoa, and failed for IgG-coated spermatozoa. An immunocolumn separation technique was performed by passage of diluted ejaculate through a column of dextran beads (Sephadex-G200,

Pharmacia) to allow subsequent separation of antibody-free sperm from antisperm antibody-coated sperm[116]. The result of column processing revealed not only increase of sperm motility, but also significant enhancement of hamster egg penetration. Moreover, adding 50% serum to semen sample collection pots, followed by rapid washing of the specimen, was suggested to increase the proportion of antibody-free spermatozoa in the sample[117]. A retrospective study has demonstrated that the addition of serum to the collection device significantly improves the oocyte fertilization rate and subsequent conception rate. *In vitro* sperm capacitation was carried out by incubating sperm in Tyrode's medium with 0.5% human serum albumin as capacitation medium[118]. By evaluating the acrosome region, sperm motility and zona binding ability, the results showed that *in vitro* capacitation was able to elute the bound antibodies from the sperm acrosome area.

Intrauterine insemination

Infertile women with cervical immunity to sperm can benefit from intrauterine insemination[119–122]. The success rates of pregnancy vary from 23% to 40% if sperm autoimmunity is the only factor found, with a nearly 80% chance that the pregnancy will occur in the first two insemination attempts. There was a significantly increased conception rate when more than 15 million motile sperm were inseminated. The head-bound antibodies level apparently reduces the success rate, whereas tail-bound antibodies seemed not to influence the chance of pregnancy. Evidently, artificial insemination of donor sperm was one of the most successful therapies for infertile couples with antisperm antibodies[123]. Theoretically, although intrauterine insemination overcomes the barrier of antibodies from cervical mucus, it cannot circumvent the damage that may be caused by antibodies in the uterine and tubal fluids.

In vitro fertilization (IVF) could be considered a useful treatment for couples with immunological infertility[124,125]. The sperm autoantibodies can interfere with fertilization, particularly when more than 80% of motile spermatozoa are antibody-bound. Data suggest IgA class antibodies may exert more deleterious effects on oocyte fertilization than IgG[126]. In females with sperm immunity, replacement of the patient's serum by donor serum or fetal cord serum was effective in improving fertilization *in vitro*[127–129]. More widely adopted today is the method of adding a sufficient number of motile sperm to provide at least 50 000 unbound sperm per oocyte[130]. It was initially reported to optimize the normal fertilization rate in IVF patients.

Van der Merwe *et al.*[131] reported that in treatment of male sperm autoimmunity by using the gamete intrafallopian transfer (GIFT) with rapidly washed spermatozoa, an ongoing pregnancy rate of 24.1% (7 of 29) per cycle was achieved. Pregnancies treated by means of the GIFT procedure are more probably due to a general improvement of semen parameters: motility and morphology, rather than a decrease in antibodies binding. Meanwhile, GIFT brings the ova into direct contact with free swimming spermatozoa, thereby excluding all the barriers from the cervical mucus upwards.

Assisted fertilization microscopic techniques have been gradually accepted in the treatment of patients with severe male factor and/or low fertilization potential. Although the results of antisperm antibodies treated by these micromanipulative procedures are yet to be reported, the beneficial effects of bypassing the zona pellucida are foreseeable.

ASA AND IVF RESULTS

The majority of the papers published in the literature on IVF results in couples with ASA in the male conclude that the fertilization rate is impaired; also, an association between ASA and low sperm motility has been mentioned.

As in the whole field of ASA in infertility, the results are clouded by several methodological difficulties. The low incidence of ASA in infertile patients does not allow the scientist to analyze statistically meaningful series. Most of the studies are retrospective and, therefore, their experimental designs are questionable. The use of different tests to investigate the presence of ASA and their application to different body materials (serum seminal plasma and sperm in the male, serum cervical mucus and follicular fluid in the female) precludes a uniform evaluation of the problem. The lack of well-proven and clinically useful ASA test result thresholds makes the interpretation of those tests difficult. The use of diverse endpoints (sperm performance in post-coital tests, pregnancy after natural reproduction, with or without other previous treatments superimposed) make a valid evaluation a very difficult task.

The Norfolk Program

Our own retrospective review of the Norfolk experience[132] based on 38 IVF cycles admitted to the program from January 1990 to June 1992, on the basis of showing positive ASA on the sperm by immunobead tests, was coupled to 56 similar patients from the Tygerberg program in South Africa. Matched controls were selected by wives' stimulation protocols and by pre-treatment basic semen analyses characteristics (concentration and motility of sperm samples from controls and patients were within a 10% variation). The differences in mean motility and concentration for both groups and subgroups were not statistically significant. Controls were also matched by type of stimulation used and type of E_2 response. The results showed that the fertilization rate was significantly lower in IVF as well as in GIFT, and the total and term pregnancy rates in IVF per cycle and per transfer, as well as in GIFT, were also lower when compared with their control counterparts. Therefore, our experience agrees with that of other centers and indicates that the presence of ASA on the sperm surface, *per se*, impairs the outcome of assisted reproduction, mainly in terms of fertilization rate of the preovulatory oocytes and possibly in terms of total and term pregnancy rates, regardless of whether IVF or GIFT is used in the treatment of these couples. This holds true regardless of the impact of other semen parameters, particularly the morphology of sperm within the semen sample.

In a second study[133] we reviewed the impact of immunoglobulin isotype and location of ASA on the human sperm surface on the results of *in vitro* fertilization. Other studies published in the literature using direct immunobead tests reported that when >70% of the spermatozoa used for insemination were covered with both immunoglobulins (IgG and IgA) the fertilization rate was significantly reduced. Other investigators showed similar results and used >80% threshold as an indicator of low fertilization mainly when IgA was involved. Unfortunately, none of them have mentioned the status of the IgM isotype and its influence on the fertilization rate, and the majority have a small number of oocytes analyzed. It has also been postulated that sera containing immunoglobulins of IgG and IgM isotypes directed primarily against the sperm head diminished the percentage of eggs penetrated by sperm. One publication noticed that antibodies reacting with the sperm tails may directly interfere with fertilization *in vitro*.

In Norfolk, from January 1990 to January 1994, 48 couples proved to be positive for male ASA by immunobead tests for IgG, IgA and IgM (of these 48, nine were tested only for IgG). These patients have undergone a total of 80 IVF cycles (series 35–53). The mean age of wives was 35.4 ± 3.4 years (mean ± SD). The average sperm concentration was 73.4 ± 55.2 million/mL, mean sperm motility was 50.2 ± 20.9, mean percentage of normal forms of spermatozoa by strict criteria was 7.8 ± 4.7%, and of slightly abnormal forms was 18.1 ± 8.9%. The total number of mature oocytes available for insemination was 574. The mean total fertilization rate was 61.3 ± 39.6%. The patients were divided into three groups according to their fertilization rates. The thresholds used were obtained from the results of the Norfolk embryology laboratory. Normal fertilization rate using normal preovulatory oocytes and normal sperm is about 90%. After subtracting two standard deviations, the minimum total fertilization rate that could be considered normal in the Norfolk program is therefore 50%[134]. Thus, patients were classified as normal fertilization when the fertilization rate was >50% (n=31); low fertilization with fertilization between 1% and 50% (n=12); and no fertilization at all (n=5). The sperm concentration, motility, percentage of normal forms and of slightly abnormal forms in each group show no significant differences. The insemination concentration of sperm during IVF showed that a significantly higher sperm number was used in the low fertilization group (Table 3). Further investigation through a linear regression analysis showed that the sperm insemination concentration had no correlation with the IgG, IgA, or IgM immunoglobulin level (P=0.342).

Our results showed no correlation between the

immunoglobulin isotype bound to the sperm surface and the fertilization rate when IgG and IgA were involved. Nevertheless, the IgM that was present in 44% of our patients had a strong correlation with the fertilization rates.

Furthermore, when IgA immunoglobulin binding was present in a high number of sperm (≥68%), the total fertilization rate dropped abruptly from 48.6% for those with <68% of the sperm predominantly bound to IgA to 14.6% for those with ≥68% of the sperm bound to IgA. When IgM immunoglobulins were found on the sperm surface, no fertilization occurred when >40% of the sperm showed IgM binding.

When we look at the importance of the location of the binding sites, IgA showed a statistical reduction in fertilization rate only when head-directed antibodies were present.

IgM, meanwhile, showed a strong correlation with the fertilization rate when binding was present at the level of the head and/or the tail tip. For those couples with ≥6% of the sperm bound to IgM over head and/or tail tip, the fertilization rate was <50% (low). When head/tail tip-directed IgM was present in >10% of the sperm, the fertilization rate dropped further to <30%.

These results seem to indicate that two male antisperm Ig isotypes significantly impair fertilization rates. IgA exerted its impact when a high level of binding was detected and only when localized on the head. IgM, present in 44% of the males, was the immunoglobulin isotype that most significantly affected fertilization rates, producing impairment when localized both at the head and at the tail tip.

CONCLUSION

ASA present on spermatozoa or in fluids of the female reproductive tract are important factors in infertility. It is estimated that 5–10% of male infertility is caused by sperm autoimmunity, and approximately 10–15% of women with unexplained infertility have circulating sperm antibodies.

The immunobead test can be used to directly quantify the sperm antibodies on the sperm surface. Immunoglobulin isotypes, binding sites on the sperm surface and proportion of spermatozoa that are antibody-bound can be accurately assessed.

The mechanism of action of sperm antibodies, although still lacking consensus, is most likely at the level of sperm binding and penetration of the zona pellucida as indicated by most studies.

Patients who acquire genitourinary tract infections, who have genital tract obstruction, who have undergone vasectomy and who have special sexual behaviors are prone to develop ASA. The real etiology of antisperm antibodies, however, remains disputed.

Of course, antisperm antibodies can reduce the chance of pregnancy but they are a relative, rather than absolute, cause of male infertility. Their sole presence will not necessarily lead to infertility. The degree of influence depends upon many factors. The total levels of antibody – the binding area on the spermatozoa, the density of binding, the type of immunoglobulins and the distribution sites in the human body – all contribute to impair the human fecundity. Our results indicate that the presence of IgG sperm antibodies is not relevant to the oocyte fertilization rate. IgA may affect fertilization only when >68% of the sperm are bound to the immunoglobulin and IgM, when present, will lower the fertilization rate remarkably. A partial explanation may be that IgM owns high valency for antigen binding (5–10 for IgM, 2 for IgG, 2–4 for IgA), and has a very efficient agglutinating ability and complement fixation. Meanwhile, there may be a concurrent infection process induced locally by the presence of IgM.

The head is the only site of binding for IgA sperm antibodies that exerts a deleterious effect on fertilization. For IgM, however, both head and tail tip bindings can drastically decrease the sperm fertilizing potential. Head status of spermatozoa has long been assumed to play a key role in fertilization due to the importance of acrosome reaction, in zona penetration and nuclear content. The tail tip, on the other hand, is important for the motility and hyperactivation that will provide spermatozoa the indispensable physiological ability for the fertilizing process to occur.

Proposed therapeutic efforts have shown a great variability in results. Sperm processing *in vitro* obviously cannot remove all the sperm antibodies, especially for those immunoglobulins already bound. Micromanipulation may offer some help. Clearly, further improvements await a better analysis and understanding of sperm autoimmunity at molecular level.

Since sperm are composed of numerous antigens many antibodies can develop, but not all of them will interfere with fertility. Meanwhile, antibodies can affect fertilization at many different sites. To define which antibodies may affect fertility, where they exert their effects and which ones may be used for contraception purposes, monoclonal antibodies have been developed. Hybridoma techniques have been used to define a number of antisperm monoclonal antibodies and the corresponding sperm antigens have been extensively investigated[135–137]. On the other hand, molecular analysis of the antigenicity and immunogenicity of sperm proteins may help to characterize the functional antigenic domains on sperm, which are beneficial in designing a safe and effective contraceptive vaccine in the future.

References

1. Baskin, M. J. (1932). Temporary sterilization by the injection of human spermatozoa: A preliminary report. *Am. J. Obstet. Gynecol.*, **24**, 892–7
2. Katsh, S. (1959). Infertility in female guinea pigs induced by injection of homologous sperm. *Am. J. Obstet. Gynecol.*, **78**, 276–8
3. Rumke, P. and Hellinger, G. (1959). Auto-antibodies against spermatozoa in sterile men. *Am. J. Clin. Pathol.*, **32**, 357–9
4. McLaren, A. (1964). Immunological control of fertility in female mice. *Nature*, **201**, 582–5
5. Bell, E. B. and McLaren, A. (1979). Reduction of fertility in female mice iso-immunized with a subcellular sperm fraction. *J. Reprod Fertil.*, **22**, 345–6
6. Yanagimachi, R., Okada, A. and Tung, K. S. K. (1981). Sperm auto-antigens and fertilization. II. Effects of anti-guinea pig serum antibodies on sperm-ovum interactions. *Biol. Reprod.* **24**, 512–18
7. Kabat, E. A. (1968). *Structural Concepts in Immunology and Immunochemistry*. (New York: Holt, Rinehart and Winston)
8. Wira, C. R. and Sandor, C. P. (1977). Sex steroid hormone regulation of IgA and IgG in rat uterine secretions. *Nature*, **268**, 534–6
9. Sullivan, D. A. and Wira, C. R. (1984). Hormonal regulation of immunoglobulins in the rat uterus. Uterine response to multiple estradiol treatments. *Endocrinology*, **114**, 650–8
10. Ogra, P. L. and Ogra, S. A. (1973). Local antibody response to polio vaccine in the human female genital tract. *J. Immunol.*, **110**, 1307–11
11. Allardyce, R. A. (1984). Effect of ingested sperm on fecundity in the rat. *J. Exp. Med.*, **159**, 1548–50
12. Tourville, D. R., Ogra, S. S., Lippes, J. and Tomasi, T. B. Jr. (1970). The human female reproductive tract. Immunohistological localizing of A, G, M secretory piece and lactoferrin. *Am. J. Obstet. Gynecol.*, **108**, 1102–4
13. Lippes, J. (1975). Applied physiology of the uterine tube. *Obstet. Gynecol. Ann.*, **4**, 119-66
14. Franklin, R. R. and Dukes, C. D. (1964). Antispermatozoal antibody and unexplained infertility. *Am. J. Obstet. Gynecol.*, **89**, 6–11
15. Kibrick, S., Belding, D.L. and Merrill, B. (1952). Methods for the detection of antibodies against mammalian spermatozoa. II. A gelatin agglutination test. *Fertil. Steril.*, **3**, 430–8
16. Rose, N. R., Hjort, T., Rumke, P., Harper, M. J. K. and Vyazov, O. (1976). Techniques for detection of iso-and auto-antibodies to human spermatozoa. *Clin. Exp. Immunol.*, **23**, 175–7
17. Bell, E. B. (1968). An immune-type agglutination of mouse spermatozoa by *Pseudomonas maltophilia*. *J. Reprod. Fertil.*, **17**, 275–6
18. Eggert-Kruse, W., Christmann, M., Gerhard, I., Pohl, S., Klinga, K. and Runnebaum, B. (1989). Circulating antisperm antibodies and fertility prognosis: a prospective study. *Hum. Reprod.*, **4**, 513–20
19. Collins, J. A., Burrows, E. A., Yeo, J. and YoungLai, E. V. (1993). Frequency and predictive value of antisperm antibodies among infertile couples. *Hum. Reprod.*, **8**, 592–8
20. Clarke, G. N., Elliot, P. G. and Smaila, C. (1985). Detection of sperm antibodies in semen using the immunobead test. A study of 813 consecutive patterns. *Am. J. Reprod. Immunol. Microbiol.*, **7**, 61–4
21. Jager, S., Kremer, J. and Van Slochteren-Draaisma, T. (1978). A simple method of screening for antisperm antibodies in the human male. Detection of spermatozoal surface IgG with the direct mixed agglutination reaction carried out in untreated fresh human semen. *Int. J. Fertil.*, **23**, 12–15
22. Haas, G. G., Cines, D. B. and Schreiber, A. D. (1980). Immunologic infertility: identification of patients with antisperm antibody. *N. Engl. J. Med.*, **303**, 722–7
23. Hancock, R. J. T. and Farakis, S. (1984). Detection of antibody-coated sperm by panning procedures. *J. Immunol. Meth.*, **66**, 149–53
24. Bronson, R. A., Cooper, G. and Hjort, T. (1985). Antisperm antibodies, detected by agglutination,

immobilization, microtoxicity and immunobead binding assays. *J. Reprod. Immunol.*, **8**, 279–82
25. Dondero, F., Lenzi, A., Gandini, L., Lombardo, F. and Culasso, F. (1991). A comparison of the direct immunobead test and other tests for sperm antibodies detection. *J. Endocrinol. Invest.*, **14**, 443–9
26. Lenzi, A., Caggiati, A., Gandini, L., Claroni, F. and Dondero, F. (1987). Scanning electron microscopy patterns in the antisperm antibodies detection with immunobead test. *Arch. Androl.*, **19**, 159–60
27. Lenzi, A., Familiari, G., Caggiati, A., Gandini, L., Claroni, F. and Dondero, F. (1988). Antisperm antibodies detection with the immunobead test as viewed by TEM. *Arch. Androl.*, **20**, 261–5
28. Hamerlynch, J. and Rumke, P. (1968). A test for the detection of cytotoxic antibodies in men. *J. Reprod. Fertil.*, **17**, 191–6
29. Isojima, S., Tsuchiya, K., Koyama, K. and Tanaka, C. (1972). Further studies on sperm-immobilizing antibody found in sera of unexplained cases of sterility in women. *Am. J. Obstet. Gynecol.*, **112**, 199–204
30. Bronson, R. A., Cooper, G. W. and Rosenfeld, D. L. (1982). Correlation between regional specificity of antisperm antibodies to the spermatozoal surface and complement-mediated sperm immobilization. *Am. J. Reprod. Immunol.*, **2**, 222–6
31. D'Cruz, O. J. and Haas, G. G. Jr (1993). The expression of the complement regulators CD46, CD55, and CD59 by human sperm does not protect them from antisperm antibody- and complement-mediated immune injury. *Fertil. Steril.*, **59**, 876–84
32. Zanchetta, R., Busolo, F. and Mastrogiacomo, I. (1982). The enzyme-linked immunosorbent assay for detection of the antispermatozoal antibodies. *Fertil. Steril.*, **38**, 730–4
33. Paul, S., Baukloh, V. and Mettler, L. (1983). Enzyme-linked immunosorbent assays for sperm antibody detection and antigenic analysis. *J. Immunol. Meth.*, **56**, 193–9
34. Itoh, M., Hiramine, C., Koseto, M. and Hojo, K. (1989). Enzyme-linked immunosorbent assay (ELISA) for detecting antisperm antibodies in mice with testicular autoimmunity. *Am. J. Reprod. Immunol.*, **21**, 9–15
35. Windt, M. L., Bouic, P. J., Lombard, C. J., Menkveld, R. and Kruger, T. F. (1989). Antisperm antibody tests: traditional methods compared to ELISA. *Arch. Androl.*, **23**, 139–45
36. Fusi, F., Vigano, P., Doldi, N., Brigante, C. and Busacca, M. (1989). Comparison between immunobead test, indirect immunofluorescence and a quantitative ELISA for the diagnosis of antisperm antibodies. *Acta Eur. Fertil.*, **20**, 23–7
37. Fichorova, R. N. and Nakov, L. S. (1993). The use of ELISA to evaluate human antibody binding to epididymal sperm from different species. *Am. J. Reprod. Immunol.*, **29**, 109–15
38. Hjort, T. and Hansen, K. B. (1971). Immunofluorescent studies on human spermatozoa. I. The detection of different spermatozoal antibodies and their occurrence in normal and infertile women. *Clin. Exp. Immunol.*, **8**, 9–23
39. Mettler, L., Czuppon, A. B. and Alexander, N. (1985). Antibodies to spermatozoa and seminal plasma antigens detected by various enzyme-linked immunosorbent (ELISA) assays. *J. Reprod. Immunol.*, **8**, 301–5
40. Fichorova, R. and Anderson, D. J. (1991). Use of sperm viability and acrosomal status assays in combination with immunofluorescence technique to ascertain surface expression of sperm antigens. *J. Reprod. Immunol.*, **20**, 1–13
41. Tung, K. S. K., Cooke, W. D. J., McCarty, T. A. and Robitaille, P. (1976). Human sperm antigens and antisperm antibodies. II. Age-related incidence of antisperm antibodies. *Clin. Exp. Immunol.*, **25**, 73–9
42. Shai, S., Bar Yoseph, N., Peer, E. and Naot, Y. (1990). A reverse (antibody capture) enzyme-linked immunosorbent assay for detection of antisperm antibodies in sera and genital tract secretions. *Fertil. Steril.*, **54**, 894–901
43. London, S. N., Haney, A. F., and Weinberg, J. B. (1985). Macrophages and infertility: enhancement of human macrophage-mediated sperm killing by antisperm antibodies. *Fertil. Steril.*, **43**, 274–8
44. Gonzales, G. F., Kortebani, G. and Mazzolli, A. B. (1992). Effect of isotypes of antisperm antibodies on semen quality. *Int. J. Androl.*, **15**, 220–8
45. Shuxiang, X., Tsai, C. C., Williamson, H. O. and Mathur, S. (1990). Time-related decline in sperm motility patterns in men with cytotoxic antibodies. *Arch. Androl.*, **24**, 267–75
46. Jager, S., Kremer, J., Kuiken, J. and Mulder, I. (1981). The significance of the Fc part of antispermatozoal antibodies for the shaking phenomenon in the sperm–cervical mucus contact test. *Fertil. Steril.*, **36**, 792–7
47. Alexander, N. J. (1984). Antibodies to human spermatozoa impede sperm penetration of cervical mucus or hamster eggs. *Fertil. Steril.*, **411**, 433–9
48. Bronson, R. A., Cooper, G. W., Rosenfeld, D. L., Gilbert, J. V. and Plaut, A. G. (1987). The effect of an IgA1 protease on immunoglobulins bound to the sperm surface and sperm cervical mucus penetrating ability. *Fertil. Steril.*, **47**, 984–90
49. Daru, J., Williamson, H. O., Rust, P. F., Homm, R. J. and Mathur, S. (1988). A computerized postcoital test sperm motility: comparison with clinical postcoital test and correlations with sperm antibodies. *Arch. Androl.*, **21**, 189–203
50. Bronson, R. A., Cooper, G. W. and Rosenfeld, D. L. (1984). Autoimmunity to spermatozoa: effect on sperm penetration of cervical mucus as reflected by postcoital testing. *Fertil. Steril.*, **41**, 609–16

51. Tung, K. S., Okada, A. and Yanagimachi, R. (1980). Sperm autoantigens and fertilization. I. Effects of antisperm autoantibodies on rouleaux formation, viability, and acrosome reaction of guinea pig spermatozoa. *Biol. Reprod.*, **23**, 877–86
52. Tsukui, S., Noda, Y., Fukuda, A., Matsumoto, H., Tatsumi, K. and Mori, T. (1988). Blocking effect of sperm immobilizing antibodies on sperm penetration of human zonae pellucidae. *J.* In Vitro *Fertil. Embryo Transf.*, **5**, 123–8
53. Francavilla, F., Romano, R. and Santucci, R. (1991). Effect of sperm-antibodies on acrosome reaction of human sperm used for the hamster egg penetration assay. *Am. J. Reprod. Immunol.*, **25**, 77–80
54. Romano, R., Santucci, R., Marrone, V. and Francavilla, F. (1993). Effect of ionophore challenge on hamster egg penetration and acrosome reaction of antibody-coated sperm. *Am. J. Reprod. Immunol.*, **29**, 56–61
55. Bronson, R. A., Cooper, G. W. and Phillips, D. M. (1989). Effects of anti-sperm antibodies on human sperm ultrastructure and function. *Hum. Reprod.*, **4**, 653–7
56. Bronson, R. A., Cooper, G. W. and Rosenfeld, D. L. (1982). Sperm-specific isoantibodies and autoantibodies inhibit the binding of human sperm to the human zona pellucida. *Fertil. Steril.*, **38**, 724–9
57. Tsukui, S., Noda, Y., Yano, J., Fukuda, A. and Mori, T. (1986). Inhibition of sperm penetration through human zona pellucida by antisperm antibodies. *Fertil. Steril.*, **46**, 92–6
58. Liu, D. Y., Clarke, G. N. and Gordon Baker, H. W. (1991). Inhibition of human sperm–zona pellucida and sperm–oolemma binding by antisperm antibodies. *Fertil. Steril.*, **55**, 440–2
59. Mahony, M. C. and Alexander, N. J. (1991). Sites of antisperm antibody action. *Hum. Reprod.*, **6**, 1426–30
60. Dubova Mihailova, M., Mollova, M., Ivanova, M., Kehayov, I. and Kyurkchiev, S. (1991). Identification and characterization of human acrosomal antigen defined by a monoclonal antibody with blocking effect on *in vitro* fertilization. *J. Reprod. Immunol.*, **19**, 251–68
61. Shibahara, H., Burkman, L. J., Isojima, S. and Alexander, N. J. (1993). Effects of sperm-immobilizing antibodies on sperm–zona pellucida tight binding. *Fertil. Steril.*, **60**, 533–9
62. Zouari, R., De Almeida, M., Rodrigues, D. and Jouannet, P. (1993). Localization of antibodies on spermatozoa and sperm movement characteristics are good predictors of *in vitro* fertilization success in cases of male autoimmune infertility. *Fertil. Steril.*, **59**, 606–12
63. Kato, M. (1990). Effect of antisperm antibodies in males on *in vitro* fertilization. *Nippon Sanka Fujinka Gakkai Zasshi*, **42**, 1613–19
64. Naz, R. K. (1992). Effects of antisperm antibodies on early cleavage of fertilized ova. *Biol. Reprod.*, **46**, 130–9
65. Braude, P., Bolton, V. and Moore, S. (1988). Human gene expression first occurs between the four- and eight-cell stages of preimplantation development. *Nature*, **332**, 459–61
66. Menge, A. C. (1979). Immune reactions and infertility. *J. Reprod Fertil.*, **10**, 171–5
67. Mathur, S., Gust, J. M., Williamson, H. O. and Fudenberg, H. H. (1980). Antigenic cross-reactivity of sperm and T lymphocytes. *Fertil Steril.*, **34**, 469–76
68. McIntyre, J. A. and Faulk, W. P. (1978). Suppression of mixed lymphocyte cultures by antibodies against human trophoblast membrane antigens. *Transplant. Proc.*, **10**, 919–25
69. Witkin, S. S. and David, S. S. (1988). Effect of sperm antibodies on pregnancy outcome in a subfertile population. *Am. J. Obstet. Gynecol.*, **158**, 59–62
70. Witkin, S. S. and Chaudhry, A. (1989). Association between recurrent spontaneous abortions and circulating IgG antibodies to sperm tails in women. *J. Reprod. Immunol.*, **15**, 151–8
71. Clarke, G.N. and Baker, H. W. G. (1993). Lack of association between sperm antibodies and recurrent spontaneous abortion. *Fertil. Steril.*, **59**, 463–4
72. Ritchie, A. W. S., Hargreave, T. B., James, K. and Chisholm, G. D. (1984). Intraepithelial lymphocytes in the normal epididymis. A mechanism for tolerance to sperm auto-antigens? *Br. J. Urol.*, **56**, 79–83
73. James, K. and Hargreave, T. B. (1984). Immunosuppression by seminal plasma and its possible clinical significance. *Immunol. Today*, **5**, 357–61
74. Anderson, D. J. and Tarter, T. H. (1982). Immunosuppressive effects of mouse seminal plasma components *in vivo* and *in vitro*. *J. Immunol.*, **128**, 535–42
75. Tung, K. S. K., Ellis, L. and Teuscher, C. (1981). The black mink (*Mustela vison*). A natural model of immunologic male infertility. *J. Exp. Med.*, **154**, 1016–18
76. Lekili, M., Tekgul, S., Ergen, A., Tasar, C. and Hascelik, G. (1992). Acute experimental unilateral orchitis in the rabbit and its effect on fertility. *Int. Urol. Nephrol.*, **24**, 291–7
77. Soffer, Y., Ron-El, R., Golan, A., Herman, A., Caspi, E. and Samra, Z. (1990). Male genital mycoplasmas and chlamydia trachomatis culture: its relationship with accessory gland function, sperm quality, and autoimmunity. *Fertil. Steril.*, **53**, 331–6
78. Toth, A., Lesser, M. L., Brooks, C. and Labriola, D. (1983). Subsequent pregnancies among 161 couples treated for T-mycoplasma genital tract infection. *N. Engl. J. Med.*, **308**, 505–7
79. Auroux, M. (1988). Urogenital infection and male fertility. *J. Gynecol. Obstet. Biol. Reprod. Paris*, **17**, 869–75
80. Micic, S., Petrovic, S. and Dotlic, R. (1990). Seminal

antisperm antibodies and genitourinary infection. *Urology*, **35**, 54–6
81. Shulman, S., Zappi, E., Ahmed, U. and Davis, J. (1972). Immunologic consequences of vasectomy. *Contraception*, **5**, 269–74
82. Fisch, H., Labor, E., BarChama, N., Witken, S. S., Tolia, B. M. and Reid, R. E. (1989). Detection of testicular endocrine abnormalities and their correlation with serum antisperm antibodies in men following vasectomy. *J. Urol.*, **141**, 1129–32
83. Naaby Hansen, S. (1990). The humoral autoimmune response to vasectomy described by immunoblotting from two-dimensional gels and demonstration of a human spermatozoal antigen immunochemically crossreactive with the D2 adhesion molecule. *J. Reprod. Immunol.*, **17**, 187–205
84. Alexander, N. J. and Anderson, D. J. (1979). Vasectomy: consequences of autoimmunity to sperm antigens. *Fertil. Steril.*, **32**, 253–60
85. Stauffer, C. W. and Parsons, C. L. (1989). Fibronectin levels in male ejaculate and evidence for its role in unexplained infertility. *Urology*, **34**, 80–5
86. Herr, J. C., Howards, S. S., Spell, D. R., Carey, P. O., Kendrick, S. J., Gallien, T. N., Handley, H. H. and Flickinger, C. J. (1989). The influence of vasovasostomy on antisperm antibodies in rats. *Biol. Reprod.*, **40**, 353–60
87. Broderlick, G. A., Tom, R. and McClure, R. D. (1989). Immunological status of patients before and after vasovasostomy as determined by the immunobead antisperm antibody test. *J. Urol.*, **142**, 752–5
88. Fuchs, E. F. and Alexander, N. J. (1983). Immunologic considerations before and after vasovasostomy. *Fertil. Steril.*, **40**, 497–9
89. Matson, P. L., Junk, S. M., Masters, J. R., Pryor, J. P. and Yovich, J. L. (1989). The incidence and influence upon fertility of antisperm antibodies in seminal fluid following vasectomy reversal. *Int. J. Androl.*, **12**, 98–103
90. D'Cruz, O. J., Haas, G. G. Jr., de la Rocha, R. and Lambert, H. (1991). Occurrence of serum antisperm antibodies in patients with cystic fibrosis. *Fertil. Steril.*, **56**, 519–27
91. Girgis, S. M., Eklandroas, E. M., Iskander, R., El-Dokhly, R. and Girgis, R. N. (1982). Sperm antibodies in serum and semen in men with bilateral congenital absence of the vas deferens. *Arch. Androl.*, **8**, 301–3
92. Hirsch, I. H., Sedor, J., Callahan, H. J. and Staas, W. E. (1992). Antisperm antibodies in seminal plasma of spinal cord-injured men. *Urology*, **39**, 243–7
93. Dahlberg, A. and Hovatta, O. (1989). Anejaculation following spinal cord injury does not induce sperm-agglutinating antibodies. *Int. J. Androl.*, **12**, 17–21
94. Chacho, K. J., Hage, C. W. and Shulman, S. (1991). The relationship between female sexual practices and the development of antisperm antibodies. *Fertil. Steril.*, **56**, 461–4
95. Wolff, H. and Schill, W. B. (1985). Antisperm antibodies in infertile and homosexual men: Relationship to serologic and clinical findings. *Fertil. Steril.*, **44**, 673–9
96. Witkin, S. S. and Sonnabend, J. (1983). Immune response to spermatozoa in homosexual men. *Fertil. Steril.*, **39**, 337–41
97. Bahraminejad, R., Kadanali, S., Erten, O. and Bahar, H. (1991). Reproductive failure and antisperm antibody production among prostitutes. *Acta Obstet. Gynecol. Scand.*, **70**, 483–5
98. Friedman, A. J., Juneau Norcross, M. and Sedensky, B. (1991). Antisperm antibody production following intrauterine insemination. *Hum. Reprod.*, **6**, 1125–8
99. Goldberg, J. M., Haering, P. L., Friedman, C. I., Dodds, W. G. and Kim, M. H. (1990). Antisperm antibodies in women undergoing intrauterine insemination. *Am. J. Obstet. Gynecol.*, **163**, 65–8
100. Horvath, P. M., Beck, M., Bohrer, M. K., Shelden, R. M. and Kemmann, E. (1989). A prospective study on the lack of development of antisperm antibodies in women undergoing intrauterine insemination. *Am. J. Obstet. Gynecol.*, **160**, 6311–17
101. Haas, G. G. (1983). Immunological infertility: which approaches are best? *Contemp. Obstet. Gynecol.*, **22**, 141–50
102. Koyama, K., Kubota, K., Ikuma, K., Shigeta, M. and Isojima, S. (1988). Application of the quantitative sperm immobilization test for follow-up study of sperm-immobilizing antibody in the sera of sterile women. *Int. J. Fertil.*, **33**, 201–6
103. Sugi, T., Makino, T., Maruyama, T., Nozawa, S. and Iizuka, R. (1993). Influence of immunotherapy on antisperm antibody titer in unexplained recurrent aborters. *Am. J. Reprod. Immunol.*, **29**, 95–9
104. Katz, M. and Newill, R. (1980). Steroid treatment for infertility associated with antisperm antibodies. *Lancet*, **1**, 1306–8
105. De Almeidia, M. and Jouannet, P. (1981). Dexamethasone therapy of infertile men with sperm auto-antibodies: immunological and sperm follow-up. *Clin. Exp. Immunol.*, **44**, 567–73
106. Shulman, S., Harlin, B., Davis, P. and Reyniak, J. V. (1978). Immune infertility and new approaches to treatment. *Fertil. Steril.*, **29**, 309–13
107. Shulman, J. F. and Shulman, S. (1982). Methylprednisolone treatment of immunologic infertility in the male. *Fertil. Steril.*, **38**, 591–6
108. Alexander, N. J., Sampson, J. H. and Fulgham, D. L. Pregnancy rates in patients treated for antisperm antibodies with prednisone. *Int. J. Fertil.*, **28**, 63–7
109. Butler, W. T. and Rossen, R. D. (1973). Effects of corticosteroids on immunity in man. I. Decreased serum IgG concentration caused by 3 to 5 days of high doses of methylprednisolone. *J. Clin. Invest.*, **52**, 2629–36
110. Ulcova-Gallova, Z., Mraz, L., Planickova, E., Macku, F. and Ulc, I. (1988). Local hydrocortisone

treatment of sperm-agglutinating antibodies in infertile women. *Int. J. Fertil.*, **33**, 421–5

111. Ulcova-Gallova, Z., Mraz, L., Planickova, E., Macku, F. and Ulc, I. (1990). Three years experience with local hydrocortisone treatment in women with immunological cause of infertility. *Zentralbl. Gynackol.*, **112**, 867–72
112. Jeulin, C., Soumah, A., Da Silva, G. and De Almeida, M. (1989). *In-vitro* processing of sperm with autoantibodies: analysis of sperm populations. *Hum. Reprod.*, **4**, 44–8
113. Mage, M. G., McHugh, L. L. and Rothstein, T. L. (1977). Mouse lymphocytes with or without surface immunoglobulins: preparative scale separation in polystyrene tissue culture dishes coated with specifically purified anti-immunoglobulin antibodies. *J. Immunol. Meth.*, **15**, 47–56
114. De Almeida, M., Gazagne, I., Jeulin, C., Herry, M., Belaisch-Allart, J., Frydman, R., Jouannet, P. and Testart, J. (1989). *In-vitro* processing of sperm with autoantibodies and *in-vitro* fertilization results. *Hum. Reprod.*, **4**, 49–53
115. Vigano, P., Fusi, F. M., Brigante, C., Busacca, M. and Vignali, M. (1991). Immunomagnetic separation of antibody-labelled from antibody-free human spermatozoa as a treatment for immunologic infertility. A preliminary report. *Andrologia*, **23**, 367–71
116. Kiser, G. C., Alexander, N. J., Fuchs, E. F. and Fulgham, D. L. (1987). *In vitro* immune absorption of antisperm antibodies with immunobead-rise, immunomagnetic, and immunocolumn separation techniques. *Fertil Steril.*, **47**, 466–74
117. Elder, K. T., Wick, K. L. and Edwards, R. G. (1990). Seminal plasma anti-sperm antibodies and IVF: the effect of semen sample collection into 50% serum. *Hum. Reprod.*, **5**, 179–84
118. Lenzi, A., Gandini, L., Lombardo, F., Micara, G., Culasso, F. and Dondero, F. (1992). *In vitro* sperm capacitation to treat antisperm antibodies bound to the sperm surface. *Am. J. Reprod. Immunol.*, **28**, 51–5
119. Kremer, J., Jager, S. and Kuiken, J. (1978). Treatment of infertility caused by antisperm antibodies. *Int. J. Fertil.*, **23**, 270–7
120. Alexander, N.J. and Ackerman, S. (1987). Therapeutic insemination. *Obstet. Gynecol. North Am.*, **14**, 905–13
121. Haas, G. G. (1987). Immunologic infertility. *Obstet. Gynecol. North Am.*, **14**, 1069–75
122. Margalioth, E. J., Sauter, E., Bronson, R. A., Rosenfeld, D. L., Scholl, G. M. and Cooper, G. W. (1988). Intrauterine insemination as treatment for antisperm antibodies in the female. *Fertil. Steril.*, **50**, 441–6
123. Smarr, S. C., Wing, R. and Hammond, M. G. (1988). Effect of therapy on infertile couples with antisperm antibodies. *Am. J. Obstet. Gynecol.*, **158**, 969–73
124. Ackerman, S. B., Graff, D., van Uem, J. F. H. M., Swanson, R. J., Veeck, L. L., Acosta, A. A. and Garcia, J. E. (1984). Immunologic infertility and *in vitro* fertilization. *Fertil. Steril.*, **42**, 474–7
125. Palermo, G., Khan, I., Devroey, P., Wisanto, A., Camus, M. and Van Steirteghem, A. C. (1989). Assisted procreation in the presence of a positive direct mixed antiglobulin reaction test. *Fertil. Steril.*, **52**, 645–9
126. Clarke, G. N., Lopata, A., McBain, J. C., Baker, H. W. G. and Johnston, W. I. H. (1985). Effect of sperm antibodies in males on human *in vitro* fertilization (IVF). *Am. J. Reprod. Immunol.*, **8**, 62–6
127. Yovich, J. L., Stanger, J. D., Kay, D. and Boettcher, B. (1984). *In vitro* fertilization of oocytes from women with serum antisperm antibodies. *Lancet*, **1**, 369–71
128. Clarke, G. N., Lopata, A. and Johnston, W. I. H. (1986). Effect of sperm antibodies in females on human *in vitro* fertilization. *Fertil. Steril.*, **46**, 435–41
129. Clarke, G. N., McBain, J. C., Lopata, A. and Johnston, W. I. H. (1985). *In vitro* fertilization results for women with sperm antibodies in plasma and follicular fluid. *Am. J. Reprod. Immunol.*, **8**, 130–1
130. Hamilton, F., Gutlay-Yeo, A. L. and Meldrum, D. R. (1989). Normal fertilization in men with high antibody sperm binding by the addition of sufficient unbound sperm *in vitro. J.* In Vitro *Fertil. Embryo Transf.*, **6**, 342–4
131. Van der Merwe, J. P., Hulme, V. A., Kruger, T. F., Menkveld, R. and Windt, M. L. (1990). Treatment of male sperm autoimmunity by using the gamete intrafallopian transfer procedure with washed spermatozoa. *Fertil. Steril.*, **53**, 682–7
132. Acosta, A. A., van der Merwe, J. P., Doncel, G., Kruger, T. F., Sayilgan, A., Franken, D. R. and Kolm, P. (1994). Fertilization efficiency of morphologically abnormal spermatozoa in assisted reproduction is further impaired by antisperm antibodies on the male partner's sperm. *Fertil. Steril.*, **62**, 826–33
133. Yeh, W.-R., Acosta, A. A. and Seltman, H. J. (1995). Impact of immunoglobulin isotype and location of antisperm antibodies on the human sperm surface on fertilization *in vitro. Fertil. Steril.*, **63**, 1287–92
134. Acosta, A. A. (1992). Male factor in assisted reproduction. *Infertil. Reprod. Med. Clin. North Am.*, **3**, 487–503
135. O'Rand, M. G., Irons, G. P. and Porter, J. P. (1984). Monoclonal antibodies to rabbit sperm autoantigens. I. Inhibition of *in vitro* fertilization and localization of the egg. *Biol. Reprod.*, **30**, 721–9
136. Wright, R. M., John, E., Klotz, K., Flickinger, C. J. and Herr, J. C. (1990). Cloning and sequencing of cDNA coding for the human intra-acrosomal antigen SP-10. *Biol. Reprod.*, **42**, 693–701
137. Kameda, K., Tsuji, Y., Koyama, K. and Isojima, S. (1992). Comparative studies of the antigens recognized by sperm-immobilizing monoclonal antibodies. *Biol. Reprod.*, **46**, 349–57

Sperm enzymes for diagnostic purposes 14

L. J. D. Zaneveld, R. S. Jeyendran, J. P. W. Vermeiden and J. W. Lens

INTRODUCTION

The standard semen analysis relies almost entirely on microscopic observations, i.e. the number, motility and morphology of the spermatozoa. However, sperm function also involves events that are not measured by these physical parameters such as capacitation, acrosome reaction, oocyte penetration and fusion, nuclear decondensation, etc. Although the standard sperm variables are important for the assessment of the fertilizing potential of a sperm sample, they are insufficient in reaching a diagnosis unless the obtained values are extremely poor[1]. When the standard sperm parameters fall into the abnormal range but are not so low that infertility is almost certain to result, one cannot come to a diagnosis except to say that fertility is 'less likely to occur'. If all functional aspects are normal in this case, the spermatozoa are probably capable of fertilizing. If one or more of the functional parameters are also seriously impaired, fertilization will more than likely not occur[2]. Similarly, if the standard sperm parameters fall into the normal range but one of the functional variables is severely abnormal, fertility is most likely impaired.

A number of biological assays are available to assess the functional activity of spermatozoa such as the cervical mucus penetration test, the zona-free hamster occyte penetration assay and the hemizona assay[2]. However, these tests are often complicated, technician-dependent, costly, produce inconsistent results and the test material may not be easy to obtain. Assays should be developed that provide the same information but are simpler and more reproducible. Biochemical assays fall into this category.

Ideally, biochemical tests should be developed for each sperm organelle[2]. The assay should be able to detect a non-functional organelle as indicated by results that fall into a pre-established 'infertile' range. For the assay to have that validity, it should measure an essential component of a organelle. A number of such assays are under development[2].

Enzymatic activity associated with an organelle is often essential for its function. To date, two enzymes have been proposed as indicators of organelle activity: acrosin for the acrosome and creatine kinase (CK) for the midpiece. Acrosin has additional importance because of its essential role in zona penetration by the oocyte. Other enzymes may also be valid as functional indicators, but presently no good data are available to substantiate their clinical relevance.

Tremendous confusion exists in the literature regarding the evaluation of new sperm assays, often resulting in the rejection of an assay even though it is perfectly valid[3]. The primary errors that are made include:

(1) Claiming that a new assay has validity when it correlates well with a standard assay (by contrast, the poorer the correlation the better because this indicates that different entities are being measured);

(2) Performing the assay on one sperm sample but performing *in vitro* penetration, fertilization or zona-binding procedures with a different sperm sample (usually obtained by a selection procedure);

(3) Attempting to establish a good correlation between a single sperm assay and penetration or fertilization outcome (sperm function involves many variables so that a single test is not likely to correlate with fertility outcome); and

(4) Trying to compare fertile and supposedly infertile men (too much overlap is present between these two groups with a single test)[3].

When these errors are not considered during a review of the literature, erroneous conclusions can be reached[4].

A logical approach in determining the diagnostic use of a new assay is to established that:

(1) It does not provide the same data as obtained by one of the standard sperm parameters; and

(2) A cutoff point is found indicative of infertility[3].

In addition, the assay should be repeatable and technically be so simple that it can readily be performed in most clinical laboratories.

ACROSIN

Background

Acrosin is a serine proteinase with many similarities to trypsin[5,6]. It appears to have an essential role in: (1) the acrosome reaction; (2) the penetration of spermatozoa through the zona pellucida; and, possibly, (3) sperm–zona binding. Acrosin is associated primarily with the acrosome proper and the inner acrosomal membrane, although some may be associated with the outer sperm membranes. Sperm acrosin is almost entirely present in an inactive form, called proacrosin. Most of the proacrosin is activated to acrosin during the acrosome reaction[5]. The proacrosin that remains bound to the inner acrosomal membrane after completion of the acrosome reaction may be activated during sperm passage through the zona pellucida but this remains to be firmly established.

Assay

A variety of assays are available to measure the activity of acrosin. These tests are primarily based on the proteolytic, esterolytic and aminolytic activity of the enzyme, or on its interaction with antibodies[7,8]. Clinically, the most frequently used assay is one of the following or a modification thereof: (1) esterolytic assay; (2) the 'clinical' aminolytic assay; (3) the proteolytic plate assay; and (4) the radioimmunoassay. Details of these assays can be found in the quoted publications.

The radioimmunoassay[9] is a competitive binding assay that utilizes antiacrosin serum and iodinated acrosin. The assay is very sensitive but only measures the total amount of acrosin/proacrosin associated with spermatozoa without considering the ability of proacrosin to be converted to acrosin. It is important to measure proacrosin conversion because fertility may be impaired if this cannot occur during the fertilization process. Immunocytochemistry has also been used to quantitate sperm acrosin but, as expected, was found to be less reliable than biochemical measurements in detecting infertile patients[10].

The proteolytic plate assay[9] estimates the amount of acrosin by placing spermatozoa on a gelatin/photographic plate and determining the size of the 'halo' formation around the sperm head. The halo is formed by released acrosin (presumably after proacrosin activation) that digests the gelatin. This assay is simple but unreliable and not quantitative.

The esterolytic assay[11] is the most accurate test and involves the dispersion of the acrosome at low pH, varying the pH of the extract so that proacrosin converts to acrosin, and/or the acrosin inhibitor separates from acrosin, assessing the esterolytic activity at each pH. In this fashion, measurements can be made of the amount of proacrosin, acrosin and acrosin inhibitor associated with spermatozoa. The assay is somewhat time-consuming and probably provides more information than necessary for clinical purposes.

The 'Kennedy' aminolytic assay[12] was specifically developed for the clinical laboratory. It involves the removal of seminal plasma from the spermatozoa by Ficoll centrifugation and incubation of the sperm pellet in a buffered medium at pH 8.0 (allows conversion of proacrosin to acrosin). The medium also contains Triton X-100 (for acrosome extraction) and *N*-α-benzoyl-D,L-argine *p*-nitroanalide (BAPNA; amide substrate to measure acrosin activity). The sperm mixture is incubated for 3 h and the amide hydrolysis products are assessed spectrophotometrically at 410 nm. The values are expressed in $\mu IU/10^6$ spermatozoa. It is recommended that a known amount of trypsin is used as positive control. This assay measures the total amount of acrosin available to spermatozoa, i.e. the free acrosin plus the convertible proacrosin. A similar assay was published for bull spermatozoa[13].

Several modifications of the Kennedy assay have been published. The assay can be simplified by using microplate wells for incubation instead of test tubes and measuring the absorbance directly with a microplate reader[14]. Another improvement is to measure the sperm numbers after Ficoll centrifugation (Mack, Kaminski and Zaneveld, unpublished) instead of before this procedure, as originally recommended[12]. A third modification[15,16] involves the separation of spermatozoa from seminal plasma by vacuum filtration rather than Ficoll centrifugation and employing a 1.5-h rather than a 3-h incubation period. The last modification has been marketed under the name of Accu-Sperm (O.E.M. Concepts, Inc.; distributed by Polymedco, Inc., Yorktown Heights, NY, USA). The outcome is expressed as an 'acrosin activity index':

$$= OD_{\text{diluted sperm}} \times 10^{12}/OD_{\text{positive control}} \times \text{no. of sperm/mL}$$

Unfortunately, it is extremely difficult to compare the results obtained from one assay to another. Even a fairly simple modification may produce different data. Cutoff points for normal and abnormal are only valid for a particular assay. Due to the large variety of acrosin assays used, it is not possible to compare the reported values from different laboratories and clinics. Therefore, qualitative statements are generally made in the following text without giving specific data. Exceptions are the fertilization data obtained with the Kennedy assay and the Accu-sperm assays since these assays are most extensively used at present.

Clinical laboratory observations

Sperm storage and cryopreservation

Ejaculates can be kept refrigerated or at 22–24°C for 24 h, or at 37°C for 6 h without loss of acrosin activity[12,17]. However, higher temperatures or freezing at –20°C cause a large reduction in the sperm's acrosin levels[12].

Cryopreservation also causes a large decrease in sperm-associated acrosin[10,18,19]. Acrosin can be used as an additional indicator of the cryosurvival of spermatozoa[20]. However, it should be noted that several studies report no decrease[17] or even an increase[10,21] in acrosin activity after cryopreservation. This is surprising, since it is known that freeze–thawing causes acrosomal damage, leading to the partial or complete release of the acrosomal contents. Furthermore, acrosin and particularly proacrosin are unstable to freeze–thawing. It is possible that the conversion of proacrosin to acrosin was inadequate during the assays used by investigators who report an increase in acrosin activity after freeze–thawing. If so, the free acrosin levels were usually measured before and after cryopreservation. Even though a large decrease in proacrosin/acrosin may have occurred overall, the freeze–thawing procedure may convert some proacrosin to acrosin so that the total amount of free acrosin appears to increase after cryopreservation if only the free acrosin is measured.

Sperm samples should not be frozen or cryopreserved if accurate acrosin values are desired.

Leukocytes

A genital tract infection can cause the entry of a large number of leukocytes into the ejaculate. Such leukocytes contain proteinases. However, even in severe infections, not enough aminolytic activity is produced by the seminal leukocytes to affect the interpretation of the assay[22].

Viscosity lowering agents

The sperm acrosin levels do not change when α-chymotrypsin is used to lower the viscosity of the ejaculate[23]. The effect of other viscosity lowering or coagulum liquefying agents has not been established.

Abstinence

The acrosin activity of spermatozoa remains similar up to 5 days of abstinence but decreases almost two-fold after 10 days of abstinence[22,24]. Therefore, the abstinence period needs to be taken into consideration when the acrosin assay is performed. It is not known why the acrosin levels decrease after prolonged abstinence, but it is possible that the acrosome deteriorates under such conditions.

Sperm selection procedures

Selection methods that improve the overall quality of spermatozoa in a sample generally also select for spermatozoa with normal or high acrosin levels. For instance, after swim-up, glass wool filtration or

Percoll centrifugation, the mean acrosin activities of the resultant spermatozoa are about 2–3-fold higher than the mean acrosin levels of the original sperm sample[16,17,25–28]. L-4 membrane filtration may produce spermatozoa with an even higher acrosin level than those obtained after swim-up[29]. Therefore, data obtained with unselected and selected spermatozoa or those obtained by different selection techniques are difficult to compare. The Ficoll centrifugation step in the Kennedy assay is used to remove seminal plasma and should not select spermatozoa because almost all spermatozoa should precipitate if the centrifugation is done correctly. Since this is not always the case, it is now recommended that the sperm number is determined after the centrifugation step (Mack, Kaminski and Zaneveld, unpublished).

Intercourse versus masturbation

The acrosin levels, as well as all other sperm variables, appear to be improved when the spermatozoa are collected by intercourse (with a pouch) as compared to masturbation[30].

Split ejaculates

The first fraction of a split ejaculate generally possesses higher quality spermatozoa than the last fraction (mostly of seminal vesicle origin). Spermatozoa from the first fraction also possess approximately twice the acrosin levels[31]. However, others have not found such differences, but this may be due to the use of frozen–thawed spermatozoa[24].

Relationship to the standard sperm parameters

A large number of studies have been performed to determine if the acrosin levels of spermatozoa are correlated to sperm numbers, sperm motility and sperm morphology[10,17,23,32–35]. From these studies, it can be concluded that the acrosin activity generally varies independently from the other sperm parameters. However, relationships can occasionally be expected and have been reported. For instance, when the ejaculate has many abnormalities, e.g. a very low sperm count or motility, or a high percentage of morphological aberrations, the acrosin levels are also likely to be abnormal. In the absence of such severe conditions, acrosin activity cannot be predicted from the standard sperm parameters.

Not surprisingly, the acrosin levels are most closely related to morphological abnormalities, particularly those of the acrosome[10,24,32]. When the acrosomes are absent from ejaculated spermatozoa, the acrosin levels are greatly decreased or absent[24,36–38]. Even though such spermatozoa can be motile, they are unable to penetrate zona-free hamster oocytes or fertilize *in vivo*[36–39]. Thus, acrosin can be used as a marker for acrosomal integrity.

Several authors have reported that polyzoospermia is associated with decreased acrosin levels[24,35]. This may be due to the increased membrane and other abnormalities of such spermatozoa[24].

Cervical mucus penetration

Spermatozoa with low acrosin activity tend to penetrate cervical mucus poorly, both *in vivo* (postcoital tests) and *in vitro* (Kremer capillary test)[35]. Since acrosin itself does not appear to be involved in cervical mucus penetration[40], these observations are likely due to morphological (e.g. acrosomal) abnormalities. Indeed, in this study, a correlation existed between reduced acrosin and increased morphological abnormalities[35].

Varicocele

Quantitative alterations in sperm acrosin occur after artificial induction of a varicocele in the rabbit[41]. The changes are restored after varicocelectomy. Such studies have not as yet been performed in the human.

Microbial infections

No significant relationship appears to exist between the acrosin activity of spermatozoa and the microbial colonization of the ejaculate[35]. However, there may be a tendency toward higher acrosin activity in the case of *Mycoplasma* and with *Chlamydia* infections. Lower acrosin activity may be associated with potentially pathogenic anaerobes in the ejaculate[35].

Age

Acrosin activity does not appear to vary with the age of the semen donor[35].

Smoking, chemical exposure and stress

Smokers have significantly lower acrosin levels than non-smokers[35]. Patients exposed to heat, chemicals or stress tend to exhibit lower acrosin levels[35].

Genital tract abnormalities

Men who, on examination, show genital tract abnormalities have the same acrosin values as those who do not[35]. Epidemic parotitis, previous inflammatory processes and andrologic operations do not significantly influence acrosin activity[35].

However, there is a tendency towards lower acrosin activity after genital traumatization[35].

In vitro fertilization

Published data

A relationship between the successful outcome of *in vitro* fertilization (IVF) and the acrosin content of spermatozoa has been established by most laboratories that studied such a relationship[12,16,23,42,43] with a few exceptions[28,33,34]. However, two of these exceptions used frozen–thawed spermatozoa and did not allow conversion of proacrosin to acrosin so that only a fraction of the sperm's acrosin activity was determined[28,33]. Since the Kennedy assay and the Accu-sperm assay are the ones most frequently used at the present time for clinical purposes, the following only describes the results obtained with these assays.

Using the Kennedy assay, De Jonge *et al.*[43] concluded that acrosin was higher in ejaculates that fertilized 70% or more of the mature oocytes than those that fertilized less than 70% of the mature oocytes. A strong correlation between pre-IVF acrosin activity and high IVF success was present.

The data by Sharma *et al.*[23] obtained with a modification of the Kennedy assay, confirm the positive correlation between total sperm acrosin and IVF outcome, particularly with spermatozoa prepared on a Percoll gradient. These investigators concluded that the number of motile spermatozoa before insemination should be adjusted so that the acrosin activity per oocyte is >7.6 μIU to ensure fertilization.

Utilizing the Accu-sperm technique, a good correlation with IVF outcome was initially reported[16]. Of all the semen parameters measured, only the acrosin activity index (AAI) was found to correlate with IVF outcome. Total acrosin was higher in cycles when one or more mature oocytes were fertilized as compared to cycles with failed fertilization of all mature oocytes. An AAI cut off of <4.5 was suggested as an indication of enzyme deficiency, contributing to sub- or infertility.

Opposite results were obtained by another group of investigators with the Accu-sperm test[34]. Although the mean AAI tended to increase with an increased percentage fertilization, the increases were not statistically significant. Much overlap also appeared to be present in the ranges of AAI activity, e.g. between those sperm samples that did not fertilize a single oocyte and those that fertilized all oocytes.

All IVF studies, with one exception[34], utilized different sperm samples for the assay (the ejaculate) and for the IVF procedure (a selected sample). When no sperm selection was performed before IVF[12], the acrosin activity of sperm samples that fertilized at least one oocyte ranged from 14 to 60 $\mu IU/10^6$ sperm (mean ± SEM: 34.4 ± 2.9), whereas those of sperm samples that did not fertilize an oocyte ranged from 7 to 35 $\mu IU/10^6$ sperm (mean ± SEM: 20.3 ± 3.2). Overlap in acrosin values between these two groups is not surprising since an inability to fertilize may be due to other factors besides acrosin. Thus, the acrosin levels of infertile sperm can be expected to range from very low to high, whereas those of fertile sperm should not drop below a certain cutoff point. Based on these data, the value of 14 $\mu IU/10^6$ sperm was tentatively suggested as the cutoff for abnormal in the Kennedy assay when no sperm selection is performed before IVF. This value is similar to the cutoff value for fertility found under natural fertility conditions (see further).

The Free University Hospital of Amsterdam experience

Since 1990, the acrosin assay has been used for the IVF program at the Free University of Amsterdam (Lens and Vermeiden, unpublished). Initially, a cutoff point of 14 $\mu IU/10^6$ sperm was used as a decision point. The acrosin assay as published by Kennedy *et al.*[12] was applied to the ejaculate if the first IVF attempt failed. If the acrosin activity fell below 14 μIU/10^6 sperm and less than four oocytes were retrieved during the first IVF cycle, the couple was discouraged from participating in a second attempt. However, if more than four oocytes were recovered during the first IVF treatment, a second IVF was performed independent of the acrosin activity of the ejaculate.

An initial study of 48 couples was performed that underwent a second IVF treatment. No fertilization occurred during this second attempt in 29 cases, whereas 19 cases fertilized. The acrosin values in the ejaculates of these two groups (infertile and fertile) were, respectively, 15.3±7.7 (mean±SD; range: 5.8–35.5) and 24.8±10.8 (range: 5.4–44.5) μIU/10^6 sperm. These differences were statistically significant (P=0.0017; Student's t-test) and confirmed the poor *in vitro* fertilizing potential of ejaculates with acrosin values below 14 μIU/10^6 sperm.

In a subsequent study, 84 couples from our routine IVF program were studied. Ejaculates were analyzed by the Kennedy acrosin assay. The ejaculates were obtained 1 month before or after the IVF procedure. The semen samples were considered fertile if at least one of four oocytes was fertilized during the first or the second IVF attempt (IVF-fertile). In addition, the acrosin levels were measured in ejaculates from 18 men who had impregnated their wives within 3 months from the analysis (natural-fertile).

Taking the results from the initial and subsequent IVF studies together, the acrosin values of the entire IVF-fertile group averaged 22.6±9.4 μIU/10^6 sperm (n=80; range: 2.0–44.5) and that of the infertile group (n=52) averaged 16.2±9.1 μIU/10^6 sperm (range: 1.9–41.1). The difference is statistically significant (P=0.0002).

The *in vivo* fertile group averaged acrosin values of 30.0±10.3 μIU/10^6 sperm (range: 12.0–59.0). These values were comparable to the acrosin activities found in the IVF-fertile ejaculates that fertilized more than 30% of the oocytes. *In vitro* fertilization patients who fertilized less than 10% of the oocytes had statistically significantly lower acrosin values (18.6±9.7 μIU/10^6 sperm) than those who fertilized more than 30% of the oocytes. These results suggest that the fertility potential of ejaculates with an acrosin activity of less than 20 μIU/10^6 sperm may be impaired.

In order to analyze these data further, the acrosin values were divided into four different groups (0–10; 11–14; 15–19; and 20 μIU/10^6 sperm or more). Seventy-one percent of the men with acrosin values between 0 and 10 μIU/10^6 sperm were infertile and the fertilization rate of the remaining men in this group was low (14±10% of the oocytes fertilized). The fertilization rate of the groups with higher acrosin values increased proportionally (chi-quadrate=17.0; P<0.001). Seventy-eight percent of the men with acrosin values above 20 μIU/10^6 sperm were fertile and the average fertilization rate was 46±29%.

At the Free University, acrosin values above 20 μIU/10^6 sperm are now considered 'normal' for IVF and for *in vivo* fertility (16 of 18 *in vivo* fertile men had acrosin values above 20 μIU/10^6 sperm). These values correspond well with those reported by Blackwell *et al.*[44] who found the minimal cutoff values for *in vivo* fertility to be 17–18 μIU/10^6 sperm (see further).

Acrosin values between 10 and 20 μIU/10^6 sperm are considered subfertile for IVF at the Free University. The fertilization potential of semen samples with acrosin activities below 10 μIU/10^6 sperm appears to be seriously impaired. In this low group, the chance of one oocyte being fertilized out of seven is only 30%. Therefore, patients are strongly advised not to try a second IVF attempt if the acrosin values are below 10 μIU/10^6 sperm.

The cutoff point of 10 μIU/10^6 sperm used by the Free University is somewhat lower than that reported by Kennedy *et al.* (14 μIU/10^6 sperm)[12]. This is expected because ejaculates were analyzed at the Free University, but selected samples (Percoll gradient) were used for IVF, whereas non-selected samples were used for IVF in the Kennedy study. Selected samples generally have higher acrosin levels than non-selected (washed, ejaculated) samples. Thus, lower ejaculate acrosin values can be expected to result in fertilization when selected samples are used instead of non-selected samples.

In vivo observations

A number of studies have been performed to compare the acrosin activity of sperm samples from presumably fertile men to those of presumably infertile/subfertile patients[9,10,17,31,35,45–48]. There is general agreement among the investigators so that these studies will not be discussed individually. Independent of the acrosin assay technique used, each study concludes that significant differences are present between presumably infertile and fertile men. The ability of men to impregnate their partners tends to increase as their sperm acrosin values increase. Low sperm acrosin levels are associated with infertility. A proportion of infertile men (estimated at 33%)[17] with unexplained infertility have low acrosin levels but normal sperm numbers, motility and morphology. These observations have led each investigator to conclude that the acrosin assay can identify subpopulations of infertile or subfertile patients that are not recognized by the standard sperm parameters.

Only one group of investigators have published data comparing the Kennedy assay and the Accu-sperm assay[48]. A fairly poor correlation existed between the two methods. In addition, the reported cutoff values for normal and abnormal in the Accu-sperm assay corresponded poorly with the presumed fertility/infertility status of the men. By contrast, a high correspondence was found with the Kennedy assay. However, at the Free University Hospital (Lens and Vermeiden, unpublished) a good correlation (r=0.87) was found between the Kennedy assay and the Accu-sperm assay.

A large overlap in acrosin values between fertile and infertile groups of men can be expected because acrosin represents only one of the many sperm parameters that can be faulty, leading to infertility. The acrosin levels can be normal, yet infertility may occur because one or more of the other sperm variables are abnormal. However, a distinct cutoff value should be present below which mostly infertile or subfertile men fall.

Cutoff values for abnormal and normal vary among the investigations because of the different assays employed. In a recent study, using the Kennedy assay, it was found that the acrosin values of normal donors (presumably fertile), varied from 17 to 45 μIU/10^6 sperm[44]. The cutoff of 17 μIU/10^6 sperm corresponds closely to that found in the previous IVF study that utilized unselected spermatozoa[12]. Thus, 14–17 μIU/10^6 sperm may represent a valid cutoff for normal if the Kennedy assay is followed exactly and if fertility is achieved under natural conditions.

A distinct cutoff value was also reported in another study[10]. The values were higher than those reported above, probably because a modification of the Kennedy assay was used. The acrosin values for presumably fertile men ranged from 30 to 254 μIU/10^6 sperm and those for presumably infertile men ranged from 5 to 15 μIU/10^6 sperm. Approximately half of the infertile men had acrosin values below 30 μIU/10^6 spermatozoa. These results confirm the presence of a distinct cutoff point for fertility under natural conditions.

CREATINE KINASE (CK)

Introduction

Adenosine triphosphate (ATP) is the substrate for tubulin–dynein interaction, i.e. for the sliding of the tail fibers and sperm motility. Therefore, it is not surprising that ATP has been proposed as a measure of sperm function. However, it does not appear to be a useful indicator. Differences between fertile men and men attending infertility clinics were initially reported[49] but could not be confirmed[50]. Furthermore, measurements of sperm-associated ATP and the ATP/ADP ratio showed no differences between normospermic and oligospermic specimens[51].

Another important substrate for fibrillar movement is creatine phosphate. Treatment with this agent can enhance the motility and velocity of human spermatozoa[52]. In mitochondria, the phosphate group of ATP is utilized for the conversion of creatine to creatine phosphate. Creatine phosphate moves to the tail fibers where the action of creatine kinase (CK; creatine phosphokinase, creatine-*N*-phosphotransferase) transfers the phosphate group to ADP to produce ATP. Dephosphorylated creatine migrates back to the mitochondria and the cycle starts over again. The potential usefulness of creatine phosphate for diagnostic purposes has not been evaluated, but a number of studies have been performed with CK.

CK was initially analyzed because it was considered to be a key enzyme in the synthesis and transport of energy. However, subsequent results indicated that little or no correlation was present between CK levels and sperm motility (see further). In addition, spermatozoa showed diminished fertilizing capacity when their CK activities were high. Further results suggested that the increased CK activity in infertile spermatozoa is due to an increase in cytoplasmic proteins including CK[53]. This has led to the suggestion that the higher CK content is related to the incomplete shedding of cytoplasm before the release of spermatozoa from the Sertoli cell. Shed cytoplasm normally forms the residual body found on epididymal spermatozoa. If so, elevated CK levels indicate a developmental defect and incomplete cellular maturity, i.e. a 'latent arrest' of the spermatozoa[53].

Two isozymes of CK have been found in spermatozoa, the B- and M-types (called CK–BB and CK–MM because they occur as dimers). In other contractile cells, only the B-type is present before birth. After birth, the M-type develops during cellular differentiation. Similar changes appear to occur during sperm maturation so that the CK isoforms may be a better indicator of sperm maturity than the CK content (see further)[54].

Assay

Details of the assay can be found in several references[54–56]. Briefly, seminal fluid is removed from the spermatozoa by centrifugation in ice-cold medium containing 0.15 M NaCl with 0.03 M imidazole, pH 7.0[54]. The sperm pellet is extracted by homogenization or vortexing for 20 s in ice-cold medium containing 0.03 M imidazole, 10% glycerol, 5 mM DTT and 0.1% Triton, at pH 7.0. This treatment causes the extraction of more than 90% of the CK from the spermatozoa. Subsequently, a three-step reaction is used to measure liberated CK activity. In the first step, CK catalyzes the synthesis of ATP from creatine phosphate and ADP. In the second step, the ATP is utilized for glucose-6-phosphate synthesis in the presence of hexokinase. In the third step, the glucose-6-phosphate is oxidized to 6-phosphogluconate with reduction of NADP to NADPH with an optical density change at 340 nM and an increase in fluorescence. The activity is expressed in IU/10^8 spermatozoa. CK test kits can be purchased. B- and M-isoform detection is done by washing and extracting the spermatozoa as described above and subjecting the sperm extract to electrophoretic separation on agarose gels. The gels are overlaid with CK substrate and the relative concentrations of the CK isoforms are detected by their enzymatic activity. The NADH fluorescence is quantified after electrophoresis by a scanning fluorometer[54].

Clinical laboratory observations

Relationship to standard semen parameters

Sperm CK levels show an inverse relationship to sperm concentration[55,57]. Spermatozoa from normospermic ($>20\times10^6$ sperm/mL) ejaculates possess much lower CK levels than spermatozoa from oligospermic or 'variablespermic' (occasionally $>20\times10^6$mL) specimens. Initially, <0.250 CK units per 10^8 spermatozoa was taken as normal or fertile[55,57], but based on the intrauterine insemination experiments (see further), this value should be lowered by several orders of magnitude.

No correlation exists between sperm motility and the sperm CK levels[55]. Also, no relationship exists between sperm CK activity, sperm morphology or the ATP levels[51,55]. Therefore, it appears that sperm CK levels are independent of the standard sperm parameters. However, more recently a high correlation between the CK content and the morphology of spermatozoa was reported[58].

Studying the isoforms, a four-fold difference in the CK–MM ratio (expressed as % CK–MM/CK–MM+CK–BB) was found between normospermic and oligospermic men[59]. A close correlation between the CK activity and CK–MM ratios appears to be present, indicating that the loss of cytoplasm and commencement of M-isoform production are related during spermatogenesis (see above). Thus, CK–MM may indicate the biochemical maturity of spermatozoa.

Selection procedures

Selection of spermatozoa by a swim-up procedure results in a sperm population that contains lower CK levels (by at least 20%) than the starting population, i.e. a relative increase in normal spermatozoa occurs[55,57,60]. The percentage of spermatozoa with normal CK levels as detected immunocytochemically doubles after swim-up[61].

Fertility observations

In vitro *fertilization*

Spermatozoa with an immature CK pattern as determined histochemically bind less successfully to human zonae than normal spermatozoa[61]. In a blinded study, the sperm CK–MM ratios (CK–MM/CK–MM+CK–BB) were found to reflect the *in vitro* fertilizing capacity of spermatozoa[54]. Both ejaculates and swim-up samples were used for analysis and the results combined. A CK–MM ratio of <10% was considered as having a low likelihood for fertilization (CK–MM-infertile). A four-fold difference in the fertilization rate (53.4% versus 14.2%) was found between the CK–MM-fertile and CK–MM-infertile groups, and 72.7% versus 25.8% failed to achieve any fertilization. All 14 pregnancies occurred in the CK–MM-fertile group. Although the sperm concentration (78.4×10^6/mL versus 31.5×10^6/mL) and the sperm motility (54.0% versus 45.6%) were also higher in the CK–MM-fertile than the infertile groups, no correlation appeared to be present between these two standard sperm variables and IVF outcome.

In vivo *fertilization*

Comparisons between oligospermic fertile and oligospermic infertile ejaculates with close to identical sperm motility and concentration were performed (fertility was established by intrauterine insemination)[60]. The infertile ejaculates averaged approximately twice the CK activity of the fertile ejaculates. A large overlap between fertile and infertile samples was present, so much so that the range of values was essentially identical between the fertile and infertile groups when the ejaculates were tested. However, after swim-up, 6/46 (13%) of the fertile samples had lower CK activity than any of the infertile samples. The CK levels of these samples were several orders of magnitude below 0.25 IU/10^6 spermatozoa. CK analysis of spermatozoa after swim-up may be of use to predict unsuccessful intrauterine insemination outcome. However, the cutoff value for fertile should be lowered by several orders of magnitude from that originally assigned (see above).

CONCLUSIONS

Whenever a new assay is developed and evaluated by different laboratories and clinics, controversy arises. Such controversy is often due to inappropriate methodology used in evaluating the assay[3]. In regard to the acrosin assay, one should not use frozen–thawed spermatozoa because this often causes a loss in acrosin/proacrosin. The extraction and assay technique has to allow for the conversion of proacrosin to acrosin otherwise only a fraction of the acrosin content of the spermatozoa is determined. Finally, factors such as abstinence have to be taken into consideration.

A single assay should normally not 'correlate' with *in vitro* fertilization outcome, i.e. with the percentage of fertilized oocytes, because fertilization depends on many factors not just the one under study. A large amount of overlap can be expected between fertile and infertile populations. If a 'correlation' with fertilization happens to occur, it is probably incidental and due to the specific donor sample employed. In addition, when such a 'correlation' is present, the *r* value is usually so low that the test is not predictive of fertility outcome even though the value may be statistically significant. A single test can only be indicative of infertility (*in vivo*) or lack of fertilization (in an IVF program), never of fertility/fertilization. To be useful, a minimal cutoff value needs to be established for an assay below which it is 95% certain that fertility/fertilization will not occur. Therefore, in evaluating an assay, only the percentage of false negatives is of concern.

Controversy also arises during *in vitro* studies because the ejaculate is normally used for analysis, whereas a selected sample is added to the oocytes. Such selected samples may or may not reflect the initial sperm population in regard to the sperm parameter under evaluation. From a practical standpoint, it is usually necessary that ejaculates are analyzed in an IVF program. This can still be useful because one can expect that poor acrosin values of ejaculated spermatozoa are generally reflected in poor acrosin values of the spermatozoa selected from such ejaculates. However, this is not always the case, so that the percentage of false negatives may be fairly high in some donor populations. In such cases, the ejaculated sperm sample may produce low acrosin values, while the selected sperm sample has normal levels and is still able to fertilize (although often poorly).

When these issues are considered carefully in the above review of the literature on the acrosin assay, it is clear that acrosin can be used as a decision-making tool for infertility. Under natural conditions, cutoff points appear to be present below which fertility is often compromised or does not occur. Almost all investigators conclude that the acrosin assay can be used to identify subgroups of infertile or subfertile men which would not be recognized by the standard sperm parameters. With assisted reproduction, the data are somewhat more controversial for the reasons mentioned above, but the data still support the use of the assay. Clear cutoff points are harder to obtain, however, because different samples are used for the assay and for IVF (see above). Several clinics are now utilizing the assay as one of the factors in deciding whether or not to recommend a second IVF procedure. Unfortunately, cutoff points will vary from clinic to clinic depending on the assay or modification employed. Ultimately, a single acrosin assay should be utilized by all clinics.

The creatine kinase (CK) assay also appears to have merit for diagnostic purposes although the data are limited as compared to the acrosin assay and have only been produced by a single laboratory. The CK isozymes are of particular interest because they appear to be a chemical marker of testicular sperm maturation. Further study of this assay is recommended.

References

1. Zaneveld, L. J. D. and Jeyendran, R. S. (1988). Modern assessment of semen for diagnostic purposes. *Semin. Reprod. Endocrinol.*, **6**, 323–8
2. Zaneveld, L. J. D. and Jeyendran, R. S. (1992). Sperm function tests. In Overstreet, J. W. (ed.) *Male Infertility*, pp. 353–71. (From Diamond, M. P. and DeCherney, A. G. (eds.) *Infertil. Reprod. Med. Clin. North Am.* Philadelphia: W. B. Saunders)
3. Jeyendran, R. S. and Zaneveld, L. J. D. (1993). Controversies in the development and validation of new sperm assays. *Fertil. Steril.*, **59**, 726–8
4. Liu, D. Y. and Baker, H. W. G. (1992). Tests of human sperm function and fertilization *in vitro. Fertil. Steril.*, **58**, 465–83
5. Zaneveld, L. J. D. and DeJonge, C. J. (1991). Mammalian sperm acrosomal enzymes and the acrosome reaction. In Dunbar, B. and O'Rand, M. (eds.) *A Comparative Overview of Mammalian Fertilization*, pp. 63–79. (New York, Plenum Press)
6. Klemm, U., Muller-Esterl, W. and Engel, W. (1991). Acrosin, the peculiar sperm-specific serine protease. *Hum. Genet.*, **87**, 635–41
7. Muller-Esterl, W. and Fritz, H. (1981). Sperm acrosin. *Meth. Enzymol.*, **80**, 621–9
8. Pleban, P., Zaneveld, L. J. D. and Jeyendran, R. S. (1990). Tests of spermatozoa function: acrosin. In Acosta, A. A., Swanson, R. J., Ackerman, S. B., Kruger, T. F., Van Zyl, J. A. and Menkveld, R. (eds.) *Human Spermatozoa in Assisted Reproduction*, pp. 96–101. (Baltimore: Williams and Wilkins)
9. Mohsenian, M., Syner, F. N. and Moghissi, K. S. (1982). A study of sperm acrosin in patients with unexplained infertility. *Fertil. Steril.*, **37**, 223–9
10. Francavilla, S., Palermo, G., Gabriele, A., Cordeschi, G. and Poccia, G. (1992). Sperm acrosin activity and fluorescence microscopic assessment of proacrosin/acrosin in ejaculates of infertile and fertile men. *Fertil. Steril.*, **57**, 1311–15
11. Goodpasture, J. D., Polakoski, K. L. and Zaneveld, L. J. D. (1980). Acrosin, proacrosin, and acrosin inhibitor of human spermatozoa: extraction, quantitation, and stability. *J. Androl.*, **1**, 16–27
12. Kennedy, W. P., Kaminski, J. M., Van der Ven, H. H., Jeyendran, R. S., Reid, D. S., Blackwell, J., Bielfeld, P. and Zaneveld, L. J. D. (1989). A simple, clinical assay to evaluate the acrosin activity of human spermatozoa. *J. Androl.*, **10**, 221–31
13. Froman, D. P., Schenk, J. J. and Amann, R. P. (1987). Sperm-bound amidase activity as a marker for acrosomal integrity of bull spermatozoa. *J. Androl.*, **8**, 162–9
14. Cross, N. L. (1990). A modified and improved assay for sperm amidase activity. *J. Androl.*, **11**, 409–15
15. Deutsch, A., Prisco, J., Melnick, H., Viscelli, T. A., Ionascu, L. and Williams, W. (1990). A simplified method for measuring acrosin activity in spermatozoa. *J. Int. Fed. Clin. Chem.*, **2**, 228–31
16. Tummon, I. S., Yuzpe, A. A., Daniel, S. A. J. and Deutsch, A. (1991). Total acrosin activity correlates with fertility potential after fertilization *in vitro. Fertil. Steril.*, **56**, 933–8
17. Koukoulis, G. N., Vantman, D., Dennison, L., Banks, S. M. and Sherins, R. J. (1989). Low acrosin activity in a subgroup of men with idiopathic infertility does not correlate with sperm density, percent motility, curvilinear velocity, or linearity. *Fertil. Steril.*, **52**, 120–7

18. Mack, S. R. and Zaneveld, L. J. D. (1987). Acrosomal enzymes and ultrastructure of unfrozen and cryo-treated human spermatozoa. *Gamete Res.*, **18**, 375–83
19. Goodpasture, J. C., Zavos, P. M., Cohen, M. R. and Zaneveld, L. J. D. (1981). Effects of various conditions of semen storage on the acrosin system of human spermatozoa. *J. Reprod. Fertil.*, **63**, 397–405
20. Jeyendran, R. S., Van der Ven, H. H., Kennedy, W., Perez-Pelaez, M. and Zaneveld, L. J. D. (1984). Comparison of glycerol and a zwitter ion buffer as cryoprotective media for human spermatozoa: motility, hamster oocyte penetration and acrosin/proacrosin. *J. Androl.*, **5**, 1–7
21. Schill, W. B. (1975). Acrosin activity of cryo-preserved human spermatozoa. *Fertil. Steril.*, **26**, 711–15
22. Blackwell, J. M. and Zaneveld, L. J. D. (1992). Effect of abstinence on sperm acrosin, hypoosmotic swelling, and other semen variables. *Fertil. Steril.*, **58**, 798–802
23. Sharma, R., Hogg, J. and Bromham, D. R. (1993). Is spermatozoan acrosin a predictor of fertilization and embryo quality in the human? *Fertil. Steril.*, **60**, 881–7
24. Schill, W. B. (1990). Determination of active, non-zymogen acrosin, proacrosin and total acrosin in different andrological patients. *Arch. Dermatol. Res.*, **282**, 335–42
25. Rhemrev, J., Jeyendran, R. S., Vermeiden, J. P. W. and Zaneveld, L. J. D. (1989). Human sperm selection by glass wool filtration and two-layer, discontinuous Percoll gradient centrifugation. *Fertil. Steril.*, **51**, 685–90
26. Van der Ven, H. H., Kennedy, W.P., Kaminski, J. M., Jeyendran, R. S. and Zaneveld, L. J. D. (1987). Human sperm acrosin as a fertility marker. *J. Androl.*, **8**, Suppl. 1, 20
27. Hoesing, K., Schwartz, J. R. and DeJonge, C. J. (1994). Acrosin activity in spermatozoa prepared using ficoll or percoll. *J. Androl.*, Suppl. 1, 27
28. Liu, D. Y. and Baker, H. W. (1990). Relationships between human sperm acrosin, acrosomes, morphology and fertilization *in vitro*. *Hum. Reprod.*, **5**, 298–303
29. Loughlin, K. R., Ikemoto, I. and Agarwal, A. (1993). Improvement in human sperm acrosin levels and membrane integrity by use of L4 membrane. *J. Androl.*, Suppl. 1, 61
30. Sofikitis, N. and Miyagawa, I. (1993). Endocrinological, biophysical and biochemical parameters of semen collected via masturbation versus sexual intercourse. *J. Androl.*, **14**, 366–73
31. Goodpasture, J. C., Zavos, P. M., Cohen, M. R. and Zaneveld, L. J. D. (1982). Relationship of human sperm acrosin and proacrosin to semen parameters. 1. Comparisons between symptomatic men of infertile couples and asymptomatic men, and between different split ejaculates. *J. Androl.*, **3**, 151–6
32. Goodpasture, J. C., Zavos, P. N. and Zaneveld, L. J. D. (1987). Relationship of human sperm acrosin and proacrosin to semen parameters. II. Correlations. *J. Androl.*, **8**, 267–71
33. Kruger, T. F., Haque, D., Acosta, A. A., Pleban, P., Swanson, R. J., Simmons, K. F., Matta, J. F., Morshedi, M. and Oehninger, S. (1988). Correlation between sperm morphology, acrosin and fertilization in a IVF program. *Arch. Androl.*, **20**, 337–45
34. Yang, Y. S., Chen, S. U., Ho, H. N., Chen, H. F., Lien, Y. R., Lin, H. R., Huang, S. C. and Lee, T. Y. (1994). Acrosin activity of human sperm did not correlate with IVF. *Arch. Androl.*, **32**, 13–19
35. Gerhard, I., Frohlich, E., Eggert-Kruse, W., Klinga, K. and Runnebaum, B. (1989). Relationship of sperm acrosin activity to semen and clinical parameters in infertile patients. *Andrologia*, **21**, 146–54
36. Florke-Gerlott, S., Topfer-Peterson, E., Muller-Esterl, W., Mansouri, A., Schatz, R., Schirren, C., Schill, W. and Engel, W. (1984). Biochemical and genetic investigations of round-headed spermatozoa in infertile men including two brothers and their father. *Andrologia*, **16**, 187–202
37. Jeyendran, R. S., Van der Ven, H. H., Kennedy, W. P., Heath, E., Perez-Pelaez, M., Sobrero, A. J. and Zaneveld, L. J. D. (1985). Acrosomeless sperm: a cause of primary male infertility. *Andrologia*, **17**, 31–4
38. Lalonde, L., Langlais, J., Antaki, P., Chapdelaine, A., Roberts, K. D. and Bleau, G. (1988). Male infertility associated with round-headed acrosomeless spermatozoa. *Fertil. Steril.*, **49**, 316–21
39. Weissenberg, R., Eshkol, A., Rudak, E. and Lunenfeld, B. (1983). Inability of round acrosomeless human spermatozoa to penetrate zona free hamster ova. *Arch. Androl.*, **11**, 167–9
40. Beyler, S. A. and Zaneveld, L. J. D. (1979). The role of acrosin in sperm penetration through human cervical mucus. *Fertil. Steril.*, **32**, 671–5
41. Sofikitis, N., Zavos, P. M., Saito, M. and Miyagowa, I. (1993). The effect of varicocele on the sperm acrosin system in rabbits. *J. Androl.*, Suppl. 1, 54
42. Burkman, L. J., Syner, F. N., Moghissi, K. S. and Acosta, A. (1984). Sperm acrosin content and semen parameters for successful *in vitro* fertilization: 'normal' and oligospermic groups. *Fertil. Steril.*, **41**, 102S
43. De Jonge, C. J., Tarchala, S. M., Rawlins, R. G., Binor, Z. and Radwanska, E. (1993). Acrosin activity in human spermatozoa in relation to semen quality and *in-vitro* fertilization. *Hum. Reprod.*, **8**, 253–7
44. Blackwell, J., Kaminski, J. M., Bielfeld, P., Mack, S. R. and Zaneveld, L. J. D. (1992). Human sperm acrosin. Further studies with the clinical assay and activity in a group of presumably fertile men. *J. Androl.*, **13**, 571–8
45. Schill, W. B., Topfer-Peterson, E. and Heissler, E. (1988). The sperm acrosome: functional and clinical aspects. *Hum. Reprod.*, **3**, 139–45
46. Schill, W. B. (1991). Some disturbances of acrosomal

development and function in human spermatozoa. *Hum. Reprod.*, **6**, 969–78

47. Zaneveld, L. J. D., Jeyendran, R. S., Kaminski, J. M. and Pleban, P. (1990). Biochemistry: acrosin. In Acosta, A. A., Swanson, R. J., Ackerman, S. B., Kruger, T. F., Van Zyl, J. A. and Menkveld, R. (eds.) *Human Spermatozoa in Assisted Reproduction*, pp. 189–94. (Baltimore: Williams and Wilkins)
48. Agarwal, A., Fanning, L., Loughlin, K. R. and Ikemoto, I. (1993). Human sperm acrosin levels: comparison of Kennedy and Accusperm methods. *J. Androl.*, Suppl. 1, 61
49. Comhaire, F., Vermeulen, L. and Ghedira, K. (1983). Adenosine triphosphate in human semen. A quantitative estimate of fertilizing potential. *Fertil. Steril.*, **40**, 500–8
50. Irvine, D. S. and Aitken, R. J. (1985). The value of adenosine triphosphate (ATP) measurements in assessing the fertilizing ability of human spermatozoa. *Fertil. Steril.*, **44**, 806–11
51. Vigue, C., Vigue, L. and Huszar, G. (1992). Adenosine triphosphate (ATP) concentrations and ATP/adenosine diphosphate ratios in human sperm of normospermic, oligospermic, and asthenospermic specimens and in their swim-up fractions: lack of correlation between ATP parameters and sperm creatine kinase concentrations. *J. Androl.*, **13**, 305–11
52. Fakih, H., MacLusky, N., DeCherney, A., Walliman, T. and Huszar, G. (1986). Enhancement of human sperm motility and velocity *in vitro*: effects of calcium and creatine phosphate. *Fertil. Steril.*, **46**, 938–44
53. Huszar, G. (1993). Spermatogenic arrest: a classical and futuristic view. *Fertil. Steril.*, **60**, 947–9
54. Huszar, G., Vigue, L. and Morshedi, M. (1992). Sperm creatine phosphokinase M-isoform ratios and fertilizing potential of men: a blinded study of 84 couples treated with *in vitro* fertilization. *Fertil. Steril.*, **57**, 882–8
55. Huszar, G., Corrales, M. and Vigue, L. (1988). Correlation between sperm creatine phosphokinase activity and sperm concentrations in normospermic and oligospermic men. *Gamete Res.*, **19**, 67–75
56. Zaneveld, L. J. D. and Jeyendran, R. S. (1990). Biochemical analysis of seminal plasma and spermatozoa. In Webster, B. W. and Keel, B. A. (eds.) *CRC Handbook of the Laboratory Diagnosis and Treatment of Infertility*, pp. 79–96. (Boca Raton: CRC Press)
57. Huszar, G., Vigue, L. and Corrales, M. (1988). Sperm creatine phosphokinase activity as a measure of sperm quality in normospermic, variablespermic and oligospermic men. *Biol. Reprod.*, **38**, 1061–6
58. Huszar, G. and Vigue, L. (1993). Incomplete development of human spermatozoa is associated with increased creatine phosphokinase concentrations and abnormal head morphology. *Mol. Reprod.*, **34**, 292–8
59. Huszar, G. and Vigue, L. (1990). Spermatogenesis-related changes in the synthesis of the creatine kinase B-type and M-type isoforms in human spermatozoa. *Mol. Reprod. Dev.*, **25**, 258–62
60. Huszar, G., Vigue, L. and Corrales, M. (1990). Sperm creatine kinase activity in fertile and infertile oligospermic men. *J. Androl.*, **11**, 40–6
61. Huszar, G., Vigue, L. and Oehninger, S. (1992). Creatine kinase-immunocytochemistry of human hemizona–sperm complexes: preferential binding of sperm with CK-staining pattern characteristic of high fertilizing potential. *Am. Fertil. Soc., New Orleans, LA.*, S35

Determination of membrane integrity and viability

15

J. C. Calamera and M. del Carmen Quiros

SPERM PLASMA MEMBRANE STRUCTURE

In order to study the integrity and viability of the mammalian spermatozoon membrane, it is necessary to know, in the first place, the characteristics of the sperm plasma membrane.

The present concept of the spermatozoon external structure is that of a highly differentiated plasma membrane or plasmalemma stretching over the entire surface (head and tail).

As regards its configuration and function, this membrane appears to be analogous to the fluid–mosaic–transmembrane system of cells, which consists of three distinct parts: (1) an external glycocalyx composed of charged glycolipid and glycoprotein residues with oligosaccharide chains extending from the cell surface; (2) a membrane matrix underneath, made up of proteins embedded within a lipid bilayer with hydrophilic ends directed outward and hydrophobic ends inward; and (3) a submembrane cytofibrillar system of microtubules (cytoskeletal elements) and microfilaments (contractile elements)[1,2].

The schematic representation of a sperm plasma membrane is based on results obtained from chemical analysis of isolated membrane components and it shows the generally accepted concept (Figure 1).

Physical techniques that allow the molecular characterization of the three selected parts of the sperm surface have been developed[3,4].

A molecular membrane model of the human incapacitated sperm plasma membrane has been described as an assembly of phospholipids and sterols in dynamic equilibrium with peripheral and integral membrane proteins[5].

More accurate determinations were made with purified plasmalemma, where it was found that phospholipids represent about 70% of the total lipids, sterols being the next most abundant lipids. Cholesterol is also abundant in human spermatozoa[6] and part of the steroid is sulfoconjugated[7]. Ejaculated human spermatozoa have a cholesterol/phospholipid ratio equal to 0.99 and a polyunsaturated/saturated fatty acid ratio equal to 1[6].

Cholesterol introduced into bilayers of phospholipids with one saturated chain and another unsaturated one greatly reduces the membrane permeability[8]. Thus, the lipid composition of the human spermatozoon plasma membrane is characteristic of highly stable biological membranes.

Proteins within these lipids are considered either intrinsic (integral and essential for structure) or extrinsic (associated with the membrane, but easily removed by mild physical treatment).

The plasmalemma, covering all the spermatozoon surface, shows very defined morphological and immunological domains[9].

The evidence that the organization and composition of the plasma membrane varied among different regions of the sperm surface led to the concept that the sperm plasma membrane is a mosaic of unrestricted domains that reflect the specialized functions of surface and cytoplasmic components[9].

The sperm surface can be divided into five domains, each of which plays a separate and specific part in the series of events which lead to fertilization. These five domains are: anterior head (acrosomal segment); equatorial segment; posterior head (post-acrosomal segment); midpiece; and principal piece[10,11].

The morphology of the mammalian spermatozoon membrane, analyzed by means of transmission electron microscopy, shows the classical organization of biological membrane units. When the membrane is analyzed by the method of the

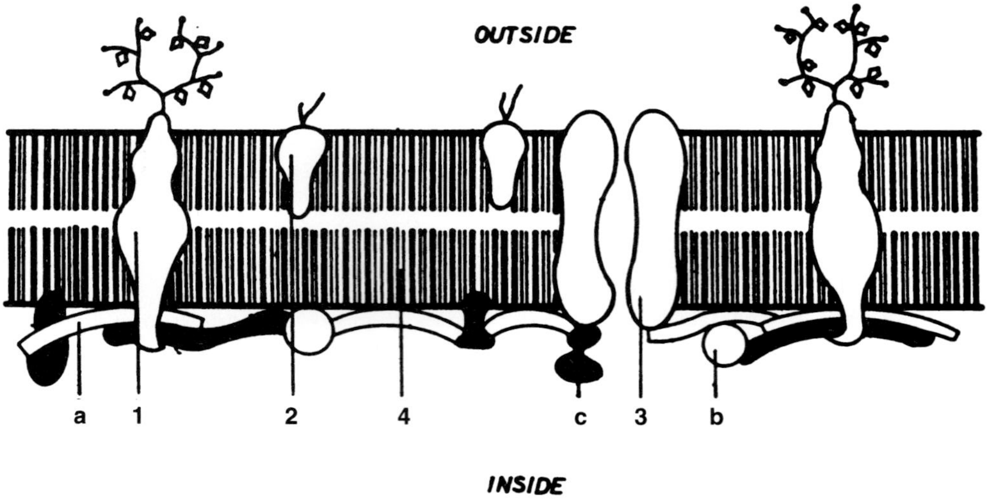

Figure 1 Schematic representation of sperm plasma membrane. 1, Non-motile glycoproteins with oligosaccharide chains; 2, motile glycoproteins; 3, transmembrane proteins; 4, lipid bilayer (a) spectrin; (b) actin; (c) enzymatic components

surface replica or by means of freeze-fracture techniques, considerable differences appear among the different regions of the spermatozoon surface.

A good description of membranes in different species was given a long time ago[12–14]. These studies have particularly reviewed the membrane characteristics and the different regions of the spermatozoon membrane appear relatively well defined.

For instance, the acrosome surface shows groups of fine particles intermingled with smooth areas devoid of particulate elements. In addition, the post-acrosomal region shows a parallel striation and the equatorial segment usually appears in a deep line with parallel depressions toward the post-acrosomal region. As regards the tail, the midpiece shows dispersed particles of 5 nm and a double line of 8 nm particles which lie adjacent to fibers 1 and 5 of the flagellum (Figure 2)[15].

When using techniques in which freeze-fracture methods are combined with cytochemical procedures, to locate glycoproteins, changes in the surface membrane of the spermatozoon in different physiological situations were observed[1]. It was established that the boar sperm head has some transmembrane glycoproteins which are particularly evident in the acrosome region[16].

The relation of distinct membrane regions with different protein components has been demon-

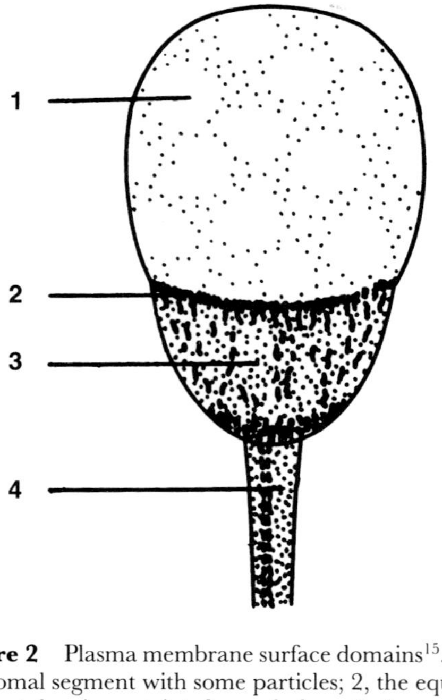

Figure 2 Plasma membrane surface domains[15]. 1, The acrosomal segment with some particles; 2, the equatorial segment showing a striated morphology; 3, the post-acrosomal segments with abundant particles; 4, the tail segment (midpiece and principal piece) with dispersed particles

strated by the use of membrane markers, particularly lectins[17,18]. Lectins have relative specific affinities with determined saccharide molecules[19,20]. They are often multimeric and can bind simultaneously with more than one saccharide ligand on a given cell or can cause agglutination by linking adjacent cells. Lectins can be tagged with fluorescent markers, enzymes, radioactive labels or materials visible through electron microscopy; however, the surface domains recognized by lectins are often not well defined and different binding patterns have been observed with identical lectins on sperm from the same species[21,22]. By using polyvalent or monoclonal antibodies, these different domains have also been clearly located.

However, it is likely that all three mechanisms for maintaining the compositional integrity of this membrane (extracellular glycocalyceal attachments, intramembranous lipid phase diffusional parameters and intracellular cytoskeletal attachments) are operative, and each mechanism regulates the movements of different components; thus, all of them act in concert to produce the mosaic of domains in the sperm[23].

This situation was particularly true when monoclonal antibodies were developed against different membrane protein components. By the use of such markers, specific antigens can be located from the early spermatogenesis stage to the mature spermatozoon[9]. In this regard, it has been shown that some antigens are acquired by the spermatozoon membrane as early as the spermatocyte stage[24], and some of such antigens persist during fertilization. Other antigens are gained during spermiogenesis as part of the membrane formation which logically occurs during this process[25]. In some cases, it has been found that antigens shared with other cell types are restricted to specific regions of the sperm surface[26,27].

Lastly, other antigens are acquired during the maturing process of the epididymis. These antigens cause the membrane to have a complicated picture of proteins, some of which show cross-reactivity with closely related species[28], but others show species specificity and are probably used during the membrane interrelationship with the female gamete phenomena.

Changes in the surface charge, lectin binding, intramembranous particle distribution, membrane fluidity, lipid and protein composition and antibody binding have been reported as the sperm travels through the epididymis[29].

Other alterations of the sperm surface composition may occur upon ejaculation. These include: changes in the surface charge[30], lectin binding[31] and possible changes in the lipid composition[32], absorption of blood antigens[33], histocompatibility antigens[34] and immunosuppressive factors[35].

METHODOLOGY

Supravital techniques

The integrity and functional activity of the sperm membrane are essential for viability and also for the physiological changes that occur on the sperm surface during the fertilization process, including capacitation, acrosome reaction and binding to the zona pellucida and oolemma.

In 1930 Moench[36], when investigating sperm motility, used a supravital staining to determine the percentage of live spermatozoa. Subsequently in 1942, MacLeod[37], using a similar methodology, found that the results were unsatisfactory.

The proportion of motile and immotile spermatozoa is routinely determined in most laboratories by direct visual microscopic estimation, supplemented by the live–dead staining. The membrane of living spermatozoa acts as a barrier to stain penetration; thus, only damaged or dead gametes are stained.

The traditional methods of assessing whether the membrane is intact or disrupted are based on the examination of the percentage of viable sperm by dye exclusion of eosin–opal blue, Blom's eosin–nigrosin or eosin alone[38–42].

The discriminatory ability of these supravital stains depends on the ability of functionally intact membranes to exclude the eosin chromophores from the nuclear compartment of spermatozoa. The capacity to differentiate between viable and non-viable spermatozoa is also important in such studies as the evaluation of sperm incubation or in different storage techniques.

The ability to evaluate the survival of spermatozoa allows the investigator to detect sublethal damage that may diminish sperm function. However, an additional problem with classical supravital stains is that they are not appropriate for assessing viability in cryopreserved spermatozoa because glycerol would interfere with the stain[43].

Nevertheless, recently three methods for the study of the effect of glycerol have been employed: motility, acrosome integrity and sperm treatment with carboxyfluorescein diacetate and propidium iodide (to assess membrane integrity). It was concluded that 4% glycerol gives maximum viability of frozen–thawed spermatozoa when these methods were employed[44].

Carboxyfluorescein diacetate is a membrane-permeable, non-fluorescent stain that is hydrolyzed by intracellular esterases, and the resulting product, 6-carboxyfluorescein, is membrane-impermeable and fluorescent; consequently spermatozoa with intact plasma membrane fluoresce bright green, while those with non-intact membrane do not. The carboxyfluorescein diacetate, therefore, permits measurement of the functional integrity of spermatozoal organelles and membranes[45].

The possibility of damage to sperm membrane as a consequence of cryopreservation might occur in spite of the maintenance of other seminal parameters[46].

Recently, the effects of various cryoprotective agents and membrane-stabilizing compounds on the sperm membrane integrity have been studied[47].

Further research on cryopreservation should focus on membrane stabilization since membrane-stabilizing compounds yield more promising results than ice-preventing agents. In addition, spermatozoa viability is difficult to assess when cells are suspended in opaque media. A method by which motile, immotile and dead (eosin-staining) spermatozoa can be differentiated simultaneously is available for human semen[48].

The supravital techniques (see Appendix) also provide a check on the accuracy of the motility evaluation, since the percentage of dead cells could be compared with the percentage of immotile spermatozoa. In the eosin–nigrosin test, live spermatozoa appear white and dead ones are pink (Figure 3).

A population of non-motile sperm that exclude the supravital dye in human semen has been known for a long time[49]. The functional significance of these spermatozoa is not known; however, if they remain immotile, they cannot participate in fertilization. Furthermore, the presence of a large proportion of viable but immotile cells may indicate structural defect in the flagellum[50].

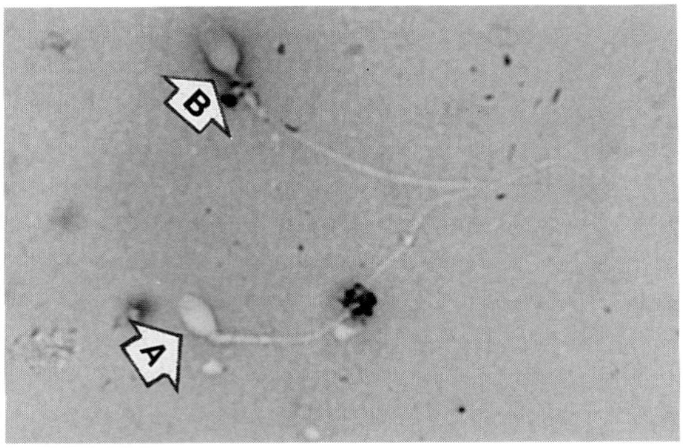

Figure 3 Supravital stain, eosin–nigrosin technique. A, Live spermatozoon; B, dead spermatozoon

The use of supravital technique allows the definitive diagnosis of true necrozoospermia (all cells dead), since biochemical changes occur immediately after the cell dies. Therefore, this test is still recommended as part of standard semen analysis by WHO[50]. Although the clinical significance of this test in evaluating male fertility should be better known, it provides diagnostic information about the spermatozoa survival, especially when sperm motility is very low[51].

It was suggested that eosin Y exclusion measures the structural integrity of the sperm membrane, whereas the hypo-osmotic swelling test evaluates the physiological integrity of the sperm membrane[52].

Combined methods that include sperm viability assessment

The idea of combining different tests to study the spermatozoal membrane is not new. For example, stains have been used to determine sperm viability in hypo-osmotic solution, then the sperm plasma membrane characteristics are analyzed by a combination of the hypo-osmotic swelling test (HOS) and the eosin test[53].

The sperm plasma membrane has also been studied recently using the HOS test and staining with either the eosin Y or propidium iodide dye. This method was proposed for a simultaneous measurement of both the functional and structural state of the sperm membrane[54]. By combining supravital staining with the HOS test, the number of false positive results can be reduced[55].

One of the most commonly used lightmicroscope cytochemical methods for the evaluation of acrosome status is the triple-stain technique[56] which, in addition to acrosome stains, involves a pre-fixation supravital staining believed to mark all dead spermatozoa. Nevertheless, there are some doubts as to its real ability to distinguish all non-viable spermatozoa. Some data indicate that cells excluding supravital dyes may not necessarily be living[52].

Spermatozoal viability and acrosomal status were also studied by introducing a dual stain procedure[57,58]. These techniques were proposed as useful in the routine evaluation of the spermatozoal fertilizing potential.

In this sense, a practical and reliable staining method was developed to distinguish the viability and acrosomal status of mammal spermatozoa. The first stain with trypan blue or congo red is rapid and avoids artefacts. This stain is precipitated by neutral red and gives a high-contrast block color that persists during the time required for staining the acrosome with Giemsa[59]. Through this methodology, it is possible to distinguish live or dead spermatozoa with intact acrosome, as well as damage or absence of acrosomes.

The addition of centrifugation steps required by some supravital staining methods reduces the yield of spermatozoa for smear preparation, which is inconvenient in cases where only a limited number of spermatozoa are available for this kind of examination.

Recently, fluorescent probes to provide quantifiable information of spermatozoal viability and fertilizing potential have been developed[45,60,61].

The endpoint of a cell's death was determined by a combination of the fluorescent dyes fluorescein diacetate and ethidium bromide. Fluorescein diacetate rapidly enters living cells and is converted into fluorescein (green) by esterases, whereas ethidium bromide is largely excluded by living cells, only effectively penetrating the plasma membrane and staining nuclear components (red) on breakdown of the permeability barrier. Three distinct populations of spermatozoa were discernible by microscopic examination: (1) viable spermatozoa; (2) moribund spermatozoa; and (3) dead cells. These populations were quantified using a flow cytometric analysis[45]. Sperm viability is an important parameter to be assessed in systems employed to study sperm capacitation and acrosome reaction.

Cell viability by propidium iodide exclusion and acrosomal integrity by FITC-conjugated *Pisum sativum* agglutinin (FITC-PSA) were also estimated using flow cytometry[62]. This combination can be used to correlate different features simultaneously upon individual spermatozoa, and at the same time assay many cells per sample without expensive preparations.

Ericsson *et al.*[63] used rhodamine 123, hydroethidine and FITC–PSA to assess the mitochondrial function, plasma membrane integrity and acrosomal characteristics of bovine sperm. This method is based on the observation that only coupled, respiring mitochondria will take up rhodamine dye. It was determined that viable spermatozoa, capable of excluding supravital dye, are also alive as evidenced by the presence of functional mitochondria[64].

The need to assess spermatozoal viability in order to differentiate physiological acrosome reaction from pathological acrosome loss has been recognized since the publications of pioneer studies[56,65].

Cross *et al.*[65] described a supravital nuclear staining test, using bis-benzamide (Hoechst N 33258) to mark sperm cells. This test was largely employed with good results. The use of a supravital stain such as Hoechst 33258 (H 258) (see Appendix) is a convenient way to obtain more information on the physiological state of individual sperm[64].

When acrosomal loss is induced by methods that simultaneously result in a significant reduction of sperm motility, for example calcium ionophore, sperm viability can alternatively be assessed by the use of supravital stain. Approximately 10% of the spermatozoa incubated with the calcium ionophore A 23187 demonstrate a loss of membrane integrity as indicated by positive H 258 staining. The majority of human spermatozoa remains viable although non-motile after calcium ionophore treatment[66].

In other studies, motility characteristics and membrane integrity of cryopreserved human spermatozoa were determined by HOS test and with the supravital fluorescent dye H 258. A considerable decline in the percentage of progressive motile spermatozoa and a significant reduction in the proportion of spermatozoa with intact plasma membrane after cryopreservation were observed; however, the results of these tests were widely variable, especially among donors[67].

Some studies were also done using fluorescence microscopy to determine the viability and acrosome status of fresh and frozen–thawed human spermatozoa[68]. This technology was compared to conventional eosin–nigrosin staining and sperm motion parameters. Replacing the H 258 with propidium iodide in combination with FITC-PSA, specimens could be excited by a single excitation source, so that the fluorescence from both the propidium iodide and the FITC-PSA could be simultaneously observed. It was concluded by using this technology that the frozen–thawed spermatozoa may undergo premature breakdown of the acrosome prior to interaction with the oocyte; thus, this would explain the reduced fertility of cryopreserved semen.

All techniques produce some sperm that are not easily classified. This is not a serious problem if the number of ambiguous sperm is low compared to the number of sperm included in identifiable classes. The level of uncertainty varies considerably among assays, and researchers may find that this is an important issue in their selection of an assay.

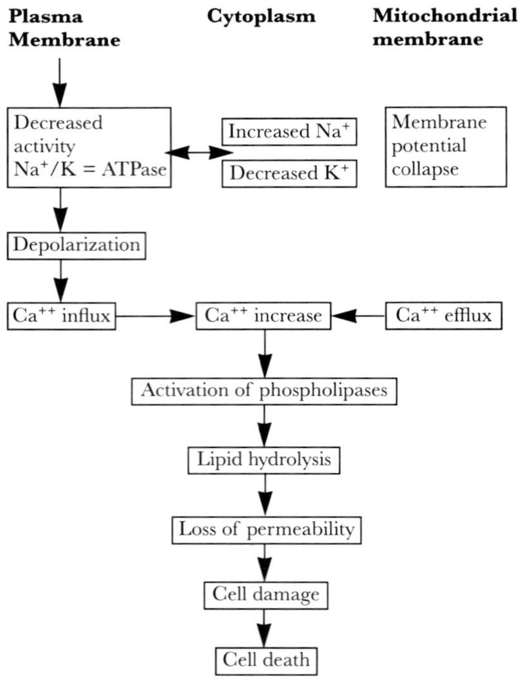

Figure 4 Progression of events associated with imbalanced ATP synthesis–degradation. Reproduced with permission of J. B. Lippincott[143]

Other methods used for the determination of membrane integrity

The functional integrity of the spermatic membrane was studied through the so-called 'water-test', a simple method of assessing sperm membrane integrity. The results of these experiences were correlated with routine semen analysis and with the eosin Y staining[69]; as a matter of fact, this method, of recent appearance, should be tested more widely.

The vital key to the cellular mechanism may be obtained by combining metabolic end-product analyses and enzyme kinetics. While the full approach to this is complex, the essential core of it is the balance between the rate of ATP generation and ATP consumption[70]. The latter is probably dominated by ion pumping and motility since little biosynthesis occurs in these cells[71]. When energy requirements are changed, the cell must be able to adjust the rates of ATP generation and consumption to establish a new ATP turnover rate, reflecting the new situation.

The intact plasma membrane of sperm is considered to be almost impermeable to ATP. Some toxic substances affect the permeability of cellular membranes, resulting in the leakage of various molecules into or out of the cell. Thus, leakage of intracellular ATP to the extracellular medium is indicative of membrane damage[72]. ATP is an excellent indicator of cellular 'health' because it is the prime energy donor[73].

On the other hand, the viable cell number correlates with the intracellular ATP level of the live cells. When the cell dies, the respiratory activity ceases and a rapid ATP depression follows[73].

When the cellular ATP content is depleted, the metabolites passing through the plasma membrane are quickly degraded by serum and the surface membrane hydrolases (Figure 4). The mechanism of ATP depletion in spermatozoa is not well known; it might result from an action of free radicals on membrane lipids (see *Lipid peroxidation test*, later in this chapter) or by inhibition of cellular enzymes acting on mitochondrial functions, anaerobic glycolysis, protein synthesis, plasma membrane adenylate cyclase, etc.[74].

Kangas *et al.*[75] reported that the intracellular ATP level significantly correlated with the number of cell, viability and (^{3}H)-thymidine incorporation. Results may be obtained in a short time and the required number of cells is low with the ATP assay.

As suggested by Wolf *et al.*[76], the most useful assay might be one that could be performed on living cells, so that the acrosomal status and the motility of each spermatozoon could be assessed simultaneously.

Hypo-osmotic swelling test (HOS)

Water permeability is a fundamental biophysical property of all living cells. It is known that a quality of the cell membrane is its ability to allow the transport of selective fluids and certain molecules through it.

Water permeability assumes widely dissimilar values among different cells even within a given cell type[77]. Some of these cells, such as the human spermatozoon, have plasma membranes that are devoid of microvilli or other forms of membrane reserves and are, therefore, fixed in area. If such cells are placed in sufficiently low concentrations of non-permeating solutes, they will swell until their fixed area of membrane encompasses the maximum value. If the attainment of osmotic equilibrium requires that they swell beyond that critical volume, they will lyse[78]. When a cell behaves as an ideal osmometer, the volume of osmotically available water contained within the plasma membrane will be reciprocally related to the osmolality of non-permeating solutes in the external medium[79].

In 1984, Jeyendran *et al.*[80] developed a simple test called the hypo-osmotic swelling test, used to determine the functional integrity of the spermatic plasma membrane. The assay is based on the fact that fluid transport occurs across an intact cell membrane under hypo-osmotic conditions until equilibrium is reached between the inside and the outside of the cell[81]. When live spermatozoa with a normal membrane function are exposed to a solution of low osmolality (150 mOsm/L), 33–80% of the spermatozoa will exhibit tail swelling (Figure 5). The authors say that when the plasma membrane balloons under hypo-osmotic conditions, the bending of the tail fibers occurs within the plasma membrane. Extra space is created in spermatozoal head and tail. Since the tail fibers are under tension, the excess space causes them to curl within the membrane[82]. The sperm tails seem to be particularly sensitive to such swelling, since the membranes are more loosely attached to the underlying structures in this region than the membrane of the sperm head. Spermatozoa that are not viable or gametes with non-functioning membranes do not swell. Figure 5 shows the various aspects that the spermatozoa may reach. Some of the tails may be either entirely disfigured or curled, while others could be less deformed. It is considered that the tail's membrane is intact if there is evidence of swelling, no matter to what extent.

By means of indirect immunofluorescence with antiboar outer acrosomal membrane antibodies and exposure to the human spermatozoa to a hypo-osmotic medium, it was possible to visualize the swelling phenomenon in the sperm head. This experience shows both the expansion capacity of the plasma membrane in the acrosomal region and the principal specificity of this antiserum for the outer acrosomal membrane[83]. (See Appendix for the HOS test technique).

It is normal for an ejaculate to possess 60% or more of swollen spermatozoa after having been subjected to the HOS test. Between 50 and 59% of swollen spermatozoa represent a gray area in which no diagnosis can be reached. Less than 50% swollen spermatozoa is abnormal.

HOS test results were correlated with different sperm parameters, such as sperm concentration, sperm motility, normal morphology and particularly with viability assessed by eosin Y exclusion. As can be observed in Table 1, the correlation coefficients are in general too low to be predictive. These results indicate that the HOS test measures a different entity than do the standard semen parameters.

Van den Saffele *et al.*[84] confirm that the HOS test gives information on the spermatozoal capacity to pump water into the cell, but they assume that the test provides the same information as does the viability stain with eosin solution.

Jeyendran *et al.*[80] found that a hypo-osmotic swelling test was highly correlated with the hamster zona-free oocyte penetration test (SPA), and they claimed that the assay is a useful and simple clinical test to study the human sperm function. However, other researchers have reported that there was no

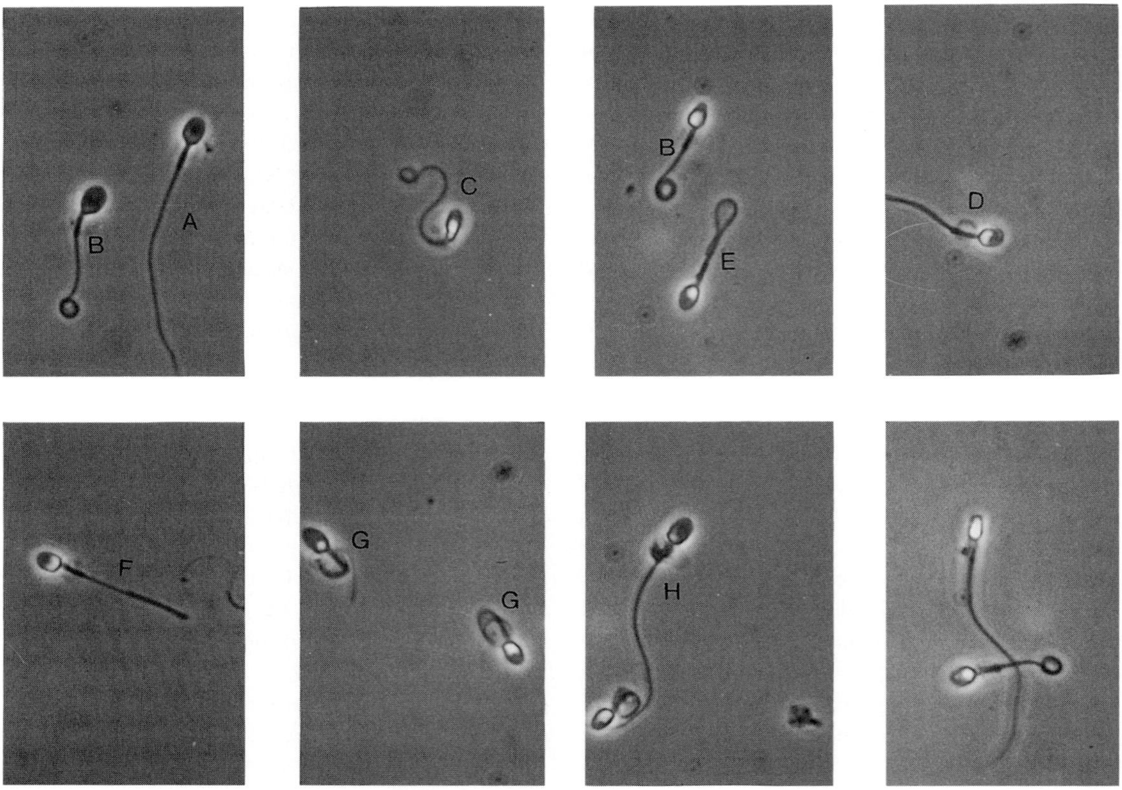

Figure 5 Different sperm tail swellings in human spermatozoa. A, Spermatozoon without changes; B–H, spermatozoa with various types of tail changes

Table 1 Correlation coefficients between the HOS test and other sperm variables

Authors	*Sperm conc.* (10^6 sp/mL)	*Motility* (%)	*Morphology* (%)	*SPA* (%)	*Live/dead* (%)
Jeyendran *et al.*[80]	—	0.61	0.30	0.90	0.52
Chan *et al.*[85]	0.02	0.22	0.32	0.05	—
Wang *et al.*[86]	0.19	0.60	0.41	0.41	—
Chan and Wang[137]	—	0.33	0.14	0.08	—
Chan *et al.*[87]	—	0.41	0.10	0.04	—
Coetzee *et al.*[138]	—	—	0.51	0.42	0.76
Rogers and Parker[139]	0.48	0.51	0.26	0.32	—
van Kooij *et al.*[140]	—	NS	NS	NS	0.70
Liu *et al.*[92]	0.23	0.48	0.25	—	0.47
van den Saffele *et al.*[84]	—	0.54	—	—	0.50
Takahashi *et al.*[141]	—	—	—	0.40	—

SPA=zona-free hamster oocyte penetration assay; NS=not significant

significant correlation between the HOS test and the SPA when performed in semen samples obtained from a large number of fertile and infertile men (Table 1)[85–88]. Nevertheless, it was claimed that the HOS test provides additional evidence in the evaluation of subfertile men as a relevant part of a comprehensive assessment of male fertility[89]. In addition, the HOS test was used to monitor other sperm procedures, such as the selection, preparation, cryosurvival and effect of toxins[90,91].

The hypo-osmotic viability parameter was correlated with the outcome of the motility of thawed sperm. The pre-freeze supravital staining for sperm viability and the hypo-osmotic sperm swelling test could not predict the thawed sperm total motility. As a result of these studies, it was found that the integrity of the sperm membrane was more important at the head than at the tail[55]. Attempts have been made to correlate the finding obtained with this test and the fertilization potential of semen samples. However, the significance of the HOS test in predicting male fertility still remains controversial.

Actually, it is very difficult to prove that a test can predict the spermatozoal fertilizing capacity. Human *in vitro* fertilization (IVF) may be used to assess the validity of an assay[92]. The HOS test was also correlated with IVF rates.

Studies have shown that samples with >62% swelling are capable of fertilizing ova, whereas <60% swelling is observed in infertile semen samples[93]. Other papers have shown that the results of this test were highly correlated with human fertilization[93,94].

Riedel *et al.*[95] found that if a penetration of more than 40% occurred in the SPA, and more than 65% of the spermatozoa reacted in the HOS test, the ejaculates were fertile for IVF even if the other spermatic parameters were abnormal. These data might indicate that fertility is generally associated with a positive HOS test.

Nevertheless, there are opposing reports showing that the test did not have a prognostic value for the fertilization rate *in vitro*[96–99]. It appears that the test is subjected to a high level of false positive results[96].

Taking into account such opposing reports, it seems that this test may be useful for the study of some aspects of the spermatic membrane physiology, but its incidence in the prediction of fertility should be reviewed[100].

Lipid peroxidation test

Since the appearance of Jones and Mann's[101,102] and Holland and Storey's[103] pioneer papers, it is known that mammalian spermatozoa are highly susceptible to lipid peroxidation. The presence of unsaturated lipids in cells is a potential threat because of the extreme lability of such lipids in the presence of oxygen and their widespread distribution in the cell membrane. For this reason, parameters related to the structure and function of the plasma membrane have proven to be popular markers of the radical-mediated cellular injury.

There are data that suggest that electrochemical potentials may provide an early marker documenting injury to cellular membranes, preceding changes in permeability and morphology[104].

Certain aspects of the spermatic lipid biochemistry, particularly the nature of different lipid constituents and their metabolism, are better understood today. The content and composition of lipids and the percentage of lipid-bound fatty acids and aldehydes have been worked out for both spermatozoa and seminal plasma[105].

Phospholipids have several possible roles. They are important for stabilizing membrane integrity and for maintaining membrane fluidity[106]; they serve as substrates for phospholipases that generate second messengers inducing intracellular response, and are responsible for the generation of prostaglandins[107]. They can also serve as a source of energy generation[108].

The oxidation of polyunsaturated fatty acids abounding in the sperm phospholipids provides a good example of reactions directly involving oxygen radicals which, by leading to the formation of the highly toxic lipid peroxidases, cause the senescence and death of cells.

The loss of membrane integrity and inactivation of enzymes[109], the swelling of mitochondria[110] and the structural damage to DNA[111] have all been correlated with the formation of lipid peroxidases.

The biophysical consequence of lipid peroxidation in biological membranes was also studied. In the lipid domains, peroxidation causes: (1) an increase in the order and 'viscosity' of the membrane bilayer, particularly at the depth around the acyl-carbon; (2) changes on the thermotropic phase behavior; (3) decreases in the electrical resistance;

and (4) facilitates phospholipid exchange between the two monolayers.

Spermatozoa are activated by a variety of stimuli to release superoxide radicals ($O_2^{-\cdot}$). Activators of $O_2^{-\cdot}$ and thus H_2O_2 formation due to either spontaneous or enzyme-catalyzed dismutation of O_2, include among others, phorbol esters and Ca^{++} ionophores[112].

The superoxide anion generated by human spermatozoa appears to derive from a NADPH oxidase system located in the sperm plasma membrane which is similar to the mechanisms responsible for the oxidative phenomenon of phagocytic macrophages and neutrophils[113].

The NADPH oxidase system becomes activated upon removal of seminal plasma or incubation in suitable conditions and the $O_2^{-\cdot}$ generated is responsible for sperm capacitation[114].

The opposite action of living cells against the intermediates of oxygen reduction depends primarily on the enzymes that dispose of these highly reactive products.

The superoxide radical is eliminated by the superoxide dismutase (SOD), which catalyzes its dismutation to hydrogen peroxide and oxygen[115,116].

$$O_2^{-}+O_2^{-\cdot}+2H^+ \rightarrow H_2O_2+O_2$$

However, unless removed by catalase ($2\ H_2O_2 \rightarrow 2H_2O+O_2$), or glutation peroxidase ($2\ GSH+H_2O_2 \rightarrow GSSG+2H_2O$) hydrogen peroxide, by interacting with $O_2^{-\cdot}$, gives rise to the formation of the second free radical, namely the hydroxyl radical.

$Fe^{++} + H_2O_2 \rightarrow Fe^{+++} + OH^- + OH\cdot$ Fenton reaction

$O_2^{-\cdot}+H_2O_2 \rightarrow O_2+OH^-+OH\cdot$ Haber–Weiss reaction.

The hydroxyl radicals, powerful initiators of the lipid peroxidation, induce changes in the membrane fluidity and integrity[117].

Three distinct types of SOD, all metalloprotein enzymes, have been described[102]. The presence of SOD and of the glutathione peroxidase/reductase system in human semen was well established[118].

Therefore, in spite of the presence of endogenous antioxidant defense mechanisms within the cell, the flux of local oxidant generation may frequently overwhelm these defenses, resulting in tissue injury, denaturation of functional (enzymatic) and structural proteins, mutagenic or lethal damage to nucleic acids and the denaturation of polysaccharide components of the interstitium and of basement membranes[119].

The evidence that spermatozoa suffer irreversible damage as a result of experimentally induced lipid peroxidation raises the possibility that analogous reactions take place as part of the natural structural decay, lessening motility and declining metabolic activity in spermatozoa which are aging, either within the reproductive tract *in vivo* or during storage *in vitro*[120].

For experimental purposes, peroxidation of the sperm cell phospholipids can be induced by aerobically incubating washed spermatozoa in the presence of catalytic amounts of ferrous ion and ascorbate.

Iron chelation by biological and artificial binding sites can decisively influence the mechanism of interaction with O_2 and its reduced derivatives, and it is essential for the initiation and propagation of the peroxidative breakdown of cellular membranes (Figure 6)[121].

The thiobarbituric acid (TBA) reaction, quantified by colorimetry or fluorimetry, is the most used method for studying lipid peroxidation in both laboratory animals and in humans[122]. The assay can be observed in the Appendix, and the progress of endogenous peroxidation for 1–2 h at 37°C can be followed quantitatively.

Liquid peroxidation was recently measured using a modified version of the TBA reaction[123]. The TBA test has been widely used to provide a convenient index of lipid peroxidation, the outcome of which correlates properly with alternative techniques for assessing peroxidation, including chemiluminescence. This follows from the fact that the thiobarbituric acid-reactive product (malondialdehyde) accumulates at a considerably faster rate in the immotile or poorly motile spermatozoa from necrozoospermic or oligozoospermic semen than in fully motile normal spermatozoa.

The high value of the energy of activation indicates that a key step in the complex peroxidation reaction sequence leading to malondialdehyde is a reaction of O_2 with a biallylic methylene group of a long chain fatty acyl moiety of a phospholipid.

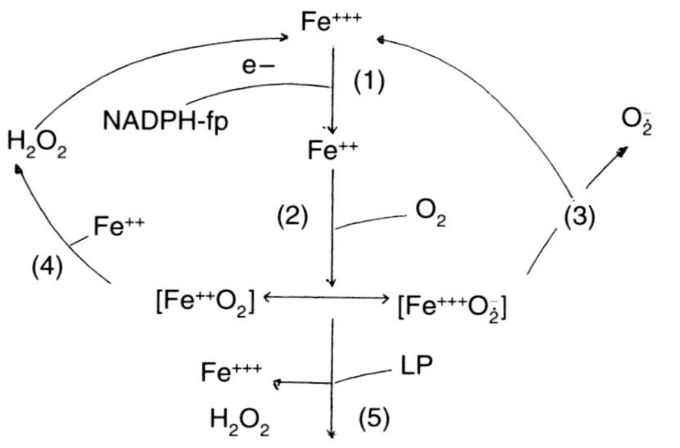

Figure 6 Pathways of iron oxygen interactions involved in the generation of lipid free radicals. Under aerobic conditions the $Fe^{++}O_2$ complex is readily formed (2). Decomposition of the $Fe^{++}O_2$ complex leads to Fe^{+++} and O_2 (3). A further decomposition pathway may arise if Fe^{+++} encounters a $Fe^{++}O_2$ complex (4). Therefore, depending on the concentration of Fe^{++}, the features of chelation and the presence of effective electron donors, the Fe^{++} can readily undergo auto-oxidation along reactions (2,4) generating $O_2^{\cdot-}$ and H_2O_2. Since both of these reduced oxygen species can interact with Fe^{+++} in the coupled Fenton–Haber–Weiss reaction, they generate $OH^{\cdot}$ radicals. Under steady state conditions, the concentration of the $Fe^{++}O_2$ complex and hence the rate of initiation of lipid peroxidation (5) depends on the relative rates of complex formation via reactions (1) and (2) and complex decomposition via reactions (3) and (4). Reproduced from DeGroot and Noll (1987)[121] with permission of Elsevier Scientific Publishers Ireland Ltd

The major drawback of the assay is that only a fraction of membrane lipids, much like cyclic endopexides, yields TBA-reactive products on peroxidation.[124].

It has been suggested that measurements of the lipid peroxide potential (LPOp) could serve as a valuable tool in the assessment of the structural integrity of human spermatozoa[125]. It was also demonstrated that human spermatozoa LPOp might be linked to the incidence of midpiece defects[126].

The polymorphonuclear neutrophils (PMN) and macrophages which are components of the early inflammatory conditions have the capacity to generate large quantities of free radical species. The oxidative burst from PMN has the potential to arrest sperm movement, but only when PMNs are properly stimulated and are present in a sufficient concentration[127]. On the other hand, a positive role for the superoxide anion in the triggering of human sperm hyperactivation and capacitation was suggested[114].

Coinciding with the lipid peroxide formation, motility and metabolism in the sperm suspension decline and certain intracellular enzymes escape from the spermatozoa through the damaged plasma membrane.

It has been shown that forced lipid peroxidation in normal and asthenozoospermic samples causes a decrease in sperm motility, velocity and linearity which is evident at different times of incubation[72,128].

When cell membranes are damaged, intracellular substances may leak into the surrounding medium. The purpose of Calamera *et al* (1989) was to study the effect of forced peroxidation upon human spermatozoa and its relation with the ATP content[72]. We know that one of the functions of the plasma membrane is to keep an appropriate ATP 'atmosphere' within the spermatozoon in order to maintain motility.

It was interesting to observe the significant decrease of spermatic ATP between control and forced lipid peroxidation groups at 120 min incubation using asthenozoospermic samples. This phenomenon was not observed in the normozoospermic group and this may suggest a lower resistance of the plasma membrane to peroxidation[72].

A frequent characteristic in the patients showing a defect of the sperm function is the spermatozoal refractoriness to calcium signal. This is certainly due to changes in the properties of the plasma membrane induced by lipid peroxidation[113].

In addition, the superoxide dismutase activity of a fresh sperm sample appears to be a good predictor of the lifetime (up to the complete loss of motility) of that particular sample; therefore, it may prove advantageous in semen analysis.

Proteins such as albumin[129] and small molecules just as glutathione[129], pyruvate[128], taurine and hypotaurine[130] and vitamins E and C[131,132] also play an important role in the protection of tissues against the oxidative stress.

Apart from the significance of ascorbic acid as a scavenger of $O_2^{\cdot-}$, vitamin C may not play a role similar to that of SOD in the intracellular defense, but it also may have a primary role as an extracellular defense against free radicals[133,134].

Aitken and Clarkson[135] presented evidence

indicating that human spermatozoa are capable of producing reactive oxygen species. The loss of sperm function in certain cases of male infertility was also demonstrated.

The confirmation that H_2O_2 and not $O_2^{\cdot -}$ is cytotoxic to human spermatozoa was observed in studies in which the direct addition of this oxidant to human spermatozoa was utilized. Its influence on the gamete movement and on the competence for oocyte fusion was also shown[136].

The purpose of this description was solely to focus the lipid peroxidation as a marker of the sperm plasma membrane permeability. The incidence of the free radicals on the sperm function will be developed in another chapter.

References

1. Koehler, J. K. (1978). The mammalian sperm surface studied with specific labeling techniques. *Int. Rev. Cytol.*, **54**, 75–108
2. Pollock, E. G. (1978). Fine structural analysis of animal cell surface: membranes and cell surface topography. *Am. Zool.*, **18**, 25–30
3. Azzi, A. and Montecucco, C. (1977). Spin labels and biological membranes. *Horizons Biochem. Biophys.*, **4**, 266–94
4. Hammerstedt, R. H., Amman, R. P., Rucinsky, T., Morse, P. D., Lepock, J., Snipes, W. and Keith, A. D. (1976). Use of spin labels and electron spin resonance spectroscopy to characterize membranes of bovine sperm. Effect of butylated hydroxytoluene and cold shock. *Biol. Reprod.*, **14**, 381–97
5. Langlais, J. and Roberts, K. D. (1985). A molecular membrane model of sperm capacitation and the acrosome reaction of mammalian spermatozoa. *Gamete Res.*, **12**, 183–224
6. Darin-Bennet, A. and White, I. G. (1977). Influence of the cholesterol content of mammalian spermatozoa on susceptibility to cold shock. *Cryobiology*, **14**, 466–70
7. Lalumiere, G., Blean, G., Chapdelaine, A. and Roberts, K. D. (1976). Cholesteryl sulfate and sterol sulfatase in the human reproductive tract. *Steroids*, **27**, 247–60
8. Demel, R. A., Geurts van Kessel, W. S. M. and van Deenen, L. L. M. (1972). The properties of polyunsaturated lecithins in monolayers and liposomes and the interactions of these lecithins with cholesterol. *Biochem. Biophys. Acta*, **166**, 26–40
9. Holt, W. V. (1984). Membrane heterogeneity in the mammalian spermatozoon. *Int. Rev. Cytol.*, **87**, 159–94
10. Bearer, E. L. and Fried, D. S. (1990). Morphology of mammalian sperm membranes during differentiation, maturation and capacitation. *J. Elect. Microsc. Tech.*, **16**, 281–97
11. Fawcett, D. W. (1975). The mammalian spermatozoon. *Dev. Biol.*, **44**, 394–436
12. Flechon, J. E. (1974). Freeze fracturing of rabbit spermatozoa. *J. Microscopy*, **19**, 59–64
13. Friend, D. S. (1982). Plasma membrane diversity in a highly polarized cell. *J. Cell Biol.*, **93**, 243–9
14. Susuki, F. (1981). Changes in intramembrane particules distribution in epididymal spermatozoa of the boar. *Anat. Rec.*, **199**, 361–76
15. Esponda, P. (1985). Spermiogenesis and spermatozoa in mammals. In Barbera-Guillen, E. (ed.), pp. 14–16. (Leioa-Vizcaya: Servicio Editorial Universidad Pais Basco)
16. Aguas, P. and Pino da Silva, P. (1993). Regionalization of transmembrane proteins in the plasma membrane of boar sperm head is revealed by fracture label. *J. Cell Biol.*, **97**, 1356–64
17. Nicolson, G. L. and Yanagimachi, R. (1974). Mobility and the restriction of mobility of plasma membrane binding components. *Science*, **184**, 1294–6
18. Bedford, J. M. and Cooper, G. W. (1978). Membrane fusion events in the fertilization of the vertebrate eggs. In Poste, F. and Nicholson, G. E. (eds). *Cell Surface Reviews*, **5**, pp. 65–125. (New York: Academic Press)
19. Sharon, N. and Lis, H. (1974). Use of lectins for the study of membranes. In Korn, E. D. (ed.) *Methods in Membrane Biology*, pp. 147–200. (New York: Academic Press)
20. Nicolson, G. L. (1974). The interactions of lectins with animal cell surface. In Bourne, G. H. and Danielli, J. F. (eds.) *International Review of Cytology*, pp. 89–190. (New York: Academic Press)
21. Koehler, J. K. (1981). Lectins as probes of the spermatozoon surface. *Arch. Androl.*, **6**, 197–217
22. Millette, C. F. (1977). Distribution and mobility of lectin binding sites on mammalian spermatozoa. In Edidin, M. and Johnson, H. H. (eds.) *Immunobiology of Gametes*, pp. 51–71. (Cambridge: Cambridge University Press)
23. Primakoff, P. and Myles, D. C. (1983). A map of the guinea pig sperm surface constructed with monoclonal antibodies. *Dev. Biol.*, **98**, 417–28
24. O'Rand, M. G. (1980). Antigens of spermatozoa and their environment. In Dhinsha, D. S. and Schumaker, G. F. (eds.) *Immunological Aspects of Infertility Regulation*, pp. 155–71. (New York: Elsevier)

25. Olson, G. E. and Hamilton, D. W. (1978). Characterization of the surface glycoproteins of rat spermatozoa. *Biol. Reprod.*, **19**, 26–35
26. O'Rand, M. D. and Romrell, L. J. (1980). Appearance of regional surface autoantigens during spermatogenesis: Comparison of antitestis and antisperm antisera. *Dev. Biol.*, **75**, 431–41
27. Tung, K. S. K., Han, L. B. P. and Evans, A. P. (1979). Differentiation autoantigen of testicular cells and spermatozoa in the guinea pig. *Dev. Biol.*, **68**, 224–38
28. Koehler, J. K. (1974). Studies on the distribution of antigenic sites on the surface of rabbit spermatozoa. *J. Cell Biol.*, **74**, 86–7
29. Moore, H. D. M. (1979). The net negative surface charge of mammalian spermatozoa as determined by isoelectric focusing. Changes following sperm maturation, ejaculation, incubation in the female tract, and after enzyme treatment. *Int. J. Androl.*, **2**, 244–62
30. Vaidya, R. A., Glass, R. W., Dandekar, P. and Johnson, K. (1971). Decrease in electrophoretic mobility of rabbit spermatozoa following intrauterine incubation. *J. Reprod. Fertil.*, **24**, 299–301
31. Nicolson, G. L., Usui, N., Yanagimachi, R., Yanagimachi, H. and Smith, J. R. (1977). Lectin-binding sites on the plasma membrane of rabbit spermatozoa. Changes in surface receptors during epididymal maturation and after ejaculation. *J. Cell Biol.*, **74**, 950–62
32. Nikolopoulau, M., Soncek, D. A. and Vary, J. C. (1985). Changes in the lipid content of boar sperm plasma membranes during epididymal maturation. *Biochem. Biophys. Acta*, **815**, 486–98
33. Boettcher, B. (1968). Correlation between human ABO blood group antigens in seminal plasma and on seminal spermatozoa. *J. Reprod. Fertil.*, **16**, 49–54
34. Kerek, G., Biberfeld, P. and Afzelius, B. A. (1973). Demonstration of HL-A antigens, 'species' and 'semen' specific antigens on human spermatozoa. *Int. J. Fertil.*, **18**, 145–55
35. James, K. and Hargreave, T. B. (1984). Immunosuppression by seminal plasma and its possible clinical significance. *Immunol. Today*, **5**, 357–63
36. Moench, G. L. (1930). Evaluation of the motility of spermatozoa. *J.A.M.A.* **94**, 478
37. MacLeod, J. (1942). An analysis in human semen of a staining method for differentiating live and dead spermatozoa. *Anat. Rec.*, **83**, 573
38. Dott, H. M. and Foster, G. C. (1972). A technique for studying the morphology of mammalian spermatozoa which are eosinophilic in a differential live/dead stain. *J. Reprod. Fertil.*, **29**, 443–8
39. Dougherty, K. A., Emilson, L. B., Cockett, A. T. K. and Urry, R. L. (1975). A comparison of subjective measurements of human sperm motility and viability with two live–dead staining techniques. *Fertil. Steril.*, **26**, 700–5
40. Eweis, A. and Schirren, C. (1972). Experimentelle fluoreszenz-mikroskopische Untersuchungen Sur Sog. Vitalfluorochromierung menschlicher spermatozoen. *Andrologie*, **4**, 129–32
41. Eliasson, R. and Treichl, L. (1971). Supravital staining of human spermatozoa. *Fertil. Steril.*, **22**, 134–8
42. Fredricsson, B., Waxegard, G., Brege, S. and Lundberg, I. (1977). On the morphology of live spermatozoa of human semen. *Fertil. Steril.*, **28**, 168–73
43. Mixner, J. P. and Saroff, J. (1954). Interference by glycerol with differential staining of bull spermatozoa. *J. Dairy Sci.*, **37**, 652–8
44. Almlid, T. and Johnson, L. A. (1988). Effects of glycerol concentration, equilibration time and temperature of glycerol addition on post-thaw viability of board spermatozoa frozen in straws. *J. Anim. Sci.*, **66**, 2899–905
45. Garner, D. L., Pinkel, D., Johnson, L. A. and Pace, M. M. (1986). Assessment of spermatozoal function using dual fluorescent staining and flow cytometric analyses. *Biol. Reprod.*, **34**, 127–38
46. Check, M. L., Check, J. H. and Long, R. (1991). Detrimental effects of cryopreservation on the structural and functional integrity of the sperm membrane. *Arch. Androl.*, **27**, 155–60
47. De-Leeuw, F. E., De-Leeuw, A. M., Den Daas, J. H., Colenbrander, B. and Verkleifj, A. J. (1993). Effects of various cryoprotective agents and membrane-stabilizing compounds on bull sperm membrane integrity after cooling and freezing. *Cryobiology*, **30**, 32–44
48. Makler, A. A. (1979). Simultaneous differentiation between motile, non-motile, live and dead human spermatozoa by combining supravital staining and multiple exposure photography procedures. *Int. J. Androl.*, **2**, 32–6
49. Burgos, M. H. and di Paola, G. (1951). Eosin test for the evaluation of sperm vitality. *Fertil. Steril.*, **2**, 542–4
50. World Health Organization. (1987). *Laboratory Manual for Examination of Human Semen and Semen–Cervical Mucus Interaction.* (Cambridge: Press Syndicate of the University of Cambridge)
51. Wilton, L. J., Temple-Smith, P. D., Baker, H. W. G. and de Kretser, D. M. (1988). Human male infertility caused by degeneration and death of sperm in the epididymis. *Fertil. Steril.*, **49**, 1052–8
52. Schrader, S. M., Plateck, S. F., Zaneveld, L. J. D., Perez Pelaez, M. and Jeyendran, R. S. (1986). Sperm viability: a comparison of analytical methods. *Andrologia*, **18**, 530–8
53. Ramirez, J. P., Carreras, A. and Mendoza, C. (1992). Sperm plasma membrane integrity in fertile and infertile men. *Andrologia*, **24**, 141–4
54. Carreras, A., Ramirez, J. P. and Mendoza, C. (1992). Sperm plasma membrane integrity measurement: a combined method. *Andrologia*, **24**, 335–40
55. Chan, P. J., Tredway, D. R., Corselli, J., Pang, S. C. and Su, B. C. (1991). Combined supravital staining and hypo-osmotic swelling test. *Hum. Reprod.*, **6**, 1115–8

56. Talbot, P. and Chacon, R. S. (1981). A triple-stain technique for evaluation of normal acrosome reaction in human sperm. *J. Exp. Zool.*, **215**, 201–8
57. Didon, B. A., Dobrinsky, J. R., Giles, J. R. and Graves, C. N. (1989). Staining procedure to detect viability and the true acrosome reaction in spermatozoa of various species. *Gamete Res.*, **22**, 51–7
58. Vigano, P., Brignate, C., Gonfrantini, C., Dordi, N. and Busacca, M. (1990). Which is the best test to evaluate the integrity of human sperm membrane? *Acta Eur. Fertil.*, **21**, 231–4
59. Kovacs, A. and Foote, R. H. (1992). Viability and acrosome staining of bull, boar and rabbit spermatozoa. *Biotech. Histochem.*, **56**, 119–24
60. Harrison, R. A. and Vickers, S. E. (1990). Use of fluorescent probes to assess membrane integrity in mammalian spermatozoa. *J. Reprod. Fertil.*, **88**, 343–52
61. Ericsson, S. A., Garner, D. L., Redelman, D. and Ahmad, K. (1989). Assessment of the viability and fertilizing potential of cryopreserved bovine spermatozoa using dual fluorescent staining and two-flow cytometric systems. *Gamete Res.*, **22**, 355–68
62. Graham, J. K., Kunze, E. and Hammerstedt, R. H. (1990). Analysis of sperm cell viability, acrosomal integrity and mitochondrial function using flow cytometry. *Biol. Reprod.*, **43**, 55–64
63. Ericsson, J. A., Kramer, R. Y., Garner, D. L. and Redelman, D. (1989). Trifunctional fluorescent staining of cryopreserved bovine spermatozoa. *J. Androl.*, **10**, 31–6
64. Casey, P. J., Hillman, R. B., Robertson, K. R., Yudin, A. I., Liu, I. K. M. and Drobnis, E. Z. (1993). Validation of cryopreserved bovine spermatozoa. *J. Androl.*, **14**, 289–97
65. Cross, N. L., Morales, P., Overstreet, J. W. and Hauson, F. W. (1986). Two simple methods for detecting acrosome-reacted human sperm. *Gamete Res.*, **15**, 213–26
66. Holden, C. A. and Trounson, A. O. (1992). Influence of a capacitation period on human sperm acrosome loss. *J. Exp. Zool.*, **264**, 468–74
67. McLaughlin, E. A., Ford, W. C. and Hull, M. G. (1992). Motility characteristics and membrane integrity of cryopreserved human spermatozoa. *J. Reprod. Fertil.*, **95**, 527–34
68. Centola, G. M., Mattox, J. H., Burde, S. and Leary, J. F. (1990). Assessment of the viability and acrosome status of fresh and frozen-thawed human spermatozoa using simple-wavelength fluorescence microscopy. *Mol. Reprod. Dev.*, **27**, 130–5
69. Lomeo, A. M. and Giambersio, A. M. (1991). 'Water test', a simple method to assess sperm membrane integrity. *Int. J. Androl.*, **14**, 278–87
70. Kemp, R. B., Cross, D. M. and Meredith, R. W. J. (1988). Comparison of cell death and adenosine triphosphate content as indicators of acute toxicity in vitro. *Xenobiotica*, **18**, 633–9
71. Inskeep, P. B. and Hammerstedt, R. H. (1985). Endogenous metabolism by sperm in response to altered cellular ATP requirements. *J. Cell Physiol.*, **123**, 180–90
72. Calamera, J. C., Giovenco, P., Quiros, M. C., Brugo, S., Dondero, F. and Nicholson, R. F. (1989). Effect of lipid peroxidation upon human spermatic adenosine triphosphate (ATP). Relationship with motility, velocity and linearity of the spermatozoa. *Andrologia*, **14**, 239–41
73. Calamera, J. C., Brugo, S. and Vilar, O. (1982). Relation between motility and adenosine triphosphate (ATP) in human spermatozoa. *Andrologia*, **14**, 239–41
74. Comporti, M. (1989). Three models of free radical-induced cell injury. *Chem. Biol. Interact.*, **72**, 1–56
75. Kangas, L., Gronroos, M. and Niemineu, A. L. (1984). Bioluminescence of cellular ATP: a new method for evaluating cytotoxic agents *in vitro*. *Med. Biol.*, **72**, 338–43
76. Wolf, D. P., Boldt, J., Byrd, W. and Bechtol, K. B. (1985). Acrosomal status evaluation in human ejaculated sperm with monoclonal antibodies. *Biol. Reprod.*, **3**, 1157–62
77. Stein, W. D. (1990). *Channels, Carriers and Pumps. An Introduction to Membrane Transport.* (New York: Academic Press)
78. Noiles, E. E., Mazur, P., Watson, P. F., Kleinhans, F. W. and Critser, J. K. (1993). Determination of water permeability coefficient for human spermatozoa and its activation energy. *Biol. Reprod.*, **48**, 99–109
79. Mazur, P. and Schneider, U. (1986). Osmotic response of preimplantation mouse and bovine embryos and their cryobiological implications. *Cell Biophys.*, **8**, 259–85
80. Jeyendran, R. S., van der Ven, H. H., Perez Pelaez, M., Crabo, B. G. and Zaneveld, L. J. D. (1984). Development of an assay to assess the functional integrity of the human sperm membrane and its relationship to other semen characteristics. *J. Reprod. Fertil.*, **70**, 219–28
81. Song, B. L., Peng, D. R., Li, H. Y., Shang, G. H., Zhang, J. and Li, L. K. (1991). Evaluation of the effect of butyl p-hydroxybenzoate on the proteolytic activity and membrane function of human spermatozoa. *J. Reprod. Fertil.*, **91**, 435–40
82. Zaneveld, L. J. D. and Jeyendran, R. S. (1988). Modern assessment of semen for diagnostic purpose. *Semin. Reprod. Endocrinol.*, **6**, 323–37
83. Sanchez, R., Concha, M., Topfer-Petersen, E. and Schill, W.-B. (1993). Demonstration of acrosomal membranes using the hypo-osmotic swelling test. *Andrologia*, **25**, 1–2
84. van den Saffele, J., Vermeulen, L., Schoonjans, F. and Comhaire, F. H. (1992). Evaluation of the hypo-osmotic swelling test in relation with advanced methods of semen analysis. *Andrologia*, **24**, 213–17
85. Chan, S. Y. W., Fox, E. J., Chan, M. M. C., Tsoi, W.,

Wang, C., Tang, L. C. M., Tang, G. W. K. and Ho, P. (1985). The relationship between the human sperm hypo-osmotic swelling test, routine semen analysis and the human sperm zona-free hamster ovum penetration assay. *Fertil. Steril.*, **44**, 668–72
86. Wang, C., Chan, S. Y. W., Ng, M., So, W. W. K., Tsoi, W., Lo, T. and Leung, A. (1988). Diagnostic value of sperm function test and routine semen analysis in fertile and infertile men. *J. Androl.*, **9**, 384–9
87. Chan, S. Y. W., Wang, C., Ng, N., So, W. W. K. and Ho, P. (1988). Multivariate discriminant analysis of the relationship between the hypo-osmotic test and the *in vitro* fertilization capacity of human sperm. *Int. J. Androl.*, **11**, 369–78
88. Fuse, H., Iwasaki, M. and Katayama, T. (1993). Correlation between the hypo-osmotic swelling test and various sperm function tests. *Int. J. Fertil.*, **38**, 311–5
89. Smith, R., Madariaga, M. and Bustos Obregon, E. (1992). Reappraisal of the hypo-osmotic swelling test to improve assessment of seminal fertility status. *Int. J. Androl.*, **15**, 5–13
90. Huszar, G., Parish, F. and Corrales, M. (1988). HOS and supravital staining in the initial and migrated sperm fractions of normospermic and oligospermic specimens. *J. Androl.*, **9**, 45–50
91. Centola, G. M. and Mattox, J. A. (1988). Preparation of frozen-thawed semen for intrauterine insemination. *Proceedings of the Annual Meeting of the American Fertility Society*, pp. 18–57
92. Liu, D. M., DuPlessis, Y. P., Nayudu, P. L., Johnston, W. I. H. and Baker, H. W. G. (1988). The use of *in vitro* fertilization to evaluate putative test of human sperm function. *Fertil. Steril.*, **49**, 272–7
93. van der Ven, H. H., Jeyendran, R. S., Al-Hasani, S., Perez Pelaez, M., Diedrich, K. and Zaneveld, L. J. D. (1986). Correlation between human sperm swelling in hypo-osmotic medium (hypo-osmotic swelling test) and *in vitro* fertilization. *J. Androl.*, **7**, 190–6
94. Check, J. H., Epstein, R., Nowroozi, K., Shanis, B. S., Wu, C. H. and Bollendorf, A. (1989). The hypo-osmotic swelling test as a useful adjunct to the semen analysis to predict fertility potential. *Fertil. Steril.*, **52**, 159–61
95. Riedel, H. H., Hubner, F., Enssler, S. C., Bieniek, K. W. and Grillo, M. (1989). Minimal andrological requirement for *in vitro* fertilization. *Hum. Reprod.*, **4**, 73–7
96. Barratt, C. L. R., Osborn, J. C., Harrison, P. E., Monks, N., Dunphy, B. C. and Cooke, I. D. (1989). The hypo-osmotic swelling test and the sperm mucus penetration test in determining fertilization of human oocytes. *Hum. Reprod.*, **4**, 430–4
97. Chan, S. Y. W., Wang, C., Chan, S. T. H. and Ho, P. (1990). Differential evaluation of human sperm hypo-osmotic swelling test and its relationship with the outcome of *in vitro* fertilization of human oocytes. *Hum. Reprod.*, **5**, 84–8
98. Avery, S., Bolton, V. M. and Mason, B. A. (1990). An evaluation of the hypo-osmotic swelling test as a predictor of fertilizing capacity *in vitro*. *Int. J. Androl.*, **13**, 93–9
99. Sjoblom, P. and Coccia, E. (1989). On the diagnostic value of the hypo-osmotic sperm swelling test in an *in vitro* fertilization (IVF) program. In Vitro *Fertil. Embryol. Transf.*, **6**, 41–3
100. Liu, D. Y. and Gordon Baker, H. W. (1992). Tests of human sperm function and fertilization *in vitro*. *Fertil. Steril.*, **58**, 465–83
101. Jones, R., Mann, T. and Sherins, R. J. (1978). Adverse effects of peroxidized lipid on human spermatozoa. *Proc. R. Soc. London (Biol)*, **201**, 413–20
102. Jones, R., Mann, T. and Sherins, R. J. (1979). Peroxidative breakdown of phospholipids in human spermatozoa, spermicidal properties of fatty acid peroxides and protective action of seminal plasma. *Fertil. Steril.*, **31**, 531–7
103. Holland, M. K. and Storey, B. T. (1981). Oxygen metabolism of mammalian spermatozoa. *Bioch. J.*, **198**, 273–80
104. Scott, J. A. and Rabito, C. A. (1988). Oxygen radicals and plasma membrane potential. *Free Rad. Biol. Med.*, **5**, 237–46
105. White, I. G., Darin-Bennett, A. and Poulos, A. (1976). Lipids of human semen. In: Hafez, E. S. E. (ed.) *Human Semen and Fertility Regulation in Men*, p. 144. (St. Louis: Mosby)
106. Hinkovskagalcher, V., Srivastava, P. N. (1992). Phosphatidylcholine and phosphatidylinositol-specific phospholipase C of bull and rabbit spermatozoa. *Mol. Reprod. Dev.*, **33**, 281–6
107. Roy, A. C. and Ratnam, S. S. (1992). Biosynthesis of prostaglandins by human spermatozoa *in vitro* and their role in acrosome reaction and fertilization. *Mol. Reprod. Dev.*, **33**, 303–6
108. Mita, M. (1992). Diacyl choline phosphoglyceride, the endogenous substrate for energy metabolism in sea urchin spermatozoa. *Zool. Sci.*, **9** 563–8
109. Roubal, W. T. and Tappel, A. L. (1966). Damage to proteins, enzymes and aminoacids by peroxidizing lipids. *Arch. Biochem. Biophys.*, **113**, 8–13
110. McKight, R. C. and Hunter, F. E. (1966). Mitochondrial membrane ghosts produced by lipid peroxidation induced by ferrous ion. *J. Biol. Chem.*, **241**, 2757–65
111. Reiss, U. and Tappel, A. L. (1973). Fluorescent product formation and changes in structure of DNA reacted with peroxidising arachidonic acid. *Lipids*, **8**, 199–202
112. Rymsa, B., Wang, J. F. and Groot, H. (1991). O_2-release by activated kupffer cells upon hypoxia-reoxygenation. *Am. J. Physiol.*, **261**, 602–7
113. Aitken, R. J., Clarkson, J. S. and Fishel, P. (1989). Generation of reactive oxygen species, lipid peroxidation and human sperm function. *Biol. Reprod.*, **40**, 183–97

114. de Lamirande, E. and Gagnon, C. (1993). Human sperm hyperactivation and capacitation as parts of an oxidative process. *Free Rad. Biol. Med.*, **14**, 156–66
115. Mannella, M. R. T. and Jones, R. (1980). Properties of spermatozoal superoxide dismutase and lack of involvement of superoxides in metal-ion-catalyzed lipid peroxidation reactions in semen. *Biochem. J.*, **191**, 289–97
116. Alvarez, J. G., Touchstone, J. C., Blasco, L. and Storey, B. T. (1987). Spontaneous lipid peroxidation and superoxide in human spermatozoa superoxide dismutase as a major enzyme product against oxygen toxicity. *J. Androl.*, **8**, 338–48
117. Slater, T. F. (1984). Free radical mechanisms in tissue injury. *Biochem. J.*, **22**, 1–15
118. Alvarez, J. and Storey, B. T. (1989). Role of glutathione peroxidase in protecting mammalian spermatozoa from loss of motility caused by spontaneous lipid peroxidation. *Gamete Res.*, **23**, 77–90
119. Bulkley, G. E. (1993). Free radicals and other reactive oxygen metabolites. Clinical relevance and the therapeutic efficacy of antioxidant therapy. *Surgery*, **113**, 479–83
120. Mann, T. and Lutwak-Mann, C. (1975). Biochemical aspects of aging in spermatozoa in relation to motility and fertilizing ability. In Blandau, R. S. (ed.) *Aging Gametes*, p. 122. (Basel: Karger)
121. DeGroot, H. and Noll, T. (1987). The role of physiological oxygen partial pressure in lipid peroxidation. Theoretical considerations and experimental evidence. *Chem. Physiol. Lipids*, **44**, 209–26
122. Mann, T., Jones, R. and Sherins, R. J. (1980). Fructolysis in human spermatozoa in normal and pathological conditions. *J. Androl.*, **1**, 229–33
123. Aitken, R. J., Harkiss, D. and Buckingham, D. (1993). Relationship between iron-catalyzed lipid peroxidation potential and human sperm function. *J. Reprod. Fertil.*, **98**, 257–65
124. Shimizu, T., Kondo, K. and Hayaishi, O. (1981). Role of prostaglandin endoperoxides in the serum thiobarbituric acid reaction. *Arch. Biochem. Biophys.*, **206**, 271–6
125. Johnsen, O., Eliasson, R. and Samuelson, U. (1982). Conditioning effect of seminal plasma on the lipid peroxide potential of washed human spermatozoa. *Acta Physiol. Scand.*, **116**, 305–7
126. Roa, B., Soufir, J. C., Martin, M. and David, B. (1989). Lipid peroxidation in human spermatozoa as related to midpiece abnormalities and motility. *Gamete Res.*, **24**, 127–34
127. Kovalski, N. N., de Lamirande, E. and Gagnon, C. (1992). Reactive oxygen species generated by human neutrophils inhibit sperm motility: protective effect of seminal plasma and scavengers. *Fertil. Steril.*, **58**, 809–16
128. de Lamirande, E. and Gagnon, C. (1992). Reactive oxygen species and human spermatozoa. II. Depletion of adenosine triphosphate plays an important role in the inhibition of sperm motility. *J. Androl.*, **13**, 379–86
129. Halliwell, B. and Gutteridge, J. M. C. (1989). *Free Radicals in Biology and Medicine*, 2nd edn, pp. 126, 152, 153. (Oxford: Clarendon Press)
130. Alvarez, J. G. and Storey, B. T. (1983). Taurine, hypotaurine, epinephrine, and albumin inhibit lipid peroxidation in rabbit spermatozoa and protect against loss of motility. *Biol. Reprod.*, **29**, 548–55
131. Chow, C. K. (1991). Vitamin E and oxidative stress. *Free Rad. Biol. Med.*, **11**, 215–32
132. Niki, E. (1991). Action of ascorbic acid as a scavenger of active and stable oxygen radicals. *Am. J. Clin. Nutr.*, **54**, 11195–245
133. Calamera, J. C., Brugo-Olmedo, S., Quiros, M. D. and Nicholson, R. F. (1990). Efecto del acido ascorbico del plasma seminal sobre la perioxidacion lipidica espermatica. *Ginecol. Reprod.*, **2**, 155–8
134. Rose, R. C. and Bode, A. M. (1993). Biology of free radical scavengers: an evaluation of ascorbate. *FASEB J.*, **7**, 1135–42
135. Aitken, R. J. and Clarkson, J. S. (1987). Cellular basis of defective sperm function and its association with the genesis of reactive oxygen species by human spermatozoa. *J. Reprod. Fertil.*, **81**, 459–69
136. Aitken, R. J., Buckingham, D. and Horkiss, D. (1993). Use of a xanthine oxidase free radical generating system to investigate the cytotoxic effects of reactive oxygen species on human spermatozoa. *J. Reprod. Fertil.*, **97**, 441–50
137. Chan, S. Y. W. and Wang, C. (1987). Correlation between semen adenosine triphosphate and sperm fertilizing capacity. *Fertil. Steril.*, **47**, 717–9
138. Coetzee, K., Kruger, T. F., Menkveld, R., Lombard, C. J. and Swanson, J. R. (1989). Hypo-osmotic swelling test in the prediction of male fertility. *Arch. Androl.*, **23**, 131–8
139. Rogers, B. J. and Parker, R. A. (1991). Relationship between the human sperm hypo-osmotic swelling test and sperm penetration assay. *J. Androl.*, **12**, 152–8
140. van Kooij, R. T., Balerna, M., Raotti, A. and Campana, Z. (1986). Oocyte penetration and acrosome reactions of human sperm. II. Correlation with other seminal parameters. *Andrologia*, **18**, 503–8
141. Takahashi, K., Uchida, A. and Kitao, M. (1990). Hypo-osmotic swelling test of sperm. *Arch. Androl.*, **25**, 225–42
142. Jeyendran, R. S., van der Ven, H. H. and Zaneveld, L. J. B. (1992). The hypo-osmotic swelling test: an update. *Arch. Androl.*, **29**, 105–16
143. Hammerstedt, R. H., Graham, J. K. and Nolan, J. P. (1990). Cryopreservation of mammalian sperm: what we ask them to survive. *J. Androl.*, **11**, 73–88

Assessment of nuclear maturity 16

H. W. G. Baker and D. Y. Liu

INTRODUCTION

Human sperm immaturity can be tested by nuclear chromatin decondensation (NCD) in 1% sodium dodecylsulfate, chromatin maturity by acidic aniline blue (AAB) staining and DNA normality by acridine orange (AO) fluorescence. The relationship between these and other sperm test results and fertilization rates were analyzed by logistic regression.

Nuclear chromatin decondensation was inversely correlated with sperm motility, but there were no significant relationships with other semen analysis variables. Also, there was no significant correlation between NCD and the proportion of oocytes fertilized *in vitro*.

AAB staining was correlated with sperm morphology and weakly related to fertilization rates in some studies. The results of AO fluorescence were related to AAB staining. The percentage of sperm with normal DNA by AO, the number of sperm bound to the zona pelludica (ZP) and the percentage of sperm with normal morphology were significantly related to fertilization rates *in vitro*. In patients with normal morphology >15% or with more than 10 sperm bound per ZP, the percentage of sperm with normal DNA, the number of sperm bound to the ZP and motility grade were significantly related to fertilization rates *in vitro*. In patients with normal morphology >15%, failure of fertilization may be due to defects of sperm-ZP penetration or abnormal DNA. Sperm with mature nuclei and normal DNA bind selectively to the ZP. It is concluded that assessment of sperm DNA normality by AO fluorescence may aid prediction of fertilization rates in addition to measurements of normal morphology and sperm–ZP penetration.

HISTORICAL CONSIDERATIONS

Although semen analysis is the basic test for predicting fertility, the standard measurements of sperm concentration, percentage motility and morphology may not reveal subtle sperm defects[1]. Results of semen analysis also relate poorly to subsequent pregnancy rates; for example, pregnancies have been noted to occur with very low numbers of normal motile sperm in follow-up studies of infertile men[2]. Even though sperm motility and normal morphology are related to fertilization rates *in vitro* and pregnancy rates with donor insemination, these appear to be less well related to pregnancy rates in subfertile couples[3–5]. There is a great need for more accurate and specific tests for predicting the fertilizing potential of human sperm. A variety of biochemical markers of sperm function have been developed including measurement of ATP in semen, creatine kinase in sperm, and generation of reactive oxygen species by abnormal spermatozoa[1,7–10]. We have no experience with these methods but suspect they provide indices of sperm maturity which would be related to the results of tests to be discussed in this chapter.

Use of the results of *in vitro* fertilization (IVF) to evaluate tests of human sperm function is a powerful approach since sperm used for insemination of oocytes can be tested and the results of sperm tests directly related to IVF rates. Logistic regression analysis allows determination of which groups of sperm characteristics are independently significantly related to fertilization rates[5]. The percentage of sperm with normal morphology assessed with strict criteria, in which all sperm with doubtfully normal shape are classified as abnormal, is one of the most significant sperm factors related to fertilization rates *in vitro*[5,6,11]. However, the accuracy of prediction of IVF rates using sperm morphology alone is currently still poor. Therefore, other sperm function tests such as assessment of sperm with normal intact acrosomes and sperm–zona pellucida (ZP) binding have been developed and used in combination with sperm morphology to improve the overall correlation with IVF rates[12–14]. Using these sperm function tests, the majority of patients with failure of fertilization are found to have defects of sperm morphology, acrosomes and ZP interaction. However, the causes of failure of fertilization for the other 25% of patients are unclear and it is necessary to investigate other defects of sperm or oocytes, particularly in those patients without severe defects of sperm morphology and sperm–ZP binding.

BASIC CONCEPTS OF SPERM NUCLEAR MATURITY

During spermiogenesis complex changes occur in the sperm nucleus involving different generations of nucleoproteins and specific regular arrangement of the chromatin in a lamellar arrangement[15]. The nuclear proteins of mature spermatids are very basic, containing abundant arginine. Cysteine residues are also abundant and these become cross-linked during sperm maturation in the testis and particularly in the epididymis. For example, in the rat 100% of the cysteine residues have free SH groups in the testis, whereas in the caput epididymis, about 50%, and in the cauda epididymis, 100% are in the disulfide form[16]. These changes in the sperm chromatin give a number of characteristics to the sperm nucleus for example, staining with various stains including reduced staining with cationic dyes and greatly enhanced resistance to DNA thermal denaturation and decondensation in detergents[15].

It is possible that defects of nuclear chromatin which are assayed by tests of sperm nuclear maturity may occur with non-specific disorders of spermatogenesis and spermiogenesis or with more specific problems. In the past, a number of reports have appeared suggesting that defects of chromatin may cause infertility[17]. More recently patients with lack of protamine P_2 have been identified[18]. It is also possible that such defects might interfere with fertilization by preventing normal intravitelline sperm processing by the oocyte.

Sperm maturation

Sperm complete maturation during passage along the genital tract, especially in the epididymis. These structural and biochemical changes are considered to be prerequisites for achieving optimal fertilizing ability[19–21]. The changes include alterations of the sperm head and principal piece by formation of disulfide bonds[19]. Formation of disulfide bonds within nuclear protamines results in an increase in the stability of sperm head. The biological importance of sperm chromatin stability is surmised; rigid sperm nuclei may aid successful transport in the female reproductive tract and penetration of the oocyte[15]. In humans, the transit time of sperm through the epididymis varies between individuals[22]. Thus, ejaculated sperm have various degrees of nuclear stability[23].

Sperm nuclear decondensation in detergent

Human sperm have various degrees of resistance to the detergent, sodium dodecylsulfate (SDS) or SDS in combination with disulphide bond-reducing agents, such as dithiothreitol (DTT)[23,24]. The decondensation of immature sperm nuclei is more rapid and complete than with mature sperm. The percentage of sperm undergoing decondensation of nuclear chromatin on exposure to DTT+SDS correlates with the number of immature sperm present in the ejaculate[25]. Reduced resistance to decondensation of sperm nuclei may be associated with male infertility in bulls, rams and men[23,26–28]. Colleu *et al.*[29] reported that asthenospermic semen contained more sperm with immature nuclei which decondensed in SDS than did normospermic semen.

Acidic aniline blue stain

Immature sperm nuclei can be detected by staining with acidic aniline blue (AAB)[30] since they contain lysine-rich histones. The persistence of lysine-rich nuclear proteins may cause defects of chromatin condensation[31]. Dadoune *et al.*[32] reported an association of AAB stained heads with morphologically abnormal sperm. However, 20% of morphologically normal sperm also have partially or totally AAB stained heads[32]. This is consistent with defects in chromatin condensation which can be observed by transmission electron microscope in some morphologically normal sperm[33]. Asthenospermic semen contains more sperm that stain with AAB[25]. Jeulin *et al.*[34] reported higher AAB staining in patients with low fertilization rates *in vitro* than in patients with high fertilization rates. Hofmann and Hilscher[35] reported that 23–78% of morphologically normal sperm had immature nuclei stained with AAB in infertile patients in whom treatment by either artificial insemination with husband's sperm or IVF was unsuccessful.

Acridine orange fluorescence

Acridine orange (AO) has been used to distinguish between sperm containing normal or abnormal nuclear chromatin[35–40]. Acridine orange has been used for many studies of nucleic acid structure *in situ*[39]. It binds to nucleic acids and other macromolecules. With the monomeric form of the dye preponderant at low AO concentrations there is orthochromatic fluorescence (green) but with high concentrations there are dye–dye interactions from aggregation and polymerization and this causes a metachromatic shift to red fluorescence. It is said that AO fluoresces green when bound to normal double-stranded deoxyribonucleic acid (DNA) and red when bound to denatured or single-stranded DNA[35–39]. It is believed one AO molecule intercalates between every third base pair of double helical DNA and under these circumstances the fluorescence is green. However, with single-stranded DNA, there is dye stacking from aggregation and dye–dye interactions following electrostatic binding of AO to the phosphate groups of the bases and the fluorescence is red[39]. Although it is said that the method is measuring single-stranded DNA or denatured DNA when red fluorescence occurs, it is hard to believe that this would be the case in the sperm head. It is known that DNA in sperm is poorly stabilized relative to nucleosomal DNA in somatic cells, and perhaps the red fluorescence occurs more as a result of heterogeneity of chromatin structure because of defects of spermiogenesis or subsequent degeneration of chromatin in dead sperm rather than actual abnormalities in the DNA. Similar fluorescence occurs in somatic cells with pyknotic nuclei[39].

There is a significant correlation between results of AO and the AAB stain and abnormal sperm morphology[33,37]. The AO test may predict fertility[36,40], but AO staining was not related to zona-free hamster oocyte penetration[37]. Le Lannou and Blanchard[41] reported that the proportion of sperm with mature or normal nuclear chromatin assessed by both AAB and AO staining methods was significantly increased by selection of motile sperm by swim-up or Percoll gradient centrifugation.

CLINICAL APPLICATION

Patients

Four investigations were performed with couples who underwent IVF: (1) 106 couples in 1986 with the AAB stain[6]; (2) 74 couples in 1987 with NCD[42]; (3) 91 couples in 1991[43]; and (4) 197 couples in 1992[44] with both AAB and AO. In each study, the wife's oocytes were inseminated with the husband's sperm. The first two studies included all patients except where there was oligospermia and insufficient semen left over after sperm preparation for examination. In the third and fourth studies, patients were selected on the basis that at least three mature oocytes were inseminated and some or all of the oocytes failed to fertilize. Consecutive patients with zero fertilization were matched with patients, treated on the same day, who had some oocytes which did not fertilize. The indications for IVF in the first two studies were tubal occlusion in 57% and male infertility in 8%, but in the third and fourth studies 21% were tubal and 36% male. Couples with sperm antibodies in either partner were excluded.

In vitro fertilization

During these studies, follicular development was induced by clomiphene and human menopausal gonadotropin (hMG) or gonadotropin-releasing hormone (GnRH) agonist and hMG. Doses of hMG were based on serum estradiol measurements and increased if necessary, and continued until the serum estradiol reached 4 nmol/L. After 1989, ovarian ultrasound replaced estradiol measurements for monitoring follicular development. Human chorionic gonadotropin (hCG) was given and oocyte collection performed laparoscopically or by vaginal ultrasound-guided aspiration 34–36 h after hCG injection or the estimated time of commencement of a spontaneous LH surge. Oocytes were scored under a dissecting microscope. Semen was collected by masturbation 2 h prior to the expected time of insemination and the sperm prepared by swim-up, Percoll or miniPercoll techniques. Approximately 100 000 sperm were added to each oocyte in 1 mL of culture medium in a plastic multiwell tray. After 1989, the concentration of motile sperm in the insemination medium was increased up to 0.5–1 M/mL if abnormal sperm morphology was >95% or if previous IVF attempts had resulted in fertilization rates <20%. Fertilization was assessed 18–20 h later and embryos transferred to the uterus or cryopreserved 2 days after insemination. The fertilization rate was the quotient of number of oocytes fertilized and the number of mature oocytes inseminated. Fertilized oocytes included those with two or more pronuclei observed at 16–20 h after insemination. Other abnormal fertilizations, such as the appearance of only one pronucleus or two pronuclei delayed until 48 h after insemination, were not included.

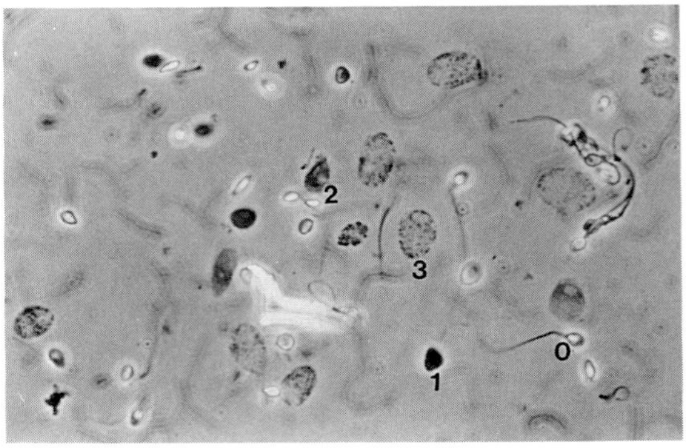

Figure 1 Different grades of nuclear swelling following treatment with DDT+SDS (see Appendix). 0 = non-decondensed nucleus; 1 = partially decondensed nucleus; 2 = markedly decondensed nucleus; 3 = completely decondensed nucleus (400× phase-contrast microscope). Reproduced from Liu *et al.*[42] with permission from the Fertility Society of Australia

Analysis of sperm in semen and media

In the first two studies, analyses were performed on semen remaining after preparation of sperm for IVF within 2–3 h of collection and on a sample of the sperm suspension for insemination. In the third and fourth studies, sperm in the insemination medium were obtained after embryos or unfertilized oocytes had been removed at 48–60 h after insemination. The insemination medium from all the culture dishes was pooled for the same patient. Sperm in semen and swim-up preparation were not examined in these studies, since many of the patients had poor semen and all the sample was used for sperm preparation for insemination of oocytes.

Sperm concentrations in semen and insemination or culture media were determined using a hemocytometer. Sperm motility was measured in semen with three grades of forward progression: 1=no progressive motility; 2=fair progressive motility; and 3=good progressive motility[45,46]. The percentage motility was calculated by counting 100 sperm. Sperm viability (% live sperm) was determined by exclusion of eosin Y[1]. Sperm morphology was assessed on stained smears prepared from semen or media after washing and adjustment of sperm concentration to approximately 80 million/mL. The sperm in semen or culture medium were washed with 10 mL of 0.9% NaCl and the sperm pellet was resuspended in 0.02–0.1 mL of 0.9% NaCl. The sperm suspension was smeared on glass slides and the density and evenness of spread of the sperm were checked microscopically before the slides were left to dry. The smears were stained with the Shorr method and 200 sperm were assessed under oil immersion with magnification of 1000× and bright-field illumination[34]. Normal sperm morphology was assessed following the World Health Organization criteria for the silhouette plus internal staining characteristics with the acrosomal region being clearly seen, regular in shape and occupying at least half of the sperm head[1,6]. The percentage of sperm with normal morphology was determined by assessing 200 sperm from more than 10 individual fields under oil immersion with magnification of 1000× and bright-field illumination. These modified criteria are similar to the Tygerberg, Kruger 'strict' criteria[5,6].

Nuclear chromatin decondensation

Tests for inducing sperm NCD *in vitro* were performed according to the method of Calvin and Bedford[24] with the modification of Rodriguez *et al.*[27] (see Appendix for details) (Figure 1).

Nuclear maturity

Maturity of nuclear chromatin was examined with the AAB, stain method described in the Appendix.

DNA normality

The normality of DNA was assessed by the AO fluorescence method described by Tejada *et al.*[36] (see Appendix).

Number of sperm bound to the ZP

In the third and fourth studies, the numbers of sperm bound to the ZP of all the unfertilized oocytes were counted with an inverted phase-contrast microscope with magnification of 250× after removing the cumulus or corona cells if present[47]. To perform this, the oocytes were pipetted (inner diameter 250 μm) gently several times to dislodge sperm not tightly bound to the ZP. When there were more than 100 sperm bound to one ZP, it was difficult to count the number of sperm accurately. In this situation the number was recorded as 100.

Sperm-ZP penetration

In the fourth study, sperm penetrating into the ZP and perivitelline space (PVS) were counted after removing sperm bound to the surface of the ZP[44]. The oocytes were aspirated in and out of a pipette of inner diameter slightly smaller than the oocyte (inner diameter 120 μm) to shear off sperm on the surface of the ZP. After this pipetting procedure sperm with heads in the ZP or PVS are easily seen and counted under the microscope.

Assessment of sperm bound to the ZP

In order to determine whether the ZP selectively binds sperm with a mature nucleus and normal DNA, oocytes with more than 20 sperm bound to the ZP from the same patient were pooled and smeared on a glass slide. These slides were stained with AAB and AO[43].

Statistical analysis

Differences between mean results of tests were examined by analysis of variance or *t*-tests. Transformations were used to normalize data where necessary. Weighted mean binding rates were calculated[48]. Correlations between sperm test results, and between sperm test results and IVF rates were performed by non-parametric (Kendall or Spearman) tests. Relationships between sperm test results and IVF rates were studied by maximum likelihood logistic regression analysis.

DIAGNOSTIC APPLICATIONS

Acid aniline blue

In the first study[6], the proportion of sperm with immature nuclei which stained with AAB averaged about 20% in semen and in insemination medium, but there was a wide range of values (2–54%). While the AAB results in semen and insemination medium were strongly correlated (r=0.683), and there were moderately strong negative correlations with percentage normal sperm morphology in semen, insemination medium and culture medium (r=–0.219–0.401), there was only a weak negative correlation with the result of the hypo-osmotic swelling test in semen (r=–0.193) and no significant correlations with other sperm variables or fertilization rate *in vitro*. There were only three significant factors in the logistic regression model of fertilization rate – percentage normal sperm morphology, sperm concentration in the insemination medium and percentage live sperm in semen[6].

Nuclear chromatin decondensation[42]

The appearance of sperm heads with different grades of nuclear decondensation is shown in Figure 1. Table 1 shows that washing with EDTA increased the proportion of sperm undergoing decondensation and the greatest proportion of sperm with NCD occurred with the combination SDS+DTT. Sperm in the insemination medium had significantly less NCD than did sperm in the original semen sample. Grades 2 and 3 of NCD were correlated within each treatment (r=0.244–0.446, P<0.01), but grade 1 was not significantly correlated with the other two grades NCD with SDS+EDTA and SDS+DTT in semen. Total NCD (the sum of grades 1, 2 and 3) was used for subsequent analysis.

There were negative relationships between SDS+DTT and sperm motility (P<0.001), motility index (P<0.01) and percentage of live sperm (P<0.05). There was no significant correlation

Table 1. Proportion of sperm showing three grades of nuclear chromatin decondensation (NCD, mean, SEM and range)

Treatment	*n*	*NCD grade*			*Total NCD*
		1	*2*	*3*	
ASDS alone	72	8.0±0.7 (1–31)	4.0±0.7 (0–31)	0.3±0.2 (0–8)	12.5±1.2 (1–50)
BSDS+EDTA	65	11.9±0.6 (4–22)	13.4±1.0 (0–38)	1.0±0.4 (0–18)	27.1±1.5 (5–68)
CSDS+DTT	74	11.0±0.8 (0–32)	20.7±1.1 (2–48)	9.7±0.8 (0–40)	40.9±1.7 (11–89)
DSDS+DTT	73	10.6±0.8 (1–35)	10.8±1.1 (0–50)	0.6±0.2 (0–9)	22.0±1.8 (3–77)

A, B, C, sperm washed from semen; D, sperm washed from insemination suspension. Differences between mean results of treatment were assessed by analysis of variance. Contrasts between A and B, A and C, and C and D were all significant ($P<0.05$) except for NCD grade 1 C and D. Reproduced from Liu *et al.*[42], with permission from the Fertility Society of Australia

between any NCD test result (grade or total) and fertilization rate. Only the percentage of sperm with normal morphology was significantly related to fertilization rate by logistic regression analysis of all semen variables including NCD[42].

These results compare with previous reports of means of 11% of sperm showing NCD with SDS alone with sperm from groups of fertile donors and normal men of unknown fertility[19,28]. A wide variation of NCD following exposure to SDS alone (1–50%) and SDS+DTT (11–89%) is also confirmed[42]. Sperm in insemination medium had significantly lower NCD than the sperm in semen, indicating that motile sperm, selected by the swim-up procedure, are likely to be more mature and more resistant to NCD. Sperm washed with EDTA had a significantly higher percentage showing NCD. The effect of washing with EDTA was studied because seminal zinc has been reported to inhibit NCD[49,50]. EDTA removes zinc more efficiently than saline washes[51].

NCD (DTT+SDS) was inversely correlated with sperm motility, motility index and viability in semen[42]. These relationships are consistent with the attainment of the capacities for progressive motility and nuclear stability through disulfide cross-linking during epididymal transit. They also suggest that some men produce sperm which have not undergone full maturation. Thus a relationship between NCD and the fertility might be expected. However, our study showed no relationship between NCD determined in four different ways and human fertilization rates *in vitro*.

Acid aniline blue and acridine orange

In the third study[43], there were significantly ($P<0.05$) lower mean percentages of sperm with mature nuclei (40, range 1–91%, versus 56, 6–95%) and normal DNA (74, 1–98%, versus 82, 15–97%) in patients with no oocytes fertilized than in those with some oocytes fertilized[43]. There was also a significantly higher proportion of patients with normal DNA <30% (43%, 18/42 versus 20%, 10/49; 2×=54, $P<0.05$) with zero fertilization rates than for those with some oocytes fertilized. There were significant correlations between mature nuclei and sperm motility in insemination medium ($P<0.01$), normal morphology ($P<0.001$) and number of sperm bound to the ZP ($P<0.05$), and between normal DNA and normal morphology ($P<0.05$) and number of sperm bound to the ZP ($P<0.05$)[43]. Percentage mature nuclei and normal DNA were also correlated ($P<0.001$). There was a highly significant correlation between the percentage of sperm with normal DNA ($r=0.302$, $P<0.001$) and IVF rates. Percentage mature nuclei ($r=0.252$, $P<0.05$) was less significant. Number of sperm bound to the ZP, the percentages of sperm with normal morphology and normal DNA, and motility grade were strongly related to IVF rates by logistic regression analysis (Table 2). In patients with normal morphology ⩾15%, number of sperm bound to the ZP, the percentages of sperm with normal DNA and mature nucleus, and motility grade were significantly related to IVF rates (Table 2). In patients

Table 2 Significant variables related to IVF rates by logistic regression analysis in the third study

Variables	*Regression coefficient*	*SE**	*z⁺*	*P*
All patients studied (*n*=91), (n=91, r^2=0.379)				
normal morphology (%)	0.046	0.007	6.57	<0.001
number of sperm bound/ZP	0.017	0.003	5.67	<0.001
normal DNA (%)	0.015	0.003	5.00	<0.001
motility grade	0.559	0.160	3.49	<0.001
Patients with normal morphology ≥15% (n=51, r^2=0.253)				
number of sperm bound/ZP	0.016	0.003	5.33	<0.001
normal DNA (%)	0.017	0.004	4.25	<0.001
motility grade	0.486	0.187	2.60	<0.01
mature nucleus (%)	0.020	0.008	2.50	<0.05
Patients with ⩾10 sperm bound/ZP (n=43, r^2=0.193)				
motility grade	0.744	0.165	4.51	<0.001
normal DNA (%)	0.014	0.004	3.50	<0.005
number of sperm bound/ZP	0.010	0.003	3.33	<0.01

*SE, standard error; ⁺ z, normal deviate (regression coefficient/SE); r^2, proportion of deviance explained by the model
Reproduced from Liu and Baker[43] with permission from the American Society of Reproductive Medicine

with ⩾10 sperm bound per ZP, motility grade, percentage of sperm with normal DNA and number of sperm bound to the ZP were related to IVF rates (Table 2).

Defects of sperm morphology and sperm–ZP binding seem to be the most common causes of failure of fertilization *in vitro*[12,14,47,52]. However, patients without severe defects of morphology and sperm–ZP binding may still have failure of fertilization. It is possible that other sperm defects or oocyte abnormalities may be involved in failure of fertilization in some of these patients. Sperm DNA normality assessed with AO stain was a significant factor related to fertilization rates in patients with either normal morphology ⩾15% in insemination medium or in patients with ⩾10 bound per ZP[43]. This suggests the failure of fertilization may be related to abnormal nuclear chromatin.

Nuclear maturity and DNA normality of sperm bound to the ZP

There were significantly higher proportions of sperm with mature nuclei (18 subjects, mean and range, 93 (71–100) on the ZP versus 83 (69–94) in insemination medium, $P<0.01$). Similarly, normal DNA was higher with sperm bound to the ZP (19 subjects, 87 (35–100)) than in the insemination medium (57 (7–95), $P<0.001$)[43]. However, some sperm with abnormal DNA or immature nuclei were bound to the ZP but the mean rates of binding of these sperm were lower than for sperm with normal DNA or mature nuclei (normal DNA=28.2; abnormal DNA=8.4; mature nucleus=21.1; immature nucleus=12.0/ZP/105/mL inseminated). This suggests that the human ZP selectively binds sperm with a mature nuclei and normal DNA.

Acridine orange and sperm ZP penetration

In the fourth study[44], there were significant differences in the percentages of sperm with normal DNA between the two groups with zero fertilization or some oocytes fertilized. There were significant correlations between most of the sperm test results. The percentage of sperm with normal DNA was significantly correlated with sperm motility ($r=0.322$, $P<0.001$) and normal morphology ($r=0.470$, $P<0.001$). There was also a significant correlation between IVF rate and the percentage of sperm with normal DNA ($r=0.406$, $P<0.001$).

When all data from the 197 patients were examined by logistic regression analysis (Table 3), only the proportion of ZP penetrated; the percentage of

Table 3 Logistic regression analysis of fertilization rates in 197 patients in the fourth study

Variables	*Regression coefficient*	*SE**	Z^+	*P*
All significant variables included (r^2=0.476)				
ZP penetrated (%)	0.029	0.002	14.5	<0.001
normal morphology (%)	0.031	0.004	7.8	<0.001
normal DNA (%)	0.012	0.002	6.0	<0.001
number of sperm bound/ZP	0.004	0.002	2.0	<0.05
ZP penetrated excluded (r^2=0.318)				
normal morphology (%)	0.041	0.004	10.2	<0.001
no. sperm bound/ZP	0.017	0.002	8.5	<0.001
normal DNA (%)	0.010	0.002	5.0	<0.001

*SE, standard error; $^+$ Z, normal deviate (regression coefficient/SE); r^2, proportion of deviance explained by the model. Reproduced from Liu and Baker[44] with permission from IRL Press Ltd

sperm with normal morphology and the percentage of sperm with normal DNA were highly significantly related to IVF rate. The number of sperm bound/ZP was less significant. All the other variables were not significant[44]. When the proportion of ZP penetrated was excluded from the logstic regression model, the number of sperm bound/ZP together with normal sperm morphology and normal DNA were most strongly related to IVF rate, but this model explained less of variance of the IVF rates (Table 3).

Subgroups of patients were analyzed separately by logistic regression (Table 4). In patients (n=51) with normal morphology ⩾30%, the proportion of ZP penetrated and normal DNA were significantly related to IVF rate. In patients (n=55) with ⩾30 sperm bound/ZP, normal morphology and the proportion of ZP penetrated were related to IVF rate. In patients (n=88) with 100% ZP penetrated, normal morphology and normal DNA were related to IVF rate.

The fourth study shows that oocytes which have failed to fertilize *in vitro* can be examined to determine the proportion which have sperm in the ZP or PVS and that the proportion of ZP penetrated is highly significantly related to IVF rate. The percentages of sperm with normal morphology and normal DNA were also significant. This result suggests that failure of sperm-ZP penetration is a major cause of failure of fertilization *in vitro*. Because the proportion of ZP penetrated was highly significantly correlated with the number of sperm bound per ZP, the latter became less significant in logistic regression models when the percentage of ZP penetrated was included. In patients with good sperm–ZP binding and good sperm morphology, either normal morphology >30% or >30 sperm bound/ZP, the proportion of ZP penetrated and normal DNA were highly significantly related to fertilization rate. Thus, in these patients, failure of fertilization appears to be mainly due to failure of sperm penetrating into the ZP. It is possible that sperm from these patients may have disorders of the ZP-induced acrosome reaction, zona lysis or secondary zona binding activity, or subtle defects of motility[53–56].

In patients with zero fertilization and all oocytes with some sperm penetrating into the ZP or PVS, IVF rates were related to percentage normal sperm morphology and percentage normal DNA. In these patients, fertilization may fail because the sperm cannot fuse with the oolemma or form male pronuclei. Although the human ZP is selective for sperm with normal morphology and normal DNA, sperm with abnormal morphology and abnormal DNA are observed on the ZP[43,57].

CONCLUSION: SIGNIFICANCE OF DEFECTS OF SPERM NUCLEAR MATURITY

At present it is difficult to understand the precise nature of defects of sperm nuclear maturity that are revealed by these tests. On one hand, they may be related to defects of spermatogenesis and spermiogenesis or sperm maturation in a rather non-specific manner. Under these circumstances, it is possible

Table 4 Logistic regression analysis of fertilization rates in subgroups of patients with the number of sperm bound/ZP ⩾30, 100% ZP penetrated and normal morphology ≥30% in the fourth study

Variables	*Regression coefficient*	*SE**	Z^{+}	*P*
Patients with ⩾30 sperm bound/ZP (n=55, r^2=0.212)				
normal morphology (%)	0.032	0.006	5.3	<0.001
ZP penetrated (%)	0.029	0.008	3.7	<0.001
Patients with 100% ZP penetrated (n=88, r^2=0.258)				
normal morphology (%)	0.032	0.005	6.4	<0.001
normal DNA (%)	0.011	0.003	3.7	<0.001
Patients with normal morphology ≥30% (n=51, r^2=0.318)				
ZP penetrated (%)	0.030	0.004	7.5	<0.001
normal DNA (%)	0.011	0.004	2.8	<0.01
normal morphology (%)	0.033	0.014	2.4	<0.05

*SE, standard error; $^{+}$Z, normal deviate (regression coefficient/SE); r^2, proportion of deviance explained by the model. Reproduced from Liu and Baker[44] with permission from IRL Press Ltd

that the results would correlate with other tests of production of immature sperm such as reactive oxygen species generation and creatine kinase measurements[7–10]. On the other hand, there may be individual patients with specific defects of sperm chromatin or other aspects of nuclear maturity which cause their infertility. These patients would appear to be rare, however, as we have only identified one man who has very low DNA normality on the basis of acridine orange fluorescence and yet has otherwise normal semen. This man has a long duration of infertility, but at this stage, has not undergone IVF. Another patient with a high proportion of sperm with abnormal DNA by acridine orange stain had a good result with ICSI. Thus we are not sure at this stage whether specific defects of sperm chromatin maturity will interfere with the intravitelline processing of the sperm genome.

These studies further emphasize that multiple sperm factors are often involved in failure of fertilization. Therefore, a group of important sperm function tests are required in order to predict fertility accurately[58]. Logistic regression analysis is useful to determine which groups of sperm function tests are independently related to fertilization rates. The study of the causes of failure of fertilization *in vitro* could provide valuable information for understanding and improving treatment of male infertility. Assessment of maturity of nuclear chromatin and normality of DNA could aid prediction of fertilization rates *in vitro* in patients with either ⩾15% of sperm with normal morphology or ⩾10 sperm bound per ZP. Thus, the tests may help in the selection of patients for microinjection of sperm into the ooplasm.

ACKNOWLEDGEMENTS

We thank Ms Mingli Liu for technical assistance and all scientists in the IVF laboratories for collecting the oocytes and sperm samples for these studies which were supported by the Royal Women's Hospital Research Committee and National Health and Medical Research Council grant number 930628.

References

1. World Health Organization. (1992). *WHO Laboratory Manual for Examination of Human Semen and Semen–Cervical Mucus Interaction.* (Cambridge: Cambridge University Press)
2. Silber, S. J. (1994). A modern view of male infertility. *Reprod. Fertil. Dev.*, **6**, 93–104
3. Hargreave, T. B. and Elton, R. A. (1983). Is conventional sperm analysis of any use? *Br. J. Urol.*, **55**, 774–9
4. Zaini, A., Jennings, M. G. and Baker, H. W. G. (1985). Are conventional sperm morphology and motility assessments of predictive value in subfertile men? *Int. J. Androl.*, **8**, 427–35

5. Kruger, T. F., Menkveld, R., Stander, F. S. H., Lombard, C. J., Van der Merwe, J. P., Van Zyl, J. A. and Smith, K. (1986). Sperm morphological features as a prognostic factor in *in vitro* fertilization. *Fertil. Steril.*, **46**, 1118–23
6. Liu, D. Y., du Plessis, Y. P., Nayudu, P. L., Johnston, W. I. H. and Baker, H. W. G. (1988). The use of *in vitro* fertilization to evaluate putative tests of human sperm function. *Fertil. Steril.*, **49**, 272–7
7. Huszar, G., Vigue, L. and Oehninger, S. (1994). Creatine kinase immunocytochemistry of human sperm–hemizona complexes: selective binding of sperm with mature creatine kinase-staining pattern. *Fertil. Steril.*, **61**, 136–42
8. Aitken, R. J. and Clarkson, J. S. (1987). Cellular basis of defective sperm function and its association with the genesis of reactive oxygen species by human spermatozoa. *J. Reprod. Fertil.*, **81**, 459–69
9. Aitken, R. J., Clarkson, J. S. and Fishel, S. (1989). Generation of reactive oxygen species, lipid peroxidation, and human sperm function. *Biol. Reprod.*, **40**, 183–97
10. Aitken, R. J., Clarkson, J. S., Hargreave, T. B., Irvine, D. S. and Wu, F. C. W. (1989). Analysis of the relationship between defective sperm function and the generation of reactive oxygen species in cases of oligospermia. *J. Androl.*, **10**, 214–20
11. Kruger, T. F., Acosta, A. A., Simmons, K. F., Swanson, R. J., Matta, J. F. and Oehninger, S. (1988). Predictive value of abnormal sperm morphology in *in vitro* fertilization. *Fertil. Steril.*, **49**, 112–7
12. Liu, D. Y. and Baker, H. W. G. (1988). The proportion of sperm with poor morphology but normal intact acrosomes detected with pisum sativum agglutinin correlates with fertilization *in vitro*. *Fertil. Steril.*, **50**, 288–93
13. Liu, D. Y., Lopata, A., Johnston, W. I. H. and Baker, H. W. G. (1988). A human sperm–zona pellucida binding test using oocytes that failed to fertilize *in vitro*. *Fertil. Steril.*, **50**, 782–8
14. Liu, D. Y., Clarke, G. N., Lopata, A., Johnston, W. I. H. and Baker, H. W. G. (1989). A sperm–zona pellucida binding test and *in vitro* fertilization. *Fertil. Steril.*, **52**, 281–7
15. Mann, T. and Lutwak-Mann, C. (1981). *Male Reproduction Function and Semen*, p. 99. (Berlin: Springer-Verlag)
16. Bedford, J. M. and Calvin, H. I. (1974). The occurrence and possible functional significance of S–S crosslinks in sperm heads, with particular reference to eutherian mammals. *J. Exp. Zool.*, **188**, 137–56
17. Gledhill, B. L. (1970). Enigma of spermatozoal deoxyribonucleic acid and male infertility: a review. *Am. J. Vet. Res.*, **31**, 539–45
18. Yebra, L. I., de Ballesca, J. L., Vanrell, J. A., Bassas, L. I. and Oliva, R. (1993). Complete selective absence of protamine P_2 in humans. *J. Biol. Chem.*, **268**, 10553–7
19. Bedford, J. M., Calvin, H. and Cooper, G. W. (1973). The maturation of spermatozoa in the human epididymis. *J. Reprod. Fertil.*, **18** (Suppl.), 199–213
20. Moore, H. D. M., Hartman, T. D. and Pryor, J. P. (1983). Development of the oocyte-penetrating capacity of spermatozoa in the human epididymis. *Int. J. Androl.*, **6**, 310–8
21. Blaquier, J. A., Cameo, M. S., Stephany, D., Piazza, A., Tezon, J. and Sherins, R. J. (1987). Abnormal distribution of epididymal androgens on spermatozoa from infertile men. *Fertil. Steril.*, **47**, 302–9
22. Rowley, M., Teshima, J. F. and Heller, C. G. (1970). Duration of transit of spermatozoa through the human male ductular system. *Fertil. Steril.*, **21**, 390–7
23. Bedford, J. M., Best, M. J. and Calvin, H. (1973). Variations in the structural character and stability of nuclear chromatin in morphologically normal human spermatozoa. *J. Reprod. Fertil.*, **33**, 19–29
24. Calvin, H. and Bedford, J. M. (1971). Formation of disulphide bonds in the nucleus and accessory structures of mammalian spermatozoa during maturation in the epididymis. *J. Reprod. Fertil.* (Suppl.), **13**, 65–75
25. Beil, R. E. and Graves, C. N. (1977). Nuclear decondensation of mammalian spermatozoa: changes during maturation and *in vitro* storage. *J. Exp. Zool.*, **202**, 235–41
26. McCosker, P. J. (1969). Abnormal spermatozoal chromatin in infertile bulls. *J. Reprod. Fertil.*, **18**, 363–7
27. Rodriguez, H., Ohanian, C. and Bustos-Obregon, E. (1985). Nuclear chromatin decondensation of spermatozoa *in vitro*: a method for evaluating the fertilizing ability of ovine semen. *Int. J. Androl.*, **8**, 147–58
28. Blazak, W. F. and Overstreet, J. W. (1982). Instability of nuclear chromatin in the ejaculated spermatozoa of fertile men. *J. Reprod. Fertil.*, **65**, 331–9
29. Colleu, D., Lescoat, D., Boujard, D. and Le Lannou, D. (1988). Human sperm nuclear maturity in normozoospermia and asthenozoospermia. *Arch. Androl.*, **21**, 155–62
30. Terquem, A. and Dadoune, J. P. (1983). Aniline blue staining of human spermatozoa chromatin: Evaluation of nuclear maturation. In Andre J. J. (ed.) *The Sperm Cell*, pp. 249–52. (The Hague: Mastinus Nijhoff Publishers)
31. Dadoune, J. P. and Alfonsi, M. F. (1986). Ultrastructural and cytochemical changes of the head components of human spermatids and spermatozoa. *Gamete Res.*, **14**, 33–46.
32. Dadoune, J. P., Mayaux, M. J. and Guihard-Moscato, M. L. (1988). Correlation between defects in chromatin condensation of human spermatozoa stained by aniline blue and semen characteristics. *Andrologia*, **20**, 211–7
33. Bartoov, B., Eltes, F., Weissenberg, R. and Lunenfeld, B. (1980). Morphological characterization of abnormal human spermatozoa using transmission electron microscopy. *Arch. Androl.*, **5**, 305–22
34. Jeulin, C., Feneux, D., Serres, C., Jouannet, P., Guillet-Rosso, F., Belaisch-Allart, J., Frydman, R. and Testart, J. (1986). Sperm factors related to failure of

human *in vitro* fertilization. *J. Reprod. Fertil.*, **76**, 735–44

35. Hofmann, N. and Hilscher, B. (1991). Use of aniline blue to assess chromatin condensation in morphological normal spermatozoa in normal and infertile men. *Hum. Reprod.*, **6**, 979–82
36. Tejada, R. I., Mitchell, C., Norman, A., Marik, J. J. and Friedman, S. (1984). A test for the practical evaluation of male fertility by acridine orange (AO) fluorescence. *Fertil. Steril.*, **42**, 87–91
37. Ibrahim, M. E. and Pedersen, H. (1988). Acridine orange fluorescence as male fertility test. *Arch. Androl.*, **20**, 125–9
38. Roux, C. and Dadoune, J. P. (1989). Use of the acridine orange staining on smears of human spermatozoa after heat treatment: Evaluation of the chromatin condensation. *Andrologia*, **21**, 275–81
39. Darzynkiewicz, Z. (1979). Acridine orange as a molecular probe in studies of nucleic acids *in situ*. In Melamed, M. R., Mullaney, P. F. and Mendelsohn, M. L. (eds.) *Flow Cytometry and Sorting*, pp. 285–316. (New York: Wiley)
40. Evenson, D. P., Darzynkiewicz, Z. and Melamed, M. R. (1980). Relation of mammalian sperm chromatin heterogeneity to fertility. *Science*, **210**, 1131–3
41. Le Lannou, D. and Blanchard, Y. (1988). Nuclear maturity and morphology of human spermatozoa selected by Percoll density gradient centrifugation or swim-up procedure. *J. Reprod. Fertil.*, **84**, 551–68
42. Liu, D. Y., Elton, R. A., Johnston, W. I. H. and Baker, H. W. G. (1987). Spermatozoal nuclear chromatin decondensation *in vitro*: A test for sperm immaturity. Comparison with results of human *in vitro* fertilization. *Clin. Reprod. Fertil.*, **5**, 191–201
43. Liu, D. Y. and Baker, H. W. G. (1992). Sperm nuclear chromatin normality: relationship with sperm morphology, sperm-zona pellucida binding, and fertilization rates *in vitro*. *Fertil. Steril.*, **58**, 1178–84
44. Liu, D. Y. and Baker, H. W. G. (1994). A new test for the assessment of sperm–zona pellucida penetration: relationship with results of other sperm tests and fertilization *in vitro*. *Hum. Reprod.*, **9**, 489–96
45. Liu, D. Y., Clarke, G. N. and Baker, H. W. G. (1986). The effect of serum on motility of human spermatozoa in culture. *Int. J. Androl.*, **9**, 109–16
46. Liu, D. Y., Jennings, M. G. and Baker, H. G. W. (1987). Correlation between defective motility (asthenospermia) and ATP reactivation of demembranated human spermatozoa. *J. Androl.*, **8**, 349–53
47. Liu, D. Y., Lopata, A., Johnston, W. I. H. and Baker, H. W. G. (1989). Human sperm–zona binding, sperm characteristics and *in-vitro* fertilization. *Hum. Reprod.*, **4**, 696–701
48. Liu, D. Y. and Baker, H. W. G. (1992). Morphology of spermatozoa bound to the zona pellucida of human oocytes that failed to fertilize *in vitro*. *J. Fertil. Reprod.*, **94**, 71–84
49. Kvist, U. (1980). Sperm nuclear decondensation ability. *Acta Physiol. Scand.*, **486** (Suppl.), 1–24
50. Kvist, U. and Eliasson, R. (1980). Influence of seminal plasma on the chromatin stability of ejaculated human spermatozoa. *Int. J. Androl.*, **3**, 130–42
51. Roomans, G. M., Lundevall, E., Bjorndahl, L. and Kvist, U. (1982). Evaluation of zinc from subcellular regions of human spermatozoa by EDTA treatment studied by X-ray microanalysis. *Int. J. Androl.*, **5**, 478–84
52. Liu, D. Y. and Baker, H. W. G. (1990). Relationships between human sperm acrosin, acrosomes, morphology and *in vitro* fertilization. *Hum. Reprod.*, **5**, 298–303
53. Katz, D. F., Diel, L. and Overstreet, J. W. (1982). Differences in the movement of morphologically normal and abnormal human seminal spermatozoa. *Biol. Reprod.*, **26**, 556–70
54. Liu, D. Y. and Baker, H. W. G. (1990). Inducing the human acrosome reaction with a calcium ionophore A23187 decrease sperm–zona pellucida binding with oocytes that failed to fertilize *in vitro*. *J. Reprod. Fertil.*, **89**, 127–34
55. Liu, D. Y. and Baker, H. W. G. (1993). Inhibition of acrosin activity with a Trypsin inhibitor blocks human sperm penetration of the zona pellucida. *Biol. Reprod.*, **48**, 340–8
56. Liu, D. Y. and Baker, H. W. G. (1994). Disordered acrosome reaction of sperm bound to the zona pellucida: a newly discovered sperm defect with reduced sperm–zona pelludica penetration and reduced fertilization *in vitro*. *Hum. Reprod.*, **9**, 1694–1700
57. Liu, D. Y. and Baker, H. W. G. (1992). Morphology of spermatozoa bound to the zona pellucida of human oocytes that failed to fertilize *in vitro*. *J. Fertil. Reprod.*, **94**, 71–84
58. Liu, D. Y. and Baker, H. W. G. (1992). Tests of human sperm function and fertilization *in vitro*. *Fertil. Steril.*, **58**, 465–83

Cervical mucus penetration assays in assisted reproduction

17

G. F. Doncel and J. W. Overstreet

INTRODUCTION

Male fertility is conventionally assessed on the basis of a semen profile which incorporates descriptive criteria, reflecting the quality of the ejaculate in terms of its overall appearance, sperm number, morphology and motility. Such descriptive criteria are adequate to identify the most severe abnormalities of male reproductive function, as in oligo- or azoospermia, but when the defects are more subtle, as manifested in idiopathic infertility, prospective studies have shown that the conventional semen profile is incapable of discriminating between fertile and infertile men[1].

The human spermatozoon is a highly specialized cell that must express a diverse array of biological functions, including elements of cell recognition, membrane fusion and movement, in order to achieve its ultimate goal of fertilizing the oocyte. Although the *in vitro* fertilization of mature human oocytes might be considered the ultimate technique for assessing the functional competence of human spermatozoa, this approach presents obvious difficulties on ethical and practical grounds as a routine diagnostic procedure. Instead, the fertilizing capacity of sperm cells must be assessed indirectly, using an integrated battery of techniques, each one of which focuses on a different aspect of sperm function. Hence, computerized image analysis techniques are now available for measuring the movement characteristics of human spermatozoa[2], zona-binding and penetration assays have been developed for assessing sperm–zona interaction[3–5], the zona-free hamster-oocyte penetration test[6] has been introduced as a measure of sperm–oocyte fusion, and conjugated lectins or monoclonal antibodies have been identified for monitoring the acrosome reaction[7,8]. Such sophisticated techniques have several drawbacks; they are technically cumbersome, do not provide an unequivocal interpretation, usually measure one sperm function and, in fact, they are not available in every laboratory supporting an assisted reproduction unit. Therefore, a simple standardized procedure for assessing the overall functional competence of human spermatozoa would be invaluable to the clinician counseling infertile couples with respect to the appropriateness of assisted reproduction techniques and their possible outcome.

After being deposited in the vagina, and in order to reach and fertilize the ovum, human spermatozoa must migrate through a complex biological fluid that fills the cervical canal known as cervical mucus (CM). Several factors govern such sperm migration *in vitro*[9]. For the spermatozoon, motion parameters, morphology and surface characteristics seem to be of crucial importance.

When human spermatozoa in semen come into contact with CM, only a small fraction succeeds in penetration[10]. Cervical mucus is a selective barrier to sperm transport, facilitates the onset of sperm capacitation and also modulates the ascent of spermatozoa to the upper female tract[11].

Taking into consideration the functional properties of CM and the factors controlling sperm migration through it, cervical mucus penetration (CMP) tests should be useful diagnostic tools to assess sperm functional capacity, as well as to predict fertility outcome both *in vivo* and *in vitro*. In fact, Hull *et al.*[12], correlating *in vitro* fertilization (IVF) rates and post-coital test (PCT) results in couples with tubal ligation or unexplained infertility, concluded that spermatozoa unable to penetrate preovulatory CM are generally also unable to fertilize the human oocyte, suggesting that the PCT has prognostic value in the context of IVF. Other groups disagree, finding no significant differences in the IVF rate whether the PCT result is positive or negative[13,14].

Part of the discrepancy may lie in the lack of standardization in methodology and interpretation of results associated with PCT. Despite multiple attempts to define normal values for this test[15–17], methodological and clinical uncertainties have led to criticism of PCT[18].

In terms of standardization and practicality, *in vitro* CMP tests should prove to be simpler and more accurate assays and, to the extent that critical sperm functions are related to interaction with CM, these tests should predict fertility outcome. In fact, they have already been applied successfully to the evaluation of male infertility and vaginal contraception[19–22].

In this chapter we will discuss the potential of *in vitro* CMP tests as diagnostic tools to be employed in the evaluation of infertile couples for whom an IVF procedure is being considered.

COMPOSITION AND STRUCTURE OF CERVICAL MUCUS

The biophysical and biochemical properties of CM are the basis for its functions, including the control of sperm entry and permeation of the mucus during the brief periovulatory period. The structural determinant of the biological functions of the mucus is its polymer phase, which is a highly glycosylated sialoglycoprotein, referred to as mucin[23,24]. The precise arrangement of the mucus microstructure is modulated primarily by cyclic variations in mucus hydration, which is generally >95%[25,26]. At midcycle, the amount of mucus increases, owing mainly to an estrogen-induced increased hydration of the gel, the mucus becomes less viscoelastic, and the penetration of spermatozoa is facilitated. In contrast, under the influence of progesterone during the luteal phase, mucus becomes less hydrated and assumes a highly viscoelastic structure which acts as a barrier to sperm.

Physicochemical studies of mucins indicate that they are linear molecules, which are arranged into a network in the whole mucus gel[27]. By electron microscopy, the macromolecules are visualized as 'threads' with a skewed and polydisperse distribution[27]. Within the mucus interior, the interstitial distance between adjacent primary elements ranges from 0.5 to 0.8 μm, and is filled with a fibrous network of secondary structural elements[28].

The mucus carbohydrate, which accounts for approximately 80% by weight of the glycoprotein, occurs mostly as a heterogeneous population of oligosaccharides, and is enriched within 'cluster'-like domains. Cervical mucus glycoproteins thus may be viewed as a linear array of oligosaccharide-rich 'clusters' alternating with structures reminiscent of a globular protein[27]. The size, shape, spacing, stiffness, surface properties and interconnections of these molecules collectively generate the intrinsic mucus resistance and selectivity to sperm.

There is variation among species in the biophysical properties of the CM. Ovulatory human mucus is less hydrated than bovine mucus and, as a consequence, the intermolecular interstices or 'pores' within human mucus are smaller, and its viscosity is higher[29]. However, human and bovine CM glycoproteins are markedly similar in sugar and amino acid composition, as well as in electrophoretic mobility, sedimentation rate and banding density in a cesium chloride density gradient[30]. Ferning patterns and viscoelastic properties also appear to be similar for human and bovine mucus[19,31].

In addition to their physicochemical similarities, results from *in vitro* bovine CMP tests have been shown to parallel test results using human CM[19,20,32,33]. In one of these reports, the ability of sperm from individual semen samples to penetrate human CM was highly correlated with their ability to penetrate a standard preparation of bovine mucus ($r=0.931$)[20].

The use of human mucus in CMP tests presents some difficulties. For instance, variation of mucus quality due to precise time of collection within the cycle requires that multiple controls be run to account for biological variability. Immunological tests of mucus donors may be required to rule out the presence of antisperm antibodies. Human CM is always a scarce material, and the laboratory may have difficulty in completely filling capillary tubes without including air bubbles. Commercially available flat-capillary tubes filled with a large pool of bovine CM may be an adequate substitute for human CM in some clinical applications. Human CMP tests, however, are very useful for the identification of mucus containing antisperm antibodies.

SPERM CHARACTERISTICS INFLUENCING CERVICAL MUCUS PENETRATION AND *IN VITRO* FERTILIZATION

Sperm passage into and through the human cervix involves mechanical interaction with the mucus and the female genital tract. Observations of sperm movement in CM have suggested that the mucus microstructure is heterogeneous and may resemble a mosaic, with regions of differing resistance to sperm penetration[25,34]. When mucus is stretched *in vitro*, its microstructure is aligned in such a way that spermatozoa swim in linear paths through the mucus interstices[9]. Because the interstices measure only a few micrometers, the spermatozoa must travel in very close proximity to the mucus macromolecules. As a result, there is substantial physical as well as hydrodynamic interaction between the sperm and mucus[35].

Several sperm characteristics have been suggested to be involved in human CM penetration, including flagellar movement, head morphology, membrane surface characteristics and capacitation status. The significance of sperm motion parameters has been emphasized in a number of different studies[20,21,36–41]. Using a multivariate statistical approach, some investigators have shown that the numbers of sperm entering mucus depend on the number of progressively motile sperm in semen, as well as their straight-line swimming velocity and amplitude of lateral head displacement[20,37,39]. Because swimming velocities and lateral head motions facilitate sperm entry into mucus, it is likely that increased sperm shearing of the mucus interface is important in reducing the initial resistance to sperm penetration[29]. Adequate lateral displacement of the sperm head also may be required for the spermatozoon to insinuate itself into the channels between the mucin chains. In addition to these biological considerations, the amplitude of sperm head displacement may indirectly reflect the efficiency of the flagellar beat pattern which, in turn, may be responsible for achieving adequate mucus penetration[37].

In a recent study, mean path velocity (VAP) was identified as the sperm movement parameter most highly correlated with CMP[38]. Straightness and linearity also were positively associated with mucus penetration.

Morphologically abnormal sperm are much more common in semen than in the oviduct[42], uterine cavity[43] or internal cervical os[44]. In comparison with semen, morphologically normal sperm predominate in cervical mucus, both *in vivo*[45] and *in vitro*[44]. Thus, it appears that abnormal sperm are less able to penetrate into and through the mucus than their morphologically normal counterparts and CM may be an important biological filter in the female tract. Sperm morphology has been repeatedly correlated with *in vitro* CMP[36,38–40].

Simultaneous assessments of sperm motility and morphology in semen have revealed that morphologically abnormal sperm in semen are less likely to be motile and even motile cells swim with lower velocity and flagellar beat frequency than normal cells[34,46]. Thus, diminished motile vigor of the abnormal sperm is likely to contribute to their diminished ability to penetrate mucus. However, the relationship between individual sperm velocity and flagellar beat parameters indicate that the heads of abnormal sperm experience greater resistance from the mucus than do normal heads[47].

Increased mucus resistance to abnormal sperm may result from surface interactions with the mucus macromolecules. Studies with capacitated sperm have indicated that more generalized cellular dysfunctions may be associated with morphological abnormalities[48]. Surface changes in the sperm cell are closely related to the functional alterations of capacitation. It is possible, therefore, that the dysfunctional state of the sperm is revealed in its earliest interaction with the CM. Seminal plasma-free human spermatozoa incubated under capacitating conditions retain their ability to penetrate mucus during the first 2–4 h of incubation. Thereafter, despite maintenance of vigorous flagellar motility, they lose the ability for sustained mucus penetration, becoming encumbered within a few body lengths of the mucus interface[49].

It is clear that the capacitation status of human spermatozoa influences their penetration in CM. However, there is also evidence that CM can induce sperm capacitation. Human sperm that are recovered from CM into a non-capacitating medium can penetrate the zona pellucida of the human oocyte[50]. The sperm's capacity to undergo the acrosome reaction in response to natural agonists is significantly accelerated by exposure to CM[51].

Furthermore, spermatozoa recovered from CM have different motility characteristics compared to control samples incubated in culture medium. Cluster analyses of sperm motion characteristics indicate that CM promotes the development of hyperactivated motility[52]. Hyperactivation is likely to confer several advantages on spermatozoa, including the development of forces necessary to detach the sperm head from epithelial adherence, the prevention of entrapment within confined spaces and the generation of increased forces to promote the penetration of viscoelastic fluids[29].

The ability of spermatozoa to fuse with zona-free hamster oocytes, which also requires capacitation, has been related to the sperm's capability for mucus penetration. In a population of patients exhibiting unexplained infertility, those with an altered CMP also had abnormal results in the hamster test[20,53].

The literature regarding the influence of sperm factors on IVF is abundant, yet sometimes confusing. Differences in testing methodology, patient background and IVF technical conditions are some of the confounding factors. In several chapters of this book, the reader can find extensive reviews on the association between IVF outcome and sperm parameters. Here, for the sake of brevity, we will mention only a few of these associations.

Multivariate regression analysis has revealed that sperm morphology, and sperm–zona binding and zona penetration are the parameters most highly correlated with IVF results[54,55]. Sperm movement characteristics, such as velocity, linearity and amplitude of lateral head displacement have also been shown to correlate with IVF[53,56]. The capacitation status of human spermatozoa, as evidenced by their ability to undergo hyperactivation, to acrosome-react, and to fuse with zona-free hamster eggs has been positively correlated with the sperm's performance in IVF as well[57–59].

Taking into account the information previously discussed, it is evident that there is a considerable overlap between the sperm characteristics contributing to CMP and those influencing IVF. Therefore it seems possible that, by assessing sperm's ability to penetrate CM, one could obtain useful information on the IVF performance of those spermatozoa. In fact, penetration of the cumulus oophorus and zona pellucida may require some of the same sperm functions involved in CMP[29].

Correlation between cervical mucus penetration and *in vitro* fertilization

Although biological reasoning suggests that *in vitro* CMP assays and IVF should give similar results, only a few studies have attempted to correlate the two outcomes. In one of the studies[60], 50 couples with bilateral tubal occlusion and six couples with unexplained infertility were evaluated. Oocytes for IVF were collected in natural cycles. Ovulatory mucus was drawn into a 7 cm flat capillary tube which was then sealed at one end. The tube was vertically incubated with the open end immersed in a 100 μL aliquot of liquefied semen (same sample used for IVF) contained in a capsule which served as a semen reservoir. After incubation at 37°C for 60 min, the tube was removed and examined under a phase-contrast microscope using a 400× magnification. The number of spermatozoa present in each of three fields at distances of 1, 4 and 7 cm along the tube was recorded. This number was corrected to give the number per 10^6 μm^2, i.e. per mm^2. These values were then used to calculate the sperm penetration test (SPT) score[61]. The SPT is one score out of 20 derived from numbers of spermatozoa per mm^2 at 1, 4 and 7 cm from the semen–mucus interface (assessed on a scale of 0–5 each), plus the distance travelled by the vanguard spermatozoa (also on a scale of 0–5). Donor sperm were included as controls.

Without exception, spermatozoa which failed to penetrate mucus failed to fertilize an oocyte. Using a score of 9 as a threshold to predict fertility, there were almost no false negatives, i.e. no fertilization was achieved if spermatozoa from an ejaculate did not sufficiently penetrate CM. Of those semen samples which did not penetrate CM, four out of five were classed as 'normal' using the World Health Organization (WHO) criteria for semen analysis[62]. All five failed to fertilize any oocyte in two IVF attempts. This finding confirms the notion that CMP can identify a subpopulation of infertile men which is not identified by basic semen analysis[40]. Five false-positive results were recorded (score >9). Such false-positive results may be due to sperm abnormalities not detected by CMP or to oocyte-related factors.

Thirty couples undergoing IVF in stimulated cycles were involved in another study[63]. Oocyte recovery was limited to a maximum of five oocytes per woman. Semen samples were evaluated following WHO guidelines[62] with a computer-assisted semen analyzer (CASA) and had characteristics ranging from normal to abnormal. Flat-capillary tubes filled with periovulatory human CM or pooled midcycle bovine CM (Penetrak®, Serono Diagnostics) were incubated for 2 h with sperm from the sample used for IVF. According to WHO[62] criteria, the *migration distance* from the semen reservoir to the foremost spermatozoon in the tube was classified into four groups as follows: 0 cm; <3 cm; >3 <4 cm; >4 cm. For *penetration density*, at a magnification of 100×, the mean number of sperm from five adjacent fields at 1 and 4.5 cm was determined. The highest penetration density was then classified into one of four groups and expressed as 0, >0 <10, >10 <50 or >50 spermatozoa per field.

The bovine CMP test was as valuable as the human CMP in evaluating sperm function. The migration distance of vanguard sperm ($P<0.001$) and the sperm penetration density ($P<0.05$) correlated most closely with the IVF results. Interestingly, there was a significant correlation of sperm penetration density in the bovine CMP test with both motility ($P<0.001$) and mean velocity ($P<0.01$) of spermatozoa recovered from the 'swim-up'. The authors suggest that the quality of a 'swim-up' preparation as well as the sperm contribution to fertilization success must be dependent upon the same combinations of sperm characteristics as those regulating the CMP test outcome.

Morrow *et al.*[64] studied 32 couples with primary infertility participating in an IVF program using stimulated cycles. Thirty-nine percent had a tubal factor, 21% endometriosis, 25% unexplained infertility, 6% anovulation and 9% abnormal semen parameters. Penetrak® tubes were placed in four drops of each fresh semen specimen and were maintained in an upright position at room temperature for 90 min in accordance with manufacturer's instructions. Results were expressed as mean of penetration length of vanguard sperm in the two tubes tested.

A statistically significant correlation ($P<0.03$) was observed between the distance travelled by spermatozoa in the mucus and the percentage of penetration of oocytes at IVF. Sperm samples with a mucus penetration ≤20 mm achieved a fertilization rate of 22.8%, while samples penetrating further than 20 mm fertilized 74.8% of the oocytes. Statistical extrapolation of the discordant results for a large series revealed that the rate of false positives (25%) and negatives (11%) could be high. However, such extrapolation should be interpreted with caution since the numbers of patients with poor or good CMP were small and considerably different from each other (4 versus 25).

In a recent study[65], 75 couples undergoing 105 stimulated cycles of IVF were investigated. The WHO[62] guidelines for sperm analysis were used to classify male patients as having the following: oligospermia, asthenospermia and teratospermia. The patients were divided into a normal group (0 or 1 anomaly), and an abnormal group (2 or 3 anomalies), on the basis of their similar fertilizing ability as demonstrated in a previous article[66]. Normal periovulatory human CM was aspirated into a 7-cm long capillary tube as described by Kremer[67]. The tubes were then incubated for 60 min at 37°C in 5% CO_2 in a semen aliquot from the same sample used for IVF. The sperm density was read at 1, 3 and 6 cm distances and results were classified according to WHO criteria[68] as *Good* when >100 motile spermatozoa were observed at 6 cm; *Fair* when between 1 and 100 motile sperm were observed at 6 cm; *Poor* when no motile sperm were observed at 6 cm, but at least one spermatozoon was seen at 3 cm; and *Negative* when no motile spermatozoa were recorded at 3 cm. The results were used to group the patients into normal (*Good*+*Fair*) and abnormal (*Poor*+*Negative*) categories.

Forty-two IVF trials associated with normal CMP test had a 51% fertilization rate and 9.5% fertilization failure rate, while 24 IVF trials associated with abnormal CMP test had a 42% fertilization rate and a 21% fertilization failure rate. Differences between fertilization rates were statistically significant ($P<0.05$). Interestingly, the results revealed the existence of a group of patients with normal semen samples and abnormal CMP test in which the fertilization rate was significantly decreased and the failure rate increased. Conversely, the test was not very informative for abnormal semen samples, since fertilization results could have been predicted with similar power by using spermiogram data.

Considering all of these data together, it can be concluded that CMP results are positively correlated with IVF rates. Such a correlation may be explained if CMP tests assess a combination of sperm characteristics that are also involved in determining IVF success. But it is also possible that the various functions of human spermatozoa, including movement, gamete recognition, acrosome reaction, and oocyte fusion are generally correlated with each other. No sperm test, including CMP, will be capable of predicting IVF rates with total accuracy because other factors, including oocyte quality, are critically involved in the fertilization process. Cervical mucus penetration tests seem to be more informative when classical semen parameters are normal, for they allow the detection of a subgroup of occult male factor cases with lower fertilization rates than expected.

It is clear that neither the assay methodology nor the interpretation of CMP results has been adequately standardized. Most of the studies on CMP and IVF utilized methodologies such as those from WHO[62] which were not designed to test the CMP assay as a predictor of IVF outcome. A careful evaluation of the laboratory procedures will be needed to establish the most appropriate protocols for the CMP test in the IVF setting. Following this standardization, a large study including other sperm test results and multiple regression analysis correlating fertilization rates to testing data will be needed to establish the real value of the CMP test in the IVF prognostic armamentarium.

NEW DEVELOPMENTS

A recently developed assay system (Tru-Trax®, Humagen, Charlottesville, VA, USA) that allows a comparison of sperm penetration in human and bovine CM on the same slide may be useful for standardizing the CMP. The Tru-Trax® system consists of a plastic slide with parallel flat linear chambers that can be filled with either human or bovine CM from luer-lock valves on the top side. The semen samples are loaded into wells located at the bottom of the slide and the distance travelled by the vanguard sperm is measured in mm directly from the calibrated grid on the slide. This system has been shown to be reliable, with reproducible results which are highly correlated with results obtained with Penetrak®[69]. The Tru-Trax® system can be used to compare donor and patient semen samples or CM and its surrogates.

Because CM, regardless of its origin, may vary from batch to batch, and is somewhat difficult to collect and store, several CM substitutes have been described. For instance, sperm penetration in fresh egg white has been shown to give relevant and unique information on male natural fertility[70]. In combination with the man's age, penetration results from this test provide an index that is predictive of the future male fertility.

An artificial CM surrogate consisting of a polyacrylamide gel has also been developed[71,72]. Human sperm ability to penetrate the synthetic medium correlated significantly with the penetration of bovine and human CM, although polyacrylamide proved to be a stronger barrier. Sperm velocity and duration of progressive motility were markedly reduced in the synthetic gel. Polyacrylamide penetration results correlated with the outcome of standard semen analyses; however, the test provided no clear prediction of subsequent natural fertility[73,74]. Further refinement of this technique may be needed before a prospective study is undertaken to ascertain its value as an IVF prognostic test.

A very interesting CM substitute is hyaluronic acid. In comparison to other proposed mucus substitutes, hyaluronate has several advantages: it is a non-biohazardous, naturally occurring polysaccharide which is readily available and from which highly purified preparations can be obtained, thus reducing the inter-batch variation. Furthermore, it has been reported that parameters of sperm motility as measured by CASA are comparable in human CM and hyaluronate[75]. Studies to determine the suitability of hyaluronate polymers as media for investigating the capacity of human spermatozoa to penetrate CM recently have been carried out[38,75,76]. In these studies, a 5 mg/mL solution of 2×10^6 molecular weight hyaluronate, or 1–4 mg/mL of hyaluronic acid (M.W.=3 and 6.8 Md, Pharmacia) or a commercially available hyaluronate preparation (Sperm Select®, Pharmacia) were used as sperm migration media. In the case of Sperm Select®, it was diluted 1:1 with HEPES buffered BWW medium and loaded into flat capillary tubes. After sealing one end, the tubes were immersed into a 50 μL aliquot of liquefied semen and incubated for 30 min at 37°C. The number of spermatozoa per high power field (40×, 0.102 mm^2) was then assessed at distances of 1.0, 3.0 and 4.5 cm from the base of the tube[38]. In the hyaluronate medium, sperm numbers decline in an exponential manner in relation to the penetration depth, such that linear regression lines can be generated by log transformation of the sperm density values. The point at which these regression lines bisect the abscissa represents the theoretical distance at which sperm density reaches zero (theoretical vanguard distance or TVD) and provides a robust measure of the overall capacity of the sperm population to penetrate a given medium[76].

The results from the above-referenced studies indicate the existence of an excellent correlation between sperm penetration into hyaluronate and human or bovine CM. The assay was clearly able to discriminate with good sensitivity (90.9%) and specificity (93.1%) between semen samples which would show normal and abnormal mucus penetrating ability. Sperm penetration into both hyaluronate media and CM were highly dependent on the number of progressively motile spermatozoa present in the ejaculate, the path velocity of these cells, and their morphology, yielding multiple regression coefficients in excess of $r=0.8$. The test results were also able to predict the outcome of the zona-free hamster oocyte penetration assay very efficiently with r values of around 0.8. These findings suggest that the relative ability of human spermatozoa to penetrate a hyaluronate polymer provides objective information on the functional competence of these cells, thus warranting its evaluation as a potential predictor of IVF results.

CONCLUSIONS

In vitro sperm penetration assays employing CM or their substitutes provide information on sperm characteristics, such as viability, number of progressively motile cells in the sample, motion parameters (e.g. velocities, linearity and amplitude of lateral head displacement), morphology and capacitation status. Indirectly, these tests may also give information on sperm capacity for acrosome reaction and hyperactivation, as well as sperm–oocyte interaction. Since many of these functions are involved in sperm fertilization, the CM penetration test should be able to predict sperm performance in IVF. It is possible that the value of these tests will be greater than the value of conventional semen parameters because IVF depends on multiple sperm properties, many of which are being evaluated in the CM penetration test.

In the few studies performed with patients undergoing IVF CM penetration test results have been significantly correlated with fertilization rates, with a low incidence of false-negative results. The test seems to be especially informative in revealing a subpopulation of infertile men with an occult male factor, not revealed by basic semen analysis, but for whom fertilization rates are lower than expected and the incidence of fertilization failures is increased.

It is important to bear in mind that no single test has been developed that is capable of accounting for 100% of the variation in IVF rates. The percentage of false-positive results obtained with the CM penetration test may be attributable to sperm properties not evaluated in the assay or to variables related to the oocyte.

Some caveats in the use of this assay are related to CM intrinsic variability, as well as lack of standardization of the methodology. The best approach has not been determined for analysis of data, and interpretation of the test results to predict IVF success. After these issues are resolved a large study, including CM penetration and other sperm test results, along with a multiple regression analysis of fertilization rates and testing data, will be needed to establish the real predictive value of the CM penetration test in assisted reproduction.

In conclusion, the CM sperm penetration test is inexpensive, reproducible and objective, and is simple to perform. If human CM is not on hand or is not preferred, commercially available substitutions can be used. Because the test evaluates a combination of sperm characteristics, it has the potential to provide much of the information generated by more sophisticated tests, such as the hamster-egg penetration assay and computer-assisted sperm motion and morphology analyses. Sperm penetration tests can have a significant clinical value in the routine diagnosis and prognosis of male factor infertility, particularly in situations where specialized expertise and facilities are limited.

References

1. Aitken, R. J., Best, F. S. M., Warner, P. and Templeton, A. (1984). A prospective study of the relationship between semen quality and fertility in cases of unexplained infertility. *J. Androl.*, **5**, 297–303
2. Davis, R. O. and Katz, D. F. (1994). Computer-aided sperm analysis: a critical review. In Getola, G. M. and Grisberg, K. A. (eds.) *Evaluation and Treatment of the Infertile Male*. (Cambridge: Cambridge University Press) in press
3. Burkman, L. J., Coddington, C. C., Franken, D. R., Kruger, T. F., Rosenwaks, Z. and Hodgen, G. D. (1988). The hemizona assay (HZA): development of a diagnostic test for the binding of human spermatozoa to the human hemizona pellucida to predict fertilization potential. *Fertil. Steril.*, **49**, 688–97
4. Liu, D. Y., Lopata, A., Johnston, W. I. H. and Baker, H. W. G. (1988). A human sperm–zona pellucida binding test using oocytes that failed to fertilize *in vitro*. *Fertil. Steril.*, **50**, 782–8
5. Overstreet, J. W., Yanagimachi, R., Katz, D. F., Hayashi, K. M. and Hanson, F. W. (1980). Penetration of human spermatozoa into the human zona pellucida and the zona-free hamster egg: a study of fertile donor and infertile patients. *Fertil. Steril.*, **33**, 534–42
6. Yanagimachi, R., Yanagimachi, H. and Rogers, B. J. (1976). The use of zona free animal ova as a test system for the assessment of the fertilizing capacity of human spermatozoa. *Biol. Reprod.*, **15**, 471–6
7. Cross, N. L., Morales, P., Overstreet, J. W. and Hanson, F. W. (1986). Two simple methods for detecting acrosome-reacted sperm. *Gamete Res.*, **15**, 213–26
8. Mortimer, D., Curtis, E. F. and Miller, R. G. (1987). Specific labelling by peanut agglutinin of the outer acrosomal membrane of the human spermatozoon. *J. Reprod. Fertil.*, **81**, 127–32
9. Overstreet, J. W., Katz, D. F. and Yudin, A. I. (1991). Cervical mucus and sperm transport in reproduction. *Sem. Perinatol.*, **15**, 149–55
10. Settlage, D. S. F., Motoshima, M. and Tredway, D. R. (1973). Sperm transport from the external cervical os to the fallopian tubes in women: a time and quantitation study. *Fertil. Steril.*, **24**, 655–61
11. Overstreet, J. W. (1983). Transport of gametes in the reproductive tract of the female mammal. In Hartman, J. F. (ed.) *Mechanism and Control of Animal Fertilization*, pp. 499–543. (New York: Academic Press)
12. Hull, M. G. R., McLeod, F. N., Yoyce, D. N. and Ray, B. D. (1984). Human *in-vitro* fertilisation, *in-vivo* sperm penetration of cervical mucus, and unexplained infertility. *Lancet*, **ii**, 245–6
13. Cohen, J., Hewitt, J. and Rowland, G. (1984). Application of *in-vitro* fertilisation, in cases of a poor post-coital test. *Lancet*, **ii**, 583
14. Matson, P. L., Tuvik, A. I., O'Halloran, F. O. and Yovich, J. L. (1986). The value of the postcoital test in predicting the fertilization of human oocytes. In Vitro *Fertil. Embryo Transf.*, **3**, 110–13
15. Moghissi, K. S. (1976). Postcoital test. Physiological basis, technique and interpretation. *Fertil. Steril.*, **27**, 117–29
16. Portuondo, J. A., Echanojauregui, A. D., Herran, C. and Augustin, A. (1982). Prognostic value of postcoital test in unexplained infertility. *Int. J. Fertil.*, **27**, 184–6
17. Collins, J. A., So, Y., Wilson, E. H., Wrixon, W. and Casper, R. F. (1984). The postcoital test as a predictor of pregnancy among 355 infertile couples. *Fertil. Steril.*, **41**, 703–8
18. Griffith, C. S. and Grimes, D. A. (1990). The validity of the postcoital test. *Am. J. Obstet. Gynecol.*, **162**, 615–20
19. Alexander, N. J. (1981). Evaluation of male infertility with an *in vitro* cervical mucus penetration test. *Fertil. Steril.*, **36**, 201–8
20. Aitken, R. J., Warner, P. E. and Reid, C. (1986). Factors influencing the success of sperm–cervical mucus interaction in patients exhibiting unexplained infertility. *J. Androl.*, **7**, 3–10
21. Menge, A. C. and Beitner, O. (1989). Interrelationships among semen characteristics, antisperm antibodies, and cervical mucus penetration assays in infertile human couples. *Fertil. Steril.*, **51**, 486–92
22. Doncel, G. F. (1994). Chemical vaginal contraceptives: preclinical evaluation. In Mauck, C. K., Cordero, M., Gabelnick, H. L., Spieler, J. M. and Rivera, R. (eds.) *Barrier Contraceptives. Current Status and Future Prospects*, pp. 147–62. (New York: Wiley-Liss)
23. Wolf, D. P., Sokoloski, J. E. and Litt, M. (1980). Composition of human cervical mucus. *Biochem. Biophys. Acta*, **630**, 545–58
24. Silberberg, A. (1987). A model for mucus glycoprotein structure. *Biorheology*, **24**, 605–14
25. Odeblad, E. (1968). The functional structure of human cervical mucus. *Acta Obstet. Gynecol. Scand. Suppl.*, **47**, 57–78
26. Litt, M., Wolf, D. P. and Khan, M. A. (1977). Functional aspects of mucus rheology. *Adv. Exp. Med. Biol.*, **89**, 191–202
27. Carlstedt, I. and Sheehan, J. K. (1989). Structure and macromolecular properties of cervical mucus glycoproteins. *Symp. Soc. Exp. Biol.*, **43**, 289–316
28. Yudin, A. I., Hanson, F. W. and Katz, D. F. (1989). Human cervical mucus and its interaction with sperm: a fine-structural view. *Biol. Reprod.*, **40**, 661–71
29. Katz, D. F., Drobnis, E. Z. and Overstreet, J. W. (1989). Factors regulating mammalian sperm migra-

tion through the female reproductive tract and oocyte vestments. *Gamete Res.*, **22**, 443–69
30. Meyer, F. A. (1977). Comparison of structural glycoproteins from mucus of different sources. *Biochim. Biophys. Acta*, **493**, 272–82
31. Lee, W. I., Verdugo, P., Blandau, R. J. and Gaddum-Rosse, P. (1977). Molecular arrangement of cervical mucus: a reevaluation based on laser light-scattering spectroscopy. *Gynecol. Invest.*, **8**, 154–66
32. Mangione, C. M., Medley, N. E. and Menge, A. C. (1981). Studies on the use of estrous bovine cervical mucus in the human sperm–cervical mucus penetration technique. *Int. J. Fertil.*, **26**, 20–4
33. Bergman, A., Amit, A., David, M. P., Homonnai, Z. T. and Paz, G. F. (1981). Penetration of human ejaculated spermatozoa into human and bovine cervical mucus. I. Correlation between penetration values. *Fertil. Steril.*, **36**, 363–7
34. Katz, D. F. and Overstreet, J. W. (1982). Mechanism and analysis of sperm migration in cervical mucus. In Chantler, E. N., Elder, J. B. and Elstein, M. (eds.) *Mucus in Health and Disease II*, pp. 319–30. (New York: Plenum Press)
35. Katz, D. F. and Berger, S. A. (1980). Flagellar propulsion of human sperm in cervical mucus. *Biorheology*, **17**, 169–75
36. David, M. P., Amit, A., Bergman, A., Yedwab, G., Paz, G. F. and Homonnai, Z. T. (1979). Sperm penetration *in vitro*: correlations between parameters of sperm quality and the penetration capacity. *Fertil. Steril.*, **32**, 676–80
37. Aitken, R. J., Sutton, M., Warner, P. and Richardson, D. W. (1985). Relationship between the movement characteristics of human spermatozoa and their ability to penetrate cervical mucus and zona-free hamster oocytes. *J. Reprod. Fertil.*, **73**, 441–9
38. Aitken, R. J., Bowie, H., Buckingham, D., Harkiss, D. and Richardson, D. W. (1992). Sperm penetration into a hyaluronic acid polymer as a means of monitoring functional competence. *J. Androl.*, **13**, 44–54
39. Mortimer, D., Pandya, I. J. and Sawers, R. S. (1986). Relationship between human sperm motility characteristics and sperm penetration into human cervical mucus *in vitro*. *J. Reprod. Fertil.*, **78**, 93–102
40. Keel, B. A. and Webster, B. W. (1988). Correlation of human sperm motility characteristics with an *in vitro* cervical mucus penetration test. *Fertil. Steril.*, **49**, 138–43
41. Ford, W. C. L., Ponting, F. A., McLaughlin, E. A., Rees, J. M. and Hull, M. G. R. (1992). Controlling the swimming speed of human sperm by varying the incubation temperature and its effect on cervical mucus penetration. *Int. J. Androl.*, **15**, 127–34
42. Ahlgren, M., Bostrom, K. and Malmquist, R. (1973). Sperm transport and survival in women with special reference to the fallopian tube. In Hafez, E. S. E. and Thibault, C. (eds.) *Biology of Spermatozoa Transport, Survival and Fertilizing Ability*, p. 63. (Basel: Karger)
43. Bergman, P. (1956). Sperm migration and its relation to the morphology and motility of spermatozoa. *Int. J. Fertil.*, **1**, 145
44. Fredricsson, B. and Björk, G. (1977). Morphology of postcoital spermatozoa in the cervical secretion and its clinical significance. *Fertil. Steril.*, **28**, 841–5
45. Hanson, F. W. and Overstreet, J. W. (1981). The interaction of human spermatozoa with cervical mucus *in vivo*. *Am. J. Obstet. Gynecol.*, **140**, 173–7
46. Morales, P., Katz, D. F., Overstreet, J. W., Samuels, S. J. and Chang, R. J. (1988). The relationship between the motility and morphology of spermatozoa in human semen. *J. Androl.*, **9**, 241–7
47. Katz, D. F., Morales, P., Samuels, S. J. and Overstreet, J. W. (1990). Mechanisms of filtration of morphologically abnormal human sperm by cervical mucus. *Fertil. Steril.*, **54**, 513–16
48. Morales, P., Overstreet, J. W. and Katz, D. F. (1988). Changes in human sperm movement during capacitation *in vitro*. *J. Reprod. Fertil.*, **83**, 119–28
49. Katz, D. G., Yudin, A. I., Drobnis, E. Z., Hanson, F. W., Cragun, J. R. and Chang, R. J. (1988). Human sperm penetration of cervical mucus and the hamster cumulus in relation to capacitation. *Society for Gynecology Investigation* (abstr.), p. 129
50. Lambert, H., Overstreet, J. W., Morales, P., *et al.* (1988). Sperm capacitation in the human female reproductive tract. *Fertil. Steril.*, **43**, 325–7
51. Zinaman, M., Drobnis, E. Z., Morales, P., Brazil, C., Kiel, M., Cross, N., Hanson, F. W. and Overstreet, J. W. (1989). The physiology of sperm recovered from the human cervix: acrosomal status and response to inducers of the acrosome reaction. *Biol. Reprod.*, **41**, 790–7
52. Zhu, J. J., Barratt, C. L. R. and Cooke, I. D. (1992). Effect of human cervical mucus on human sperm motion and hyperactivation *in vitro*. *Hum. Reprod.*, **7**, 1402–6
53. Schats, R., Aitken, R. J., Templeton, A. A. and Djahanbakhch, O. (1984). The role of cervical mucus–semen interaction in infertility of unknown aetiology. *Br. J. Obstet. Gynaecol.*, **91**, 371–6
54. Liu, D. Y. and Baker, H. W. G. (1992). Tests of human sperm function and fertilization *in vitro*. *Fertil. Steril.*, **58**, 465–83
55. Duncan, W. W., Glew, M. J., Wang, X. J., Flaherty, S. P. and Matthews, C. D. (1993). Prediction of *in vitro* fertilization rates from semen variables. *Fertil. Steril.*, **59**, 1233–8
56. Jeulin, C., Feneux, D., Serres, C., Jouannet, P., Guillet-Rosso, F., Belaisch-Allart, J., Frydman, R. and Testart, J. (1986). Sperm factors related to failure of human *in vitro* fertilization. *J. Reprod. Fertil.*, **76**, 735–44
57. Karande, V., Mbizvo, M. T., Burkman, L. J., Alexander, N. J. and Hodgen, G. D. (1990). Hyperactivation (HA) of human sperm is a prognostic indication of fertilization during IVF. *Am. Soc. Androl.* (Abstr.), 6 April

58. Cummins, J. M., Pember, S. M., Jequier, A. M., Yovich, J. L. and Hartmann, P. E. (1991). A test of the human sperm acrosome reaction following ionophore challenge. Relationship to fertility and other seminal parameters. *J. Androl.*, **12**, 98–103
59. Wolf, D. P., Sokoloski, J. E. and Quigley, M. M. (1983). Correlation of human *in vitro* fertilization with the hamster egg bioassay. *Fertil. Steril.*, **40**, 53–9
60. Barratt, C. L. R., Osborn, J. C., Harrison, P. E., Monks, N., Dumphy, B. C., Lenton, E. A. and Cooke, I. D. (1989). The hypo-osmotic swelling test and the sperm mucus penetration test in determining fertilization of the human oocyte. *Hum. Reprod.*, **4**, 430–4
61. Pandya, I. J., Mortimer, D. and Sawers, R. S. (1986). A standardized approach for evaluating the penetration of human spermatozoa into cervical mucus *in vitro*. *Fertil. Steril.*, **45**, 357–65
62. World Health Organization. (1987). *Laboratory Manual for the Examination of Human Semen and Semen–Cervical Mucus Interaction.* (Cambridge: Cambridge University Press)
63. De Geyter, Ch., Bals-Pratsch, M., Doeren, M., Yeung, C. H., Grunert, J. H., Bordt, J., Schneider, H. P. G. and Nieschlag, E. (1989). Human and bovine cervical mucus penetration as a test of sperm function for *in vitro* fertilization. *Hum. Reprod.*, **3**, 949–54
64. Morrow, A., Drudy, L., Gordon, A. and Harrison, R. F. (1992). Evaluation of bovine cervical mucus penetration as a test of human spermatozoal function for an *in vitro* fertilization programme. *Andrologia*, **24**, 323–6
65. Berberoglugil, P., Englert, Y., Van den Bergh, M., Rodesch, C., Bertrand, E. and Biramane, J. (1993). Abnormal sperm–mucus penetration test predicts low *in vitro* fertilization ability of apparently normal semen. *Fertil. Steril.*, **59**, 1128–32
66. Englert, Y., Vekemans, M., Lejeune, B., Van Rysselberghe, M., Puissant, F., Degueldre, M., Leroy, F. (1987). Higher pregnancy rates after *in vitro* fertilization and embryo transfer in cases with sperm defects. *Fertil. Steril.*, **48**, 254–7
67. Kremer, J. (1965). A simple sperm penetration test. *Int. J. Fertil.*, **10**, 209–15
68. World Health Organization. (1980). *Laboratory Manual for the Examination of Human Sperm and Semen–Cervical Mucus Interaction.* In Besley, M. A., Eliasson, R., Gallegos, A. J., Moghissi, K. S., Paulson, C. A. and Prasad, M. R. N. (eds.) (Singapore: Press Concern)
69. Niederberger, C. S., Lamb, D. J., Glintz, M., Lipshultz, L. I. and Scully, N. F. (1993). Tests of sperm function for evaluation of the male: Penetrak and Tru-Trax. *Fertil. Steril.*, **60**, 319–23
70. Bostofte, E., Bagger, P., Michael, A. and Stakemann, G. (1992). The sperm penetration test (P-test) can predict fecundability in the male partner from infertile couples. *Andrologia*, **24**, 125–9
71. Bissett, D. L. (1980). Development of a model of human cervical mucus. *Fertil. Steril.*, **33**, 211–12
72. Lorton, S. P., Kummerfeld, H. L., Foote, R. H., Feldschuh, R. and Feldschuh, J. (1981). Polyacrylamide as a substitute for cervical mucus in sperm migration tests. *Fertil. Steril.*, **35**, 222–5
73. Urry, R. L., Middleton, R. G. and Mayo, D. (1986). A comparison of the penetration of human sperm into bovine and artificial cervical mucus. *Fertil. Steril.*, **45**, 135–7
74. Eggert-Kruse, W., Schwalbach, B., Rohr, G., Klinga, K., Tilgen, W. and Runnebaum, B. (1993). Evaluation of polyacrylamide gel as substitute for human cervical mucus in the sperm penetration test. *Fertil. Steril.*, **60**, 540–9
75. Neuwinger, J., Cooper, T. G., Knuth, U. A. and Nieschlag, E. (1991). Hyaluronic acid as a medium for human sperm migration tests. *Hum. Reprod.*, **6**, 396–400
76. Mortimer, D., Mortimer, S. T., Shu, M. A. and Swart, R. (1990). A simplified approach to sperm–cervical mucus interaction testing using a hyaluronate migration test. *Hum. Reprod.*, **5**, 835–41

The human sperm acrosome reaction 18

K. Coetzee and R. R. Henkel

INTRODUCTION

For successful fertilization of oocytes by spermatozoa, a set of functionally normal parameters with regard to oocytes and spermatozoa maturity are of paramount importance. In the spermatozoon, besides motility and zona binding, the occurrence of the acrosome reaction (AR) is of primary importance in the development of functional capability. However, before spermatozoa are able to undergo acrosome reaction essential modifications in cell physiology of the sperm, called capacitation, must occur. Numerous studies have tried to elucidate the precise biochemical and biophysical changes involved in the process of determining the fertilizing capacity of the spermatozoa. The normal progress of these changes may display important markers of fertilizing ability. For example, the ability of the sperm to penetrate the cumulus oophorus, the corona radiata, the zona pellucida and the vitelline membrane.

The ability to evaluate the human AR is, however, restricted by a practical limitation. The loss of the human acrosome cannot be observed on living sperm, by phase contrast or differential interference contrast microscopy, because of its relatively small size compared to other mammalian species. Initially the best results were obtained by electronmicroscopy; this method, however, is not suited for routine analysis because of its expense and complexity. The need thus arose for a relatively simple test by which the human AR could be quantified at the lightmicroscope level. In addition, the labile nature of the human sperm acrosome makes the analysis of the reaction problematic. The chosen procedure must therefore be able to distinguish between normal and degenerative reactions.

In addition to the above limitations, the existence of a multifactorial induction and regulating system and the individual perspectives and methods of measurement chosen by laboratories contribute to the uncertainty that still exists on the subject.

THE BIOCHEMISTRY OF CAPACITATION AND ACROSOME REACTION

The acrosome of a human spermatozoa is a membrane-bound organelle which appears during spermatogenesis as a product of the Golgi complex. It surrounds the anterior portion of the sperm nucleus and can be divided into the following components:

(1) Plasma membrane;

(2) Outer acrosomal membrane;

(3) Acrosomal matrix;

(4) Inner acrosomal membrane; and

(5) Equatorial segment.

Factors inhibiting capacitation are incorporated into the membranes of sperm during maturation in the epididymis[1,2]. These factors include sialoglycoproteins, sulfoglycerolipids and steroid sulfates which induce a significant increase in the net negative charge of the outer acrosomal membrane[3]. This state of decapacitation (stability) is maintained after ejaculation by the presence of inhibitory macromolecules in the seminal plasma[4] and lower reaches of the female reproductive tract[1]. A specific glycoprotein has been identified as the primary decapacitator[1]; bound to the outer acrosomal membrane it can prevent the interaction with extracellular signals, inhibit ion channels activity and/or enzymes[5]. This stability is further enhanced by the incorporation of cholesterol into the acrosomal membrane complex, preferentially into the plasma membrane.

Sperm acquire their fertilizing ability *in vivo* during their migration through the female genital tract. Capacitation can also be induced *in vitro* in chemically defined media[6]. The complete process, however, is not yet fully understood, but is thought to involve major biochemical and biophysical changes in the membrane complex, energy metabolism and ion permeability.

(1) Modification, redistribution and/or loss of the epididymal seminal plasma and cervical decapacitation factors – by exogenous or endogenous proteases specifically activated (plasmin, kallikrein, and acrosin)[1,2].

(2) The net negative charge is decreased by endogenous hydrolases (sterol sulfatase)[3].

(3) The fluidity is increased by the efflux of cholesterol, altering the cholesterol:phospholipid ratio and the influx of unsaturated fatty acids. These changes are thought to be serum albumin-mediated[3,7].

(4) The altered permeability allows the increased uptake of calcium ions, glucose and oxygen, resulting in an elevated energy state, inducing hyperactivated motility and the ability to undergo acrosome reaction[8,9].

Notwithstanding the extent of these changes, capacitation is also thought to be a reversible event. The exact threshold of irreversibility, however, remains undefined, i.e. what constitutes the boundary between capacitation and the acrosome reaction? Many of these structural changes proposed to constitute capacitation may, however, be irreversible, which may lead to an untimely acrosome reaction. The acrosome reaction can, therefore, be seen as the endpoint of capacitation.

Initiation of AR

The signals for the initiation of the AR are most likely received by one or more receptors on the plasma membrane surface, which transmits them across the membrane. Zaneveld *et al.*[5] proposed a mechanism by which membrane receptor activation of GTP-binding proteins stimulates second messenger systems, which regulate ion transport. An endogenous calcium ion threshold concentration has long been thought of as the primary inducer of the acrosome reaction[8,10]. Yanagimachi and Usui[11] showed that on the addition of calcium, but not magnesium, guinea pig sperm incubated for several hours in calcium-free medium underwent the acrosome reaction within 10 min. Since then, calcium has been implicated in many reactions leading to the complete loss of the acrosome and eventually fertilization[10]:

(1) Activation of many enzymes (acrosin, hyaluronidase, phospholipase A2).

(2) Enzyme systems (adenylate cyclase).

(3) Neutralization of the net negative charge.

(4) Induction of hyperactivated motility[3].

Stock and Fraser[12], examining the extracellular Ca^{2+} requirements for the support of capacitation and the spontaneous acrosome reaction in human spermatozoa, concluded that the optimal conditions for capacitation and the acrosome reaction in human spermatozoa require extracellular Ca^{2+} at 1.80 mM. Calcium channels providing a means of calcium entry. In contrast, White *et al.*[13] found that the acrosome reaction rates at 4 h and 20 h were little different in media with or without calcium, although the absence of calcium did have a significant effect on the quality of motility.

The human sperm acrosome reaction is an exocytotic event characterized by significant ultrastructural changes leading to the complete loss of the outer acrosomal cap:

(1) Decondensation of the acrosomal matrix.

(2) Fenestration and vesiculation of the plasma membrane and outer acrosomal membrane.

(3) Dispersion of the vesicles.

(4) Release of the acrosomal content.

Nagae[14] proposed a unique morphological sequence for this acrosome reaction. Vesicles formed in the intermediate stage were formed by the invagination and pinching off of the outer acrosomal membrane and the plasma membrane. Similar characterization was found by Stock *et al.*[15]. In contrast, Yudin *et al.*[16] found that human sperm undergo an acrosome reaction similar to that of other mammals, in which the outer acrosomal and plasma membranes initially fuse by fenestration followed by vesiculation. The dispersion of these vesicles leaves the spermatozoon

Table 1 Human acrosome reaction evaluation, methods and critera

Authors	*Method*	*Criteria*
Talbot and Chacon[55]	FITC-RCA	Acrosomal contents, toxic
Talbot and Chacon[22]	Triple Stain	Viable AR
Cross[23]	FITC-PSA, Hoechst 33258	Viable AR, acrosomal content
Nagae[14]	TEM	Ultrastructural
Mortimer[56]	FITC-PNA	Outer acrosomal membrane
Lee[57]	Chlortetracycline	Plasma membrane
Yudin[16]	TEM	Ultrastructural
Byrd[58]	HS21	Intact acrosomal cap antigens
Okabe[59]	MH61	Acrosome membrane
Aitken and Brindle[21]	FITC-PNA, FITC-PSA, CRB9	Outer acrosomal membrane, acrosomal content
Aitken[18]	FITC-PNA, HOS-TEST	Viable AR

FITC: fluorescein isothiocyanate; RCA: *Ricinus communis* agglutinin-60; PSA: *Pisum sativum* agglutinin; PNA: *Arachis hypogea* (peanut) agglutinin; TEM: transmission electron microscopy; HS21: monoclonal antibody; MH61: monoclonal antibody; CRB9: monoclonal antibody; HOS: hypo-osmotic swelling test

surrounded by a single, continuous membrane, i.e. the inner acrosomal membrane. In addition to these changes, the membrane proteins of the plasma membrane overlying the equatorial/post-acrosomal region of the sperm head undergoes a conformational change, resulting in activation[3]. This activation may facilitate the fusion of the sperm with the oocyte vitelline membrane.

The loss of the membranes also releases or exposes activated lysins assisting the sperm penetration of the zona pellucida[2]. Acrosin, a trypsin-like serine protease found in the acrosome, has been shown to be implicated in a number of events leading to fertilization: assisting the sperm penetration of the zona pellucida, the triggering of the acrosome reaction[2] and the activation of regulatory enzymes involved in Ca^{2+} transport[5]. Studies using *p*-aminobenzamidine (PABA)[17], an inhibitor of mouse sperm acrosin, have shown that acrosin is a necessary factor for the dispersal of the acrosomal matrix, probably through the activation of proacrosin. In the presence of PABA the membranes undergo normal vesiculation, but zona pellucida penetration is inhibited.

THE MEASUREMENT OF THE AR IN HUMAN SPERMATOZOA

Capacitation and the acrosome reaction can be induced chemically, providing a controlled means for the evaluation of the acrosome reaction; calcium ionophore A23187[18], pentoxifylline[19], or low temperature[20]. There are, however, inherent negative side-effects that must be taken into account: the possible negative effect on motility and the means of induction overrides the normal processes involved in the acrosome reaction; for example, using calcium ionophore, a toxic chemical substance, as the inducer the time required for capacitation is minimized. The addition of complex biological fluids or cell cultures, such as maternal cord serum, follicular fluid (FF), granulosa cells, cumulus oophorus and zonae pellucida, even though uncontrolled in nature, is physiologically more correct. This is of particular relevance when future improvements of treatment in male infertility are to be introduced into an assisted reproduction program and for furthering of our knowledge of the *in vivo* regulatory system.

Several techniques have been employed to detect the acrosome reaction, each with its own level of characterization (Table 1). Aitken and Brindle[21], however, showed that probes targeting different components involved in the acrosome reaction measure acrosomal loss at different rates. The labile nature of the acrosomal vesicle also requires a means of determining sperm viability to be included, to distinguish between 'normal' and degenerative reactions. In the triple stain technique, according to Talbot and Chacon[22], trypan blue is used. Cross *et al.*[23] included the supravital stain Hoechst 33258, while Aitken *et al.*[18], in their protocol for assessing the ability of viable human spermatozoa to acrosome-react in response to A23187, employed a fluorescein-conjugated lectin in concert with the hypo-osmotic swelling test. The use of these different techniques may have a significant influence on the interpretation and comparison of results. This is illustrated by the often equivocal results obtained in acrosome reaction studies.

PHYSIOLOGICAL INDUCERS AND REGULATORS OF THE AR

Stock *et al.*[15] found that 32% of sperm coincubated with oocyte–cumulus complexes for 14–18 h had initiated or completed the acrosome reaction. The effect of a number of female reproductive tract products on sperm fertilizing capacity was evaluated by coincubating fertile sperm samples with endometrial, oviductal, granulosa and cumulus cells, FF and maternal serum by Bastias *et al.*[24]. Compared to control samples, endometrial and oviductal cell cultures did not alter sperm fertilizing capacity or their movement characteristics. Sperm coincubated with FF, granulosa or cumulus cells, however, exhibited a significantly higher ability to penetrate zona-free hamster ova. It is, therefore, reasonable to propose that secretions of cumulus cells could be involved in the regulation of the sperm acrosome reaction.

Siegel *et al.*[25] concluded from their study that components within follicular fluid (FF) may influence sperm physiology and enhance sperm fertilizing capacity by activating sperm proteinase systems involved in sperm reaction and interaction. An active Sephadex G-75 fraction identified in FF was found to stimulate a rapid, transient increase in the intracellular free Ca^{2+} in human spermatozoa[26]. The ability of this fraction to induce the AR led the authors to conclude that this influx of Ca^{2+} is responsible for the initiation of the AR. Using indirect immunofluorescence, FF was found to rapidly induce the acrosome reaction after the sperm had been incubated for at least 10 h[27]. The induction of the human AR by whole FF and/or the active Sephadex G-75 component was found to satisfy the ultrastructural criteria known for physiological reactions, as shown by transmission electron microscopy[16]. Yudin *et al.*[16] also showed that human sperm capacitated for 6 h at 40°C and then incubated with FF for 180 s resulted in 40% of the sperm reacting. Sperm incubated for 22 h before FF treatment had their acrosome reaction rate enhanced six fold[28], illustrating the potential effect of FF. An adequate preincubation period followed by FF treatment therefore seems to result in the synchronization of capacitation and the facilitation of the AR. In contrast Stock *et al.*[29], examining the incidence of spontaneous acrosome reactions in human spermatozoa exposed to FF, found that FF can stimulate the acrosome reaction, but only after a continuous exposure (>6 h) to 50% FF:medium. A short exposure (1 h), even after 24-h preincubation, did not induce the reaction.

The role of progesterone

Recent studies have shown that the human sperm acrosome reaction-inducing activity in FF can be attributed to progesterone. Osman *et al.*[30] purified an active fraction from the fluid aspirated from preovulatory human follicles and identified it as 4-pregnen-3,20-dione (progesterone) and 4-pregnen-17α-ol-3,20-dione (17-hydroxyprogesterone). This was confirmed by Blackmore *et al.*[31], Foresta *et al.*[32] and Baldi *et al.*[33], who found that only progesterone and 17-hydroxyprogesterone were able to induce a rapid, long-lasting dose-dependent increase of intracellular free calcium, maximum effect being obtained with 1.0 μg/mL. Sueldo *et al.*[34], however, found that 1.0 μg/mL of progesterone enhanced the acrosome reaction only after 24 h incubation.

Siegel *et al.*[25] also found that FF obtained from different women under different stimulation regimens did not affect the fertilizing potential differently. Morales *et al.*[35], however, found that there was a positive, highly significant ($r=0.72$, $P>0.005$) correlation between the acrosome reaction-inducing activity and the progesterone level of each follicular fluid sample.

However, recent reports on the chemical nature of the acrosome reaction-inducing molecule present in follicular fluid have been contradictory. In contrast to the authors who attributed the acrosome reaction-inducing activity present in human follicular fluid to progesterone, Miska *et al.*[36] found evidence to suggest that this substance is a protein. These authors identified a protein with a molecular mass of about 50 kDa and demonstrated the substance's sensitivity to unspecific proteases, increased temperature and pH changes. In a further study[37], the same authors identified the acrosome reaction-inducing substance (ARIS) as the progesterone-binding protein corticoid-binding globulin (CBG). Using anti-human CBG antibodies and dextran-coated charcoal they showed that only progesterone bound to CBG can induce the AR, CBG being a member of the serpin (serin proteinase inhibitors) superfamily which binds progesterone tightly. Proteolysis by serine proteinases results in the release of this steroid hormone. This mechanism is thought to be essential in activation of neutrophils by delivering high local concentrations of corticoids in inflammatory processes. The serine proteinase involved in the spermatozoon is acrosin, which is localized at the plasma membrane, with inactive proacrosin located within the acrosome. During capacitation proacrosin and acrosin are exposed at the plasma membrane. The CBG–progesterone complex, which may become bound on the plasma membrane, will therefore be proteolytically cleaved by exposed acrosin, leading to high local concentrations of progesterone and subsequent induction of acrosome reaction and confirming the important role of acrosin in physiological AR. The exact mechanism underlying progesterone-stimulated calcium entry in human sperm, however, has not been fully established. Another question to be answered concerns the source of CBG. Whether it comes from liver, where it is known to be produced, and then is accumulated in follicular fluid, or whether the cumulus or granulosa cells can synthesize this protein, still has to be established.

The role of the zona pellucida

The importance of the zona pellucida (ZP) for induction of acrosome reaction, however, is without doubt, since spermatozoa must penetrate this last barrier in the reacted state before they can enter and fertilize the oocyte. *In vitro* studies by Saling and Storey[38] using mouse sperm were the first to demonstrate a role for the ZP in the acrosome reaction. They incubated cumulus-free eggs with sperm suspensions in which >50% of the population had undergone the acrosome reaction. After gradient centrifugation, only acrosome-intact sperm were detected on the zona pellucida. They concluded that the acrosome reaction of a fertilizing mouse sperm occurs on the zona pellucida. Saling *et al.*[39] and Bleil and Wasserman[40] maintained that, at least in the mouse, the acrosome reaction is induced by a zona pellucida constituent, the glycoprotein ZP3. They proposed the following concept:

(1) Attachment to ZP;

(2) Binding to the ZP; and

(3) Induction of the acrosome reaction.

Cross *et al.*[41] used two approaches to test the ability of the human zona pellucida to induce acrosome reactions in human sperm. Non-viable human oocytes and acid-disaggregated zonae were used; both the binding to, and exposure to, induced the acrosome reactions in human sperm. Using the monoclonal antibody T-6, Coddington *et al.*[42] found that 93% of sperm bound to hemisected human zonae pellucida exhibited immunofluorescent patterns indicative of the acrosome reaction. Hoshi *et al.*[43] observed that the acrosome reaction rate after sperm attachment to the zona for 6 h was 35.7% ± 17.7% which was higher than the controls (2.8% ± 1.9%). The results so far indicate that spermatozoal ability to migrate to the zona pellucida is a closely regulated process, ensuring that only the sperm at the correct stage attach to and penetrate the zona pellucida.

Species differences may account for the disparity in the results published, but the major differences among researchers are probably caused by the different experimental conditions and the varied assessment criteria. The *in vitro* conditions under which the work is performed can have a dramatic effect on the normal biochemical (metabolic and acrosomal) reactions of sperm; so do the maturity of the oocyte–cumulus complexes and the molecules trapped in the complexes. In this respect, attention should be drawn not only to spermatozoal function, but also to the maintenance of the functional competence of the zona pellucida (Henkel *et al.*, unpublished).

THE AR SITE

The precise site of the acrosome reaction still remains clouded by controversy. Three possible sites have been proposed[3]:

(1) When the sperm are in the oviductal fluid of the ampulla;

(2) When the sperm are in the cumulus matrix; and

(3) When the sperm are on the surface of the zona pellucida.

The majority of the initial sperm acrosome reaction site studies were performed on the cauda epididymal sperm of the golden hamster because of its relatively large acrosomal cap. The progress of the acrosome reaction can, therefore, be followed by phase contrast microscopy. Data from the oviductal studies are, however, equivocal. Cummings and Yanagimachi[44] studied the ampullary contents of female hamsters by phase contrast microscopy 4–10 h after insemination with golden hamster caudal epididymal sperm and observed that 93 of 96 sperm swimming freely had modified and swollen acrosomal caps. In an earlier study, Yanagimachi and Phillips[45], also using phase contrast microscopy, found that only four of 14 free swimming golden hamster sperm had modified acrosomal caps.

In looking at the cumulus matrix as the site of acrosomal reaction, Cummings and Yanagimachi[44] reported that all 25 motile golden hamster sperm detected in the cumuli from oviducts had undergone or were undergoing the acrosome reaction. Yanagimachi and Phillips[45] reported that eight of 11 motile sperm within cumuli of golden hamster cumulus intact complexes from the ampulla had modified acrosomes. However, in a videotaped study, Cherr *et al.*[46] found that only 3–6% of sperm had actually completed the acrosome reaction within the cumulus matrix, which was comparable to the control levels of the acrosome reaction occurring in free-swimming sperm. Their study included both cumulus-intact and cumulus-free eggs, with a higher percentage of reacted sperm found in association with the zona pellucida of cumulus-intact eggs than with the zona pellucida of cumulus-free eggs.

Tesarik[47] undertook a study to determine the site of the acrosome reaction of spermatozoa penetrating into freshly inseminated human oocytes. The inseminated oocytes were treated with an anti-acrosin monoclonal antibody and the bound antibody visualized at the ultrastructural level with the use of a second peroxidase-conjugated antibody. His findings indicate that the acrosome reaction of the fertilizing spermatozoon must be exactly synchronized with its penetration through the egg vestments by the action of specific acrosome reaction-promoting substances in the oocyte–cumulus complex. Quantitative analysis of the results showed that the number of spermatozoa within the zona pellucida corresponds to the number of acrosin deposits associated with acrosomal ghosts on the zona pellucida surface. Using the triple stain technique the acrosomal status of sperm outside and within cumulus during *in vitro* fertilization was examined[48]. The percentage of sperm undergoing the acrosome reaction significantly increased ($P<0.05$) from 14.5 ± 15 to 24.5 ± 1.9 when incubated with a cumulus mass, and further increased to 49 ± 3.3 when incubated with mature expanded cumulus tissue containing an oocyte. White *et al.*[13] exposed prepared spermatozoa for 20–30 min to large pieces of human cumulus oophorus, while these spermatozoa were able to penetrate deep into the cumulus mass. None, however, were found to have clearly undergone the acrosome reaction. From this study they also concluded the spermatozoa did not require a capacitation period for penetration.

The cumulus matrix as a selection barrier

In an *in vitro* system, depolymerization (softening) of the cumulus matrix may occur because of the high sperm concentration used. This may allow sperm to reach the zona pellucida with intact acrosomes. Cummings and Yanagimachi[44], therefore, studied the ability of hamster sperm to penetrate intact cumulus matrices at low (3:1) sperm:egg ratios. Uncapacitated sperm were unable to penetrate the cumuli; at least 2 h of preincubation were required. Of the 628 *in vitro* capacitated sperm seen in and on the cumuli, 270 could penetrate, of which only 10 had intact unmodified acrosomes. They concluded that penetration of the cumuli was limited to a phase in capacitation before the completion of the acrosome reaction, since sperm that had lost the acrosomal cap penetrated poorly and showed reduced viability. Corselli and Talbot[49] also developed a system in which physiological sperm numbers (1–100) were used to challenge fresh hamster oocyte–cumulus complexes in capillary tubes. Their results showed that capacitated acrosome-intact hamster sperm can penetrate the extracellular matrix between the cumulus cells and can ultimately bind to the zona pellucida. The results obtained by these two groups indicate that uncapacitated sperm tend to adhere to the cumulus cells on the periphery, unable to penetrate, and that sperm that have lost the acrosomal cap also penetrate poorly.

The cumulus matrix may, therefore, be seen as a selection barrier, allowing only morphologically normal sperm that can undergo a normal acrosome reaction to penetrate to the zona pellucida, and/or it may contain molecules that influence the ability of sperm to undergo the reaction. CBG and progesterone, which is present in high concentrations in the cumulus matrix, have been proposed as the physiological stimulus for the initiation of the acrosome reaction.

THE AR AND *IN VITRO* FERTILIZATION

In two independent experiments, Barros *et al.*[50] and Singer *et al.*[51], using golden hamster sperm and human sperm, found that sperm became infertile with prolonged incubation, as judged by their ability to bind and penetrate the zona pellucida. The reason for this decline in penetration with increasing incubation was attributed to an increase in the percentage of acrosome-reacted sperm. In contrast, an increase in the penetration of zona-free hamster eggs was seen with increasing incubation time (increase in the acrosome-reacted population). Thus 'old' sperm are prevented from penetrating the zona pellucida. These results indicate that the fertilizing ability of spermatozoa is a time-dependent process.

Although only acrosome-reacted spermatozoa are capable of fusing with zona-free oocytes, there is no significant correlation between the proportion of acrosome-reacted cells and the levels of sperm–oocyte fusion observed. Thus, the two assays are measuring two different aspects of the sperm's ability to acrosome react. White *et al.*[13] similarly concluded that there was no relationship between the acrosome reaction rate and fertilization of normal human oocytes *in vitro*. In a study to assess whether patients who do not fertilize human oocytes *in vitro* can be identified by a lack of acrosomal response of their spermatozoa, Pampiglione *et al.*[52] found that patients who fertilized oocytes responded like donors. It was also calculated that a result of <31.3% predicts fertilization failure in 100% of cases. While spontaneous reactions bore no relation to fertility, the inducibility (i.e. difference between induced AR after induction and spontaneous AR) of acrosome reaction, which describes the ability of viable sperm to undergo acrosome reaction, was significantly reduced or absent in subfertile men, indicating acrosomal dysfunction as a likely cause of fertilization failure[53,54]. Henkel *et al.*[54] showed that inducibility should be at least 7.5% to be indicative of good fertilization. A level of >13% acrosome-reacted sperm after induction of AR was also shown to have predictive value for fertilizing potential, because elevated levels of sperm able to lose their acrosome are necessary for successful fertilization. For diagnostic purposes the kind of induction, be it physiological by means of the zona pellucida glycoproteins or non-physiological by the application of calcium-ionophore or low temperature, is apparently not important. However, inducibility[54] and appropriate timing of the acrosome reaction with the penetration of the zona pellucida[47] are prerequisites for good fertilization.

CONCLUSIONS

The fertilizing spermatozoon undergoes a continuous reactionary process, responding to signals during specific transformation stages at specific sites, that will ensure the binding to and the penetration of the zona pellucida. To allow for maximal control there are specific and non-specific inducers that may act synergistically or as an intricate backup system[2]. The following sequence of events is an attempt to describe the *in vivo* acrosome reaction:

(1) Capacitation during the passage through the female reproductive tract to the oocyte–cumulus complex.

(2) Initiation of the acrosome reaction near the periphery of, on, or in the cumulus matrix.

(3) Penetration of the cumulus matrix, during which the acrosome reaction continues.

(4) Attachment of the sperm to the ZP.

(5) Loss of the acrosomal cap and binding to the ZP (remnants of the acrosome must be present).

(6) Penetration of the ZP.

The asynchronous nature of the reaction may result in large-scale redundancy, because only the sperm at the right place and at the right time will be able to penetrate the zona pellucida and fertilize the oocyte. The *in vivo* situation does, however, seem to promote the probability of fertilization by ensuring that the maximum possible number of sperm reach the egg at the correct stage of capacitation.

References

1. Oliphant, G., Reynolds, A. L. B. and Thomas, T. S. (1985). Sperm surface components involved in the control of the acrosome reaction. *Am. J. Anat.*, **174**, 269–83
2. Meizel, S. (1985). Molecules that initiate or help stimulate the acrosome reaction by their interaction with mammalian sperm surface. *Am. J. Anat.*, **174**, 285–302
3. Langlais, J. and Roberts, K. D. (1985). A molecular membrane model of sperm capacitation and the acrosome reaction of mammalian spermatozoa. *Gamete Res.*, **12**, 183–224
4. Kanwar, K. C., Yanagimachi, R. and Lopata, A. (1979). Effects of human seminal plasma on fertilization capacity of human spermatozoa. *Fertil. Steril.*, **31**, 321–7
5. Zaneveld, L. J. D., De Jonge, C. J., Anderson, R. A. and Mack, S. R. (1991). Human sperm capacitation and the acrosome reaction. *Hum. Reprod.*, **6**, 1265–74
6. Yanagimachi, R. (1982). *In vitro* sperm capacitation and fertilization of golden hamster eggs in a chemically defined medium in *in vitro* fertilization and embryo transfer. In Hafez, E. S. E. and Semm, K. (eds.) In Vitro *Fertilization and Embryo Transfer*, pp. 65–75. (New York: Alan Liss)
7. Fleming, A. D. and Yanagimachi, R. (1981). Effect of various lipids on the acrosome reaction and fertilizing capacity of guinea pig spermatozoa, with special reference to the possible involvement of lysophospholipids in the acrosome reaction. *Gamete Res.*, **4**, 253–73
8. Murphy, S. J., Roldan, E. R. S. and Yanagimachi, R. (1986). Effects of extracellular cations and energy substrates on the acrosome reaction of precapacitated guinea pig spermatozoa. *Gamete Res.*, **14**, 1–10
9. Katz, O. F., Cherr, G. N. and Lambert, H. (1986). The evolution of hamster sperm motility during capacitation and interaction with the ovum vestments *in vitro*. *Gamete Res.*, **14**, 333–46
10. Yanagimachi, R. (1978). Calcium requirements for sperm–egg fusion in mammals. *Biol. Reprod.*, **19**, 949–58
11. Yanagimachi, R. and Usui, N. (1974). Calcium dependence of the acrosome reaction and activation of guinea pig spermatozoa. *Exp. Cell. Res.*, **89**, 161–74
12. Stock, C. E. and Fraser, L. R. (1989). Divalent cations, capacitation and the acrosome reaction in human spermatozoa. *J. Reprod. Fertil.*, **87**, 463–78
13. White, D. R., Phillips, D. M. and Bedford, J. M. (1990). Factors affecting the acrosome reaction in human spermatozoa. *J. Reprod. Fertil.*, **90**, 71–80
14. Nagae, T., Yanagimachi, R., Drivastava, P. N. and Yanagimachi, H. (1986). Acrosome reaction in human spermatozoa. *Fertil. Steril.*, **45**, 701–7
15. Stock, C. E., Bates, R., Lindsay, K. S., Edmonds, D. K. and Fraser, L. R. (1989). Human oocyte–cumulus complexes stimulate the acrosome reaction. *J. Reprod. Fertil.*, **86**, 723–30
16. Yudin, A. I., Gottlieb, W. and Meizel, S. (1988). Ultrastructural studies of the early events of the human sperm acrosome reaction as initiated by human follicular fluid. *Gamete Res.*, **20**, 11–24
17. Fraser, L. (1982). *p*-aminobenzamidine, an acrosin inhibitor, inhibits mouse sperm penetration of the zona pellucida but not the acrosome reaction. *J. Reprod. Fertil.*, **66**, 185–302
18. Aitken, R. J., Buckingham, D. W. and Fang, H. G. (1993). Analysis of the response of human spermatozoa to A23187 employing a novel technique for assessing the acrosome reaction. *J. Androl.*, **14**, 132–41
19. Tesarik, J. and Mendoza, C. (1993). Sperm treatment with pentoxifylline improves the fertilizing ability in patients with acrosome reaction insufficiency. *Fertil. Steril.*, **60**, 141–8
20. Sanchez, R., Töpfer-Petersen, E., Aitken, R. J. and Schill, W.-B. (1991). A new method for evaluation of the acrosome reaction in viable human spermatozoa. *Andrologia*, **23**, 197–203
21. Aitken, R. J. and Brindle, J. P. (1993). Analysis of the ability of three probes targeting the outer acrosomal membrane or acrosomal contents to detect the acrosome reaction in human spermatozoa. *Hum. Reprod.*, **8**, 1663–9
22. Talbot, P. and Chacon, R. S. (1981). A triple-stain technique for evaluating normal acrosome reactions of human sperm. *J. Exp. Zool.*, **215**, 201–8
23. Cross, N. L., Morales, P., Overstreet, J. W. and Hanson, F. W. (1986). Two simple methods for detecting acrosome-reacted human sperm. *Gamete Res.*, **15**, 213–26
24. Bastias, M. C., Kamijo, H. and Osteen, K. G. (1993). Assessment of human sperm functional changes after *in vitro* coincubation with cells retrieved from the

human female reproductive tract. *Hum. Reprod.*, **8**, 1670–7
25. Siegel, M. S., Paulson, R. J. and Graczykowski, J. W. (1990). The influence of human follicular fluid on the acrosome reaction, fertilizing capacity and proteinase activity of human spermatozoa. *Hum. Reprod.*, **5**, 975–80
26. Thomas, P. and Meizel, S. (1988). An influx of extracellular calcium is required for the initiation of the human sperm acrosome reaction induced by human follicular fluid. *Gamete Res.*, **20**, 397–411
27. Suarez, S. S., Wolf, D. P. and Meizel, S. (1986). Induction of the acrosome reaction in human spermatozoa by a fraction of human follicular fluid. *Gamete Res.*, **14**, 107–21
28. Fukuda, M., Cross, N. L., Cummings-Paulson, L. and Yee, B. (1989). Correlation of the acrosomal status and sperm performance in the sperm penetration assay. *Fertil. Steril.*, **52**, 836–41
29. Stock, C. E., Bates, R., Lindsay, K. S., Edmonds, D. K. and Fraser, L. R. (1989). Extended exposure to follicular fluid is required for significant stimulation of the acrosome reaction in human spermatozoa. *J. Reprod. Fertil.*, **86**, 401–11
30. Osman, R. A., Andria, M. L., Jones, A. D. and Meizel, S. (1989). Steroid induced exocytosis: The human sperm acrosome reaction. *Biochem. Biophys. Res. Commun.*, **160**, 828–33
31. Blackmore, P. F., Beebe, S. J., Danforth, D. R. and Alexander, N. (1990). Progesterone and 17-hydroxyprogesterone: Novel stimulators of calcium influx in human sperm. *J. Biol. Chem.*, **265**, 1376–80
32. Foresta, C. Rossata, M., Mioni, R. and Zorzi, M. (1991). Progesterone induces capacitation in human spermatozoa. *Andrologia*, **24**, 33–5
33. Baldi, E., Casano, R., Falstti, C., Krausz, C., Maggi, M. and Forti, G. (1991). Intracellular calcium accumulation and responsiveness to progesterone in capacitating human spermatozoa. *J. Androl.*, **12**, 323–30
34. Sueldo, C. E., Oehninger, S., Subias, E., Mahony, M., Alexander, N. J., Burkman, L. J. and Acosta, A. A. (1993). Effect of progesterone on human zona pellucida sperm binding and oocyte penetrating capacity. *Fertil. Steril.*, **60**, 137–40
35. Morales, P., Llanos, M., Guiterrez, G., Kohen, P., Vigil, P. and Vantman, D. (1992). The acrosome reaction-inducing activity of individual human follicular fluid samples is highly variable and is related to the steroid content. *Hum. Reprod.*, **7**, 646–51
36. Miska, W., Henkel, R. and Fehl, P. (1994). Recent studies on the structure of the acrosome reaction-inducing substance (ARIS) in human follicular fluid. *Int. J. Androl.*, unpublished
37. Miska, W., Fehl, P. and Henkel, R. (1994). Biochemical and immunological characterization of the acrosome reaction inducing substance (ARIS) of hFF. *Biochem. Biophys. Res. Commun.*, **199**(1), 125–9
38. Saling, P. M. and Storey, B. T. (1979). Mouse gamete interactions during fertilization *in vitro*: chlortetracycline as a fluorescent probe for the mouse acrosome reaction. *J. Cell. Biol.*, **83**, 544–55
39. Saling, P. M., Irons, G. and Waibel, R. (1985). Mouse sperm antigens that participate in fertilization. I. Inhibition of sperm fusion with the egg plasma membrane using monoclonal antibodies. *Biol. Reprod.*, **33**, 515–26
40. Bleil, D. J. and Wassarman, P. M. (1983). Sperm–egg interactions in the mouse: sequence of events and induction of the acrosome reaction by a zona pellucida glycoprotein. *Dev. Biol.*, **95**, 317–24
41. Cross, N. L., Morales, P., Overstreet, J. W. and Hanson, F. W. (1988). Induction of acrosome reactions by the human zona pellucida. *Biol. Reprod.*, **38**, 235–44
42. Coddington, C. C., Fulgam, D. L., Alexander, N. J., Johnson, D., Herr, J. C. and Hodgen, G. D. (1990). Sperm bound to zona pellucida in hemizona assay demonstrate acrosome reaction when stained with T-6 antibody. *Fertil. Steril.*, **54**, 504–8
43. Hoshi, K. H., Sugano, T., Endo, C., Yoshimatsu, N., Yanagida, K. and Sato, A. (1993). Induction of the acrosome reaction in human spermatozoa by human pellucida and effect of cervical mucus on zona-induced acrosome reaction. *Fertil. Steril.*, **60**, 149–53
44. Cummings, J. M. and Yanagimachi, R. (1986). Development of the ability to penetrate the cumulus oophorus by hamster spermatozoa capacitated *in vitro* in relation to the timing of the acrosome reaction. *Gamete Res.*, **15**, 187–212
45. Yanagimachi, R. and Phillips, D. M. (1984). The status of acrosomal caps of hamster spermatozoa immediately before fertilization *in vivo*. *Gamete Res.*, **9**, 1–19
46. Cherr, G. N., Lambert, H. and Katz, D. (1984). Completion of the hamster sperm acrosome reaction on the zona-pellucida *in vivo*. *J. Cell. Biol.*, **99**, 261A
47. Tesarik, J. (1989). Appropriate timing of the acrosome reaction is a major requirement for the fertilizing spermatozoon. *Hum. Reprod.*, **4**, 957–61
48. Carrell, D. T., Middelton, R. G., Peterson, C. M., Jones, K. P. and Urry, R. L. (1993). Role of the cumulus in the selection of morphologically normal sperm and induction of the acrosome reaction during human *in vitro* fertilization. *Arch. Androl.*, **31**, 133–7
49. Corselli, J., Talbot, P. (1986). An *in vitro* technique to study penetration of hamster oocyte–cumulus complexes by using physiological numbers of sperm. *Gamete Res.*, **13**, 293–308
50. Barros, C., Jedlicki, A., Bize, I. and Aguire, E. (1984). Relationship between the length of sperm preincubation and zona penetration in the golden hamster: A scanning electron microscopy study. *Gamete Res.*, **9**, 31–43
51. Singer, S. L., Lambert, H., Overstreet, J. W., Hanson, F. W. and Yanagimachi, R. (1985). The kinetics of

human sperm binding to the human zona pellucida and zona-free hamster oocyte *in vitro*. *Gamete Res.*, **12**, 29–39
52. Pampiglione, J. S., Tan, S. and Campbell, S. (1993). The use of the stimulated acrosome reaction test as a test of fertilizing ability in human spermatozoa. *Fertil. Steril.*, **59**, 1280–4
53. Cummins, J. M., Pember, S. M., Jequier, A. M., Yovich, J. L. and Hartmann, P. E. (1991). A test of the human sperm acrosome reaction following ionophore challenge: Relationship to fertility and other seminal parameters. *J. Androl.*, **12**, 98–103
54. Henkel, R., Müller, C., Miska, W., Gips, H. and Schill, W.-B. (1993). Determination of the acrosome reaction in human spermatozoa is predictive of fertilization *in vitro*. *Hum. Reprod.*, **8**, 2128–32
55. Talbot, P. and Chacon, R. (1980). A new procedure for rapidly scoring acrosome reactions of human sperm. *Gamete Res.*, **3**, 211–6
56. Mortimer, D., Curtis, E. F. and Miller, R. G. (1987). Specific labelling by peanut agglutinin of the outer acrosomal membrane of the human spermatozoon. *J. Reprod. Fertil.*, **81**, 127–35
57. Lee, M. A., Trucco, G. S., Bechtol, K. B., Wummer, N., Kopf, G. S., Blasco, L. and Storey, B. T. (1987). Capacitation and acrosome reactions in human spermatozoa monitored by chlortetracycline fluorescence assay. *Fertil. Steril.*, **48**, 649–58
58. Byrd, W., Tsu, J. and Wolf, D. P. (1989). Kinetics of spontaneous and induced acrosomal loss in human sperm incubated under capacitating and noncapacitating conditions. *Gamete Res.*, **22**, 109–22
59. Okabe, M., Nagira, M., Kawai, Y., Matzno, S., Mimura, T. and Mayumi, T. (1990). A human sperm antigen possibly involved in binding and/or fusion with zona-free hamster eggs. *Fertil. Steril.*, **54**, 1121–6

The zona-free hamster egg sperm penetration assay

19

K. Coetzee

INTRODUCTION

Male factor infertility in humans has become one of the primary indications for treatment by assisted reproduction techniques. Although the advent of *in vitro* fertilization programs has contributed to the solution of a number of male and female factors, the precise pathophysiology underlying sperm dysfunction is not usually well defined. In most instances patients may be classified as having abnormalities of sperm locomotion, of energy-source utilization, of capacitation and of sperm/oocyte recognition and interaction. An *in vitro* system using mature human oocytes would fulfill the majority of the requirements for the expansion of our understanding of fertilization. The ultimate endpoint still remains the establishment of a normal term pregnancy. Ethical and moral considerations, however, preclude the use of human gametes for these purposes. No single bioassay available is able to determine the fertilizing capacity of the human sperm, making the accurate diagnostic and prognostic evaluation of human sperm difficult. The following are some of the currently available sperm evaluation techniques:

(1) Standard (basic) semen analysis;

(2) Computer-assisted sperm analysis (CASA);

(3) Sperm penetration assay (SPA);

(4) Hemizona assay (HZA);

(5) Hypoosmotic swelling test (HOS);

(6) Sperm decondensation assay;

(7) Acrosome reaction analysis (AR); and

(8) ATP determination.

The zona-free hamster egg sperm penetration assay, or sperm penetration assay (SPA), provides the only means of measuring a sequential, multifactorial process essential for fertilization. The golden hamster is unique in that, on the removal of the zona pellucida, all species specificity is lost, allowing the hamster ovum to be penetrated by sperm of other species[1–3]. The zona-free hamster eggs have, therefore, been used extensively in the determination of the fertilizing capacity of human sperm under specific conditions. The concept of the SPA was introduced by Yanagimachi[1] in 1972 and perfected for the use in humans[3] in 1976. Since then the SPA has been widely used in the diagnosis of male infertility, for developing improved methods of sperm processing and cryopreservation, for fertilization and contraceptive research and to analyze sperm chromosomes. It is able to measure sperm capacitation and the acrosome reaction, sperm plasmalemma/oolemma fusion, sperm incorporation into the ooplasm and the decondensation of the sperm chromatin. The SPA may, therefore, be able to quantify the proportion of sperm per ejaculate which have fertilizing ability to a limited extent.

Capacitation and the subsequent acrosome reaction are essential for normal fertilization in all mammalian species and they are also a precondition for a normal SPA. These changes can be induced under the appropriate culture conditions, forcing the sperm to develop all necessary qualities to be recognized and engulfed by the hamster ovum. These reactions are, therefore, assumed to have taken place in the SPA if spermatozoa undergo nuclear decondensation after penetration of zona-free ova. Although only acrosome-reacted spermatozoa are capable of fusing with zona-free hamster oocytes no significant correlation between the proportion of acrosome-reacted cells and the levels of sperm–oocyte fusion has been observed[4], indicating that these bioassays are measuring different aspects of human sperm function.

The predictive value of SPA is limited because of its inherent shortcomings; thus it is susceptible to both false-positive and false-negative results, the latter being of the greatest clinical significance. This limited predictive value is due mainly to the multifactorial nature of the fertilization process compared to the narrow testing capabilities of the SPA and the always unknown status of the associated female factors.

The limited acceptance of the SPA in assessing male fertility is also due to the fact that no consensus has been achieved on a specific protocol for the assay, in spite of the efforts of the World Health Organization.

SPERM PENETRATION ASSAY: METHODOLOGY

Patient sexual abstinence

The length of abstinence is an important variable, with >48 h required for maximum results. An abstinence of <48 h has been shown to significantly depress the fertilizing capacity of the ejaculate[5]. This reduction may be due to the reduced number of mature sperm and/or to a depletion of functional seminal plasma[6].

Semen liquefaction

Native seminal plasma is believed to contain macromolecules, or factors associated with macromolecules, which can inhibit capacitation and/or the acrosome reaction[7,8]. Certain motility parameters are also inhibited by the viscosity of the seminal plasma. Kinetic studies have shown that maximum penetration of hamster ova is obtained with exposure times between 30 and 90 min[5,9]. Long exposure times (>90 min) may irreversibly inhibit fertilization. A normal semen sample should liquefy within 60 min at room temperature[10]. The process can be facilitated by incubation at 37°C or enzymatically with α-amylase[11].

Semen preparation

After allowing 30–90 min for full liquefaction, an initial count and motility (including forward progression, 1–4) estimation is made. A morphology slide is simultaneously prepared for later assessment. The need to separate human sperm from seminal plasma and its inhibitory effects is essential for the expression of spermatozoa's intrinsic fertilizing potential. The standard swim-up procedure has been the most extensively used technique to obtain a sperm preparation relatively free of dead sperm, non-cellular debris and non-sperm cells. The recovery rate from cryopreserved, oligozoospermic and asthenozoospermic samples is, however, relatively poor. The centrifugation of unselected sperm has also been associated with iatrogenic sperm damage, due to mechanical stress and the generation of reactive oxygen species[12], which may compromise sperm function. Other procedures, such as Percoll gradient centrifugation[13], glass wool filtration[14] and post-swim-up centrifugation methods[10], are now commonly used to prevent sperm damage and to maximize recovery from problem semen samples. The standard swim-up procedure is routinely used at Tygerberg Hospital, with glass wool filtration used when encountering problematic semen samples, such as mentioned above. After the preparation procedure the sperm concentration in the sample is adjusted to 1×10^7 cells/mL. This requirement results in the exclusion of many oligozoospermic samples from optimal evaluation.

The preincubation period also constitutes an important variable and has therefore been another point of dispute. Preincubation times have varied from 1 h[15] to 24 h[16], the convenience of laboratory procedures often being a major determining factor. A confounding factor is, however, the interdonor variability in capacitation patterns[17]. There is a significant number of men whose sperm can penetrate the hamster oolemma after 6–10 h, but not after 18–24 h of incubation and vice versa. An incubation period allowing most samples to attain maximum levels of capacitation and acrosome reactions must be chosen[6,18,19]. It may be advisable, however, to evaluate patients after a different capacitation period if a negative result is obtained at first. The World Health Organization[10] prescribes a period of 18–24 h at 37°C in an atmosphere of 5% CO_2, 95% air, which is followed at Tygerberg Hospital. If a CO_2 incubator is not available the sperm can be stored in tightly capped tubes at 37°C in air. The tubes are placed at a 20° angle to prevent pelleting of the sperm and to increase the surface area for gaseous exchange in a 5% CO_2 environment.

After the capacitation period, one of the following procedures is followed:

(1) The sample is mixed well, the motility and forward progression measured and two aliquots (50–100 μL) of sperm adjusted to 1×10^7 cells/mL are placed in the center of a Petri dish and covered with mineral oil[16].

(2) The tube is carefully returned to the vertical position for 20 min to allow settlement of any immotile cells. The motile spermatozoa are then aspirated in the supernatant and adjusted to 3.5×10^6 motile cells/mL[10]. Sperm are then placed under mineral oil, as in the method above.

Sperm concentration, percentage and quality of motility in the insemination medium can have a significant effect on the outcome of the SPA, especially the number of motile acrosome-reacted spermatozoa. The chosen method may have a significant effect on the end results, the second method thus being optimal, because it eliminates collision interference and possible penetrations by immotile spermatozoa. Maximal penetration requires an insemination mixture with a minimum of 4–6% motile sperm, if the concentration is adjusted to 1×10^7 cells/mL[20].

Egg recruitment

Hamster egg recruitment and processing is one aspect of the SPA that has remained reasonably well standardized. Oocytes can be obtained from immature hamsters injected at random or from mature hamsters injected on day 1 of their estrous cycle[10]. Day 1 is characterized by a viscous, stringy (5–20 cm), visible vaginal discharge[21]. Pregnant mare serum gonadotropin (PMS) and human chorionic gonadotropin (hCG) are given by intraperitoneal injection at a dose of 30–40 IU, 48–72 h apart. The hamsters are then killed by cervical dislocation 15–18 h after the hCG injection. The cumulus masses are removed from the dissected oviducts and treated with 0.1% (1 g/L) hyaluronidase and 0.1% (1 g/L) trypsin to remove the cumulus cells and the zonae pellucidae, respectively. After each enzyme treatment the oocytes are washed at least twice in medium. From 25 to 60 zona-free eggs can be collected from each stimulated hamster. The eggs have a limited viability period[22] and the time between recovery and insemination must therefore be as short as possible. Egg viability can be extended by storage at 4°C[22] or by cryopreservation.

Insemination

Between 15 and 30 zona-free eggs can be placed within the sperm-containing droplets. The gametes are then coincubated for 3 h at 37°C in air or in 5% CO_2.

Evaluation

After the 3-h coincubation period the level of penetration is assessed by carefully removing the eggs from the insemination droplets and washing them free of loosely attached spermatozoa. The eggs are placed on a clean microscope slide with petroleum jelly/paraffin wax (15:1) supports on the corners, and are then compressed to a depth of 30 μm beneath a 22 mm×22 mm coverslip and examined by phase-contrast microscopy. Exposure of the eggs to 5% formalin solution prior to mounting, however, resulted in fewer ruptured eggs[23]. To allow future evaluation the eggs can be fixed in 1% glutaraldehyde, stained with lacmoid or aceto-orcein[6,24], and the edges sealed with fingernail polish. Significantly fewer penetrated eggs and penetrations per egg were noted when eggs were read as fresh mounts compared to eggs that were fixed and stained prior to evaluation[23]. Penetration had occurred if a decondensed sperm head was seen within the cytoplasm of the ovum. A tail must be attached or associated with the decondensed sperm head as confirmation of the event and to distinguish it from the egg pronucleus. The percentage of ova penetrated and the mean number of spermatozoa per ovum (penetration index) were then calculated. A donor sample run simultaneously must penetrate a minimum of 20% of the ova for the test to be considered valid. The number of sperm remaining attached to the ova after washing may also be recorded.

Medium

The medium most often used for the SPA is Biggers, Whitten and Whittingham's (BWW)[10]. Numerous modifications to the standard BWW medium have been developed in an attempt to eliminate false-positive and false-negative results.

One of the major variables in the medium used for the SPA is the protein source, human serum albumin (HSA) or bovine serum albumin (BSA), and its concentration. The protein source is essential for normal evolution of sperm activation. Rogers[6] preferred HSA, Gould *et al.*[25] preferred BSA, while Van Kooij *et al.*[26] found no advantage in using HSA over BSA. A complicating factor is the variable ability of different batches of the reagent from the same manufacturer and from different manufacturers to activate spermatozoa. The World Health Organization (WHO)[10] manual prescribes the use of BSA for the SPA. The concentration of the protein source has varied between 0.3% and 3.5%. Barros *et al.*[15] used 35 mg HSA/mL for 1 h capacitation period. Aitken *et al.*[27] used 18 mg HSA/mL for a 6–7 h incubation period, while Rogers *et al.*[16] used 3 mg/mL for a period of 18–20 h. An increased albumin concentration, therefore, seems to be associated with an increase in the rate of capacitation[28]. This association has not been found by all investigators[29]. In its protocol, the WHO[10] prescribes the longer period (18–24 h) supplemented with 3.5 mg/mL of albumin, which is adhered to at Tygerberg Hospital.

Inorganic ions such as calcium, sodium and potassium have been shown by several investigators[30–34] to be essential for the natural progress of events leading to fertilization. Of these ions calcium is the most important, being implicated with capacitation, the acrosome reaction, hyperactivated motility, fusion of the sperm plasmalemma with the oocyte plasma membrane, and development of pronuclear oocytes into two-cell pre-embryos[35]. These ions must be present in the medium at optimal concentrations to have maximal effect[31]. For example, a higher percentage of acrosome reactions and penetrations was observed in spermatozoa incubated in 25 mM K when compared with 4.7 mM K[36]. Mortimer *et al.*[37] showed that calcium can be replaced by strontium. The presence and the concentration of the ions mentioned above is determined by the particular outcome being investigated – standard, enhanced or inhibited penetration.

Organic energy sources added to the medium play an important role not only in the metabolism of the sperm, but also in its ability to undergo the activation processes required for fertilization[38,31]. It has been proposed that certain levels of organic metabolites needed for the initiation of the acrosome reaction may be present within the sperm. The additional energy sources in the medium may only be needed to maintain motility and to maximize the acrosome reaction rate.

The standard medium used has an osmolarity of 305 mOsm/L. Aitken *et al.*[39] and Ibrahim *et al.*[40] raised the osmolarity to 410 mOsm/L, which increases the penetration rate. This higher osmolarity increases the efficiency with which the decapacitating factors are removed. Murphy *et al.*[31] found that precapacitated sperm could undergo the acrosome reaction in a medium with a osmolarity of 160–500 mOsm/L. The osmolarity range within which most sperm are able to undergo the acrosome reaction, while still retaining a degree of motility, was found to be 220–380 mOsm/L. A medium of more physiological osmolarity, but ensuring an adequate penetration rate, should be preferred. We found that an osmolarity of 305mOsm/L provided such an outcome.

The pH of the medium can also influence the outcome of the test significantly. While a pH of <7 may prevent or greatly retard capacitation, exposure to a higher pH can increase the rate of capacitation, the acrosome reaction and penetration[41]. However, prolonged exposure to this unphysiologically high pH may be stressful to the sperm. The pH of the BWW medium ($NaHCO_3$-buffered) commonly used by us was 7.4–7.6 under 5% CO_2 conditions, but 8.1–8.3 under air. The WHO[10] prescribes the use of BWW medium within the physiological ranges of pH and osmolarity, with the addition of 20 mM of HEPES buffer. The inclusion of HEPES stabilizes the pH under both 5% CO_2 and pure air conditions[42].

CORRELATION OF THE SPA WITH CONVENTIONAL SEMEN PARAMETERS

The correlation between the SPA and the conventional semen parameters has been examined by numerous authors, without achieving any real consensus. This can be attributed to the different criteria of normality for semen parameters used by different laboratories. In fact, the WHO[10] states that it is preferable for each laboratory to determine its own normal ranges. A confounding factor is that these parameters have changed in accordance with our increasing understanding of fertilization and with the technological advances in the assessment of the critical factors required for fertilization. An illustration of this is the change in the reference normal value adopted by the WHO in regard to the percentage of normal forms: 50% or more in 1987 to 30% or more in 1992. The uncertainty about the normal ranges for semen parameters makes comparative studies difficult.

The majority of early investigations[43–46] found no significant correlations between the SPA and any of the traditional semen parameters: sperm density, motility and morphology. Cohen *et al.*[47,48] found low but significant correlations with the total motile sperm count and the percentage of morphologically normal sperm, with the former as the better predictor of SPA. Rogers *et al.*[49] also reported a correlation with motility and morphology, but found the latter to be more important. Aitken *et al.*[27] conducted a number of studies in which the semen parameters and motility characteristics, analyzed by time–exposure photomicrography, were compared with the SPA. In examining normally fertile men he found that the only factors which correlated positively were the percentage of progressively motile sperm (>25 μm/s) and the sperm amplitude of lateral head displacement >10 μm. In a group of patients with unexplained infertility[50], the majority of the semen parameters and motility characteristics were depressed compared to fertile donors; a reduction in normal morphology was the most significant finding. Aitken *et al.*[51], using seven post-capacitation characteristics of motility in a multivariate discrminate analysis, could predict correctly 91% of samples exhibiting normal penetration rates. However, only 60% of the samples with impaired penetration capacity were correctly identified. In order to develop a standard protocol for the SPA, Aitken and Elton[20] applied the Poisson–Gamma model to determine the correct number of gametes present (number of oocytes and number of motile sperm concentration) for the assay to be valid, when comparing different fertility population groups.

More recent studies have also provided contradictory results. Van Kooij *et al.*[52] found no correlation between semen parameters and SPA values, while others found correlation with motility and sperm density, amplitude of lateral head displacement, the percentage of abnormal acrosomes[53,54] and all semen parameters, especially motility[55].

The overall results so far indicate that of all the semen parameters, motility and morphology seem to show the best correlation with the SPA.

In vivo, the quality of motility (forward progression) is of paramount importance in the fertilization process, since only progressively motile sperm can pass through the cervical mucus and migrate to the ampulla. Logically, this characteristic is not as important under *in vitro* conditions. Nonetheless, the concentration of motile sperm in the incubation medium significantly influences the penetration rate, because the greater the percentage motility, the greater the number of possible collisions with the eggs and resultant penetrations. This direct correlation between the percentage of motility and penetration has been shown with the SPA[20,27]. However, in the hamster system the quality of motility is not a significant factor, because sperm do not have to traverse the cumulus cells and the zona pellucida, immotile sperm thus being able to penetrate zona-free hamster ova. There is also a difference between the penetrating potential of different fertile donors at a fixed motile concentration[48,56]. Under standardized conditions the possible reasons for these discrepancies would be the differences in: (1) quality of motility and concentration of motile sperm; (2) biochemical status of the sperm; (3) biochemical status of the ova; and/or (4) the experimental conditions.

The importance of morphology in the prediction of penetration and fertilization potential has been greatly underestimated. The morphology of spermatozoa may be a reflection of their underlying biochemical and biophysical status. In our laboratory, we use a modified classification system (strict criteria)[57,58]. Two studies using these criteria have found that a statistically significant correlation exists between normal sperm morphology and the SPA[59,60].

CORRELATION OF SPA WITH NATURAL REPRODUCTION AND ASSISTED REPRODUCTION RESULTS IN THE HUMAN

Human IVF must be considered the ultimate test for measuring the fertilization potential of sperm. A correlation between SPA and IVF would thus emphasize the importance of the SPA as a screening test for male fertility. Before comparisons with IVF were possible Overstreet *et al.*[43] inseminated non-living zona-intact human ova with the same semen sample used in the SPA. A positive correlation was seen in 85% (n=27) of the inseminations with both hamster and human ova, whether penetrated or not. A false-positive result was obtained in four cases (15%). Since then numerous studies have shown significant correlations between SPA and IVF[61–63].

The majority of investigators then started to apply a classification system whereby ≤10% penetrations is considered negative, 11% to 20% uncertain and >20% fertile. Other studies continued to report significant correlations[6,64]. An absolute lower limit of hamster egg penetration to define male infertility could not be determined, however, since a poor SPA was not always indicative of the inability of the sperm to fertilize a human oocyte. Margalioth *et al.*[65] conducted a thorough investigation of 134 couples, divided into groups according to their indications for IVF (tubal disease, unexplained infertility, male factor and male/female factors). The SPA was a good predictor of IVF success in 91 of 107. Of these four groups, tubal disease and unexplained infertility had the highest correlation with the SPA (94% and 76%, respectively). In 38 simultaneous inseminations of human and hamster eggs, no false-negative assessments were found by Nahas and Blumenfeld[66]; seven false-positive assessments were obtained which were attributed to egg immaturity and equipment failure.

Foreman *et al.*[67] and Rudak *et al.*[68], however, found no evidence that the SPA had any usefulness in predicting IVF outcome. Even though the proportion of hamster eggs penetrated were significantly lower for men who could not fertilize their wives' eggs than for those who could. Their conclusions with regard to the false-negative rate of the SPA were contradictory. Foreman *et al.*[67] reported that the occurrence of false negatives was rare, but Rudak *et al.*[68] reported a false-negative rate of 85.7%. This high incidence of false-negative results was confirmed by two studies using the same semen parameter criteria, but different preincubation periods. Coetzee *et al.*[60], utilizing an 18–20-h preincubation period found a false-negative rate of 64.5%, while Kruger *et al.*[59] obtained a false-negative rate of 66.7% for a 6-h preincubation.

The question to be answered, therefore, is whether the SPA has the potential to distinguish categorically between clinically infertile and fertile men. Is there an absolute threshold that distinguishes between these two groups? Yanagimachi[41] compared all published data and reported that sperm of men with proven fertility generally penetrate >10% of eggs, with an overall average of 57%. Sperm of clinically infertile men penetrated a significantly lower percentage of eggs, with an overall average of 17%. The wide range of penetration levels found among proven fertile donors poses a problem with the interpretation of the SPA results. Aitken[69], following patients with unexplained infertility for 2–3 years, found that patients with scores of 1 to 10% were not incompatible with the initiation of a pregnancy. Margalioth *et al.*[70], studying 40 normal infertile men, came to the same conclusion.

This inability to correlate the SPA with fertility may mean that there are fertility determinants which cannot be evaluated, but which impact on the sperm's ability to penetrate zona-free hamster eggs; for example, the percentage of reacted sperm.

MODIFIED SPERM PENETRATION ASSAY

Many investigators have modified the SPA in a bid to increase the efficiency and effectiveness of its diagnostic potential. The majority of these methods produce enhanced penetration of the zona-free hamster ova. The mechanism by which the majority of these methods produce the enhancement probably involves the synchronization of capacitation and the subsequent increase in the acrosome reaction rate, overcoming the principal defect of the hamster oocyte system, the lack of physiological *in vivo* stimulants, such as cumulus cells and the zona pellucida. The primary goal of these modifications

Table 1 The predictive value of the SPA

Authors	*False positives (%)*	*False negatives (%)*	*Negative SPA (%)*	*Variation*
Wolf[61]	26	11	≤10	LI
Margalioth[62]	23	0	<20	LI
Foreman[67]	29	9	<14	LI
Ausmanas[64]	0	100	≤15	SI, pregnancy
	14	80	≤15	SI, Abn SA
	13	86	≤15	SI, N SA
Margalioth[65]	15	22	<20	LI
Rudak[68]	13	75	<10	SI
Aitken[76]	16	60	0	Hyperosm Independ
	15	4	0	Ionophore Independ
	17	86	0	Hyperosm Simult
	5	0	0	Ionophore Simult
Kruger[59]	18	67	≤10	SI
Coetzee[60]	5	65	≤10	LI
Ibrahim[40]	16	26	≤10	Hyperosm
McClure[71]	25	7	≤10	hFF
Soffer[74]	18	26	<20	TEST-Y

The different SPA variations employed are: short (SI, 2–7 h); long (LI, overnight) incubation periods; calcium ionophore A23187 (ionophore); human follicular fluid (hFF); TEST-yolk buffer (TEST-Y); and hyperosmotic (hyperosm, 410 mOsmol/kg) stimulation

is the elimination of the false-negative outcomes of the SPA. These are of the greatest clinical importance when counseling patients considering *in vitro* fertilization.

The modifications used include: hyperosmotic (410 mOsm) medium[39,40] and medium additions, such as human follicular fluid[71–73], TEST-yolk buffer[74,75], pentoxifylline[72] and ionophore A23187[4,76]. Other methods include the exposure to cold shock at 4°C[77], Percoll separation[13] and glass wool filtration[14]. The WHO[10] has now included a protocol incorporating Ca-ionophore in its *Manual on the Examination of Human Semen and Sperm–Cervical Mucus Interaction*[10]. These variations to the standard SPA have had a significant effect on the results of the SPA and consequently on their interpretation. The above modifications are all able to enhance the penetrating ability of human spermatozoa, some up to 1000-fold.

The relevance of the comparison of many of these with IVF success can be questioned because of their unphysiological means of induction. Solely as a predictor of fertilizing potential, if the specificity and sensitivity of the assay can be improved, the modified assay can be an invaluable tool for the evaluation of male fertility (Table 1). A number of authors have shown that these modifications are able to increase the predictive value of the SPA[71,74,76].

Johnson *et al.*[78] also developed a microsperm penetration assay suitable for oligospermic samples. They combined the preincubation of sperm in TEST-yolk buffer at 4°C for 42 h with the coincubation of sperm and ova occurring in a microfuge tube, in which the sperm had previously been concentrated. Their results showed that 25 000 sperm were optimal.

DISCUSSION

When comparing SPA, IVF and/or pregnancy, one must keep a number of factors in mind. First, a man rarely ejaculates two identical samples; thus, if the same sample is not used for comparison, it must be noted whether the samples were at least comparable in their semen parameters. For standardization, ejaculates should probably be no more than 4 weeks apart. It is also preferable to repeat an individual patient analysis, especially if a zero penetration score is obtained. Secondly, not all oocytes aspirated from a woman are of equal quality, especially at the molecular level and, therefore, they are not equally amenable to fertilization. In contrast, large numbers of zona-free hamster ova can be obtained with relatively equal quality. For statistical accuracy only preovulatory, mature metaphase II human ova with an extruded polar body should be used to compare IVF results with the SPA. Thirdly, the SPA lacks the stimulatory effects of the cumulus cells and zona pellucida. Finally, pregnancy adds an additional dimension with its own variables.

The sperm penetration assay, however, remains an expensive, time-consuming method and an assay subject to great variability. Thus, it is advisable to consider the complete semen profile by means of, for example, the conventional semen parameters, biochemical analyses and other functional assays when trying to establish a prognosis on fertility based on semen samples.

References

1. Yanagimachi, R. (1972). Penetration of guinea-pig spermatozoa into hamster eggs *in vitro*. *J. Reprod. Fertil.*, **28**, 477–80
2. Hanada, A. and Chang, M. L. (1978). Penetration of the zona-free or intact eggs by foreign spermatozoa and the fertilization of deer mouse eggs *in vitro*. *J. Exp. Biol.*, **203**, 277–86
3. Yanagimachi, R., Yanagimachi, H. and Rogers, B. J. (1976). The use of zona-free animal ova as a test-system for the assessment of the fertilizing capacity of human spermatozoa. *Biol. Reprod.*, **15**, 471–6
4. Aitken, R. J., Buckingham, D. W. and Fang, H. G. (1993). Analysis of the responses of human spermatozoa to A 23187 employing a novel technique for assessing the acrosome reaction. *J. Androl.*, **14**, 132–41
5. Rogers, B. J., Perreault, S. D., Bentwood, B. J., McCarville, C., Hale, R. W. and Soderdahl, D. W. (1983). Variability in the human–hamster *in vitro* assay for fertility evaluation. *Fertil. Steril.*, **39**, 204–11
6. Rogers, B. J. (1985). The sperm penetration assay: its usefulness reevaluated. *Fertil. Steril.*, **43**, 821–40
7. Kanwar, K. C., Yanagimachi, R. and Lopata, A. (1979). Effects of human seminal plasma on fertilizing capacity of human spermatozoa. *Fertil. Steril.*, **31**, 321–7
8. Van der Ven, H., Bhattacharyya, A. K., Binor, Z., Leto, S. and Zaneveld, L. J. D. (1982). Inhibition of human sperm capacitation by a high-molecular-weight factor from human seminal plasma. *Fertil. Steril.*, **38**, 753–5
9. Wolf, D. P. (1986). The hamster egg bioassay in studies of sperm–egg interaction at fertilization. *Int. J. Androl.*, **6S**, 49–58
10. World Health Organization. (1992). *World Health Organization Manual for the Examination of Human Semen and Semen–Cervical Mucus Interaction.* (London: Cambridge University Press)
11. Vermeiden, J. P. W., Bernardus, R. E., ten Brug, C. S., Statema-Lohmeijer, C. H. and Willemsen-Brugma Schoemaker, J. (1989). Pregnancy rate is significantly higher in *in vitro* fertilization procedure with spermatozoa isolated from nonliquefying semen in which liquefaction is induced by α-amylase. *Fertil. Steril.*, **51**, 149–52
12. Mortimer, D. (1991). Sperm preparation techniques and iatrogenic failures of *in vitro* fertilization. *Hum. Reprod.*, **6**, 173–6
13. Chan, S. Y. W. and Tucker, M. J. (1992). Differential sperm performance as judged by the zona-free hamster egg penetration test relative to differing sperm penetration techniques. *Hum. Reprod.*, **7**, 255–60
14. Holmgren, W. J. and Jeyendran, R. S. (1993). Synergistic effect of TEST–yolk buffer treatment and glass wool filtration of spermatozoa on the outcome of the hamster oocyte penetration assay. *Hum. Reprod.*, **8**, 425–7
15. Barros, L., Gonzalez, J., Herrera, E. and Bustos-Obregon, E. (1979). Human sperm penetration into zona-free hamster oocytes as a test to evaluate the sperm fertilizing ability. *Andrologia*, **11**, 197–210
16. Rogers, B. J., Van Campen, H., Ueno, M., Lambert, H., Bronson, R. and Hale, R. (1979). Analysis of human spermatozoal fertilizing ability using zona-free ova. *Fertil. Steril.*, **32**, 664–70
17. Perreault, S. D. and Rogers, B. J. (1982). Capacitation pattern of human spermatozoa. *Fertil. Steril.*, **38**, 258–60
18. Singer, S. L., Lambert, H., Overstreet, J. W., Hanson, F. W. and Yanagimachi, R. (1985). The kinetics of human sperm binding to the human zona pellucida and zona-free hamster oocyte *in vitro*. *Gamete Res.*, **12**, 29–39
19. Johnson, J. P. and Alexander, N. J. (1984). Hamster egg penetration: comparison of preincubation periods. *Fertil. Steril.*, **41**, 599–602
20. Aitken, R. J. and Elton, R. A. (1986). Quantitative analysis of sperm–egg interaction in the zona-free hamster penetration test. *Int. J. Androl.*, **6S**, 14–30
21. Mizoguchi, H. and Dukelow, W. R. (1981). Fertilizability of ova from young or old hamsters after spontaneous or induced ovulation. *Fertil. Steril.*, **35**, 79–83

22. Syms, A. J., Johnson, A. R., Lipshultz, L. I. and Smith, R. G. (1985). Effect of aging and cold storage of hamster ova as assessed in the sperm penetration assay. *Fertil. Steril.*, **43**, 766–72
23. Hammitt, D. G., Anchenbrenner, D. W., Syrop, C. H. and Heinkel, D. D. (1991). Techniques for improving the accuracy and the efficiency of the sperm penetration assay. *Andrologia*, **23**, 11–15
24. Campana, A., Gatti, M. Y., Ruspa, M., Van Kooij, R., Buetti, C., Eppenberger, U. and Balerna, M. (1983). Relationship between fertility, semen analysis and human sperm penetration of zona-free hamster eggs. *Acta Eur. Fertil.*, **14**, 331–6
25. Gould, J. E., Overstreet, J. W., Yanagimachi, H., Yanagimachi, R., Katz, D. F. and Hanson, F. W. (1983). What functions of the sperm cell are measured by *in vitro* fertilization of zona-free hamster eggs? *Fertil. Steril.*, **40**, 344–52
26. Van Kooij, R. J., Balerna, M., Roatti, A. and Campana, A. (1986). Oocyte penetration and acrosome reactions of human spermatozoa. I. Influence of incubation time and medium composition. *Andrologia*, **18**, 152–60
27. Aitken, R. J., Best, F. S. M., Richardson, D. W., Djahanbakhch, O. and Lees, M. M. (1982). The correlate of fertilizing capacity in normal fertile men. *Fertil. Steril.*, **38**, 68–76
28. Wolf, D. P. and Sokoloski, J. E. (1982). Characterization of the sperm penetration bioassay. *J. Androl.*, **3**, 445–51
29. Plachot, M., Mandelbaum, J. and Junca, A.-M. (1984). Acrosome reaction of human sperm used for *in vitro* fertilization. *Fertil. Steril.*, **42**, 418
30. Yanagimachi, R. and Usui, N. (1974). Calcium dependence of the acrosome reaction and activation of guinea pig spermatozoa. *Exp. Cell Res.*, **89**, 161–74
31. Murphy, S. J., Roldan, E. R. S. and Yanagimachi, R. (1986). Effects of extracellular cations and energy substrates on the acrosome reaction of precapacitated guinea pig spermatozoa. *Gamete Res.*, **14**, 1–10
32. Hyne, R. V., Higginson, R. E., Kohlman, D. and Lopata, A. (1984). Sodium requirement for capacitation and membrane fusion during the guinea-pig sperm acrosome reaction. *J. Reprod. Fertil.*, **70**, 83–94
33. Fraser, L. R. (1983). Potassium ions modulate expression of mouse sperm fertilizing ability, acrosome and hyperactivated motility *in vitro*. *J. Reprod. Fertil.*, **69**, 539–53
34. Mortimer, D., Courtot, A. M., Giovangrandi, Y., Jeulin, C. and David, G. (1984). Human sperm motility after migration into, and incubation in, synthetic media. *Gamete Res.*, **9**, 131–44
35. Yanagimachi, R. (1982). *In vitro* sperm capacitation and fertilization of golden hamster eggs in a chemically defined medium in *in vitro* fertilization and embryo transfer. In Hafez, E. S. E. and Semm, K. (eds.) *In Vitro Fertilization and Embryo Transfer*, pp. 65–75. (New York: Alan Liss)
36. Roblero, L. S., Guadarrama, A., Ortiz, M. E., Fernandez, E. and Zegers-Hochschild, F. (1990). High potassium concentration and the cumulus corona oocyte complex stimulate the fertilizing capacity of human spermatozoa. *Fertil. Steril.*, **54**, 328–32
37. Mortimer, D., Curtis, E. F. and Dravland, J. E. (1986). The use of strontium-substituted media for capacitating human spermatozoa: an improved sperm penetration method for the zona-free hamster egg penetration test. *Fertil. Steril.*, **46**, 97–103
38. Perreault, S. D. and Rogers, B. J. (1981). Effects of various sugars on the course of human spermatozoal capacitation *in vitro*. *J. Androl.*, **2**, 22–3
39. Aitken, R. J., Wang, Y. F., Liu, J., Best, F. and Richardson, D. W. (1983). The influence of medium composition, osmolarity and albumin content on the acrosome reaction and fertilizing capacity of human spermatozoa: development of an improved zona-free hamster egg penetration test. *Int. J. Androl.*, **6**, 180–93
40. Ibrahim, M. E., Moussa, M. A. A. and Pedersen, H. (1989). Efficacy of zona-free hamster egg sperm penetration assay as a predictor of *in vitro* fertilization. *Arch. Androl.*, **23**, 267–74
41. Yanagimachi, R. (1984). Zona-free hamster eggs: their use in assessing fertilizing capacity and examining chromosomes of human spermatozoa. *Gamete Res.*, **10**, 187–233
42. Martin, R. H. and Taylor, P. J. (1982). Reliability and accuracy of the zona-free hamster ova assay in the assessment of male fertility. *Br. J. Obstet. Gynaecol.*, **89**, 951–6
43. Overstreet, J. W., Yanagimachi, R., Katz, D. F., Hayashi, K. and Hanson, F. W. (1980). Penetration of human spermatozoa into the human zona pellucida and the zona-free hamster egg: a study of fertile donors and infertile patients. *Fertil. Steril.*, **33**, 534–42
44. Hall, J. L. (1981). Relationship between semen quality and human sperm penetration of zona-free hamster ova. *Fertil. Steril.*, **35**, 457–63
45. Zausner-Guelman, B., Blasco, L. and Wolf, D. P. (1981). Zona-free hamster eggs and human sperm penetration capacity: a comparative study of proven fertile donors and infertility patients. *Fertil. Steril.*, **36**, 771–7
46. Tyler, J. P. P., Pryor, J. P. and Collins, W. P. (1981). Heterologous ovum penetration by human spermatozoa. *J. Reprod. Fertil.*, **63**, 499–508
47. Cohen, J., Weber, R. F. A., Van Der Vijver, J. C. M. and Zeilmaker, G. H. (1982). *In vitro* fertilizing capacity of human spermatozoa with the use of zona-free hamster ova: interassay variation and prognostic value. *Fertil. Steril.*, **37**, 565–72
48. Cohen, J., Edwards, R., Fehilly, C., Fishel, S., Hewitt, J., Purdy, J., Rowlands, G., Steptoe, P. and Webster, J. (1985). *In vitro* fertilization: a treatment for male infertility. *Fertil. Steril.*, **43**, 422–32
49. Rogers, B. J., Bentwood, B. J., Van Campen, H.,

Helmbrecht, G., Soderdahl, D. and Hale, R. W. (1983). Sperm morphology assessment as an indicator of human fertilizing capacity. *J. Androl.*, **4**, 119–25
50. Aitken, R. J., Best, F. S. M., Richardson, D. W., Djahanbakhch, O., Mortimer, D., Templeton, A. A. and Lees, M. M. (1982). An analysis of sperm function in cases of unexplained infertility: conventional criteria, movement characteristics, and fertilizing capacity. *Fertil. Steril.*, **38**, 212–21
51. Aitken, R. J., Warner, P., Best, F. S. M., Templeton, A. A., Djahanbakhch, O., Mortimer, D. and Lees, M. M. (1983). The predictability of subnormal penetrating capacity of sperm in cases of unexplained infertility. *Int. J. Androl.*, **6**, 212–20
52. Van Kooij, R. J., Balerna, M., Roatti, A. and Campana, A. (1985). Oocyte penetration and acrosome reactions of human sperm. II. Correlation with other semen parameters. *Andrologia*, **18**, 503–8
53. Hirch, I., Gibbons, W. E., Lipshultz, L. I., Rossavik, K. K., Young, R. L., Poindexter, A. N., Dobson, M. and Findley, W. E. (1986). *In vitro* fertilization in couples with male factor infertility. *Fertil. Steril.*, **45**, 659–64
54. Jeulin, C., Feneux, D., Serres, C., Jouannet, P., Guillet-Rosso, F., Belaisch-Allart, J., Frydman, R. and Testart, J. (1986). Sperm factors related to failure of human *in vitro* fertilization. *J. Reprod. Fertil.*, **76**, 735–44
55. Van Duren, D. B. P. J., Vemer, H. M., Bastiaans, B. L. A., Doesburg, W. H., Willemsen, W. N. P. and Rolland, R. (1987). Importance of sperm motility after capacitation in interpreting the hamster ovum sperm penetration assay. *Fertil. Steril.*, **47**, 456–9
56. Albert, M., Bailly, M. A. and Roussel, L. (1986). Influence of the concentration of motile sperm inseminated on the ovum penetration assay results: towards a standardized method. *Andrologia*, **18**, 161–70
57. Kruger, T. F., Menkveld, R., Stander, F. S. H., Lombard, C. J., Van der Merwe, J. P., van Zyl, J. and Smith, K. (1986). Sperm morphologic features as a prognostic factor in *in vitro* fertilization. *Fertil. Steril.*, **46**, 1118–22
58. Menkveld, R. (1987). An investigation of environmental influences on spermatogenesis and semen parameters. *Ph.D. dissertation, University of Stellenbosch, Tygerberg, South Africa*
59. Kruger, T. F., Swanson, R. J., Hamilton, M., Simmons, K. F., Acosta, A. A., Matta, J. F., Oehninger, S. and Morshedi, M. (1988). Abnormal sperm morphology and other semen parameters related to the outcome of the hamster oocyte human sperm penetration assay. *Int. J. Androl.*, **11**, 107–13
60. Coetzee, K., Kruger, T. F., Menkveld, R., Swanson, R. J., Lombard, C. J. and Acosta, A. A. (1989). Usefulness of sperm penetration assay in fertility predictions. *Arch. Androl.*, **23**, 207–12
61. Wolf, D. P., Sokoloski, J. E. and Quigley, M. M. (1983). Correlation of human *in vitro* fertilization with the hamster egg bioassay. *Fertil. Steril.*, **40**, 53–9
62. Margalioth, E. J., Navot, D., Laufer, N., Yosef, S. M., Rabinowitz, R., Yarkoni, S. and Schenker, J. G. (1983). Zona-free hamster ovum penetration assay as a screening procedure for *in vitro* fertilization. *Fertil. Steril.*, **40**, 386–8
63. Hall, J. L., Engel, D., Berger, G. S., Dingfelder, J. K. and Marik, J. (1984). Use of the hamster zona-free ovum test in human *in vitro* fertilization program. *Fertil. Steril.*, **41(S)**, 105–6
64. Ausmanas, M., Tureik, R. W., Blasco, L., Kopf, G. S., Ribas, J. and Mastroianni, L. (1985). The zona-free hamster egg penetration assay as a prognostic indicator in a human *in vitro* fertilization program. *Fertil. Steril.*, **43**, 433–7
65. Margalioth, E. J., Navot, D., Laufer, N., Lewin, A., Rabinowitz, R. and Schenker, J. G. (1986). Correlation between the zona-free hamster egg sperm penetration assay and human *in vitro* fertilization. *Fertil. Steril.*, **45**, 665–70
66. Nahhas, F. and Blumenfeld, Z. (1989). Zona-free hamster egg penetration assay: Prognostic indicator in an IVF program. *Arch. Androl.*, **23**, 33–7
67. Foreman, R., Cohen, J., Fehilly, C. B. and Edwards, R. B. (1984). The application of the zona-free hamster egg test for the prognosis of human *in vitro* fertilization. *J.* In Vitro *Fertil. Embryo Transf.*, **1**, 166–71
68. Rudak, E., Dor, J., Nebel, L., Maschiach, S. and Goldman, B. (1986). Assessment of the predictive ability of the zona-free hamster egg penetration test for the outcome of treatment by IVF-ET. *Int. J. Androl.*, **6S**, 131–42
69. Aitken, R. J. (1983). The zona-free hamster egg penetration test. In Hargreave, T. B. (ed.) *Male Infertility*, p. 75. (Berlin: Springer-Verlag)
70. Margalioth, E. J., Laufer, N., Navot, D., Voss, R. and Schenker, J. G. (1983). Reduced fertilization ability of zona-free hamster ova by spermatozoa from male partners of normal infertile couples. *Arch. Androl.*, **10**, 67–71
71. McClure, R. D., Tom, R. A. and Dandekar, P. V. (1990). Optimizing the sperm penetration assay with human follicular fluid. *Fertil. Steril.*, **53**, 546–50
72. Lambert, H., Steinleitner, A., Eiserman, J., Serpa, N. and Cantor, B. (1992). Enhanced gamete interaction in the sperm penetration assay after coincubation with pentoxifylline and human follicular fluid. *Fertil. Steril.*, **58**, 1025–8
73. Fukuda, M., Cross, N. L., Cummings-Paulson, L. and Yee, B. (1989). Correlation of acrosomal status and sperm performance in the sperm penetration assay. *Fertil. Steril.*, **52**, 836–41
74. Soffer, Y., Golan, A., Herman, A., Pansky, M., Caspi, E. and Ron-el, R. (1992). Prediction of *in vitro* fertilization outcome by sperm penetration assay with TEST–yolk buffer preincubation. *Fertil. Steril.*, **58**, 556–62

75. Falk, R. M., Silverberg, K. M., Fetterolf, P. M., Kirchner, F. K. and Rogers, B. J. (1990). Establishment of TEST-yolk buffer enhanced sperm penetration assay limits for fertile males. *Fertil. Steril.*, **54**, 121–6
76. Aitken, R. J., Thatcher, S., Glasier, A. F., Clarkson, J. S., Wu, F. C. W. and Baird, D. T. (1987). Relative ability of modified versions of the hamster oocyte penetration test, incorporating hyperosmotic medium or the ionophore A 23187 to predict IVF outcome. *Hum. Reprod.*, **2**, 227–31
77. Sanchez, R. and Schill, W.-B. (1991). Influence of incubation time/temperature on the acrosome reaction/sperm penetration assay. *Arch. Androl.*, **27**, 35–42
78. Johnson, A., Smith, R. G., Bassham, B., Lipshultz, L. I. and Lamb, D. J. (1991). The microsperm penetration assay: development of a sperm penetration assay suitable for oligospermic males. *Fertil. Steril.*, **56**, 528–34

Sperm–zona pellucida binding and penetration assays

20

D. R. Franken, S. Oehninger, K. Kaskar, T. F. Kruger and G. D. Hodgen

INTRODUCTION

Perhaps the most remarkable journey made by any cell is that of the mammalian spermatozoon as it passes from the vas deferens of the male to the fertilization site. At this site the sperm will subsequently go across the cumulus oophorus and corona radiata cells and bind to the zona pellucida, from where it will start its second intriguing journey progressing through the zona pellucida to the oolemma. The correct sequence of the different events leading to fertilization is imperative and critical analysis of sperm–oocyte interacting functions (sperm binding, penetration and fusion) forms the cornerstone of modern assisted reproductive programs. Failure of sperm–zona pellucida binding may be associated with certain cases of male infertility[1,2]. The development of a sperm–zona binding assay, therefore, received research prominence among scientists and clinicians. However, difficulties were encountered during the developing stages of such a test, namely: (1) human sperm do not bind adequately to any other zona pellucida due the species-specificity of the sperm–zona receptors; (2) availability of human oocytes; (3) inter-oocyte variability; and (4) ethical problems in using fresh viable human oocytes.

Tight binding of human spermatozoa to the human zona pellucida is an early critical event in gamete interaction leading to fertilization. This binding step may provide unique information predictive of ultimate sperm fertilizing potential. Due to species specificity, human spermatozoa will bind firmly to no other zonae pellucidae except the human[3]. The feasibility of tight human sperm binding to the zonae pellucidae of non-living human oocytes has previously been described[4].

Sperm binding and zona penetration were tested using oocytes recovered from *post mortem* ovarian tissue and later from ovaries removed for surgical indications[1]. These studies, however, did not investigate the kinetics of zona binding or the specific relationship between the binding event and male fertility.

The original sperm–oocyte assay as proposed by Overstreet *et al.*[4] was initially developed as a zona penetration assay; sperm binding to the zona was not the endpoint for the assay. Two sperm–zona binding tests currently used are the hemizona assay (HZA)[5], and a zona pellucida-binding test[2,6]. Both bioassays have the advantage of providing a functional homologous test for sperm binding to the zona pellucida, comparing populations of fertile and infertile spermatozoa in the same assay.

It is known that a human spermatozoon's ability to fertilize an egg is dependent on sperm structure, the quality of sperm motility and capacitation. The current high incidence of human infertility caused by the so-called male factor has promoted an intense search for reliable means to predict human sperm fertilizing potential *in vivo* and *in vitro*. The optimum human assay would ideally utilize living, fertilizable human oocytes. Ethical reasons, however, prevent scientists and physicians from performing such direct diagnostic functional assessments[4]. However, reliable and discriminating prognostic assays are needed to determine which infertile men are likely to achieve fertilization *in vitro* or *in vivo*. The hemizona assay[5], the zona pellucida binding test[6] and the human zona-free oocyte penetration assay[7] are frequently used as diagnostic tools in IVF treatment programs. Lanzendorf *et al.*[8] recorded the penetration potential of human spermatozoa through the human zona pellucida of non-viable human oocytes. As previously discussed all these tests have unique characteristics and fundamental utilities in that all evaluate sperm quality and performance in relation to the human oocyte.

The scarcity of human oocytes inspired several workers to develop means to amplify the limited number of human oocytes available for these sperm binding studies. The first reports to expand the possibilities of using these oocytes were focused on alternative storing facilities.

We have developed a new sperm function assay based on the relative binding of patient versus control spermatozoa to the matching halves of a bisected human oocyte[5,9–12]. This hemizona assay (HZA) assessed tight binding of sperm to the outer surface of the zona pellucida hemisphere. The HZA has three clear advantages: (1) the two halves (hemizonae) are functionally (qualitatively) equal zona surfaces, allowing a controlled comparison of binding; (2) the very limited number of recovered human oocytes is amplified, since an internally controlled test can be carried out on a single oocyte; and (3) ethical objections to possible inadvertent fertilization of a viable oocyte are eliminated by first cutting the egg into halves.

During the developmental stages of the hemizona assay, we first investigated the feasibility of cutting the zonae and then obtaining normal sperm binding to the zona pellucida. It was imperative to examine the time-dependent pattern of sperm binding to the hemizonae and establishing an optimal assay protocol. The most recent work has methodically tested HZA results against known *in vitro* fertilization (IVF) outcomes for the same patients. The results of these studies are discussed under the heading 'Clinical application'.

LABORATORY PROCEDURES

Hemizona assay: bisecting the oocytes

Oocytes were bisected using a micromanipulating system after retrieval from storage. Salt-stored oocytes, especially the prophase I oocytes, should be allowed to desalt for at least 24 h prior to testing. The micromanipulating system (Narishige, model MO 102; Research Instruments, Johannesburg, South Africa, model MO 102) was fitted to an inverted phase contrast microscope (Nikon Diaphot, Garden City, NY, USA) equipped with a pair of Narishige micromanipulators. A one-piece ophthalmological blade assembly (Beaver, no. 1767; Katena Products, Denville, NJ, USA) was placed in the holding arm of the micromanipulator. Oocytes can also be bisected by hand using a microsurgical scalpel and dissecting microscope (Morales, personal communication). Following the bisecting procedures the ooplasm inside was dislodged by pipetting the hemizona through a small-bore tip. Each hemizona pair was placed in a separate 50 μL droplet of medium in a Petri dish, covered with mineral oil (Fisher Scientific, Springfield, NJ, USA) and stored overnight at +4°C. Zona binding results obtained with (1) 7.5% fetal cord serum, (2) 10% human blood serum, and (3) 7.5% human serum albumin (Sigma A8763 St. Louis, MO, USA) as supplement to Ham's F10 culture medium were compared during a follow-up study. No significant difference could be illustrated in zona binding potential of spermatozoa in the presence of the mentioned supplements.

Preparation of spermatozoa

For all semen samples examined by the HZA, a basic semen analysis was performed using a (1) computerized analysis system (CellSoft Semen Analysis System, Labsoft Division of Cryo Resources, Ltd., New York, NY, USA); and (2) methods previously described[13,14]. In short, the latter method encompasses the evaluation of the percentage of motile spermatozoa and visual assessment of the speed of forward progression (on a scale 0–4) under phase contrast microscopy, while sperm concentrations were determined using an improved Neubauer hemocytometer. Thin smears were prepared for morphological evaluation. Smears were air-dried and stained with a modified Papanicolaou method[15]. In all cases with extremely low sperm counts or decreased motility, the sperm concentration was calculated using a hemocytometer. Percentage of motility was assessed by scoring 100 spermatozoa per microscopic slide.

Both the computerized and manual methods recorded the following parameters: sperm concentration, percentage of normal motility and percentage of normal morphology. Semen was classified as normal when (1) sperm concentration was $>20\times10^6$ cells/mL; (2) sperm motility exceeded 40%, and (3) normal sperm morphology exceeded 14% according to the new strict criteria[16,17]. It is important to note that even proven fertile men did not score equally in any assay. It was, therefore, best to screen six to eight potential control donors by testing the binding of their spermatozoa to two pairs of hemizonae. For each man, the range for the number of bound sperm per hemizona was examined. Following the semen analysis, an aliqot of semen (0.5 mL) was mixed with 1 mL of Ham's F-10 culture medium, supplemented with 7.5% heat-inactivated human fetal cord serum. Motile sperm fractions were retrieved following a standard double wash and swim-up method[18].

Hemizona assay index (HZI)

Within each experiment objective comparisons of the matching hemizona data were made possible by calculating the ratio of tightly bound sperm between the two hemizonae:

$$\text{HZ} = \frac{\text{Number of sperm bound from patient}}{\text{Number of sperm bound from fertile male}} \times \frac{100}{1}$$

During a recent study ($n=80$) we compared the HZI with the fertilization rates obtained in the IVF laboratory. With the HZI, we found and calculated a HZI threshold of 35%[19,20,22] to be of clinical importance.

Defining the valid hemizona assays

During fertility testing the variability in egg quality as well as donor semen quality has frequently confounded *in vitro* assay interpretation. Using a homologous rodent fertilization model[24,25] where eggs are easily obtained, inter-egg variation is the principal reason for placing multiple ova (5–20) in each co-incubation droplet. Similarly, the zona-free hamster egg sperm penetration assay utilized 10–20 ova per dish[26]. Cross *et al.*[24] have calculated that oocyte–oocyte differences represent one of the two most significant sources of experimental variability in a zona-binding study.

It has been frequently observed in our laboratory that the hemizonae from a particular oocyte will bind surprisingly few sperm from a proven fertile semen preparation. Due to this source of assay error, we have specifically addressed the issue of defining a 'bad zona pellucida' and subsequently, an invalid experiment[27].

In addition to the inconsistency of egg quality, the sperm from individual semen donors exhibit different capacitation or egg-interaction potential. The time course and peak levels of hamster egg penetrations[28], as well as the time course for hyperactivated motility[27], show donor-dependent variation. In our laboratory we have similarly observed differences within proven fertile men concerning the time of maximal sperm binding to the hemizona pellucida (3.5–5.5 h) and the peak number of sperm bound at that time (42–215, and 27–142). Optimal utilization of the HZA will, therefore, depend on a better understanding of the variables which influence data interpretation and clinical correlations.

During a series of experiments, we reported (1) zona binding results for men with severe teratozoospermia (<4% normal forms) to establish the upper limit of their zona binding potential; (2) oocyte–oocyte variability in sperm binding capacity among 15 zonae using a single fertile male; (3) between-assay variability among different men; and (4) sperm binding variability within each man over 90 days. The studies indicate that the upper limit for sperm binding in the presence of sperm populations with known zona binding defects and possibly poor zonae is 34 sperm per hemizona. We decided to use 34 bound sperm as the lower cutoff value for sperm populations with normal (>14% normal forms) morphological features and zona binding potential. Proven fertile sperm samples unavoidably include results with zona pellucida showing inferior sperm binding capacity. One reason for the large standard deviation encountered among fertile control men might be the unavoidable inclusion of data obtained from experiments where the sperm binding quality of the zonae were not optimal[45].

The simultaneous assays in the second study, using 15 germinal vesicle stage eggs from a single female and the same sperm suspension throughout, demonstrated great variability which was clearly due to zona quality alone. Sperm binding to the hemizonae in experiments 2, 8 and 15 was much lower than in the other 12 experiments (Table 1). Using 34 again as a lower cutoff value for morphologically normal sperm populations,

Table 1 Number of sperm tightly bound to matching hemizonae: measuring the variability in sperm binding capacity to different zonae pellucidae in the HZA. Simultaneous HZA's were performed using 15 hemizona pairs allocated in tandem with the sperm from one fertile man and one infertile man

	Fertile male (control) sperm droplet	*Subfertile male sperm droplet*
1	132	61
2	15	6
3	200	[b]
4	106	79
5	99	72
6	101	63
7	218	54
8	24	18
9	145	[b]
10	101	[b]
11	66	42
12	128	31
13	82	42
14	125	58
15	8	9
n	15	12
Mean	103.3	44.6[a]
SD	±58.4	±23.2

[a] Mean significantly lower than control ($P<0.05$); [b] data not obtained

the data in study 2 would indicate that 20% (3/15) of the zonae pellucidae from germinal vesicle stage oocytes have demonstrably impaired sperm binding potential.

At the Norfolk laboratory (Virginia, USA), using the current threshold value of 34 bound sperm, any HZA which yields <34 for the control hemizona is invalid and must be repeated. A binding value of <34 indicates that either the zona pellucida utilized was inferior or the control semen was subnormal that day. On occasion, an assay may show that the control hemizona bound fewer than 34 sperm but the matching (test) hemizona bound more than 34 of the patient's spermatozoa. In this particular instance, it is clear that the zona pellucida has normal sperm binding potential, but the control sperm was inferior in that instance.

The current findings provide guidelines for the appropriate interpretation of the hemizona assay. Within the limits stated in this chapter, the HZA is able to control for the intrinsic variability in zona pellucida binding capacity because of its use of the matching halves of a single egg. In contrast to assays utilizing an intact zona pellucida and fluorescent sperm labels,[2,29] the two hemizona halves can specifically accommodate study designs involving two different incubation protocols or zona pre-treatments. For these latter purposes, the hemizona assay remains uniquely appropriate. In this chapter, results of the HZA will be reported either as the number of sperm bound per hemizona or as HZI as previously described.

Development of sperm–zona pellucida binding assay (whole egg assay)

Liu *et al.*[6] developed a sperm–zona pellucida binding ratio using oocytes that failed to fertilize *in vitro*. Oocytes that showed no evidence of either two pronuclei or cleavage 48–60 h after insemination were placed in 1 M ammonium sulfate solution and stored at 4°C for 2–8 weeks. Eighty percent of these fresh or salt-stored oocytes were able to bind sperm. The test is based on competitive binding of two sperm populations (test patient and fertile control sperm donor) to several oocytes. Test and control sperm are labeled with different fluorochrome suspensions, namely FITC (green) and tetramethyl rhodamine isothiocyanate (red).

Fluorochrome labeling

Labeling of sperm was achieved using 1 mg fluorescein isothiocyanate (FITC, Sigma Chemical Co, St Louis, MO, USA) or 0.5 mg of tetramethylrhodamine B isothiocyanate (TRITC, Sigma Chemicals, St Louis, MO, USA) was dissolved in 0.1 mL of 0.1 M KOH and diluted within 15 s to 5 mL with sterile Dulbecco phosphate buffered saline containing 55.5 mM glucose and stored at 4°C in a plastic tube wrapped in aluminium foil for up to 1 week. Sperm pellets were prepared by centrifuging 0.4 mL of semen at 600***g*** for 5 min, and these were labeled by suspending them in 0.3 mL of the fluorochrome solution. The suspension was incubated at 37°C for 15 min and the sperm recovered by centrifugation at 600***g*** for 5 min. The sperm pellet was washed with 10 mL of Tyrode's solution and after further centrifugation diluted to a final concentration of 10×10^6 cells/mL with Ham's F10 culture medium containing 10% heat inactivated human serum.

Heterospermic insemination

Salt-stored human oocytes were washed with 1 mL of Ham's F10 culture medium. A mixture of equal numbers (1×10^5/mL) motile sperm from normal fertile donors and test samples, labeled with either FITC or TRITC, were added to each oocyte in a plastic multiwell tray containing 1 mL of Ham's F10 medium with 10% human serum. The zonae and sperm were incubated at 37°C in 5% CO_2 for 4 h and then the zonae were washed in three changes of Tyrode's solution with vigorous pipetting to dislodge sperm that are loosely attached to the zona. Zonae were then placed on a glass slide, covered with a coverslip, flattened and counted for bound sperm. A light fluorescent microscope (Dialux 20, Leitz Wetzlar, Germany) was used at a magnification of 160× or 250× with excitation at 450–490 mm for FITC and 546 nm for TRITC. Results were calculated as sperm binding ratios of the total number of tests to fertile sperm bound among five oocytes.

Clinical application

Significantly more sperm bound to zonae of oocytes that were removed from the batches where some fertilization was reported (mean 13.7, range 0–90, $n=60$, 31 patients) compared to those where no fertilization occurred (mean 2.4, range 0–50, $n=80$, 14 patients). Table 2 illustrates the mean values for semen parameters, sperm–zona binding among patients where >50% and <50% fertilization were reported during *in vitro* fertilization.

As shown in Table 2, 10 men who had achieved fertilization of >50% of oocytes in IVF had higher sperm–zona pellucida (ZP) binding ratios (test/control) than did 10 men whose sperm failed to fertilize or fertilized a low proportion of oocytes *in vitro*. The test failed in one man in the high fertilization rate group as no test or donor sperm bound to any of the five ZP used. One man in the low fertilization rate group had a normal ZP binding ratio (0.88).

Human sperm–oocyte penetration assays

Overstreet and colleagues[1,4] were the first to propose the use of an *in vitro* assay for human sperm function in order to evaluate two initial stages of sperm oocyte interaction: penetration through the zona pellucida using human oocytes recovered from cadavers and evaluate sperm entry into the ooplasma with zona-free hamster oocytes. Sperm penetration was assessed with immature human oocytes and ooplasmic reactions were recorded with mature oocytes. Dysfunctional aspects that were identified included: (1) inability of sperm to bind to the zona pellucida; (2) zona binding without penetration; (3) incomplete zona penetration; and (4) zona penetration with poor sperm entry into the ooplasma. The success of gamete interaction *in vitro* could not be correlated with any of the classic parameters of semen quality. Some of the men with so called 'normal' semen and unexplained infertility had apparent dysfunction of gamete interaction[1,4].

Lanzendorf *et al.*[8] recorded whether intact zonae from non-viable oocytes could be consistently penetrated by the human sperm and, if so, under which conditions could an *in vitro* bioassay be developed. During their study, they evaluated four different storage methods, as well as the optimal time for gamete coincubation in order to standardize the conditions of the assay for future use in infertility and contraceptive studies.

Oocyte collection

Immature (prophase I) oocytes used were obtained from surgically derived ovarian tissue from consenting patients. Immature, germinal vesicle bearing zona-intact oocytes were identified using a dissecting microscope, washed in fresh saline and then prepared for storage using one of four methods, namely:

Table 2 Mean and range (in parentheses) of sperm parameters and zona binding ratios among patients with <50% and >50% oocytes fertilized during IVF

	IVF rate	
	<50%	*>50%*
n	10	10
IVF rate (%)	7 (0–33)	80 (57–100)
Sperm concentration	113 (29–333)	105 (15–200)
Motility (%)	55 (31–71)	54 (36–70)
Normal morphology	24 (9–50)	46 (31–70)
Sperm–zona binding ratio	0.16 (0–0.88)	0.88 (0.56–1.3)

(1) Storage at −196°C in 1.5 M 1,2 propanediol (PrOH method);

(2) Storage at −70°C in 2.0 M dimethylsulfoxide (DMSO method);

(3) Storage at 4°C in a hypertonic salt solution (salt storage method); and

(4) Storage at 4°C in Ham's F-10 medium (Gibco, Grand Island, NY) supplemented with 7.5% heat inactivated human cord serum (fresh method).

For the PrOH method of storage, zona-intact oocytes were cryopreserved in a programmable controlled-rate freezing machine (Planar Series II, Kryo 10, T.S. Scientific, Perkasie, PA, USA). For storage using the DMSO method, oocytes were added to cryovials containing 0.5 mL of 2.0 M dimethylsulfoxide in phosphate buffered saline and allowed to equilibrate at room temperature for 15 min. Cryovials were then placed in a −70°C freezer for storage.

Thawing was performed at room temperature until ice crystals disappeared, at which time the contents of the vial were added to 5.0 mL Ham's medium supplemented with 7.5% human cord serum. For the salt storage method, oocytes were added to plastic vials containing 0.5 mL of a hypertonic salt solution 9 and stored at 4°C for up to 30 days. In the fresh storage method, oocytes were stored in Ham's F10 at 4°C for up to 48 h.

For all four methods, oocytes were only utilized for zona penetration if they were non-viable. Degenerate, non-viable oocytes had dark, granular cytoplasm and/or ruptured ooplasm. Oocytes with ruptured zona were not used in the study and were discarded.

Sperm samples from seven fertile men were prepared as described above under the heading 'Sperm Preparation'. Following incubation, the supernatants were removed and the samples adjusted to 500 000 motile sperm/mL. Samples were stored in the incubator until used in the assay.

Zona insemination and evaluation

Upon removal from storage, zonae were washed and then added to 100 μL drops of the sperm suspensions covered with heavy mineral oil. Zonae were examined at 5 h and then again at 20 h post-insemination for the presence of penetrating sperm. At both times, loosely bound sperm were removed by rapidly pipetting the zonae through a drawn pipette. For evaluation, zonae were placed in a fresh drop of medium and examined at 200× magnification. It was often necessary to roll the zonae using negative and positive pressure through a drawn pipette to visualize all areas of the perivitelline space. Only those sperm seen with heads clearly in the perivitelline space were considered to have penetrated the zona. A zona was considered penetrated if it contained one or more penetrating sperm heads. The number of sperm penetrated per zona was also recorded. Table 3 presents the effects zona storage has on sperm penetration. The use of the fresh method provided the highest penetration rate (50.9%) followed by the PrOH method for a penetration rate of 33%. The poorest penetration rate was observed in zona which were frozen with the DMSO method (2×4 contingency table, 2×=13.4, P=0.0004).

Table 3 Effect of storage conditions on zona penetration

Storage method	*n*	*Number of zonae*
Fresh	53	27 (50.9)^{ab}
PrOH	49	16 (32.7)^{c}
Salt	30	7 (23.3)^{a}
DMSO	20	2 (10.0)^{b,c}

$^{a}P<0.02$; $^{b}P<0.003$; $^{c}P<0.04$

Table 4 Effect of incubation time on zona penetration

	5 h	*20 h*
Number of sperm bound	0.8±1	3.8±0.2
Number of zona penetrated	31.2%	37.6%

The effect of gamete coincubation time on zona penetration is presented in Table 4. After 5 h, 0.8 sperm were visible in the perivitelline space per zona. However, after 20 h, the same oocytes had 3.8 sperm visible per zona and this increase was significant. However, the number of zona penetrated by one or more sperm at 5 h and 20 h was not significant (31% and 38%, respectively; P>0.5).

Abnormalities in zona binding represent a frequent finding in severe cases of male infertility as demonstrated both in the HZA and other sperm–zona binding assays[10,12,30–32]. Defects in sperm–oocyte fusion and sperm decondensation can also be directly tested using the sperm penetration assay (SPA)[26,34]. However, defects in sperm–zona penetration are difficult to diagnose using an *in vitro* bioassay for both practical and ethical reasons.

We have previously introduced the concept of a sequential diagnostic scheme for the evaluation of clinical cases with recurrent failed IVF[34]. Using predictive bioassays such as the HZA, the SPA and now the zona penetration assay (ZPA), in combination with IVF treatment and fertile donor cross-match tests, one can sequentially evaluate sperm binding ability to the zona pellucida, sperm–zona penetration capacity and fusion with the oolemma. This information can then be used to establish a pathophysiological diagnosis for specific sperm and oocyte functional defects that assist the clinician in the management of the infertile couple.

Tesarik[7,35] introduced a sperm penetration assay using human oocytes that failed to fertilize in a clinical IVF program; they were freed from the zona pellucida and reinseminated with spermatozoa from subfertile patients or from sperm donors. Penetration results were significantly worse when patients' spermatozoa were used as compared with donor spermatozoa. When inseminated with donor sperm, oocytes from cases of male infertility gave better penetration results as compared with those cases of idiopathic infertility with no apparent sperm defect. No differences in penetration results were found between oocytes aged 1 day and 2 days in culture before zona removal and reinsemination. Tesarik, however, cautioned the use of zona penetration as an indicator of sperm function, since oocyte maturity did not influence zona penetration[35]. Zona and ooplasmic penetration assays, nevertheless, can become an integral part of a sequential analytic profile when used with donor spermatozoa, especially in cases where oocyte failure is suspected.

Oocyte sources for zona binding and penetration experiments

Although the results described in this section report only on findings from HZA studies, all the information on the oocytes is applicable to the whole egg assays (zona pellucida binding assays) and oocyte penetration assays[2,6–8]. We have investigated a variety of oocyte sources and generally

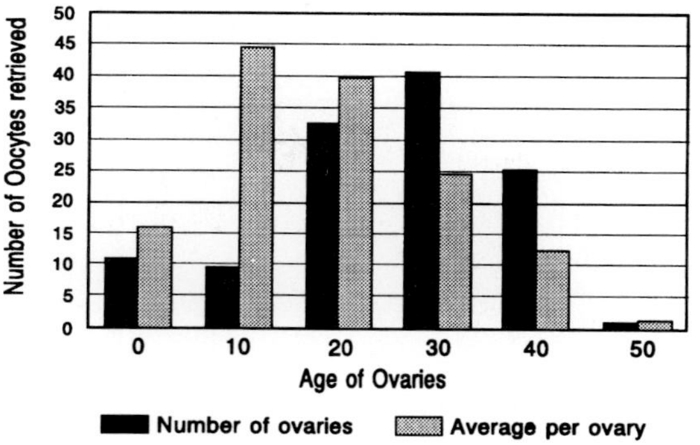

Figure 1 Number of oocytes retrieved according to patient's age

the following sources are frequently utilized to obtain non-viable oocytes: (1) *post mortem* ovarian tissue; (2) surgically removed ovarian tissue; (3) oocytes donated by *in vitro* fertilization (IVF) patients; (4) inseminated, but non-fertilized IVF oocytes; and (5) oocytes that have been used in previous hemizona assays. All oocytes used in HZA were non-living, with no developmental potential.

Post-mortem derived oocytes

After all legal and ethical guidelines had been fulfilled, the ovaries were removed. Ovarian tissue was excised within 24 h of death or surgery and stored at +4°C in phosphate-buffered saline (PBS; Gibco, Grand Island, NY, USA). Manual dissection was carried out following described protocols[1].

During a prospective study from January to October 1993, a total of 3639 prophase I oocytes were retrieved from 134 ovaries collected at different medico-legal mortuaries. Extreme care was taken at all times to ensure that ethical and legal guidelines were followed during the collection of the oocytes. A comparison between age and mean number of oocytes retrieved illustrated ovaries between age 10 and 20 years to be superior (Figure 1). Since we received ovarian tissue of females from different age groups, we addressed the sperm binding capacity of human zona pellucida. A total of 100 prophase 1 oocytes were obtained from ovaries with the following ages: 7 months ($n=20$); 5 years ($n=20$); 7 years ($n=16$); 12 years ($n=22$); and 30 years ($n=22$). Zona-intact oocytes denuded of

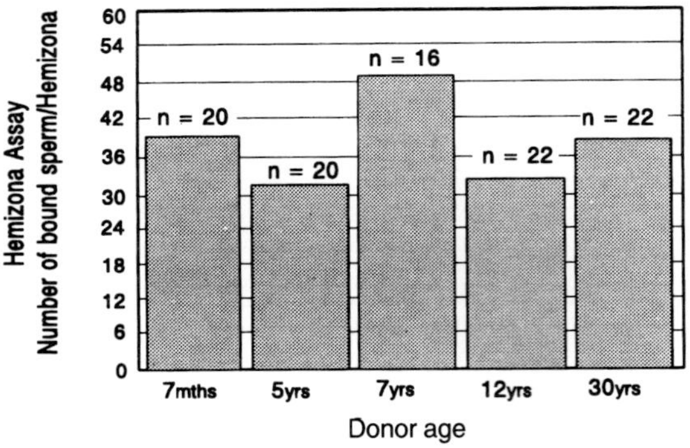

Figure 2 Sperm binding to zonae pellucidae derived from human ovaries according to female age

granulosa cells were recovered and placed in a hyperosmotic $MgCl_2$ solution[9,36] under mineral oil at +4°C until tested.

The sperm-binding capacity of zona pellucidae obtained from prophase I oocytes from ovaries of females of varying ages did not differ significantly (Figure 2). All binding results obtained for zonae from different age groups were within the limits described for normal sperm binding[25]. The functional integrity of the human zona pellucida, therefore, seems to be operational even at an early age at least for tight binding. Whether this is also true for penetration and induction of an acrosome reaction remains to be investigated.

In vitro *fertilization laboratory oocytes*

We studied extensively the use of mature, immature and inseminated non-fertilized oocytes obtained from the IVF laboratory. This section will address in detail all the results from various studies, where we used zonae pellucidae derived from IVF donated oocytes. Apart from their use in homologous bioassays, zonae pellucidae are often used in studies focusing on the glycoprotein components of the zona pellucida, especially the sperm-binding proteins[6,37–40]. Adequate numbers of zonae pellucidae are, therefore, essential to ensure ongoing and future research in the field. Additional oocyte sources, other than donated or excess *in vitro* fertilization (IVF) or gamete intrafallopian transfer (GIFT) material and surgically removed ovarian tissue were, therefore, explored.

Recycled zona pellucida

First, we evaluated during a prospective study sperm binding potential of inseminated metaphase I and II oocytes (n=14) after exposure to sperm in different hemizona assays. We therefore addressed the possibility of using 'recycled hemizonae'. These oocytes failed to fertilize as judged by the absence of pronuclear formation and extrusion of polar body[41], and were collected 50 h post-insemination. At this time, no fertilization or cleavage could be demonstrated. These oocytes were denuded of granulosa cells and salt-stored until tested. On the day of testing, two hemizona assays were performed using the same hemizonae during separate assays. The first HZA was set up and incubated with sperm from a fertile control male. After assessing the number of bound sperm to the hemizonae during HZA 1, all bound sperm were removed using a hand-drawn glass micro-pipette, slightly smaller than the size of the hemizona with a diameter of 90 μm. This sheared sperm off the hemizonae surface, leaving only a few (<10 sperm) with part of the head or entire head embedded in the zona pellucida[30]. Hemizonae were thoroughly evaluated under phase contrast microscopy (400×) for signs of remaining bound sperm. If sperm were still present, the hemizonae were pipetted for the second time. These sperm-stripped hemizonae were then reinseminated during HZA 2 with a sperm population prepared from a different fertile control male. Once again, after a second 4-h co-incubation, the number of hemizona bound sperm were reassessed.

Results for HZAs 1 and 2 performed with inseminated–unfertilized oocytes are depicted in Figure 3. The mean number of sperm bound for HZAs 1 and 2 was 117.8±37 and 113.6±35, respectively (P>0.05). No differences could be detected between the results obtained for HZA 1 and 2. Results obtained are encouraging for sperm–oocyte diagnostic tests. The exposure to and initial binding of spermatozoa to the hemizonae does not seem to influence the moieties responsible for sperm binding at least under hemizona assay conditions. The successful removal of sperm cells from the zona pellucida introduces new fields for future research in assisted reproductive technologies.

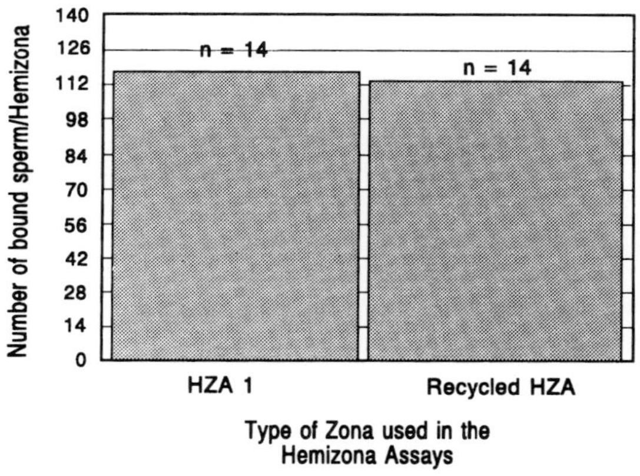

Figure 3 Hemizona assay results using non-recycled and recycled zonae pellucidae

Inseminated non-fertilized oocytes

Three groups of oocytes were evaluated: (1) uninseminated; (2) inseminated, unfertilized; and (3) fertilized, uncleaved. All oocytes had undergone germinal vesicle breakdown at the time of retrieval and were salt-stored (pH 7.2) for not more than 30 days. Sperm binding was recorded under HZA conditions using spermatozoa from eight fertile men (HZA control) and from teratozoospermic men. First, the mean number (±SD) of sperm tightly bound for fertile controls and teratozoospermic men to hemizonae from uninseminated oocytes were 69.7±16 and 14.5±7, respectively ($P<0.02$). Similarly, hemizonae from uninseminated oocytes bound 102.0±19 and 114.0±28, respectively, for fertile controls and normozoospermic men ($P<0.5$). Secondly, hemizonae obtained from inseminated, unfertilized IVF oocytes bound 44.2±12 and 19.7±6 for fertile controls and teratozoospermic men, respectively ($P<0.02$). This category of oocytes bound 100.5±7 and 108.5±11 sperm, respectively, for fertile controls and normozoospermic semen ($P<0.3$). We felt confident to use inseminated unfertilized oocytes, since these oocytes retained their ability to discriminate between terato- and normozoospermic sperm. Third, HZA results of fertilized but uncleaved oocytes showed a mean number of tightly bound sperm of 6.0±4 compared to 65.0±1 in control, uninseminated oocytes using fertile sperm. Fertilized uncleaved oocytes, therefore, cannot be utilized during zona binding experiments.

The ability of salt-stored, inseminated but unfertilized human oocytes to distinguish between zona binding potential of spermatozoa from fertile donors and subfertile men opens a new research field in the study of sperm–zona interactions. These results, however, contradict the report of Tesarik[35], who reported that the zona pellucida of metaphase I and II oocytes aged in insemination medium and stored in salt solution showed high penetrability as compared to non-treated oocytes. However, the zona binding results presented here show that if these oocytes are stored in 1.5 M MgCl, supplemented with HEPES buffer (pH 7.2), they give reliable information for sperm–zona studies[9,36,43,44]. The pH value of a unbuffered $MgCl_2$ solution decreased progressively with time until pH<5.0 was reached, thus causing salt solution to be unsuitable as a storage medium for human oocytes[10].

These results demonstrate that the use of uninseminated and inseminated (unfertilized) human oocytes, salt-stored under controlled pH conditions, give reliable information regarding sperm binding potential of human spermatozoa under HZA conditions.

Immature IVF oocytes

A total of 52 IVF donated immature (prophase I) oocytes (informed consent was obtained) had been collected by follicular aspiration following ovarian stimulation using the different exogenous stimulation therapies, i.e. (1) natural unstimulated menstrual cycles ($n=12$); (2) 100 mg clomiphene citrate from days 4 to 8 of the menstrual cycle in combination with two daily ampules of human menopausal gonadotropin (hMG) (Humegon Sci-Pharm Serono, South Africa) from days 7 to 9 of the patient's menstrual cycle ($n=20$); (3) two ampules daily of hMG starting on day 3. Human chorionic gonadotropin (10 000 IU) (Pregnal, Sci-Pharm Serono, South Africa) was given when the leading follicle reached 18 mm diameter with two other follicles measuring 16 mm in diameter ($n=20$). Results of oocytes derived from different ovulation induction regimens (phase 2) are shown in Figure 4. The sperm characteristics of the samples that were used as hemizona assay controls were (mean±SD): sperm concentration $89\pm16\times10^6$ cells/mL, percentage motile cells

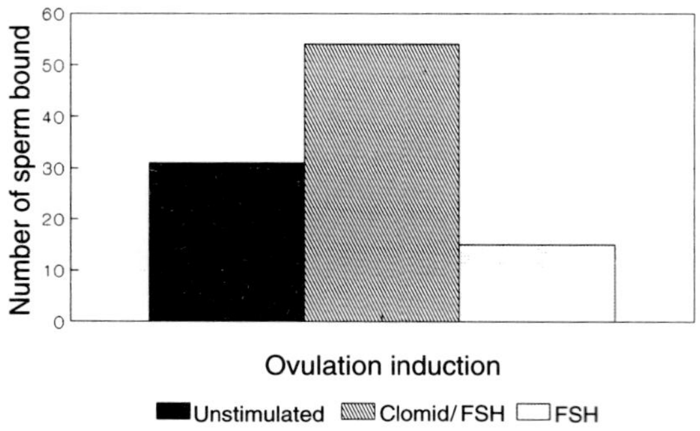

Figure 4 Hemizona assay results using oocytes derived from non-stimulated and stimulated ovaries using different protocols

60±7% and normal morphology 16±2%. The mean number sperm bound (±SD) to zonae from prophase I oocytes obtained from unstimulated ovarian tissue, clomiphene citrate/hMG and hMG stimulated cycles were 31.0±20, 54.4±12 and 15.3±9, respectively. The mean (±SD) number of sperm bound to zonae obtained from hMG derived oocytes were significantly lower compared to that of the clomiphene citrate/hMG combination therapy, i.e. 15.3±9 versus 54.40±12 (P=0.002). Significant differences (P<0.05) were reported between zona binding results of oocytes obtained from natural cycles (15.3±9) compared to stimulated cycles (54.4±12 and 31.0±20).

The sperm binding data recorded for prophase I oocytes obtained from different ovulation induction regimens showed a clear difference among those oocytes which were stimulated only with hMG. During an earlier report, we described a threshold value of 20 zona bound spermatozoa after 4 h of coincubation to be the lower 95% threshold value for a 'normal' zona pellucida and a valid HZA. Therefore, the sperm binding capacity of prophase I oocytes derived from natural unstimulated cycles were thought to be inferior compared to the oocytes derived from unstimulated and Clomid/hMG combination. Prophase I oocytes often have a higher incidence of poor zona binding capacity compared to the more mature metaphase I and II oocytes. Although we did not measure the morphological features of the prophase I oocytes, we are aware that variation in the diameter of the immature human oocyte (140–210 μm)[5], in the appearance of the zona surface[46] and in zona thickness may be linked to differences in zona function, including tight sperm binding[46].

OOCYTE STORAGE

A solution of 2 M DMSO in phosphate buffered saline was initially used to store zona-intact oocytes denuded of granulosa cells that were placed in cryopreservation tubes. The tube ends are sealed with Critoseal (Fisher Scientific, Springfield, NJ, USA) and immediately frozen at −70°C. Dimethylsulfoxide-treated oocytes were stored for 1–6 months before use.

In a well designed study, Hammit *et al.*[21] evaluated the differences in sperm binding to the zona and the recovery of oocytes from the storage vessel after oocyte preservation for the hemizona assay. They compared salt storage with a new method using DMSO/sucrose in liquid nitrogen. The results indicated the DMSO/sucrose procedure to be superior for long-term storage.

Previous studies indicated the successful storage of oocytes in small plastic vials, each containing 0.5 mL of 1.5 M magnesium chloride (Mallinckrodt Chemical Works, St. Louis, MO, USA) with 0.1% polyvinylpyrrolidone (PVP, MW 36 000, Sigma Chemical Co., St Louis, MO, USA) and 40 mM HEPES buffer at pH 7.22[1,9,36]. Acrosome-intact, partially reacted and fully reacted spermatozoa entered salt-stored hemizonae 4 h after insemination, but only fully reacted spermatozoa were seen in the inner zona area. We observed pathways or tunnels created by spermatozoa as they penetrated through the zona pellucida. Comparing sperm binding potential of salt-stored and fresh oocytes, we have demonstrated that the former method of storage can differentiate between fertile and subfertile sperm populations. Salt-stored human oocytes (pH 7.0) therefore contribute reliable information regarding sperm binding potential under HZA conditions[47]. Salt storage is, therefore, the preferred technique for short-term storage of oocytes. If longer storage periods (>3 months) are required, the DMSO/sucrose method is recommended.

Table 5 Number of sperm tightly bound in HZA at each time point (one fertile and one proven subfertile man tested in each HZA)

	Fertile specimens				*Subfertile specimens*			
Exp	*2*	*4*	*6*	*24*	*2*	*4*	*6*	*24*
1	26	55	65	60	21	33	39	39
2	20	54	64	61	4	13	16	18
3	48	125	146	142	16	27	34	30
4	26	78	91	89	6	30	30	39
5	67	188	219	218	8	14	21	20
6	18	48	56	54	10	17	38	30
7	22	64	74	70	10	15	31	20
Mean	32	87[a,b]	102	99	10	21	31	29
SD	18	51	59	60	6	8	9	8

[a] Value is significantly greater than the 2-h mean, $P<0.05$; [b] value is not significantly less than the 24-h mean, $P>0.05$

Functional aspects related to zona binding

The hemizona assay has facilitated investigations of sperm function in relation to zona pellucida binding and we have reported that the zona binding capacity of sperm from subfertile men is diminished in the HZA[9,10,48]. During a series of experiments, we evaluated whether the nature of this impairment includes temporal shifts in sperm binding, i.e. whether subfertile sperm exhibit a premature or delayed peak in zona binding relative to fertile specimens or impaired HZA binding throughout. Seven fertile men and seven subfertile men, who failed to fertilize oocytes during an *in vitro* fertilization therapeutic attempt, were put through the test.

Assessments of tight sperm binding were carried out after 2, 4, 6 and 24 h of coincubation for each hemizona. The results are depicted in Table 5. The HZA provides the strongest differential of all the measured sperm parameters for distinguishing fertile from subfertile men. Each of the seven fertile control sperm suspensions showed near maximum zona binding at the 4-h observation time with a small increase at 6 h. Six of the seven subfertile cases also demonstrated peak binding at 6 h. In contrast to the fertile controls, the subfertile group's curve showed a very slow and ultimately limited cumulative increase in zona binding that peaked at a mean of 31 sperm. There was no significant difference between the mean values at 2 and 4 h. Within the seven subfertile cases, the 6-h binding varied between 16 and 39 sperm, which is well below the range for the fertile men at 6 h (56 and 219 sperm bound) ($P<0.05$).

The influence of sperm freezing and thawing on zona binding

In order to extend our knowledge and information on zona binding we used a series of experiments to study the damage resulting from freeze–thawing procedures of human spermatozoa. A decreased zona binding potential of thawed specimens would be consistent with reports of altered motility[48] and morphology[49,50].

Five men who had fathered a child during the previous 2 years served as subjects. During seven experiments, two of the donors were used twice. Each man provided an initial semen sample that was divided into two aliquots. One portion was held aside for freezing and the second portion of the same fresh aliquot was tested the same day in the HZA to assess zona binding capacity.

The portion of semen to be frozen was mixed with an equal volume of cryopreservation medium and dispersed into straws. The straws were cooled to –90°C (Planar Kryo 10 Instruments, Biomed Inc., Middlesex, UK). After 30 days, the straws were thawed at room temperature. Within the same hour, a second semen specimen was provided by the donor of the frozen sample to be used as a matched control. This fresh specimen was used for comparison, because neither the initial fresh sperm nor the bisected hemizona would be functional 30 days later when the frozen sample was thawed for use. Both thawed and fresh specimen were washed twice with Ham's F10 medium and prepared for a 1-h swim-up. After the sperm swim-up, supernatant sperm were examined to assign the grade of motility and

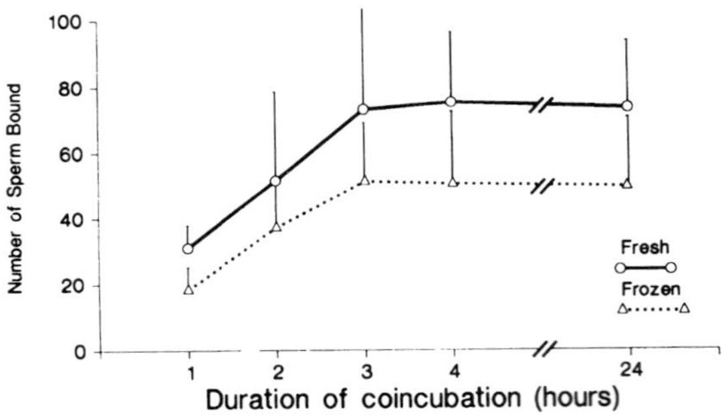

Figure 5 Kinetics of zona binding by fresh versus frozen–thawed spermatozoa from proven fertile men

then diluted with Ham's F10 medium to yield 0.5×10^6 motile cells/mL for use in the HZA.

One 50 μL droplet was taken from each of the two samples and placed under oil. One hemizona from a matching pair was transferred to each drop. After 1, 2, 4, 6 and 24 h of coincubation the number of tightly bound sperm was counted. At each time, the value of the HZI was calculated.

The initial test of binding capacity showed that fresh sperm in the first semen sample from known fertile men bound to hemizonae very well. After 24 h of coincubation the number of bound sperm varied between 40 and 225 (mean ± SD, 115 ± 58). Fresh sperm from the same control subjects 1 month later bound with a mean of 73 ± 19 (range 50–100), again indicating high rates of tight binding. As illustrated in Figure 5, the frozen–thawed sperm showed diminished binding efficiency compared with matched fresh sperm, although the kinetics of hemizona binding curves for fresh and thawed sperm were parallel. The freezing and thawing of human spermatozoa produce a measurable loss in their capacity to bind to the zona pellucida. As indicated in Figure 5, the post-thawed sperm exhibit about 30% less binding. Among the remaining functional sperm, however, the time course of tight binding followed the fresh curve.

Reliance on frozen sperm for reproductive therapies has increased for several reasons: (1) controlled screening for semen that carries the human immunodeficiency virus (HIV) antibody; (2) immediate accessibility of the desired donor semen; (3) prospective sperm banking for men undergoing an orchiectomy or chemotherapy; and (4) provision for a back-up specimen in case a fresh one is not forthcoming.

Clinical application of the hemizona assay

The fundamental utility of the HZA stems from its unique characteristics of being a functional, homologous bioassay of sperm quality and performance in relation to the oocyte zona pellucida. The HZA was developed to estimate sperm fertilizing potential, based on the relative binding of spermatozoa from a test patient versus a known fertile control using the matching halves of a non-living, bisected (hemi) human zona pellucida. The availability of control versus experimental hemispheres from the same zona pellucida has almost solved the problem of zona–zona variations in binding capacity often encountered during whole egg experiments.

Hemizona assay and normozoospermia

Sperm–zona interaction followed a dose–response curve during experiments when spermatozoa from normozoospermic men were added in increasing concentrations to the coincubation droplets (Figure 6).

The number of sperm bound to the zona decreased markedly when the concentration of spermatozoa was <250 000 sperm/mL. At a sperm concentration of 250 000 sperm/mL, the number of tightly bound sperm to the zona pellucida was 35.4 ± 5.6 (mean ± SD) compared with 8.6 ± 4 at a sperm concentration of 125 000 sperm/mL.

In contrast to many animal species, human semen is virtually unique because of its heterogeneity in sperm morphology (pleomorphism); both fertile and infertile men produce high numbers of morphologically abnormal spermatozoa[13,52–54]. This phenomenon is of paramount clinical importance as sperm morphology is regarded by both scientists and medical practitioners as an important prognostic factor in regard to pregnancy outcome. Negative correlations have been reported between the percentage of morphologically abnormal spermatozoa and natural and assisted reproduction[41,53]. Current information on the biology of human reproduction is derived from clinical observations obtained from fertilization *in vitro* directly[55–57], and associated evaluations of human gametes[1,5].

The percentage of normal spermatozoa bound to the zona pellucida reported for both normo- and teratozoospermic men showed significant improve-

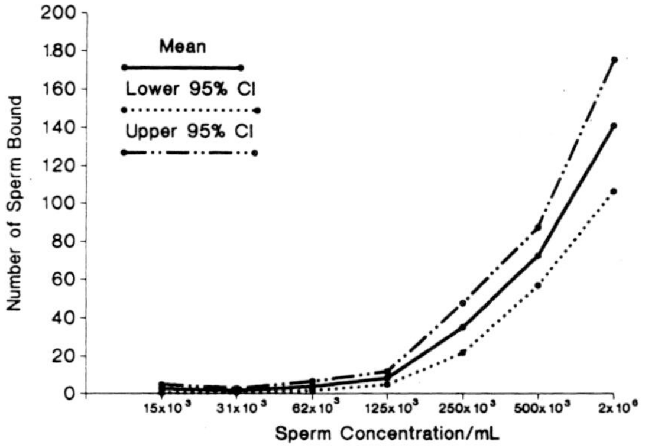

Figure 6 Hemizona assay results using increasing sperm concentration at insemination (pooled data from two fertile males)

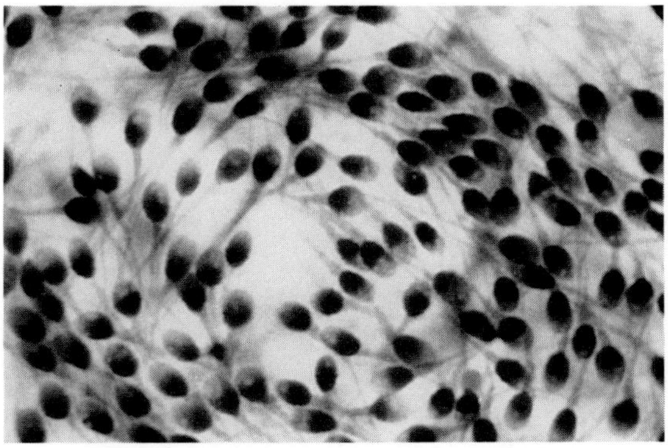

Figure 7 Human sperm bound to the hemizona (6000×); notice the uniform normal morphology exhibited by the sperm

ment when compared to the percentage of normal spermatozoa found after the swim-up procedure. The mean (±SEM) percentages of normal forms for normozoospermic men in the fresh semen specimen, after swim-up and after zona binding, were 21.5±1.6, 27.5±2.9 and 44.8±3.4, respectively. A significantly higher percentage of normal forms were found among zona-bound sperm, compared to swim-up forms (P=0.02) and seminal spermatozoa (P=0.02). The mean percentages of normal sperm forms present in fresh semen sample, after swim-up and after zona pellucida binding for teratozoospermic men, were 3.7±0.9, 5.8±1.6 and 15.6±3.1, respectively. Significant differences existed between the percentage of normal forms found in the swim-up and zona-bound spermatozoa (P<0.01 and P<0.0003, respectively), compared to the original ejaculates[42]. Figure 7 illustrates human spermatozoa tightly bound to the hemizona (notice the high quantity of normal sperm forms present).

We reported a significant linear relationship between the number of sperm tightly bound to the hemizona and the percentage of spermatozoa with normal morphology in the semen evaluated according to strict criteria[9–11,14]. These findings suggest: (1) that the zona pellucida may play a natural selective role against morphologically abnormal spermatozoa; or (2) that the abnormal spermatozoa are simply dysfunctional and unable to bind to the zona pellucida. In previous reports[8], all semen samples were assigned to samples with <4% normal spermatozoa, with 4–14% normal spermatozoa and with >14% perfectly normal spermatozoa (Table 6).

Hemizona assay and teratozoospermia

Sperm binding kinetics indicated that 250 000 motile spermatozoa/mL was the minimum number of sperm required to sustain a valid hemizona

Table 6 Comparison between zona pellucida binding potential of sperm according to sperm morphology by strict criteria (n=63 men)

Parameters	*Morphological classification*		
	Normal (n=16)	*P pattern (n=17)*	*G Pattern (n=30)*
Concentration	88.8±13	37.8±7	71.8±101
Motility (%)	50.8±2	44.1±3	49.6±2
Normal morphology (%)	19.0±2[a,b]	2.8±0.2[a]	9.5±0.5[b]
HZA binding (sperm/HZA*)	59.6±9[c,d]	23.5±4[c]	36.0±6[d]
HZA index	54.5±17[e,f]	24.3±3[e]	37.7±6[f]

[a–f] Differ significantly (P<0.0001); * sperm concentration used

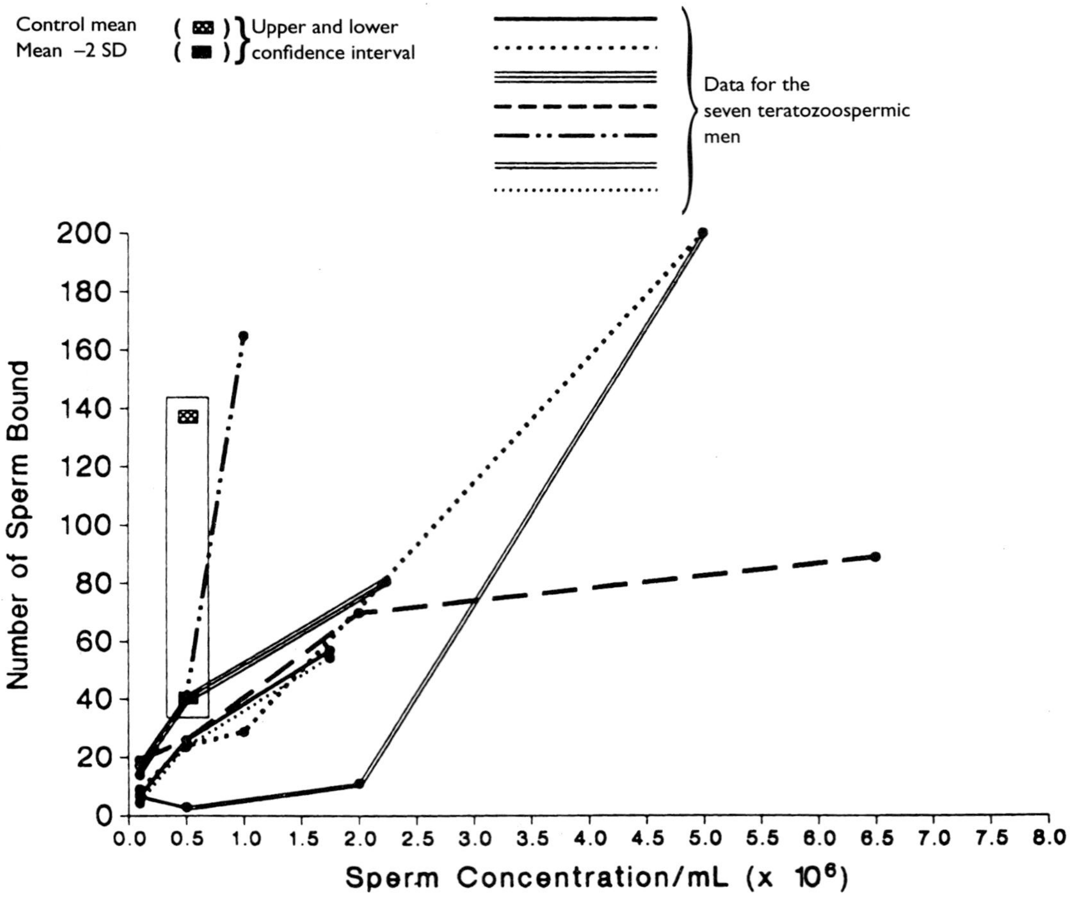

Figure 8 Hemizona assay results using spermatozoa from seven infertile teratozoospermic men in increasing (mean and lower 95% confidence interval for the fertile controls used for comparison)

assay[31,36]. Zona binding and subsequent fertilization *in vitro* are known to be impaired among men with teratozoospermia[9,55,56,58]. By increasing the number of spermatozoa/mL each teratozoospermic man revealed a specific sperm concentration necessary to achieve to zona binding parity compared to the number of bound sperm representing the lower 95% confidence interval for the control sample with the matching hemizona.

A standard hemizona sperm concentration of 500 000 motile sperm/mL was maintained for the fertile control in all experiments. The mean ± SEM for pooled zona binding data obtained from matching control hemizonae in each experiment was 133.5 ± 6. The calculated lower 95% confidence interval for the mean number of bound sperm was 40. The lower 95% confidence interval obtained from the fertile control at 500 000 sperm/mL and the zona binding results of each infertile individual at increasing insemination densities are shown in Figure 8.

At a standard concentration of 500 000 sperm/mL, fertile controls had a significantly higher number of tightly bound sperm than teratozoospermic patients (133.5 ± 6 versus 32.1 ± 2, $P<0.00001$). Three patients (numbers 1, 4 and 6) matched or exceeded the number of bound sperm calculated as the lower 95% confidence interval of the fertile control sample (that is, 40.1) at a concentration of 500 000 sperm/mL. The remaining four men (numbers 2, 3, 5 and 7) achieved parity with the fertile control at insemination concentrations/mL of 2.0×10^6, 1.25×10^6, 1.0×10^6 and 2.0×10^6. Three patients (3, 6, 7) matched the mean number of tightly bound sperm for controls (that is 133.5±6) at densities of 3.0×10^6, 1.0×10^6 and 4×10^6 sperm/mL, respectively. The remaining infertile men (1, 2, 4 and 5) were not able to reach that parity even at concentrations $>4\times10^6$ sperm/mL.

Therefore, the HZA can be used as a diagnostic indicator for the insemination concentrations during IVF procedures. The data indicate that teratozoospermic men might need a much higher insemination concentration to reach binding parity compared to that of the fertile controls.

Hemizona assay and its relationship to IVF results

Several studies were designed to compare HZA results with IVF outcome[9–11]. The principal objective of these studies was to compare the number of sperm bound to the hemizonae for patients with and without fertilization during IVF treatment. Semen was classified as normal if, in addition to the other sperm characteristics, the morphological assessment using strict criteria[56] was also normal. First, among 36 patients participating in the Norfolk IVF program, seven men had previously shown normal semen profiles; the remaining 29 had teratozoospermia, that is, <14% morphologically normal spermatozoa. All patients exhibited normal plasma endocrine profiles (follicle-stimulating hormone [FSH], luteinizing hormone [LH], prolactin, testosterone and estradiol). Each IVF couple had also been evaluated for the presence of antisperm antibodies in the semen or in the female serum. No patients with immunological problems were included in the study. Data were compiled for preovulatory oocytes only (metaphase I and II); all patients had at least one preovulatory oocyte for insemination. For oocyte insemination a concentration of 500 000 motile spermatozoa/mL was used for 17 of the 36 cases. The insemination concentration varied from 0.5×10^6 to 1×10^6 motile spermatozoa/mL for the other 19 cases. All patients were asked to provide a second semen sample for the HZA at 48 h after insemination of the oocytes.

The data for sperm binding to the hemizonae were first analyzed after assigning all IVF patients to one of two groups: the IVF fertilization group (≥1 oocyte fertilized) or the IVF failure group (0% fertilization). Spermatozoa from patients in the fertilization group showed an enhanced capacity for tight binding to the hemizonae (Table 7). The mean number (±SEM) of bound sperm was significantly greater ($P<0.05$) than the mean for the failure group (36.1±7 versus 10.4±4, respectively). The mean data for sperm concentration and percentage of motility showed no significant differences. However, clearly oligozoospermic or asthenozoospermic patients had already been excluded from this study.

Table 7 Hemizona assay results (number of tightly bound sperm to hemizonae – x±SEM) in patients who fertilized and did not fertilize in the IVF system

Parameters	*Group with fertilization (n=27)*	*Group with no fertilization (n=9)*
HZA: (tightly bound sperm/hemizona)	36±7	10±3
Normal spermatozoa (%)	12±1	3±0.9
Sperm concentration ($\times10^6$)	74±10	54±7
Motility (%)	45±4	33±6

Mean±SEM

Further insight into sperm factors that might influence zona binding was sought by running between-factor correlations. Pearson correlation coefficients were obtained for a matrix with 17 parameters. Significant linear relationships were observed between the number of sperm tightly bound to the hemizona and (1) the percentage of motile sperm in semen ($P<0.0001$); (2) the percentage of seminal sperm with normal morphology by strict criteria ($P<0.001$); and (3) the seminal sperm concentration per milliliter ($P<0.01$).

Oehninger *et al.*[11] reported that tight sperm binding to the hemizonae averaged 59.5 for the controls, compared to 72.2 ($P>0.05$) for IVF patients with normal semen characteristics and 16.7 ($P=0.05$) for IVF patients with terato/oligo/asthenozoospermic semen. Mean binding was significantly greater for IVF cases with ≥65% fertilization of mature oocytes. Based on the HZI index values, the HZA accurately predicted IVF fertilization in 21 of 22 cases.

In a study at Tygerberg hospital, 32 men were used to evaluate the clinical significance of zona pellucida binding and fertilization outcome among

Table 8 Results of hemizona assays, fertilization rates and semen parameters of 32 GIFT/IVF patients at Tygerberg Hospital

	Group with fertilization (P values) (n = 17)	*Group with no fertilization (n=15)*
Number of excess MII oocytes	47	65
Number of excess MII fertilized	9	54
Fertilization rate (%)	19	83
HZA binding (tightly bound sperm/hemizona	28.8±5	51.8±2 (0.01)
HZI	29.6±4	53.9±4 (0.006)
Sperm concentration (× 10^6/mL)	56.1±1	89.5±23 (0.01)
Sperm motility (%)	48.8±3	48.6±3 (0.8)
Normal morphology (%)	7.5±2	13.0±1 (0.0008)

Hemizona assay results (number of tightly bound sperm to hemizona x±SEM and HZI) in patients who fertilized and did not fertilize in the GIFT/IFS system at Tygerberg

Table 9 Semen parameters and fertilization rates of excess oocytes in GIFT patients with normal (≥36) and low (<36) HZI

	Hemizona index		
	≥36	*<36*	*(P value)*
Number of patients	27	36	
HZI	81.5±10	18.9±3	(0.0001)
Sperm concentration (× 10^6)	85.9±11	61.4±10	(0.08)
Motility (%)	48.5±3	48.3±2	(0.9)
Normal morphology (%)	14.±1	8.0±1	(0.001)
Fertilization rates			
metaphase I	28/62	21/72	(0.01)
metaphase II	49/72	20/46	(0.01)

excess oocytes obtained during GIFT procedures. The results were divided into two groups, namely fertilization rate of >65% and <65% of excess metaphase II oocytes (Table 8). The scattering of data provided a natural breakpoint at an HZA index value of 36, allowing us to evaluate the HZA as a predictor of IVF results. We divided the data of 63 patients participating in the Tygerberg GIFT/IVF program according to their hemizona index values into two groups, namely >36 and <36 (Table 9). During this study, we were convinced that the HZA can be used as a indicator for fertilization potential of a specific sperm sample.

During a collaborative study, Oehninger *et al.*[51] provided further evidence of the ability of the HZA to predict IVF outcome. With a sensitivity of 83%, a specificity of 95% and an incidence of one false positive and one false negative among 28, the HZA discriminated by identifying patients at risk for poor or failed fertilization. More experiments are needed to establish the threshold HZA index value and the intra-assay variation.

Zona pellucida binding potential of antibody-coated human sperm

The influence of sperm autoantibodies, particularly those of the IgA immunoglobulin class, can interfere with IVF. Generally, poor fertilization rates are obtained when 80% or more of the motile spermatozoa are coated with antibodies of the IgG and IgA immunoglobulin classes. Good fertilization rates, however, were obtained in those cases where 90–100% of sperm were coated with IgG-class anti-

Table 10 Antisperm antibody test and hemizona assay results in nine subfertile men

Patient	*Direct IgG (%)*	*IBT IgA*	*MAR %IgG*	*TAT (serum titer)*	*HZA binding sperm/hemizona*	*control test*	*HZI*
1	10TT	90TT	100	256M	55	33	60
2	100M	99H	100	256M	54	13	24
3	100H	100H	95	512M	125	27	22
4	99M	95H	100	1024M	78	30	38
5	100H	95H	100	1024M	188	14	7
6	95H	100H	100	512M	48	17	22
7	50T	50H	40	32	64	15	23
8	80H	80H	40	n/a	34	11	32
9	90H	0	95	1024M	48	16	30

Agglutination types: H=head; T=tail; M=mixed; TT=tailtip; n/a=not available. IBT=Direct immunobead test; MAR=mixed antiglobulin reaction test; TAT=tray agglutination test

bodies, but <70% coated with IgA class antibodies. This suggests that IgG-class antibodies alone are not usually capable of blocking fertilization[48]. That is, their specific antigenic recognitions and titer may be principal factors in determining whether fertilization is impaired, either following coitus or interventions using assisted reproductive technologies. We postulated that inhibition of tight binding to the zona pellucida may be correlated with high titers of either IgG or IgA.

Spermatozoa antibodies are associated with a reduced chance of conception following unprotected intercourse and act primarily by preventing spermatozoa transport through the female reproductive tract. However, there is some evidence to suggest that these antibodies may also influence the fertilization of the oocyte[49,59,61]. The HZA offers a technical advance that does assist in both diagnosis and prognosis. Given the increased attention to treatment, the HZA may be an important and useful technique to monitor the progress of therapeutic regimes.

The zona pellucida binding properties of spermatozoa from nine men, who had previously tested positive for sperm antibodies in their blood serum and on their spermatozoa, were tested. The direct immunobead test (IBT)[49,61], mixed antiglobulin reaction (MAR)[62] and the tray agglutination test (TAT)[63] were employed to evaluate the sperm antibody activity among the men.

The IVF data were confirmed in the HZA, suggesting that this may be a way to quantify the effect of the antibody on binding. Qualification of the antibody's effect on zona binding might be an important contribution in cases where total inhibition of binding occurs. We have previously found that the zona binding properties of a given semen sample indicated the fertilization outcome during *in vitro* fertilization treatment programs[20,22,64]. However, the presence of antibodies does not necessarily mean that conception could not occur; eight of nine of these couples eventually had a successful fertilization: one by natural coital insemination (number 7, Table 10), five by gamete intrafallopian transfer (GIFT), and two by intrauterine insemination. All pregnancies went to term except one of the GIFT conceptions, which miscarried at 8 weeks.

It appears that there is significantly decreased tight binding of sperm to the zona pellucida in the patients with antisperm antibodies (ASA) (19.5 ± 8 (mean ± SD) sperm bound, compared to 77.1 ± 49 (mean ± SD) sperm bound in the control male patient). The HZA was originally devised to assess the zona binding potential of a given semen sample, comparing sperm from a fertile male to that of subfertile male[5].

From these observations it appears that assisted reproduction, since a high percentage of the treated cases became pregnant, may have minimized the effects of these antibodies. The specific locus where these antibodies may influence fertilization has been averted when using the assisted reproductive methods. Such an immune effect may have been minimized by introduction of gametes into sites beyond the vaginal and cervical milieu. In addition, note that for each specimen only 1–2% of the spermatozoa in the ejaculate were evaluated. Legitimate questions remain about the representative nature of such samples. The limited population of patients studied here should also be recognized, and greater caution should be used when linking ASA with absolute infertility.

The role of zona pellucida binding in identifying male factor infertility in assisted reproduction

A pure male factor is diagnosed in roughly one-third of infertile couples, and in another 20% a multifactorial infertility involving the male is found. The advent of assisted reproduction allowed us to observe gamete interaction for the first time *in vitro* and evaluate the performance of abnormal sperm in this system. The time has come to look for new criteria to define normal sperm and gamete performance in the *in vitro* system, and to use these parameters to define sperm with fertilization potential[56,58]. It is also necessary to determine whether anyone of the tests of sperm function can help in defining and diagnosing the male factor in assisted reproduction.

A retrospective study was undertaken to investigate the performance of normal gametes in assisted reproduction, of abnormal sperm in that system, and to determine the efficiency of the HZA to predict those performances. The study proceeded in two parts to (1) calculate the total and normal fertilization rates recorded in our IVF program using normal gametes; and (2) address the questions concerning the importance of HZI as a prognostic indicator of fertilization potential in an assisted reproduction program.

Ovarian stimulation was performed according to standard protocols and in all cases at least three mature metaphase II oocytes were inseminated with the husband's sperm. In patients where all the semen parameters were within the normal limits (non-male factors), oocyte insemination was performed with standard sperm concentration of 100 000 motile sperm/mL/oocyte in 3 mL. In male factor patients (terato-, astheno- or oligozoospermia), whenever possible, insemination concentration was increased up to 500 000 sperm/mL/oocyte. Normal fertilization was diagnosed when two pronuclei were present 16–20 h post-insemination; if more than two pronuclei were present, abnormal fertilization (polyspermia) was diagnosed and, if fertilization occurred after that period, it was considered abnormal (delayed).

A standard HZA protocol (see laboratory procedures on page 238) was followed to determine zona binding potential of the men used in the study. In each assay, one hemizona was placed in a droplet containing sperm from an infertile patient, while the matching half was incubated with control sperm. Hemizona assay results were expressed in two ways: (1) absolute number of tightly bound sperm for patient and control; and (2) HZI was calculated.

Total and normal fertilization rates

To establish the total and normal fertilization rates in the normal gamete population at the Tygerberg IVF program, a total of 99 couples fulfilling the following criteria were selected:

(1) Females classified as tubal factor;

(2) Having a normal FSH/LH ratio on day 3 of the menstrual cycle;

(3) Producing three or more normal pre-ovulatory oocytes at retrieval; and

(4) Having husbands with normal sperm parameters.

Five hundred and eighty-nine oocytes were inseminated in this group. The total fertilization rate (total number of pre-ovulatory oocytes fertilized/total number of pre-ovulatory oocytes inseminated) and the normal fertilization rate (total number of pre-ovulatory oocytes with normal fertilization/total number of pre-ovulatory oocytes inseminated) were calculated (mean±SD). Minimum total and normal fertilization rates for this gamete population was defined as the mean minus 2SD.

For the 99 couples (589 oocytes) the total fertilization rate (see above) was 88.6 ± 17% (mean ± SD) and the normal fertilization rate (see above) was 81.3 ± 22% (mean ± SD). The minimum total fertilization rate (mean minus 2SD) that can be considered normal in the Tygerberg program is, therefore, 55% and the minimum normal fertilization rate 37%. Total and normal fertilization values below 55% and 37%, respectively, should be considered abnormal and in the presence of normal stimula-

Table 11 Linear discriminant analysis of 48 selected IVF patients with normal (≥30) and low (<30) hemizona indices

HZI	*≥55%*	*≤55%*	*Total*
>30	21	5	26
<30	7	15	22
Total	28	22	48

Sensitivity: 21/28=75%; specificity: 15/22=68%; negative predictive value: 15/22=68%; positive predictive value: 21/26=81%

tion and morphologically normal oocytes with sperm abnormalities (mainly teratozoospermia present) should be ascribed to a male factor in assisted reproduction.

Correlation of HZI with IVF

Correlation between HZI and IVF results in 48 couples from the IVF program were used in this part of the study. All females provided normal gametes and fulfilled the criteria set forth in phase 1. The 48 partners included normal and abnormal male factors. Because oocyte sperm binding variability, as well as sperm quality of the controls, can play a role in the result of the HZA, the previously described guidelines for the appropriate interpretation of the assay[27] were used. Based on the definition of normal fertilization and, more specifically, definition of male factor infertility in assisted reproduction described in Phase 1, 20 patients were allocated in the <55% total fertilization group, whereas 28 patients were put on the >55% total fertilization rate (Table 11). In both these groups, all the female partners adhered to the selection criteria. The zona binding results and sperm parameters of the 48 men are depicted in Table 12. Comparison

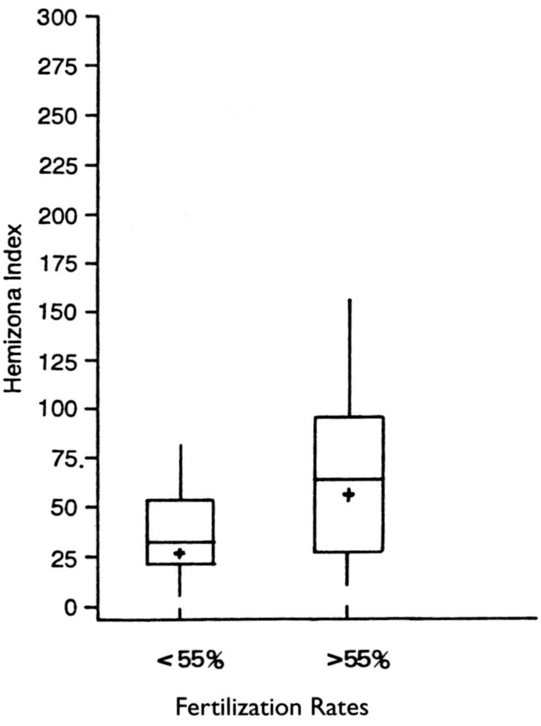

Figure 9 Hemizona index in patients with low (<55%) and normal (>55%) fertilization rates in IVF

between the hemizona indices of the <55% and >55% normal fertilization rate groups are illustrated by the boxplots (Figure 9). The fertilization rates recorded for the oocytes of each individual classified (<55% or >55%) in Table 11 are represented in Table 13.

The predictive ability of the hemizona index was calculated by a linear discriminant analysis. The mean number of the sperm bound (mean±SD) for each group in Phase 2 was calculated. The data

Table 12 Hemizona assay results (number of tightly bound sperm to hemizona – x±SEM and HZI) and semen parameters in 48 men with normal (≥55%) and low (<55%) fertilization rates

	No. Sperm bound	*HZI*	*Conc.* (x10⁶/mL)*	*Sperm parameters*		
				Motility (%)	*Morphology (%)*	*Fertilization rate (%)*
>55%	52.9±36	69.4±56	80.5±55	50.2±10	14.0±5	78.8±20
<55%	24.1±22	30.5±32	50.2±33	45.0±13	6.6±3	13.5±15
P-values	0.001	0.001	0.001	0.02	0.001	0.001

*Conc.=concentration

Table 13 Linear discriminant analysis of the number of oocytes fertilized from 48 selected IVF patients with normal (≥30) and low (<30) hemizona indices

HZI	*≥55%*	*≤55%*	*Total*
>30	167	56	223
<30	68	100	168
Total	235	156	391

Sensitivity: 167/235=71%; specificity: 100/156=64%; negative predictive value: 100/168=59%; positive predictive value: 167/223=75%; overall predictive ability: 267/391=68%

were then compared using Wilcoxon *t*-test for nonparametric analysis. The sensitivity was 71%, specificity 65% negative and positive predictive values were 59% and 75%, respectively.

The traditional approach to the diagnosis and treatment of human infertility is based on a battery of clinical and laboratory examinations, the results of which indicate the most likely cause of the problem and the most efficient manner for its alleviation. Because of the high incidence of male factor infertility, an andrological consultation of complete semen evaluation are mandatory for all couples consulting for infertility. Assisted reproduction has become the final test and one of the most successful therapeutic modalities for a wide variety of sperm dysfunction disorders.

The investigation of gamete performance in the IVF system in the normal population is quite relevant to interpret the sperm fertilizing ability of an abnormal sample under these laboratory conditions. Only sperm with fertilizing potential below normal should be considered as a male factor in assisted reproduction. Other abnormal samples that still have normal capacity for fertilization could be considered as male factors from a clinical point of view because they do not fulfill the World Health Organization criteria for semen and sperm normality, but from an assisted reproduction standpoint they should not be included within the male factor category because they are able to fertilize within the normal range. To include those specimens within the male factor in assisted reproduction will certainly distort the results obtained with these methods and make them much better than when proper criteria for identification and inclusion are used. At the present time, there is no laboratory method of sperm analysis able to separate these two groups (clinical male factor and male factor in assisted reproduction) in an adequate prospective manner.

After defining these categories in the Tygerberg program by using the fertilization rate threshold, as performed in this chapter, the investigation of the HZA and the HZI as one of the potential tests of sperm function for identification and separation of the two populations seems to be a logical approach.

The ability to predict fertilization failure was 68% when we used fertilization per patient (Table 11) and 59% per oocyte (Table 13). The specificity (68%) stresses the complexity of the fertilization process. False positive hemizona assay results can occur since the fertilization defect may be in functional steps beyond the tight binding of the sperm to the zona pellucida. Therefore, although binding is crucial for fertilization to occur, it does not guarantee that the rest of the fertilization process will proceed normally. However, tight binding to the zona pellucida is an absolute requisite for fertilization. The overall accuracy of 71% shows that the hemizona index has discriminatory power. The 29% error rate of the hemizona index is to be expected, since the hemizona assay is a biological test using gamete interaction to predict fertility. The cutoff value of the hemizona index that was used was 30%, implying that hemizona index <30% is indicative of low fertilization potential, while an index >30% indicates higher fertilization capability. Shifting the cutoff value of the hemizona index from 30 to 50–60% made no difference in terms of accuracy of discrimination. The overall accuracy with these cutoff values was, in all cases, 71%. This might be an indication that HZI values between 30 and 60 must be regarded as equal insofar as the predictive ability is concerned. The sensitivity and specificity of these HZIs do not differ as fertilization predictors.

Although the mean HZI results are above threshold in the normal population and below it in the abnormal one, the distribution overlap indicates a low discriminating power. The frequency distribution of the population with low and normal fertilization rates shows a shift in means and medians of the HZI ratio, with the better fertilization group (>55%) having a higher assay ratio. From the distribution overlap, it can be predicted that the discriminating power of the HZI will not be very good because the >55% group covers the whole range with respect to the HZI. Both groups have very skew ratio distributions with SD exceeding or nearly equaling the mean. The highest SD may be caused by some extreme values as indicated in the plots. Although bioassays such as the HZA have limitations, they still provide useful information regarding the first step in fertilization, namely, tight binding of the sperm to the ZP. The relatively low discriminating power of the HZA reported in the study is not surprising because, in general, bioassays are often limited by gray areas in a given sample population. This stresses the importance of the development of a multifactorial evaluation approach in assisted reproductive programs to add valuable information to the clinical situation. It therefore seems more logical for the clinician to depend on the results of several functional tests to supply data on gametes and their interaction.

Efforts to understand sperm function and performance in the human *in vitro* fertilization system do not answer all the questions to identify and treat the male factor in assisted reproduction. Defects of sperm–oocyte interactions are recognized as one of the underlying causes of failure in *in vitro* fertilization, and probably in natural reproduction. It is accepted that before a spermatozoon can penetrate the zona pellucida, firm attachment between the two gametes should occur. The hemizona assay has been developed as an internally controlled bioassay to measure tight binding of human sperm to human zona pellucida. Previous clinical testing has demonstrated a positive correlation between the numbers of sperm bound to the hemizona and the success during IVF[10,65,66].

Failure to fertilize normal pre-ovulatory human oocytes *in vitro* by severely abnormal sperm have already been reported[55]. These samples with high percentages of abnormal spermatozoa (severe teratozoospermia) also showed significantly lower binding to the zona pellucida under HZA conditions than normal samples[11]. However, if in these cases the concentration of spermatozoa is increased at the time of coincubation with the hemizona, significant improvement in binding can be observed. Thus, the hemizona assay has a potential use not only as a prognostic tool for IVF results, but also to determine the ideal number of spermatozoa that should be incubated with the oocyte at the time of IVF[27,59].

The minimal control zona binding of 20 sperm per hemizona should be used in order to ensure the optimal utilization of HZA results[50]. Interpretation of these results depends largely on a good understanding of the variables that influence laboratory data and their correlation with the clinical results. During fertility testing, the variability in oocyte quality, as well as sperm donor quality, has frequently confounded in the *in vitro* assay interpretation. Using a homologous rodent fertilization model[22,23], in which oocytes are easily obtained, inter-egg variation is the principal reason for placing multiple ova (5–20) in each coincubation droplet. Similarly, the zona-free hamster oocyte sperm penetration assay used 10–20 oocytes/dish[24]. Cross *et al.* have concluded that oocyte–oocyte differences represent one of the two most significant sources of experimental variability in a zona-binding study. Apart from the inconsistency of oocyte quality, the sperm from individual semen donors exhibit different capacitation abilities and potential for sperm–oocyte interaction.

The recorded sensitivity of 75% is of clinical importance, since corrective measures can be applied on these cases with low fertilizing potential. These results indicate a usefulness of utilization of the HZI as the predictor of human sperm fertilizing potential in conjunction with other tests in our infertility treatment program. Apart from influences of dysmorphic and dyskinetic spermatozoa, the HZI can disclose functional defects in a given sperm population.

The ability of zona pellucida binding to predict human fertilization in different and consecutive *in vitro* fertilization cycles

Clinicians are often troubled by the question whether the result of a specific functional assay is representative of a given sperm population over time. The zona binding potential of different sperm populations was studied in order to assess the power of HZA to prognosticate fertilization results in the same and subsequent (consecutive) IVF cycles of those same patients. We were able to evaluate a large number of patients ($n = 112$) who underwent a total of 233 IVF cycles.

A total of 112 consecutive patients who participated in the IVF/GIFT program at Tygerberg Hospital ($n=62$) and Norfolk IVF program ($n=50$) were studied. Patients were selected on the only basis of having >6 pre-ovulatory oocytes (metaphase II at aspiration) retrieved after ovarian stimulation (at Tygerberg) or >2 pre-ovulatory oocytes at the Norfolk program. Patients from the Tygerberg program were diagnosed as non-tubal infertility: unexplained infertility 23% and male-factor cases 77%. Patients from the Norfolk program were diagnosed as tubal infertility (50%), endometriosis (11%), unexplained (9%) and male-factor (30%).

GIFT was performed in the 62 couples from the Tygerberg program using four oocytes to be transferred to the Fallopian tubes. Of the excess oocytes, one was donated by the couple in order to perform a HZA (fresh oocytes). The rest of the oocytes were inseminated with the husband's sperm for the purpose of IVF. If fertilization occurred, pre-embryos were cryopreserved at the pronuclear stage using 1, 2 propanediol. Results of cryopreserved/thawed pre-embryos are not included in this study. Standard IVF procedures were performed on the 50 couples in the Norfolk program using previously described methods.

The 62 GIFT couples from Tygerberg Hospital underwent a total of 121 IVF/GIFT cycles from the period of October, 1991 to June, 1992. In all subsequent cycles following the first attempt, excess oocytes were available for IVF (in addition to the GIFT procedure). The results of the HZA performed with the wife's fresh oocytes in the first cycle were used to analyze the relationship between sperm–zona pellucida binding and fertilization rates under IVF conditions in the HZA–IVF cycle and subsequent IVF cycles. The 50 couples from the Norfolk program underwent IVF treatment in 112 cycles during a similar period and HZA–IVF results obtained for the metaphase II oocytes were segregated into: (1) fertilization rates observed during the cycle where the HZA was performed (HZA–IVF cycle); and (2) fertilization rates recorded during all subsequent cycles of the same patients (subsequent IVF cycles). Institutional Review Board approval was obtained prior to the initiation of the study in both institutions.

Controlled ovarian hyperstimulation was accomplished at Tygerberg using a combination of clomiphene citrate and human menopausal gonadotropin (hMG) following established guidelines. GIFT was performed by laparoscopy under general anaesthesia with a total of four oocytes transferred to the tubes (two oocytes randomly selected transferred per tube). Oocytes were loaded into the transfer catheter together with 1×10^5 motile sperm (after wash-swim-up). The number of sperm was increased to 5×10^5 motile sperm in the case of male-factor patients (if possible) whenever sperm morphology was <14% normal forms (strict criteria), sperm density $<10 \times 10^6$/mL and or % motility <30%[31,33,67–69]. Excess oocytes were allocated for the HZA (fresh oocyte) and for IVF. For IVF, oocytes were inseminated 5 h after retrieval[41,67]. Insemination was performed at a standard concentration of 1×10^5 motile sperm/mL/egg and, where possible, at 5×10^5 motile sperm/mL/egg in male-factor cases[68]. Fertilization was reported when two pronuclei were observed 16–20 h post-insemination. Ovarian stimulation was performed at Norfolk using a combination of GnRH agonist (leuprolide acetate) and gonadotropins (FSH and hMG) following established guidelines. Oocyte classification and insemination followed published protocols[41] and were similar to those performed at Tygerberg. Uterine transfer was performed 40–44 h after oocyte insemination (up to four embryos), with surplus oocytes being cryopreserved at the pronuclear stage.

Semen samples were collected by masturbation, and prepared and evaluated according to the methods described in this chapter[14,17,55]. The same sample was used for insemination of the eggs for IVF and HZA as well as for the GIFT procedure. In some cases, however, and due to the low sperm recovery, semen samples obtained 3 h apart were pooled with the initial sample (after sperm separation). Hemizona control sperm samples had previously been tested in the HZA showing consistently good sperm–zona binding capacity[19,23]. HZA results were calculated as: (1) absolute number of tightly bound sperm for patient and control and (2) hemizona assay index.

Linear discrminant analysis was used to determine the sensitivity, specificity and predictive value of the hemizona index as a prognostic index of fer-

Table 14 Linear discriminant analysis of fertilization rate versus hemizona index in 112 couples from the Tygerberg and Norfolk programs

HZI	*>50%*	*<50%*	*Total*
>30	61	11	72
<30	12	28	40
Total	73	39	112

Table 16 Comparison between fertilization rate of metaphase II oocytes from the Tygerberg and Norfolk programs for HZA–IVF cycle and subsequent IVF cycles in patients with HZI <30 and ⩾30

HZI category	*HZA–IVF cycles*	*Subsequent IVF cycles*
HZI⩾30	281/383 (73%)[a]	239/313 (76%)[b]
HZI<30	38/126 (30%)[c]	79/216 (36)[d]

[a,b] $P>0.05$; [a,c] $P=0.001$; [c,d] $P>0.05$; [b,d] $P=0.003$

tilization outcome. Once the most predictive hemizona index was determined, this value was used to compare fertilization results of metaphase II oocytes in the HZA–IVF cycle and subsequent IVF cycles performing chi-square analysis. Fertilization rate was calculated as the number of pre-ovulatory oocytes fertilized/inseminated. Results are expressed as mean ± standard error. $P<0.05$ was considered significant.

Analysis of the distribution of HZI among the 112 cases showed that HZI was not linear. Discriminant analysis revealed a HZI value of 30 as the most predictive index of overall fertilization results. A 2×2 contingency table using 50% as the minimum total fertilization rate (mean minus 2SD of the total fertilization rate for a large normal gamete population) showed that the HZA's ability to predict fertilization had a sensitivity of 84%, specificity of 72%, and a positive and negative predictive value of 85% and 70%, respectively (overall accuracy of 79%) (Table 14). A comparison of the semen parameters of the patients segregated according to a HZI >30 ($n=72$) and HZI <30 ($n=40$), showed significant differences among all of the sperm parameters recorded for these two groups (Table 15).

The fertilization results for metaphase II oocytes in the HZA–IVF cycle and in subsequent IVF cycles for patients with HZI >30 and <30 were 75% (520/696) and 35% (117/342), respectively. This difference was statistically significant ($P=0.0001$). Table 16 depicts the fertilization rates for patients with HZI >30 and HZI <30 segregated according to the first IVF cycle (HZA–IVF cycle) and subsequent IVF cycles. Again, results were significantly different for these two groups of patients; however, fertilization rates were very similar in subsequent cycles for the same group (HZI >30 or <30) of individuals.

The study provides additional compelling evidence of the capacity of the HZA to predict fertilization outcome of preovulatory oocytes (metaphase II) with a high frequency. Defects of sperm–oocyte interaction are now recognized as one of the underlying causes of reproductive failure in IVF and probably in natural reproduction[67]. Here, the HZA discriminated by identifying patients at high risk for poor fertilization. Although our understanding of sperm–oocyte interactions is not complete, the dynamics of sperm–zona pellucida interaction under HZA conditions are of high specificity[19,23,58,59].

Linear discriminant analysis demonstrated a most predictive hemizona index of approximately 30 for distinguishing subpopulations of patients with good versus poor fertilization rates. This hemizona index is very similar to the cutoff hemizona index levels published in prior studies[59,61] and to recently presented data evaluated by logistic regression analysis[67,68], and receiving operating characteristics[60] in the HZA. This hemizona index is, therefore, a main adjuvant in the evaluation of

Table 15 Semen parameters of patients with normal (⩾30) and low (<30) hemizona indices

HZI	*Conc. (×10⁶/mL)*	*Motility (%)*	*Forward progression (rated 0–4)*	*Normal morphology (%)*	*HZA (x±SD)*
HZI⩾30	82±52	49±10	2.5±0.3	14.0±6	63.8±56
HZI<30	52±45	44±12	2.7±0.3	7.9±6	17.1±9
P-value	0.006	0.04	0.01	0.0001	0.001

male-factor infertility. Its predictability for IVF cycles performed subsequently supports its use in the clinical setting.

Others have shown that the HZA may be useful in predicting fertilization outcome using oocyte microinsemination methods[68] and potentially applicable in immunological infertility. The utility of the HZA has also been expanded into the contraception technology as an antifertility assay[57]. Other sperm–zona binding tests have shown similar trends when exploring male infertility and IVF outcome[2]. Moreover, Oehninger *et al.*[57] signaled the role of the HZA to diagnose specific sperm defects when utilized in a sequential fashion with other sperm bioassays in the IVF setting.

FUTURE DEVELOPMENTS AND CONCLUSIONS

Defects of sperm–ooctye interaction are well recognized as underlying causes of human reproductive failure in assisted reproductive programs. The functional assays described in this chapter have been introduced as diagnostic tools to predict fertilization: the hemizona assay and the whole egg assay to record tight binding of human sperm to the human zona pellucida; the zona penetration assay to report on the ability of the sperm to capacitate and interact with and subsequently penetrate the zona pellucida; the zona-free penetration assay to evaluate the ability of oocytes that failed fertilization *in vitro*, to interact with fertile donor spermatozoa.

The complexity of the human fertilization process has led to the understanding and need for the development of a sequential analytical profile of those patients with unexplained fertilization failure[20,22]. The process is marked by multiple physiological steps that include sperm binding to the zona pellucida, sperm passage through the zona, binding to the oolemma, penetration into the oocyte, sperm nuclear decondensation and, finally, pronuclei formation and embryo cleavage. False positive results are likely to occur in the binding and penetration assays; however, in our experience, the incidence is low. This suggests that sperm binding to the zona is a critical step, and that post-binding defects might be in the minority.

We have shown that binding of sperm to hemizonae was significantly greater for men who succeeded in fertilization during IVF than in men who did not. Based on group data, we found that tight binding of spermatozoa to hemizonae correlated well with IVF performance. Our findings demonstrate no significant differences in sperm binding function when using hemizonae that were treated with high salt versus DMSO during storage. Furthermore, the kinetics of sperm binding were essentially the same regardless of the oocyte storage.

Abnormal sperm morphology is known to be a significant factor in failed fertilization. Semen specimens that were classified as morphologically poor by the strict Kruger method exhibited a significant impairment of sperm binding to the zona pellucida. Kruger reported that such semen, with $<4\%$ normal forms, were associated with a very low IVF fertilization rate (7.6% per oocyte) when using 0.05×10^6 sperm/mL.

Our present observations support the argument that the HZA can identify individual patients who are likely to encounter fertilization difficulties during IVF treatment. A diminished capacity for tight binding to the zona pellucida is implicated as a principal cause of fertilization failure in certain male-factor patients.

In summary, the bioassays discussed in this chapter seem to be useful diagnostic tests for estimating the fertilizing potential of human sperm. Other potential applications of the binding include:

(1) Sperm injection for fertilization, whereby sperm attached to the zona pellucida can be picked up into the micropipette (such sperm may be superior to other sperm picked at random without demonstrated affinity for the zona surface);

(2) Determining whether residual spermatogenesis (induced oligozoospermia) during male contraceptive therapy (such as gonadotropin-releasing hormone antagonist with testosterone treatment) is likely to lead to unwanted pregnancy; and

(3) Development of contraceptive vaccines, derived from either zona or sperm antigens, that can be titered on the ability to inhibit sperm–egg interaction in the HZA.

References

1. Overstreet, J. W., Yanagimachi, R., Katz, D. F., Hayashi, K. and Hanson, F. W. (1980). Penetration of human spermatozoa into the human zona pellucida and the zona-free hamster egg: a study of fertile donors and infertile patients. *Fertil. Steril.*, **33**, 534–42
2. Liu, D. Y., Clarke, G. N., Lopata, A., Johnston, W. I. H. and Baker, H. W. G. (1989). A sperm–zona pellucida binding test and *in vitro* fertilization. *Fertil. Steril.*, **52**, 281–7
3. Bedford, J. M. (1977). Sperm/egg interaction: the specificity of human spermatozoa. *Anat. Rec.*, **188**, 477–88
4. Overstreet, J. W. and Hembree, W. C. (1976). Penetration of zona pellucida of non-living human oocytes by human spermatozoa *in vitro*. *Fertil. Steril.*, **27**, 815–31
5. Burkman, L. J., Coddington, C. C., Franken, D. R., Kruger, T., Rosenwaks, Z. and Hodgen, G. (1988). The hemizona assay (HZA): development of a diagnostic test for the binding of human spermatozoa to human hemizona pellucida to predict fertilization potential. *Fertil. Steril.*, **49**, 688–93
6. Liu, D. Y. and Baker, H. W. G. (1988). The proportion of human sperm with poor morphology but normal intact acrosomes detected with *Pisum sativum* agglutinin correlates with fertilization *in vitro*. *Fertil. Steril.*, **50**, 288–93
7. Tesarik, J. (1989). The potential diagnostic use of human zona-free eggs prepared from oocytes that failed to fertilize *in vitro*. *Fertil. Steril.*, **52**, 821–4
8. Lanzendorf, S. E., Oehninger, S., Scott, R., Whitelock and Hodgen, G. D. (1994). Penetration of human spermatozoa through the zona pellucida of non-viable human oocytes. *J. Soc. Gynecol. Invest.*.,**1**, 69–73
9. Franken, D. R., Burkman, L. J., Oehninger, S., Veeck, L. L., Kruger, T. F., Coddington, C. C. and Hodgen, G. D. (1989). The hemizona assay using salt stored human oocytes: evaluation of zona pellucida capacity for binding human spermatozoa. *Gamete Res.*, **22**, 15–26
10. Franken, D. R., Oehninger, S., Burkman, L. J., Coddington, C. C., Kruger, T. F., Rosenwaks, Z., Acosta, A. A. and Hodgen, G. D. (1989). The hemizona assay (HZA): a predictor of human sperm fertilizing potential in *in vitro* fertilization (IVF) treatment. *J. In Vitro Fertil. Embryo Transf.*, **6**, 44–9
11. Franken, D. R., Burkman, L. J., Oehninger, S., Coddington, C. C. and Hodgen, G. (1989). In Acosta, A. A., Swanson, R. J., Ackerman, S. B., Kruger, T. F., van Zyl, J. A. and Menkveld, R. (eds.) *Human Hemizona Attachment Assay (HZA) in Human Spermatozoa in Assisted Reproduction.* (USA: Williams and Wilkins)
12. Oehninger, S., Coddington, C. C., Scott, R., Franken, D. R., Burkman, L. J., Acosta, A. A. and Hodgen, G. D. (1989). Hemizona assay: assessment of sperm dysfunction and prediction of *in vitro* fertilization outcome. *Fertil. Steril.*, **51**, 665–70
13. Van Zyl, J. A. (1980). The infertile couple. Part II. Examination and evaluation of semen. *S. Afr. Med. J.*, **57**, 485–9
14. Menkveld, R., Stander, F. S. H., Kotze, T. J. v.W., Kruger, T. F. and van Zyl, J. A. (1990). The evaluation of morphological characteristics of human spermatozoa according to stricter criteria. *Hum. Reprod.*, **5**, 586–92
15. World Health Organization. (1987). *WHO Laboratory Manual for the Examination of Human Semen and Semen–Cervical Mucus Interaction*, pp. 55–80. (Cambridge: The Press Syndicate of the University of Cambridge)
16. Kruger, T. F., Ackerman, S. B., Simmons, K. F., Swanson, R. J., Brugo, S. and Acosta, A. A. (1987). A quick reliable staining technique for sperm morphology. *Arch. Androl.*, **18**, 275–8
17. Kruger, T. F., Acosta, A. A., Simmons, F. F., Swanson, R. J., Matta, J. F. and Oehninger, S. (1988). Predictive value of abnormal sperm morphology in *in vitro* fertilization. *Fertil. Steril.*, **49**, 112–17
18. McDowell, J. S. (1986). Preparation of spermatozoa for insemination *in vitro*. In Jones, H. W. Jr, Jones, G. S., Hodgen, G. D. and Rosenwaks, Z. (eds.) *In Vitro Fertilization*, p. 162. (Norfolk, Baltimore: Williams and Wilkins)
19. Franken, D. R., Kruger, T. F., Lombard, C., Oehninger, S. C., Acosta, A. A. and Hodgen, G. D. (1993). The ability of the hemizona assay to predict human fertilization *in vitro* in different IVF/GIFT cycles. *Hum. Reprod.*, **8**, 1240–4
20. Oehninger, S., Coddington, C. C., Scott, R., Franken, D. R., Burkman, L. J., Acosta, A. A. and Hodgen, G. D. (1989). Hemizona assay: assessment of sperm dysfunction and prediction of IVF outcome. *Fertil. Steril.*, **51**, 665–70
21. Hammit, D. G., Syrop, C. H., Walker, D. L. and Bennet, M. R. (1993). Conditions of oocyte storage and use of noninseminated as compared with inseminated, nonfertilized oocytes for the hemizona assay. *Fertil. Steril.*, **60**, 131–6
22. Oehninger, S., Acosta, A., Veeck, L., Brzyski, R., Kruger, T. F., Muasher, S. J. and Hodgen, G. D. (1991). Recurrent failure of *in vitro* fertilization: role of the hemizona assay in the sequential diagnosis of specific sperm–oocyte defects. *Am. J. Obstet. Gynecol.*, **164**, 1210–5
23. Kruger, T. F., Oehninger, S., Franken, D. R. and Hodgen, G. D. (1991). Hemizona assay: use of fresh versus salt-stored human oocytes to evaluate sperm binding potential to the zona pellucida. *J.* In Vitro *Fertil. Embryo Transf.*, **8**, 154–6
24. Cross, N. L., Lambert, H. and Samuels, S. (1986).

Sperm binding activity of the zona pellucida of immature mouse oocytes. *Cell Biol. Reprod.*, **10**, 545–54

25. Bavister, D. B. (1989). A consistently successful procedure for *in vitro* fertilization of golden hamster eggs. *Gamete Res.*, **23**, 139–58
26. Yanagimachi, R., Yanagimachi, H. and Rogers, B. J. (1986). The use of zona-free animal ova as a test system for the assessment of the fertilizing capacity of human spermatozoa. *Biol. Reprod.*, **15**, 471–6
27. Franken, D. R., Coddington, C. C., Burkman, L. J., Oosthuizen, W. T., Oehninger, S., Kruger, T. F. and Hodgen, G. D. (1991). Defining the valid hemizona assay: accounting for binding variability within zonae pellucidae and within semen samples from fertile males. *Fertil. Steril.*, **56**, 1156–61
28. Perreault, S. and Rogers, B. J. (1982). Capacitation pattern of human spermatozoa. *Fertil. Steril.*, **38**, 258–60
29. Blazak, W. F., Overstreet, J. W., Katz, D. F. and Hanson, F. W. (1982). A competitive *in vitro* assay of human sperm fertilizing ability utilizing contrasting fluorescent sperm markers. *J. Androl.*, **3**, 165–71
30. Liu, D. Y. and Baker, H. W. G. (1993). Inhibition of acrosin activity with a Trypsin inhibitor blocks human sperm penetration of the zona pellucida. *Biol. Reprod.*, **48**, 340–8
31. Liu, D. Y., Lopata, A., Leung, A., Johnston, W. H. and Gordon Baker, W. H. (1988). A human sperm–zona pellucida binding test using oocytes that failed to fertilize *in vitro*. *Fertil. Steril.*, **50**, 782–8
32. Oehninger, S., Toner, J. P., Muasher, S. J., Coddington, C. C., Acosta, A. A. and Hodgen, G. D. (1992). Prediction of fertilization *in vitro* with human gametes: Is there a litmus test? *Am. J. Obstet. Gynecol.*, **167**, 1760–7.
33. Hammit, D. G., Walker, D. L., Syrop, C. H., Miller, T. M. and Bennet, M. A. (1991). Treatment of severe male-factor infertility with high concentration of motile sperm by microinsemination in embryo cryopreservation straws. *J. In Vitro Fertil Embryo Transf.*, **8**, 101–10
34. Barros, C., Jedlicki, A. and Vigil, P. (1988). The gamete membrane fusion test to assay the fertilizing ability of human spermatozoa. *Hum. Reprod.*, **3**, 637–44
35. Tesarik, J. (1990). Zona pellucida penetrability of metaphase I and II human oocytes after aging and salt treatment. *Fertil. Steril.*, **54**, 346–50
36. Franken, D. R., Oosthuizen, W. T., Cooper, S., Kruger, T. F., Burkman, L. J., Coddington, C. C. and Hodgen, G. D. (1991). Electron microscopic evidence on the acrosomal status of bound sperm and their penetration into human hemizonae pellucida after storage in a buffered salt solution. *Andrologia*, **23**, 205–8
37. Bleil, J. D. and Wasserman, P. M. (1980). Structure and function of the zona pellucida: Identification and characterization of the proteins of the mouse oocyte's zona pellucida. *Dev. Biol.*, **76**, 185–203
38. O'Rand, M. G., Matthews, J. E., Welch, J. E. and Fisher, S. J. (1985). Identification of zona binding proteins of rabbit, pig, human and mouse spermatozoa on nitrocellulose blots. *J. Exp. Zool.*, **235**, 423–8
39. O'Rand, M. G. (1988). Sperm–egg recognition and barriers to interspecies fertilization. *Gamete Res.*, **19**, 315–28
40. Shabanowitz, R. B. and O'Rand, M. G. (1988). Characterization of the human zona pellucida from fertilized and unfertilized oocytes. *J. Reprod. Fertil.*, **82**, 151–61
41. Veeck, L. L. (1988). Oocyte assessment and biological performance. *Ann. N.Y. Acad. Sci.*, **541**, 259–74
42. Menkveld, R., Franken, D. R., Kruger, T. F., Oehninger, S. C. and Hodgen, G. D. (1991). Sperm selection capacity of the human zona pellucida. *Mol. Reprod. Dev.*, **30**, 346–52
43. Yoshimatsu, N., Yanagimachi, R. and Lopata, A. (1988). Zona pellucidae of salt-stored hamster and human eggs: their penetrability by homologous and heterologous spermatozoa. *Gamete Res.*, **21**, 115–26
44. Yanagimachi, R., Lopata, A., Odom, C. B., Bronson, R. A., Mahi, C. A. and Nicolson, G. L. (1979). Retention of biologic characteristics of zona pellucida in highly concentrated salt solution: the use of salt-stored eggs for assessing the fertilizing capacity of spermatozoa. *Fertil. Steril.*, **31**, 562–74
45. Familiari, G., Nottola, S. A., Micara, G., Aragona, C. and Motta, P. M. (1988). Is the sperm binding capacity of the zona pellucida linked to its surface structure: A scanning electron microscopic study of human *in vitro* fertilization. *J.* In Vitro *Fertil. Embryo Transf.*, **3**, 134–43
46. Chen, C. and Sathananthan, A. H. (1986). Early penetration of human sperm through the vestments of human eggs *in vitro*. *Arch. Androl.*, **16**, 183–7
47. Clarke, G. N., Lopata, A., McBain, J. C., Baker, H. W. G. and Johnston, W. I. H. (1985). Effect of sperm antibodies in males on human *in vitro* fertilization (IVF). *Am. J. Reprod. Immunol.*, **8**, 62–6
48. Cohen, J., Edwards, R. G., Fehilly, C. B., Fishel, S. B., Hewitt, J., Rowland, G. F., Steptoe, P. C., Walters, D. E. and Webster, J. (1985). *In vitro* fertilization using cryopreserved donor semen in cases when both partners are infertile. *Fertil. Steril.*, **43**, 570–4
49. Mahadevan, M. M. and Trounson, A. O. (1984). Relationship of fine structure of head to fertility of frozen semen. *Fertil. Steril.*, **41**, 287–93
50. Critser, J., Huse-Benda, A., Aakar, D., Arneson, B. and Ball, G. (1987). Cryopreservation of human spermatozoa. I. Effects of holding procedure and seeding on motility, fertilizability and acrosome reaction. *Fertil. Steril.*, **47**, 656–63
51. Oehninger, S. C., Franken, D. R., Kruger, T. F., Toner, J. P., Acosta, A. A. and Hodgen, G. D. (1991). Hemizona assay: sperm defect analysis, a diagnostic

method for assessment of human sperm–oocyte interactions, and predictive value for fertilization outcome. In Seppala, M. and Hamberger, L. (eds.) *Frontiers in Human Reproduction*, pp. 111–24. (New York: Academy of Science)
52. Fredricsson, B., Waxegård, G., Brege, S. and Lundberg, I. (1977). On the morphology of live spermatozoa in human semen. *Fertil. Steril.*, **28**, 168–74
53. Katz, D. F., Diel, L. and Overstreet, J. W. (1982). Differences in the movement of morphologically normal and abnormal human seminal spermatozoa. *Biol. Reprod.*, **26**, 566–70
54. Kruger, T. F., Menkveld, R., Stander, F. S. H., Lombard, C. J., van der Merwe, J. P., van Zyl, J. A. and Smith, K. (1986). Sperm morphologic features as a prognostic factor in *in vitro* fertilization. *Fertil. Steril.*, **46**, 1118–23
55. Mahadevan, M. D., Trounson, A. O., Wood, C. and Leeton, J. F. (1987). Effect of oocyte quality and sperm characteristics on the number of spermatozoa bound to the zona pellucida of human oocytes inseminated *in vitro*. *J.* In Vitro *Fertil. Embryo Transf.*, **4**, 223–7
56. Liu, D. Y., Lopata, A., Johnston, W. I. H. and Baker, H. W. G. (1989). Human sperm–zona pellucida binding, sperm characteristics and *in vitro* fertilization. *Hum. Reprod.*, **4**, 696–701
57. Franken, D. R., Kruger, T. F., Menkveld, R., Oehninger, S. C., Coddington, C. C. and Hodgen, G. D. (1990). Hemizona assay and teratozoospermia: increasing sperm insemination concentrations to enhance zona pellucida binding. *Fertil. Steril.*, **54**, 497–503
58. Testart, J., Lasalle, B., Frydman, R. and Belaisch, J. C. (1983). A study of factors affecting the success of human fertilization *in vitro*. II. Influence of semen quality and oocyte maturity on fertilization and cleavage. *Biol. Reprod.*, **28**, 425–31
59. Bronson, R., Cooper, G. and Rosenfeld, D. (1982). Sperm-specific isoantibodies and autoantibodies inhibit the binding of human sperm to the human zona pellucida. *Fertil. Steril.*, **38**, 724–9
60. Coddington, C. C., Olive, D., Toner, J. P. and Acosta, A. A. (1992). Predictability of sperm fertilization capacity is excellent in IVF patients using the hemizona index (HZI). *J. Androl.*
61. Clarke, G. N., Lopata, A. and Johnston, W. I. H. (1986). Effect of sperm antibodies in females on human *in vitro* fertilization. *Fertil. Steril.*, **46**, 435–41
62. Jager, S., Kremer, J. and Van Slochteren-Draaisma, T. (1978). A simple method of screening for antisperm antibodies in the human male. Detection of spermatozoal surface IgG with the direct mixed antiglobulin reaction test on untreated fresh human semen. *Int. J. Fertil.*, **23**, 12–21
64. Friberg, J. (1974). A simple and sensitive micromethod for demonstration of sperm agglutinating activity in serum from infertile men and women. *Acta Obstet. Gynecol. Scand. Suppl.*, **36**, 21–9
65. Oehninger, S. and Hodgen, G. D. (1991). How to evaluate spermatozoa for assisted reproduction. In Decherney, A. (ed.). *Assisted Reproduction Review*, pp. 15–17. (Baltimore: Williams and Wilkins)
66. Oehninger, S., Alexander, N. J., Franken, D. R., Coddington, C. C., Burkman, L. J., Kruger, T. F., Acosta, A. A. and Hodgen, G. D. (1989). Antifertilization assays. In Alexander, N. J., Griffin, D., Spieler, J. M. and Waistes, G. (eds.) *Gamete Interaction: Prospects for Immunocontraception*, pp. 283–7. (New York: Wiley-Liss)
67. Van der Merwe, J. P., Kruger, T. F., Windt, M. L., Hulme, V. A. and Menkveld, R. (1990). Treatment of male sperm autoimmunity by using the gamete intrafallopian transfer procedure with washed spermatozoa. *Fertil. Steril.*, **53**, 682–7
68. Oehninger, S. C., Acosta, A. A., Morshedi, M., Veeck, L. L., Swanson, R. J., Simmons, K. F. and Rosenwaks, Z. (1988). Corrective measures and pregnancy outcome in IVF in patients with severe morphology abnormalities. *Fertil. Steril.*, **50**, 283–97
69. Oehninger, S., Veeck, L. L., Franken, D. R., Kruger, T. F., Acosta, A. A. and Hodgen, G. D. (1991). Human preovulatory oocytes have a higher sperm-binding ability than immature oocytes under hemizona assay conditions: evidence supporting the concept of 'zona maturation'. *Fertil. Steril.*, **55**, 1165–70
70. Oehninger, S. (1992). Diagnostic significance of sperm–zona pellucida interaction. In Smith, K. (ed.) *Reproductive Medicine Review*, pp. 57–81. (England: Hodder and Stoughton)

Reactive oxygen species in the context of diagnostic andrology

21

D. S. Irvine and R. J. Aitken

INTRODUCTION

The past decade has seen considerable progress in our understanding of testicular function and of the process of sperm production, spermatogenesis. We have begun to understand the basis of some cases of male infertility at molecular[1] and genomic[2] levels, and have started to unravel the biochemistry of sperm cell dysfunction[3]. However, a recent editorial in *The International Journal of Andrology*[4] summarized the current state of the art with regard to the clinical investigation and treatment of male infertility thus: 'Despite all this frenetic activity, the stark reality is that there have been virtually no advances in the clinical practice of male infertility. Where advances have occurred, they have affected relatively few patients.' However, in the past few years, the development and successful application of techniques of micro-assisted fertilization have revolutionized the therapeutic prospects for infertile men[5,6]. Indeed, the development of intracytoplasmic sperm injection (ICSI) has led some commentators to speculate that striving to diagnose sperm dysfunction or to understand the causation of male infertility is now futile, because ICSI provides the solution, whatever the problem might be.

While there can be little doubt that ICSI represents a major breakthrough in the treatment of male infertility, male infertility or even sperm dysfunction are symptoms, not diagnoses and thus, *in vitro* fertilization (IVF) and ICSI represent symptomatic, albeit successful, treatments. In addition to the genuine clinical problems of a treatment which is not predicated upon a diagnosis, one of the principal long-term goals for any clinician working with infertile patients must be primary prevention of the condition, which will remain unattainable if we fail to uncover the etiology of male infertility, most of which is currently unexplained[7].

The prevalence of subfertility in Europe has been estimated to be between 14% and 17% of couples, that is, one couple in six[8–10]. Within this population of infertile couples, defective sperm function is commonly identified as the single most common cause[8,9], accounting for some 25% of couples attending clinics. Moreover, studies using bioassays of sperm–oocyte fusion have suggested that, in cases of so-called unexplained infertility, defective sperm function may be present in about one-third of couples, even though the conventional semen profile is normal[11]. Similarly, among couples in which the male partner has oligozoospermia, available evidence suggests that sperm function is intact in some 30% of cases[12]. Despite this high prevalence of male subfertility until recently there were very few, if any, effective treatments, a situation which directly reflects our lack of knowledge of the fundamental cell biology of the human spermatozoon, and our poor understanding of the defects present in the spermatozoa of infertile men at the level of cell and molecular biology.

In a significant proportion of men whose spermatozoa fail to fuse with zona-free hamster oocytes, this failure persists even when a calcium influx and cellular alkalinization is induced by the ionophore A23187[13,14] suggesting that, in many patients, the molecular defects in sperm function lie downstream from calcium influx. The early observation that human spermatozoa are susceptible to lipid peroxidation[15–17], and that the spermatozoa of some animal species are capable of generating reactive oxygen species, led to the hypothesis that peroxidative damage to the plasma membrane of the human spermatozoon may contribute to the origins of male subfertility[3].

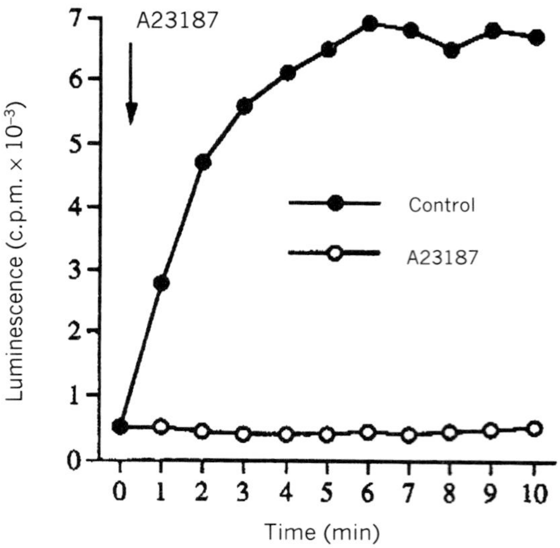

Figure 1 Generation of reactive oxygen species by human spermatozoa in response to the divalent cation ionophore A23187. Reproduced with permission of Journals of Reproduction and Fertility Ltd[3]. ●, Control; ○, A23187

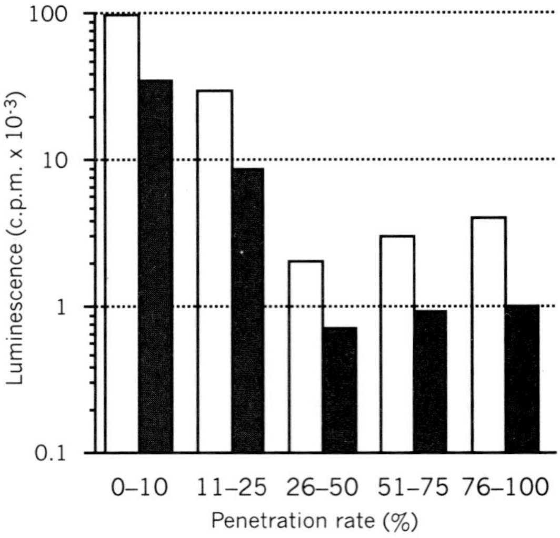

Figure 2 Generation of reactive oxygen species by human spermatozoa and their functional competence expressed in zona-free hamster oocyte penetration. Samples with high mean levels of reactive oxygen species production show low levels of sperm oocyte fusion. Data modified from Aitken and Clarkson (1987)[3] (note logarithmic axis). ■, A23187; □, control

REACTIVE OXYGEN SPECIES GENERATION BY HUMAN SPERMATOZOA

In 1987 independent studies by Aitken and Clarkson[3] and Alvarez *et al.*[18] confirmed a suggestion made half a century before by John MacLeod[19], that human spermatozoa have the capacity to generate reactive oxygen species (ROS) (Figure 1). It was subsequently demonstrated that seminal leukocytes, particularly neutrophils, were also frequently present as cellular contaminants in human sperm suspensions, and could make an additional contribution to the levels of ROS generation recorded[20]. The clinical significance of this ROS production by the human ejaculate became apparent when it was demonstrated that the intensity of this activity was positively correlated with the incidence of defective sperm function as assessed *in vivo* and *in vitro* (Figure 2)[3,21,22].

The mechanism by which ROS damage spermatozoa appears to involve an oxidative attack on the lipids present in the sperm plasma membrane leading to the initiation of a lipid peroxidation cascade. As a consequence of this pathological process, the spermatozoa lose their capacity for movement, acrosome reaction and sperm–oocyte fusion[15,23]. The reactive oxygen intermediate that appears to be cytotoxic toward human spermatozoa is hydrogen peroxide (H_2O_2)[24,25]. H_2O_2 also appears to be the major oxygen metabolite detected in chemiluminescence assays of ROS generation by human spermatozoa[26] and derives from the intracellular dismutation of superoxide anion ($O_2^{-}\cdot$) under the influence of superoxide dismutase. In addition to H_2O_2, the lipid peroxides generated as a consequence of the peroxidation process also appear to be profoundly cytotoxic, as do their degradation products, such as (*E*) 4-hydroxy-2-nonenal[27–29].

ANTIOXIDANT DEFENSE

If H_2O_2 is damaging to human spermatozoa, then enzymes that scavenge this powerful oxidant, such as catalase or glutathione peroxidase, ought to be an important part of the anti-oxidant defenses employed by human spermatozoa[30,31]. There is evidence to support the presence of both of these enzymes in human spermatozoa with particular importance being attached to the glutathione peroxidase content of these cells[31]. In addition, human spermatozoa contain superoxide dismutase, an enzyme that catalyzes the dismutation of the $O_2^{-\cdot}$ to H_2O_2 and may be part of the interactive network of defense mechanisms employed by these cells against oxidative stress.

However, whether antioxidant enzymes can ever make a profound contribution to the protection of human spermatozoa is questionable because these enzymes appear to be confined to the cytoplasm localized in the sperm midpiece. From this position, they would be unable to protect the plasma membrane covering the vulnerable regions of the sperm head and tail. Indeed, the lack of cytoplasmic space is a particularly striking feature of spermatozoa in general, which contributes significantly to their vulnerability to oxidative stress. Nature's solution to this problem has been to transfer the responsibility for protecting spermatozoa against free radical attack from the cytoplasm to the extracellular fluids that bathe these cells. It is for this reason that seminal plasma has been shown to be such a potent source of antioxidants, including superoxide dismutase, uric acid, α-tocopherol and vitamin E[15,30]. Moreover, spermatozoa are known to be coated in lactoferrin, an iron-binding protein that plays a significant role in removing this important transition metal from sites where it may catalyze peroxidative damage.

Seminal plasma is not the only extracellular fluid in the male reproductive tract to possess antioxidant factors. Recent reports of unique secreted forms of glutathione peroxidase and superoxide dismutase in the mammalian epididymis emphasize the importance of epididymal plasma in the protection of spermatozoa from peroxidative damage during their prolonged storage in the cauda epididymis[32,33].

LIPID PEROXIDATION

The susceptibility of human spermatozoa to oxidative stress stems from the abundance of unsaturated fatty acids in the sperm plasma membrane, the presence of which gives this structure the fluidity it needs to engage in the membrane fusion events associated with fertilization. Unfortunately, the presence of double bonds in these molecules makes them vulnerable to free radical attack and the initiation of a peroxidation cascade (Figure 3). Recent studies concerning the chemistry of lipid peroxidation in human spermatozoa[29,34] suggest that once this process has been initiated its propagation is impeded, leading to the accumulation of lipid peroxides in the sperm plasma membrane. Addition of ferrous ions to the spermatozoa causes these lipid peroxides to break down and generate small molecular mass metabolites, such as malondialdehyde, that can be readily detected in simple biochemical assays. As a consequence, the iron-promoted malondialdehyde assay can be used to give an indication of the oxidative stress that a given sperm population has suffered during its life history. The malondialdehyde assay therefore constitutes a useful diagnostic tool, the outcome of which correlates significantly with the motility of these cells and their competence for sperm–oocyte fusion (Figures 4,5)[23]. This loss of sperm function as a result of lipid peroxidation reflects the negative impact that lipid peroxides have on membrane fluidity and the activity of key membrane-bound enzymes, such as Ca^{2+}/Mg^{2+} ATPases, that are involved in maintaining calcium homeostasis within these cells.

LEUKOCYTES

In view of the fact that leukocytes represent a powerful source of ROS in the human ejaculate, a number of studies have been conducted into the relationships between the presence of these cells, peroxidative damage to human spermatozoa and the potential for fertilization. In general, these studies have indicated that the fertility of human spermatozoa *in vivo* and *in vitro* is unrelated to the size and the composition of the seminal leukocyte population. Even samples that possess more leukocytes than the WHO threshold for leukocytospermia (10^7/mL) have been shown to have normal sperm function *in vitro* and to be capable of establishing pregnancies *in vivo*[35].

The major reason why leukocytes do not damage human spermatozoa is presumably because the latter are protected in semen by the powerful antioxidant properties exhibited by seminal plasma. If the sites of leukocytic infiltration are the secondary sexual glands and the urethra, then the first time the spermatozoa will make contact with these cells will be at the moment of ejaculation. At this moment, the spermatozoa will be protected from the damaging effects of leukocyte-derived ROS by seminal plasma.

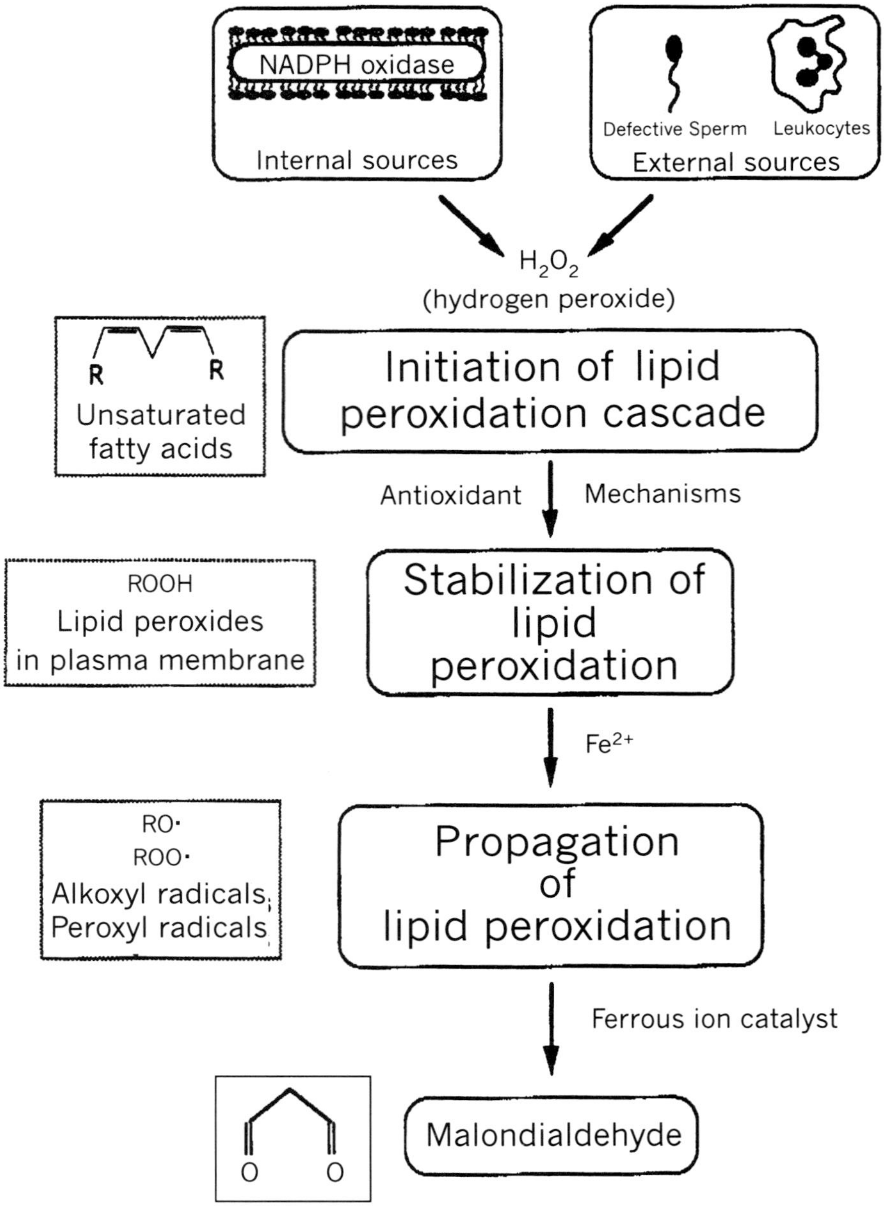

Figure 3 Pathways of lipid peroxidation in human spermatozoa. Peroxidation is initiated either through the intrinsic generation of ROS by spermatozoa or by exposure to exogenous sources of ROS such as leukocytes. Lipid peroxidases subsequently accumulate in the plasma membrane and disrupt sperm function. On addition of ferrous ions, these lipid peroxides break down and propagate the damage through the membrane, generating small carbonyl compounds such as malondialdehyde in the process. This by-product may be measured and used as an indication of the degree of peroxidative damage experienced by the spermatozoa during their life history. Malondialdehyde can be used as an endpoint for assessing the peroxidative damage sustained by human sperm suspensions

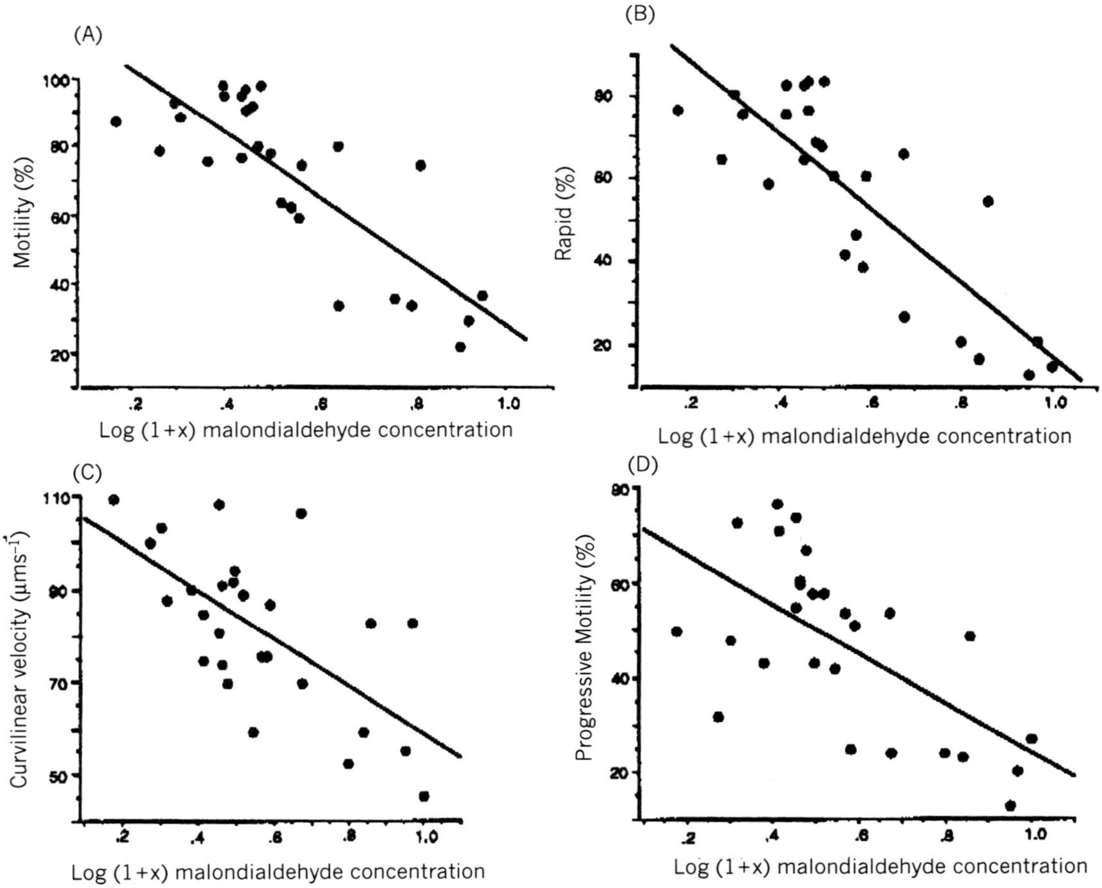

Figure 4 Measurement of malondialdehyde generation in the presence of ferrous ions exhibits a negative correlation with sperm movement as illustrated by (A) percentage motility, (B) percentage of rapid cells moving at >25 μm/s, (C) curvilinear velocity, and (D) percentage of progressive cells. Data from Aitken *et al.* (1993)[76] with permission of Journals of Reproduction and Fertility Ltd

This protection breaks down during the preparation of spermatozoa for assisted reproduction therapy. Thus, if the spermatozoa are prepared by washing the cells free of seminal plasma and then allowing the most motile spermatozoa to 'swim-up', there is ample opportunity for the normal spermatozoa to become damaged by ROS emanating from the defective gametes and/or leukocytes present in the same compacted pellet. It is for this reason that spermatozoa prepared by procedures that involve the centrifugation and compaction of unfractionated semen are potentially so damaging to the spermatozoa[36]. In contrast, sperm selection procedures that involve isolation of the most functional cells while they are still protected by seminal plasma, such as swim-up from semen or Percoll gradient centrifugation, generate populations of purified cells that, in comparative trials, are demonstrably superior to those involving sperm isolation from a washed, compacted pellet[36].

Since the presence of leukocytes will be a major factor in determining whether spermatozoa might suffer peroxidative damage during their preparation, it is important to determine the level of leukocyte infiltration[37]. This strategy has been used to demonstrate that even sperm suspensions purified by centrifugation through isotonic Percoll are frequently contaminated with leukocytes[37]. If these residual leukocytes are removed with magnetic beads, then the responses to N-formyl-methionyl-

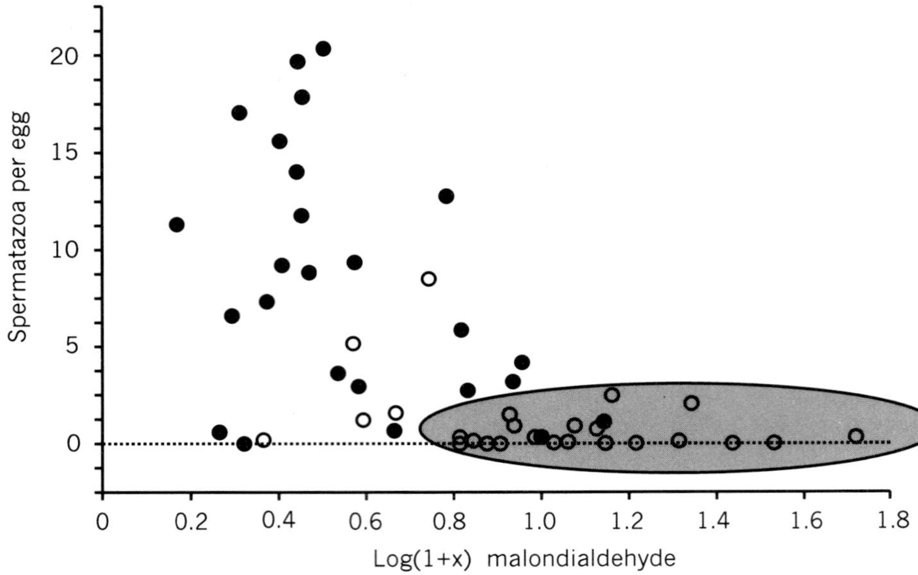

Figure 5 Inverse correlation between malondialdehyde generation and sperm–oocyte fusion. Samples exhibiting low levels of sperm–oocyte fusion in association with high levels of lipid peroxidation have been ringed. Data from Aitken *et al.* (1993) with permission of Journals of Reproduction and Fertility Ltd[76]

leucyl-phenylalanine (FMLP) stimulation are no longer observed, although approximately half of such samples still retain the ability to respond to phorbol ester stimulation. In such cases, the ROS must be originating from the spermatozoa[37].

Since the contamination of human sperm suspensions with neutrophils creates a condition of oxidative stress associated with the loss of sperm motility[38], the detection and removal of these cells would seem an important objective to achieve in the context of IVF therapy. Indeed, recent studies have shown that the use of antibody-coated magnetic beads to effect the rapid removal of leukocytes from Percoll-purified human sperm preparations leads to a significant increase in sperm function[39]. Moreover, in a recent analysis of the attributes of semen quality that best predicted IVF success, the presence of contaminating leukocytes was found to be a powerful prognostic factor that was significantly associated with a reduction in fertilization rates.

REACTIVE OXYGEN SPECIES IN THE DIAGNOSIS OF MALE INFERTILITY

While the traditional semen profile can be regarded as the foundation on which diagnostic andrology has been built, it is important to appreciate the limitations of this form of descriptive analysis. In the small percentage of cases exhibiting azoospermia or severe oligospermia, there can be no doubt that the semen profile is providing definitive diagnostic information. However, among those patients with less severe oligozoospermia the available evidence suggests that about one in three will possess functionally competent spermatozoa[13,40]. Conversely, among patients with apparently normal semen, about one in three will have demonstrably defective sperm function[41]. Repeatedly, in prospective studies of infertile couples[40,42–44], and in retrospective studies of semen used in donor insemination[45], the conventional criteria of semen quality have proven to be of limited value in predicting the achievement of pregnancy. This lack of prognostic value is due to the fact that one of the basic tenets of the conventional semen profile, namely that fertility requires the presence of more than a certain critical number of motile, morphologically normal spermatozoa, is misleading. It is misleading because it places the emphasis on *number*. A large number of spermatozoa is not required to initiate a pregnancy. It is not so much the *number* of spermatozoa that is critical, it is their *function*. Realization of this fact initiated an important phase in the evolution of diagnostic andrology, characterized by the development of a complex range of bioassays with which to assess the functional competence of human spermatozoa.

SPERM FUNCTION

The diagnosis of defective sperm function is a difficult issue because the spermatozoon is such a sophisticated cell. In order to achieve its objective of fertilizing the ovum, the male gamete has to display a wide variety of diverse properties involving differential patterns of movement, membrane restructuring during capacitation, zona recognition, signal transduction, acrosomal exocytosis, the concomitant processing of recognition and fusion molecules on the sperm head and, ultimately, fusion with the vitelline membrane of the oocyte itself. In view of this complexity, it follows that the functional assessment of human spermatozoa cannot be achieved on the basis of any single global test. Instead, a range of bioassays has been developed, each one of which focuses on a different aspect of sperm function. These include assessment of sperm–cervical mucus interaction[46–49], hyperactivated motility[50,51], sperm–zona interaction[52], the acrosome reaction[14] and sperm–oocyte interaction[45,53,54].

BIOCHEMICAL CRITERIA OF SPERM FUNCTION

The functional bioassays outlined above are perhaps best viewed as research tools with which to examine the facets of normal and abnormal sperm function at biochemical and molecular levels, leading not only to an improved understanding of the causes of sperm dysfunction, but to more widely applicable assays. The observation that dysfunctional spermatozoa often produce excessive reactive oxygen species[55] constitutes the first implementation of this approach. This problem appears to be particularly common among men with oligozoospermia[56], although it is also clear that, in a significant number of cases, the excessive production of reactive oxygen species observed is a consequence of leukocyte infiltration[37,57]. The causes and clinical consequences of this remain to be elucidated.

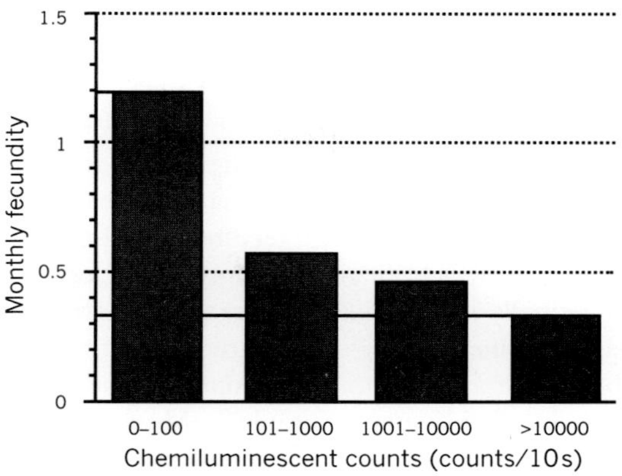

Figure 6 Monthly fecundity in relation to reactive oxygen species production in a prospective study of 139 couples with a normal female partner. Data from Aitken *et al.* (1991)[54] with permission of Mosby – Year Book Inc.

In a series of prospective studies of couples with unexplained infertility[43] and oligozoospermia[40], and in retrospective studies of semen used in donor insemination[45], we have previously shown that data on sperm motion, together with the zona-free hamster oocyte penetration test, provide clinically useful data in predicting *in vivo* fertilizing ability. However, in a recent prospective study of 139 couples attending the Infertility Clinic in Edinburgh Royal Infirmary[54], the diagnostic value of the conventional semen profile, the zona-free hamster oocyte penetration test and the generation of reactive oxygen species were examined. In all cases, the female partner was normal and the couples were followed for up to 4 years after assessment to determine the incidence of spontaneous pregnancy. Using life table analysis, it was observed that the zona-free hamster oocyte penetration test in the presence of the ionophore A23187 was highly positively correlated with fertility, and conversely, the generation of reactive oxygen species was negatively associated with fertility, while the conventional semen profile was of no diagnostic value (Figure 6).

More recently, an examination of the relationship between various attributes of sperm function and the outcomes of human *in vitro* fertilization has observed important relationships between reactive oxygen species generation in response to both FMLP and phorbol miristate acetate (PMA) and the outcome of human IVF.

REACTIVE OXYGEN SPECIES AND THE TREATMENT OF MALE INFERTILITY

Treatment of infertile male patients has generally been unrewarding because of a lack of clear scientific justification for many interventions. The conditions for which logical treatments exist are individually uncommon, and treatments are often relatively ineffective – reconstructive surgery for obstructive azoospermia secondary to epididymal occlusion being one example[59]. Most forms of medical treatment have not been of proven benefit, while corticosteroid treatment of men with antisperm antibodies[60] and the diagnosis and treatment of varicocele remain matters of controversy[61]. The case for intrauterine insemination (with or without superovulation) also remains controversial, with some authors reporting benefit[62] and others not[63]. For many couples, the only approach to treatment with a realistic chance of producing a pregnancy has been to resort to donor insemination[64,65]. Because of the relative lack of success of treatment of male infertility, and the significant impact of coincidental female factors, assisted reproductive technologies have become very important in dealing with couples with 'male factor' infertility.

The recognition of the role of reactive oxygen species in the etiology of male infertility raises, almost for the first time, the possibility of devising rational strategies of treatment. At present the potential value of treating infertile men with antioxidants, for example, remains to be formally explored. Lenzi and colleagues have examined the impact of treatment with parenteral glutathione in men with abnormal semen quality[66,67], and have observed effects on sperm motility, suggesting that the antioxidant effect may be exerted at the level of the epididymis. Other workers have demonstrated that the oral administration of the chain breaking anti-oxidant α-tocopherol (vitamin E) leads to increased amounts of this antioxidant in seminal plasma[68]. Moreover, the observation of reactive oxygen species production by seminal leukocytes and the recognition that classical techniques for quantifying these cells are inadequate raises the need for detailed work into the diagnosis and treatment of seminal leukocytosis[69], for example, with antibiotics.

REACTIVE OXYGEN SPECIES AND IMPLICATIONS FOR ASSISTED REPRODUCTION

All techniques of assisted reproduction involve the separation of motile spermatozoa from seminal plasma. The earliest techniques involved repeated cycles of centrifugation and resuspension of spermatozoa in culture media, and while this approach effectively separates spermatozoa from seminal plasma there is no element of cell selection, and suspensions prepared in this way will retain any contaminating leukocytes, non-cellular debris and epithelial cells that were present in the original sample. Selection of spermatozoa can be achieved by allowing sperm to swim-up from a centrifuged pellet, or directly from seminal plasma into culture media[70]. These approaches all rely on the motility of the spermatozoa and are thus not applicable to sperm preparation of suboptimal semen samples. More recent approaches have relied on the use of buoyant density gradient centrifugation using media such as Percoll[71–73] to select functional spermatozoa actively by virtue of their enhanced velocity and relatively high density. It has been shown that cells prepared by this approach have an enhanced capacity for fertilization[72] and Aitken and Clarkson[36] have shown that the deleterious effects of centrifugation are related to a burst of reactive oxygen species produced by a discrete subpopulation of cells which can be separated from the normal and functional cells by buoyant density gradient centrifugation.

In a recent study of the relationship between lipid peroxidation and human sperm function, it was observed that the way in which individual ejaculate fractionated on discontinuous Percoll gradients was highly positively correlated with the lipoperoxidation status of the spermatozoa, the greater the potential for malondialdehyde formation, the higher the proportion of cells entering the low density portion of the Percoll gradient. In addition, the lipoperoxidation potential was strongly associated with the capacity of the sperm movement, sperm–oocyte fusion in response to A23187 and was associated with the presence of midpiece abnormalities[23]. In further studies, the correlation between the degree of lipid peroxidation experienced by the spermatozoon and their fertilizing potential *in vitro* and *in vivo* needs to be ascertained. In diagnostic terms, there may be significant advantages to be gained from using lipid peroxidation rather than reactive oxygen species generation as the endpoint, because the former directly measures the damage sustained by these cells and is not so subject to the confounding effects of leukocyte contamination as the chemiluminescent detection of ROS. The latter can, however, be used as an extremely sensitive method for detecting leukocytes in sperm preparations used for IVF[37]. This is clinically significant, because the adverse effects of even a modest degree of leukocytic contamination is now apparent, and attention must be focused on strategies of sperm preparation which either remove leukocytes[37] or minimize the adverse consequences of the reactive oxygen species they produce[35,38].

CONCLUSION

In summary, a major new advance in our understanding of defective sperm function has been the discovery that ROS-induced lipid peroxidation is involved in the mechanisms by which spermatozoa are damaged in many cases of male infertility. These findings have implications in terms of fundamental cell biology of human spermatozoa, the diagnosis of male infertility and the treatment of this condition.

In terms of diagnostics, the use of simple biochemical tests to detect peroxidative damage in human spermatozoa, the development of extremely sensitive chemiluminescence assays to screen human suspensions for ROS generation and the introduction of protocols for differentiating between leukocytes and spermatozoa as the source of oxidative stress are all of interest. The ultimate objective of this research, however, is to convert our appreciation of the role of peroxidative mechanisms in the etiology of defective sperm function into a viable form of therapy. If leukocyte contamination of the sperm preparations is a major source of oxidative stress, then the selective removal of these cells using magnetic beads is a possible therapeutic option. Alternatively, antioxidants might be incorporated into the IVF culture media. Recent studies have already shown how the inclusion of iron-chelating agents into the incubation medium can promote embryonic development by limiting the generation of harmful oxygen radicals[74], while addition of superoxide dismutase has been found to promote sperm movement[75].

References

1. Sharpe, R. M., Maddocks, S., Millar, M., Kerr, J. B. and Saunders, P. T. (1992). Testosterone and spermatogenesis. Identification of stage-specific, androgen-regulated proteins secreted by adult rat seminiferous tubules. *J. Androl.*, **13**, 172–84
2. Ma, K., Inglis, J. D., Sharkey, A., Bickmore, W. A., Hill, R. E., Prosser, E. J., Speed, R. M., Thomson, E. J., Jobling, M., Taylor, K., Wolf, J., Cooke, H. J., Hargreave, T. B. and Chandley, A. C. (1993). A Y-chromosome gene family with RNA-binding protein homology – candidates for the azoospermia factor AZF controlling human spermatogenesis. *Cell*, **75**, 1287–95
3. Aitken, R. J. and Clarkson, J. S. (1987). Cellular basis of defective sperm function and its association with the genesis of reactive oxygen species by human spermatozoa. *J. Reprod. Fertil.*, **81**, 459–69
4. Baker, H. W. G. (1993). Treatment of male infertility – what does the future hold? *Int. J. Androl.*, **16**, 343–8
5. Van Steirteghem, A. C., Liu, J., Joris, H., Nagy, Z., Janssenswillen, C., Tournaye, H., Derde, M.-P., Van Asche, E. and Devroey, P. (1993). Higher success rate by intracytoplasmic sperm injection than by subzonal insemination. Report of a second series of 300 consecutive treatment cycles. *Hum. Reprod.*, **8**, 1055–60
6. Van Steirteghem, A. C., Nagy, Z., Joris, H., Liu, J., Staessen, C., Smitz, J., Wisanto, A. and Devroey, P. (1993). High fertilization and implantation rates after intracytoplasmic sperm injection. *Hum. Reprod.*, **8**, 1061–6
7. Thonneau, P., Quesnot, S., Ducot, B., Marchand, S., Fignon, A., Lansac, J. and Spira, A. (1992). Risk factors for female and male infertility: results of a case–control study. *Hum. Reprod.*, **7**, 55–8
8. Hull, M. G. R., Glazener, C. M. A., Kelly, N. J., Conway, D. I., Foster, P. A., Hinton, R. A., Coulson, C., Lambert, P. A., Watt, E. M. and Desai, K. M. (1985). Population study of causes, treatment and outcome of infertility. *Br. Med. J.*, **291**, 1693–7

9. Templeton, A., Fraser, C. and Thompson, B. (1990). The epidemiology of infertility in Aberdeen. *Br. Med. J.*, **301**, 148–52
10. Thonneau, P., Marchand, S., Tallec, A., Ferial, M.-L., Ducot, B., Lansac, J., Lopes, P., Tabaste, J.-M. and Spira, A. (1991). Incidence and main causes of infertility in a resident population (1 850 000) of three French regions (1988–1989). *Hum. Reprod.*, **6**, 811–16
11. Aitken, R. J., Best, F. S. M., Richardson, D. W., Djahanbakheh, O., Mortimer, D., Templeton, A. A. and Lees, M. M. (1982). An analysis of sperm function in cases of unexplained infertility: conventional criteria, movement characteristics and fertilizing capacity. *Fertil. Steril.*, **38**, 212–21
12. Aitken, R. J., Best, F. S. M., Richardson, D. W., Djahanbakhch, O., Templeton, A. and Lees, M. M. (1982). An analysis of semen quality and sperm function in cases of oligozoospermia. *Fertil. Steril.*, **38**, 705–11
13. Aitken, R. J., Ross, A., Hargreave, T., Richardson, D. and Best, F. (1984). Analysis of human sperm function following exposure to the ionophore A23187. Comparison of normospermic and oligozoospermic men. *J. Androl.*, **5**, 321–29
14. Aitken, R. J., Buckingham, D. W. and Fang, H. G. (1993). Analysis of the responses of human spermatozoa to A23187 employing a novel technique for assessing the acrosome reaction. *J. Androl.*, **14**, 132–41
15. Jones, R., Mann, T. and Sherins, R. (1979). Peroxidative breakdown of phospholipids in human spermatozoa, spermicidal properties of fatty acid peroxidases, and protective action of seminal plasma. *Fertil. Steril.*, **31**, 531–7
16. Jones, R., Mann, T. and Sherins, R. J. (1978). Adverse effects of peroxidized lipid on human spermatozoa. *Proc. Roy. Soc. Lond. – Ser. B: Biol. Sci.*, **201**, 413–17
17. Jones, R. and Mann, T. (1973). Lipid peroxidation in spermatozoa. *Proc. Roy. Soc. Lond. – Ser. B: Biol. Sci.*, **184**, 103–7
18. Alvarez, J. G., Touchstone, J. C., Blasco, L. and Storey, B. T. (1987). Spontaneous lipid peroxidation and production of hydrogen peroxide and superoxide in human spermatozoa. Superoxide dismutase as major enzyme protectant against oxygen toxicity. *J. Androl.*, **8**, 338–48
19. MacLeod, J. (1943). The role of oxygen in the metabolism and motility of human spermatozoa. *Am. J. Physiol.*, **138**, 512–18
20. Aitken, R. J., Buckingham, D., West, K., Wu, F. C., Zikopoulos, K. and Richardson, D. W. (1992). Differential contribution of leukocytes and spermatozoa to the generation of reactive oxygen species in the ejaculates of oligozoospermic patients and fertile donors. *J. Reprod. Fertil.*, **94**, 451–62
21. Weese, D. L., Peaster, M. L., Himsl, K. K., Leach, G. E., Lad, P. M. and Zimmern, P. E. (1993). Stimulated reactive oxygen species generation in the spermatozoa of infertile men. *J. Urol.*, **149**, 64–7
22. Iwasaki, A. and Gagnon, C. (1992). Formation of reactive oxygen species in spermatozoa of infertile patients. *Fertil. Steril.*, **57**, 409–16
23. Aitken, R. J., Harkiss, D. and Buckingham, D. (1993). Relationship between iron-catalyzed lipid peroxidation and human sperm function. *J. Reprod. Fertil.*, **98**, 257–65
24. Aitken, R. J., Buckingham, D. and Harkiss, D. (1993). Use of a xanthine oxidase radical generating system to investigate the cytotoxic effects of reactive oxygen species on human spermatozoa. *J. Reprod. Fertil.*, **97**, 441–50
25. DeLamirande, E. and Gagnon, C. (1992). Reactive oxygen species and human spermatozoa. I. Effects on the motility of intact spermatozoa and on sperm axonemes. *J. Androl.*, **13**, 368–78
26. Aitken, R. J., Buckingham, D. W. and West, K. M. (1992). Reactive oxygen species and human spermatozoa: analysis of the cellular mechanisms involved in luminol- and lucigenin-dependent chemiluminescence. *J. Cell Physiol.*, **151**, 466–77
27. Selley, M. L., Lacey, M. J., Bartlett, M. R., Copeland, C. M. and Ardlie, N. G. (1991). Content of significant amounts of a cytotoxic end-product of lipid peroxidation in human semen. *J. Reprod. Fertil.*, **92**, 291–8
28. DeLamirande, E. and Gagnon, C. (1992). Reactive oxygen species and human spermatozoa. II. Depletion of adenosine triphosphate plays an important role in the inhibition of sperm motility. *J. Androl.*, **13**, 379–86
29. Aitken, R. J., Harkiss, D. and Buckingham, D. W. (1993). Analysis of lipid peroxidation mechanisms in human spermatozoa. *Mol. Reprod. Dev.*, **35**, 302–15
30. Zini, A., DeLamirande, E. and Gagnon, C. (1993). Reactive oxygen species in semen of infertile patients: levels of superoxide dismutase- and catalase-like activities in seminal plasma and spermatozoa. *Int. J. Androl.* **16**, 183–8
31. Alvarez, J. G. and Storey, B. T. (1989). Role of glutathione peroxidase in protecting mammalian spermatozoa from loss of motility caused by spontaneous lipid peroxidation. *Gamete Res.*, **13**, 77–90
32. Perry, A. C., Jones, R., Niang, L. S., Jackson, R. M. and Hall, L. (1992). Genetic evidence for an androgen-regulated epididymal secretory glutathione peroxidase whose transcript does not contain a selenocysteine codon. *Biochem. J.*, **285**, 863–70
33. Perry, A. C., Jones, R. and Hall, L. (1993). Isolation and characterization of a rat cDNA clone encoding a secreted superoxide dismutase reveals the epididymis to be a major site of its expression. *Biochem. J.*, **293**, 21–25
34. Comaschi, V., Lindner, L., Farruggia, G., Gesmundo, N., Colombi, L. and Masotti, L. (1989). An investigation on lipoperoxidation mechanisms in boar spermatozoa. *Biochem. Biophys. Res. Commun.*, **158**, 769–75

35. Aitken, R. J., West, K. and Buckingham, D. (1994). Leukocytic infiltration into the human ejaculate and its association with semen quality, oxidative stress, and sperm function. *J. Androl.*, **61**, 1103–8
36. Aitken, R. J. and Clarkson, J. S. (1988). Significance of reactive oxygen species and antioxidants in defining the efficacy of sperm preparation techniques. *J. Androl.*, **9**, 367–76
37. Krausz, C., West, K., Buckingham, D. and Aitken, R. J. (1992). Development of a technique for monitoring the contamination of human semen samples with leukocytes. *Fertil. Steril.*, **57**, 1317–25
38. Aitken, R. J., Buckingham, D., West, K. and Brindle, J. (1995). On the use of paramagnetic beads and ferrofluids to assess and eliminate the leukocytic contribution to oxygen radical generation by human sperm suspensions. *Am. J. Reprod. Immunol.*, in press
39. Krausz, C., Mills, C., Rogers, S., Tan, S. L. and Aitken, R. J. (1994). Stimulation of oxidant generation by human sperm suspensions using phorbol esters and formyl peptides: relationship with motility and fertilization *in vitro*. *Fertil. Steril.*, **62**, 599–605
40. Aitken, R. J. (1985). Diagnostic value of the zona-free hamster oocyte penetration test and sperm movement characteristics in oligozoospermia. *Int. J. Androl.*, **8**, 348–56
41. Templeton, A., Aitken, J., Mortimer, D. and Best, F. (1982). Sperm function in patients with unexplained infertility. *Br. J. Obstet. Gynaecol.*, **89**, 550–4
42. Tan, K. H. and Lim, P. H. (1991). Testicular biopsy and scrotal exploration in the management of male infertility. *Singapore Med. J.*, **32**, 41–6
43. Aitken, R. J., Best, F. S. M., Warner, P. and Templeton, A. (1984). A prospective study of the relationship between semen quality and fertility in cases of unexplained infertility. *J. Androl.*, **5**, 297–303
44. Irvine, D. S., MacLeod, I. C., Templeton, A. A., Masterton, A. and Taylor, A. (1994). A prospective clinical study of the relationship between the computer assisted assessment of human semen quality and the achievement of pregnancy *in vivo*. *Hum. Reprod.*, **9**, 2324–34
45. Irvine, D. S. and Aitken, R. J. (1986). Predictive value of *in vitro* sperm function tests in the context of an AID service. *Hum. Reprod.*, **8**, 539–45
46. Hull, M. G. R., Joyce, D. N., McLeod, F. N., Ray, B. D. and McDermott, A. (1984). Human *in vitro* fertilization, *in vivo* sperm penetration of cervical mucus, and unexplained infertility. *Lancet* **ii**, 245–6
47. Hull, M. G. R., Savage, P. E. and Bromham, D. R. (1982). Prognostic value of the postcoital test: prospective study based on time-specific conception rates. *Br. J. Obstet. Gynaecol.*, **89**, 299–305
48. Aitken, R. J., Warner, P. E. and Reid, C. (1986). Factors influencing the success of sperm–cervical mucus interaction in patients exhibiting unexplained infertility. *J. Androl.*, **7**, 3–10
49. Aitken, R. J., Bowie, H., Buckingham, D., Harkiss, D., Richardson, D. W. and West, K. M. (1992). Sperm penetration into a hyaluronic acid polymer as a means of monitoring functional competence. *J. Androl.*, **13**, 44–54
50. Davis, R. O., Overstreet, J. W., Asch, R. H., Ord, T. and Silber, S. J. (1991). Movement characteristics of human epididymal sperm used for fertilization in human oocytes *in vitro*. *Fertil. Steril.*, **56**, 1128–35
51. Suarez, S. S., Katz, D. F., Owen, D. H., Andrews, J. B. and Powell, R. L. (1991). Evidence for the function of hyperactivated motility in sperm. *Biol. Reprod.*, **44**, 375–81
52. Oehninger, S., Franken, D., Alexander, N. and Hodgen, G. D. (1992). Hemizona assay and its impact on the identification and treatment of human sperm dysfunctions. *Andrologia*, **24**, 307–21
53. Irvine, D. S. and Aitken, R. J. (1986). Clinical evaluation of the zona-free hamster egg penetration test in the management of the infertile couple: prospective and retrospective studies. *Int. J. Androl.* (Suppl.), **6**, 97–112
54. Aitken, R. J., Irvine, D. S. and Wu, F. C. (1991). Prospective analysis of sperm–oocyte fusion and reactive oxygen species generation as criteria for the diagnosis of infertility. *Am. J. Obstet. Gynecol.*, **164**, 542–51
55. Aitken, R. J. and Clarkson, J. S. (1987). Cellular basis of defective sperm function and its association with the genesis of reactive oxygen species by human spermatozoa. *J. Reprod. Fertil.*, **81**, 459–69
56. Aitken, R. J., Clarkson, J. S., Hargreave, T. B., Irvine, D. S. and Wu, F. C. W. (1989). Analysis of the relationship between defective sperm function and the generation of reactive oxygen species in cases of oligozoospermia. *J. Androl.*, **10**, 214–20
57. Aitken, R. J. and West, K. M. (1990). Analysis of the relationship between reactive oxygen species production and leukocyte infiltration in fractions of human semen separated on Percoll gradients. *Int. J. Androl.*, **13**, 433–51
58. Sukcharoen, N., Keith, J., Irvine, O. S. and Aitken, R. J. (1995). Importance of sperm morphology and leukocyte contamination. *Fertil. Steril.* **63**, 1293–1300
59. Silber, S. J. (1989). Results of microsurgical vasoepididymostomy: role of epididymis in sperm maturation. *Hum. Reprod.*, **4**, 298–303
60. Hendry, W. F., Hughes, L., Scammell, G., Pryor, J. P. and Hargreave, T. B. (1990). Comparison of prednisolone and placebo in subfertile men with antibodies to spermatozoa. *Lancet*, **335**, 85–8
61. Laven, J. S., Haans, L. C., Mali, W. P., te Velde, E. R., Wensing, C. J. and Eimers, J. M. (1992). Effects of varicocele treatment in adolescents: a randomized study. *Fertil. Steril.*, **58**, 756–62
62. Hurd, W. W., Randolph, J. F. J., Ansbacher, R., Menge, A. C., Ohl, D. A. and Brown, A. N. (1993). Comparison of intracervical, intrauterine and intratubal techniques for donor insemination. *Fertil. Steril.*, **59**, 339–42

63. Zikopoulos, K., West, C. P., Wen-Thong, P., Kacser, E. M., Morrison, J. and Wu, F. C. W. (1993). Homologous intrauterine insemination has no advantage over timed natural intercourse when used in combination with ovulation induction for the treatment of unexplained infertility. *Hum. Reprod.*, **8**, 563–7
64. Irvine, D. S. and Templeton, A. A. (1994). Donor insemination. In Hargreave, T. B. (ed.) *Male Infertility*, 2nd edn, pp. 427–51. (Edinburgh: Churchill Livingstone)
65. Barratt, C. L. R. and Cooke, I. D. (1993). *Donor Insemination*, pp. 1–231. (Cambridge: Cambridge University Press)
66. Lenzi, A., Lombardo, F., Gandini, L., Culasso, F. and Dondero, F. (1992). Glutathione therapy for male infertility. *Arch. Androl.*, **29**, 65–8
67. Lenzi, A., Culasso, F., Gandini, L., Lombardo, F. and Dondero, F. (1993). Placebo-controlled, double-blind, cross-over trial of glutathione therapy in male infertility. *Hum. Reprod.*, **8**, 1657–62
68. Moilanen, J., Hovatta, O. and Lindroth, L. (1993). Vitamin E levels in seminal plasma can be elevated by oral administration of vitamin E in infertile men. *Int. J. Androl.*, **16**, 165–6
69. Hillier, S. L., Rabe, L. K., Muller, C. H., Zarutskie, P., Kuzan, F. B. and Stenchever, M. A. (1990). Relationship of bacteriologic characteristics to semen indices in men attending an infertility clinic. *Obstet. Gynecol.*, **75**, 800–4
70. Mortimer, D. (1990). Semen analysis and sperm washing techniques. In Gagnon, C. (ed.) *Controls of Sperm Motility: Biological and Clinical Aspects*, pp. 263–84. (Boston: CRC Press)
71. Chan, S. Y., Chan, Y. M. and Tucker, M. J. (1991). Comparison of characteristics of human spermatozoa selected by the multiple-tube swim-up and simple discontinuous Percoll gradient centrifugation. *Andrologia*, **23**, 213–28
72. Jaroudi, K. A., Carver-Ward, J. A., Hamilton, C. J. C. M., Siek, U. V. and Sheth, K. V. (1993). Percoll semen preparation enhances human oocyte fertilization in male factor infertility as shown by a randomized cross-over study. *Hum. Reprod.*, **8**, 1438–42
73. Sapienza, F., Verheyen, G., Tournaye, H., Janssens, R., Pletincx, I., Derde, M. and Van Steirteghem, A. (1993). An auto-controlled study in *in vitro* fertilization reveals the benefit of Percoll centrifugation to swim-up in the preparation of poor quality semen. *Hum. Reprod.*, **8**, 1856–62
74. Nasr-Esfahani, M., Johnson, M. H. and Aitken, R. J. (1990). The effect of iron and iron chelators on the *in vitro* block to development of the mouse preimplantation embryo: BAT6 a new medium for improved culture of mouse embryos *in vitro*. *Hum. Reprod.*, **5**, 997–1003
75. Kobayashi, T., Miyazaki, T., Natori, M. and Nozawa, S. (1991). Protective role of superoxide dismutase in human sperm motility: superoxide dismutase activity and lipid peroxide in human seminal plasma and spermatozoa. *Hum. Reprod.*, **6**, 987–91
76. Aitken, R. J., Harkiss, D. and Buckingham, D. (1993). Relationship between iron-catalyzed lipid peroxidation potential and human sperm function. *J. Reprod. Fertil.*, **98**, 257–65

Sperm preparation techniques and X/Y chromosome separation

22

D. R. Franken, O. E. Claassens and R. R. Henkel

INTRODUCTION

Under *in vivo* conditions spermatozoa with potentially functional characteristics are separated from semen following coitus, by active migration into cervical mucus[1]. As a result of this phenomenon, sperm separation techniques involving a self-migration step are widely used. Many clinical programs around the world use the so-called 'classical' sperm preparation technique involving multiple cycles of sperm washing followed by a swim-up step to prepare and recover a subpopulation of highly motile spermatozoa. However, examination of the earliest reports of human *in vitro* fertilization (IVF) successes reveals the swim-up step to be a later addition[2].

Furthermore, the need to separate human spermatozoa from seminal plasma to allow capacitation and expression of their intrinsic fertilizing ability is a fundamental requirement of IVF, gamete intrafallopian transfer (GIFT), intrauterine insemination (IUI) and *in vitro* tests of sperm fertilizing ability such as the zona-free hamster egg penetration test (HEPT), sperm–hemizona binding test[3] and assessment of the acrosome reaction[2,4].

The ideal separation technique should: (1) be rapid, simple, and inexpensive; (2) recover all motile sperm in the specimen; (3) result in no damage or physiological alteration of the separated sperm; (4) remove dead sperm and other cells, including microorganisms; (5) remove toxic and bioactive substances; and (6) process large volumes of semen. Depending on the application, these criteria differ in their importance.

MIGRATION TECHNIQUES

In vivo, the potentially functional sperm population is separated from liquefied semen by virtue of their migration into cervical mucus[1]. Consequently, sperm preparation techniques involving a self-migration step are widely used. Variations on this theme are numerous, including the classical 'swim-up' from liquefied semen into an overlay of culture medium (which may or may not contain other substances to help stabilize the interface), the migration–sedimentation approach which uses a combination of migration and gravitational sedimentation, or swimming through porous membranes, or swimming up into a medium containing highly purified sodium hyaluronate.

Swim-up from a washed pellet

Edwards and his colleagues described a simple one-step washing procedure in the first report of the fertilization of a human oocyte *in vitro*[5], and a two-step washing procedure for the first clinical IVF success[6,7].

The washed pellet method was highly successful in producing sperm preparations for IVF in cases where no male factor was present. These sperm preparations were characterized by extremely high proportions of motile spermatozoa, a preferential selection for morphologically normal spermatozoa, and an absence of the other cell types, anucleate cytoplasmic masses and particulate debris commonly seen in human ejaculates. Excellent fertilization rates were reported when these sperm preparations were used to inseminate human oocytes *in vitro*. However, as the indications for IVF treatment were expanded beyond simple tubal factor cases to couples with idiopathic infertility and, ultimately, to male factor cases, the problem of fertilization failure appeared[8–10].

Typically this procedure involves two- or threefold dilutions with culture medium, followed by repeated centrifugation. This produces a pellet of spermatozoa on the bottom of a centrifuge tube which is then overlayered with a volume of culture medium and the tube, or tubes, incubated at 37°C to allow the spermatozoa to swim-up from the pellet.

Although postmigration preparations are without cellular debris, reactive oxygen species produced in these sperm pellets have a marked deleterious effect[11]. In addition, in our own experience we found the technique to render a very low yield, since many of the spermatozoa in the lower levels of the pellet never reach the interface with the culture medium layer.

Overall, although many men's spermatozoa may not be impaired to the extent of inhibiting fertilization, some couples' chances of successful IVF will certainly be compromised. Clearly, one cannot continue to use a technique, such as swim-up from pelleted semen, incorporating steps known to cause irrevocable damage to spermatozoa prejudicial to a desired functional endpoint.

Swim-up from semen

The basis of successful separation for this method is the area of the interface between a semen layer and the overlaid culture medium. During this procedure, several aliquots of liquefied semen are taken from a sample and placed in tubes underneath an overlay of culture medium. Round-bottom tubes or four-well dishes should be used to optimize the surface area of the interface between the semen layer and the culture medium. The tubes may also be prepared by gently layering culture medium over the liquefied semen. The placing of semen underneath the culture medium, however, provides a much cleaner interface zone.

The methodology during this process, in brief, entails the following: semen is gently aspirated into a 1 mL sterile plastic syringe with a 19G needle attached. Care is taken to expel the air that might be trapped in the syringe by gently depressing the syringe plunger. The needle tip is then passed through the culture medium layer to the bottom of the tube. Viscous semen samples should be mixed with a small amount of culture medium prior to loading into the syringe; repeated aspiration of viscous semen (i.e. its forceful expulsion one or more times through a 19G or 22G needle) should be avoided[2].

Maximum recovery is obtained using multiple tubes with small volumes of semen per tube, thus maximizing the combined total interface area between semen and culture medium. Mortimer[2] suggested using 250 μl of semen under 500–600 μl of culture medium per tube. Tubes are then generally incubated at 20–45°C. After the incubation period at 37°C – the longer the period of incubation, the greater the yield – most of the upper culture medium layer is removed. This is done extremely carefully, working from the upper meniscus downwards, using a sterile pipette. Typically, 75% or 80% of the culture medium layer is removed, taking great care not to aspirate directly from the interface region. Separate tubes are harvested individually and the separate preparations are combined. This combined preparation is then usually centrifuged at 600***g*** for 6–10 min and resuspended into fresh culture medium at the desired concentration of motile spermatozoa.

Migration–sedimentation

This type of approach combines swim-up from semen with gravitational settling of spermatozoa from the upper medium layer[11]. Basically, spermatozoa migrate from semen contained in a ring-shaped well which is completely overlaid with a layer of culture medium. The central hole of the ring constitutes the collection well into which motile spermatozoa settle. As yet, it remains an interesting approach which may represent a useful method for dealing with male factor semen samples. Spermatozoa recovered by this method are highly motile, and compared to semen the percentage of normal morphology according to strict criteria[13] is improved; however, the yield using migration–sedimentation is relatively low.

Sperm Select

This commercial product is a highly purified preparation of sodium hyaluronate (Pharmacia, Uppsala, Sweden), with an average molecular weight of 3 000 000 Da, used at a final concentration of 1 mg/mL in culture medium. When used in a clinical IVF program, swim-up from semen into hyaluronate solution gave a significantly higher percentage of motile spermatozoa compared with the traditional swim-up from a washed pellet method[14] and, ultimately, the achievement of a higher pregnancy rate[15]. However, whether these improved results were due specifically to the use of the hyaluronate or to the use of a method which did not involve the initial pelleting of unselected spermatozoa was not ascertained.

DENSITY GRADIENT SEPARATION

The wide variety of methods described in the literature are all based on the use of density – gradient centrifugation to fractionate subpopulations of spermatozoa. Ficoll has initially been used as gradient material for preparating spermatozoa[16], but by far the most widely used has been Percoll. A commercial product known as Nycodenz is lately being used as a density gradient material for preparing human spermatozoa.

For any of these methods, the gradients may be continuous or discontinuous. With continuous gradients, there is a gradual increase in density from the top of the gradient to its bottom, but the layers of a discontinuous gradient are allowed to diffuse into each other to a limited degree. A discontinuous gradient is composed of several layers with more or less clear boundaries between them.

Percoll

A wide variety of Percoll-based gradients has been described for both the continuous[17] and discontinuous[18] types. Some reports dealt with deleterious effects of Percoll-gradient centrifugation upon the ultrastructural integrity of human spermatozoa[20], as well as upon their longevity as measured by motility maintenance[21]. However, normal sperm function as assessed in the zona pellucida-free hamster egg penetration test[22], as well as in human IVF (both routine and following sperm microinjection into the perivitelline space[23]), clearly indicate differences between Percoll-gradient methods.

Probably the most practical Percoll-gradient procedure is that developed by Dravlandá[19,24]. The yield of this method can be extremely high with normal semen samples, ranging from 15% to 96% of motile spermatozoa applied to the gradient[19]. Yield is apparently dependent only upon the motility of the spermatozoa in the original semen sample[25]. There is variable morphological selection of spermatozoa in the prepared population, with tail and/or midpiece defects being primarily excluded.

Another study using a modification of this gradient which reported the selection of spermatozoa devoid of 'coating envelopes' is extremely difficult to understand since the published electromicrographs of cells with these 'coating envelopes' are clearly only of morphologically abnormal spermatozoa with distended midpiece regions. The removal of such structures during Percoll-gradient centrifugation would not be compatible with sperm survival; nor have the structures been identified in any other studies on human sperm ultrastructure[26]. A far simpler, and more reasonable, explanation is simply that the spermatozoa in the selected population were the morphologically normal subpopulation originally present in the semen, i.e. they were selected rather than changed[27].

Sperm populations prepared by Percoll gradients, while having the advantage of being essentially free of any bacteria that were present in the original semen[28], may contain small quantities of Percoll particles. There has been great concern over the possible dangers of using such preparations for intrauterine insemination (IUI) since Percoll consists of polyvinylpyrrolidone-coated silica particles, silica being an established tissue irritant. However, this preparation method has been used for some time by IUI programs with no untoward effects[29]. This concern, in conjunction with the low yields usually seen with Percoll gradients for abnormal semen samples (especially those with low sperm motility), has led to the investigation of alternative gradient materials[21].

MiniPercoll

Since normal Percoll gradients are not very effective in treatment of oligoasthenozoospermia, Ord and coworkers[30] developed a density gradient consisting of a reduced volume of a discontinuous Percoll gradient. This MiniPercoll gradient gave significantly higher fertilization rates for this specific group of male patients.

Following centrifugation, pellets are resuspended in 0.3 mL of medium and layered on a discontinuous Percoll gradient consisting of 0.3 mL each of

50%, 70% and 95% isotonic Percoll (MiniPercoll). An isotonic solution of Percoll is obtained by mixing nine parts of Percoll (Pharmacia, Sweden) with one part Ham's F-10 (10×) (Gibco, RI) or an equivalent medium, and adding 2.1 g/L of sodium bicarbonate. To obtain the 95%, 70% and 50% layers, this isotonic solution is diluted with normal concentrated medium (1×)+HEPES. The discontinuous gradient is established by carefully pipetting 0.3 mL of 95%, 70%, 50% isotonic Percoll, and finally the pellet resuspended in 0.3 mL medium in a 15 mL centrifuge tube. The gradient is centrifuged at 300***g*** for 30–45 min. Following centrifugation of the gradient, the 95% Percoll layer was removed, washed twice and resuspended in 1 mL of medium supplemented with 10% human cord serum and incubated until the time of insemination.

At Tygerberg Hospital we use a MiniPercoll technique consisting of 80% and 40% isotonic Percoll overlaid by liquefied semen. The gradient is centrifuged for 30 min at 300***g***.

Nycodenz

The concern over the possible inflammatory responses that could be induced by the insemination of sperm populations contaminated with Percoll (Percoll being approved for *in vitro* use only) and the poor yields obtained from male factor semen samples on Percoll gradients prompted the evaluation of possible alternative gradient materials. Nycodenz (Nyegaard & Co., Oslo, Norway) is the same molecule, iohexol, as used in the X-ray contrast medium Omni-paque, and studies have revealed a low incidence of adverse reactions during angiography[21]. Both continuous and discontinuous Nycodenz gradients were evaluated, but a four-layer discontinuous gradient was found to produce populations of highly motile spermatozoa with better yields, and survival, than either swim-up or Percoll gradients from oligozoospermic and asthenozoospermic semen samples[21]. Compared to the swim-up procedure from a pelleted population Nycodenz also seems to be superior at penetrating zona-free hamster eggs[31]. Thus, this technique clearly has great potential in the preparation of motile spermatozoa from poor quality semen for IVF use and warrants further investigation.

FILTRATION TECHNIQUES

Glass wool column filtration

The use of a glass wool column, prepared by filling sterile 1 mL plastic syringes or Pasteur pipettes with 15 mg glass wool fibers, has been reported to remove the majority of debris as well as agglutinated and dead spermatozoa from semen samples[32]. While this simple procedure was considered to have potential clinical significance, a subsequent report indicated that filtration by glass wool could induce damage to the sperm plasma membrane and acrosome in some spermatozoa[33]. Furthermore, the very real danger of glass wool fragments in the final sperm population urges caution in the use of such preparations for artificial insemination. This, however, is dependent on the kind of glass wool used for sperm preparation.

In our experience, a commercially available glass wool filtration kit (SpermFertil, Mello Ltd., Exeter, UK) has been shown not to release glass wool fragments into the medium when it is pre-washed carefully.

Recently, it has been reported that glass wool column filtration yields a significantly higher recovery of viable spermatozoa than the swim-up procedure and that the sperm preparations retain their ability to fertilize human oocytes *in vitro*. Moreover, it has been shown that glass wool filtration improves sperm quality even in men with oligo- and/or asthenozoospermia[34–36]. In addition, spermatozoa separated by means of glass wool filtration have a higher potential to penetrate zona-free hamster ova[37] and there is evidence for a selective capacity of glass wool for normal chromatin condensed human spermatozoa[36].

This technique, therefore, has clear application in clinical IVF, perhaps especially in cases of poor quality semen, because of its high yield[34]. Application of this technique to gamete intrafallopian tube insemination (GIFT) procedures must, however, be viewed with concern.

Generally liquefied semen, or in the case of viscous ejaculate, diluted semen, should be filtered through the glass wool column. Previous washing steps of the sperm should be avoided, because of the extremely deleterious influence of reactive oxygen species which cause irreversible damage to the sperm membrane[38]. In extreme cases, especially men with already reduced semen quality, this may lead to complete loss of motility, and consequently to failure of fertilization[39]. The only exception to this rule should be sperm separation from men with retrograde ejaculation in whom the spermatozoa should be separated first from the urine or the mixture of urine and medium. This is to prevent the spermatozoa from experiencing the detrimental effects of the urine. In our own experience, however, the addition of 1 mg/mL pentoxifylline to the mixture of urine and medium prior to centrifugation is useful (Henkel *et al.*, unpublished), because of the radical scavenging effect of this xanthine derivative[40]. Afterward, the pellet is resuspended in 1–2 mL fresh medium and filtered through glass wool.

Glass beads

This method, which is used for the preparation of hamster spermatozoa for *in vitro* capacitation[41], has been shown to select motile human spermatozoa efficiently from semen, with high yields[42]. Because of the relatively large size of the glass beads concerns regarding their possible carry over into an insemination preparation were lessened. Our practice, however, has shown that glass beads are still present in the filtrate. Thus, using glass beads for effective sperm preparation, even for assisted reproduction, has not been widely accepted.

Sephadex columns

Recently, a commercial sperm separation kit based on the use of Sephadex beads (SpermPrep) has become available. Compared to migration–sedimentation and swim-up from pelleted semen it has produced significantly higher yields. Moreover, morphologically normal sperm cells could be enriched in filtrate after SpermPrep separation[43].

Apart from the encouraging results in research, however, practicality of this method in assisted reproduction has still to be shown.

Transmembrane migration

This technique uses an apparatus in which a motile sperm population is separated from culture medium by a Nucleopore membrane filter. These filters are unusual in that their pores are cylindrical and at right angles to the plane of the membrane[44]. The spermatozoa, therefore, have straight channels in which to swim through the membrane. Unfortunately, these membranes have a very low transparency (transparency = ratio of the total cross-sectional area of the pores to the overall membrane area) and, as a consequence, the yield is extremely low. Primarily, this method has been used for testing the motility of sperm populations treated with various pharmacological agents, not as a preparation method[45].

Another approach to separating viable human spermatozoa by means of membranes was undertaken by Agarwal *et al.*[46] using a membrane which had been developed for selective removal of leukocytes (L4 membrane; Pall). Besides a significant increase of motility ejaculates filtered through this membrane have been shown to contain less leukocytes[46]. This fact is, of course, of importance in those cases who, due to infections, have increased number of leukocytes in the ejaculate.

Moreover, this membrane seems to be selective for spermatozoa with normal membrane integrity[47] and sperm producing low amounts of reactive oxygen species[48].

CLINICAL APPLICATIONS

It is extremely important that sperm preparations for clinical use (IVF or IUI) or long-term incubation *in vitro*, should be free of microbiological contaminants that may be present in semen[49,50]. Several studies have examined the carry-over of bacterial contaminants during sperm washing and have concluded that both sperm migration and Percoll-gradient procedures yield sperm preparations essentially free of bacteria[28,50,51]. The use of culture medium supplemented with antibiotics is certainly advantageous in this respect[50,51], although problems may be encountered when preparing spermatozoa for IUI in patients allergic to, for example, penicillin. For this reason antibiotics can be omitted and media should be used immediately after preparation. To prevent viral infections, in particular HIV, patients should be tested for HIV before performing any technique of assisted reproduction. For protein supplement for the media only maternal serum or commercially available human serum albumin preparations for medication should be used, which are HIV-free due to the technical processing.

Sperm functional tests

Although recent studies pointed out the detrimental effect of pelleting sperm cells[11,39], and other sperm separation techniques have been found to be superior in maintaining spermatozoal function[36–38], WHO still recommends swim-up from a pelleted semen sample to be used as the preparation technique to perform sperm functional testing[52]. This might be for historical as well as for reasons of simplicity in andrological laboratories around the world. This method can also be employed when working with normal semen samples containing large concentrations of highly motile spermatozoa. The two-layer discontinuous Percoll gradient for normal semen samples provides a rapid and relatively simple method, resulting in an excellent yield.

Abnormal semen samples, especially those with increased viscosity, may benefit from a prior filtration on a glass wool or glass bead column. The initial motile sperm preparation should be washed and pelleted once (perhaps twice) to ensure minimum seminal plasma contamination of the final preparation. Among asthenozoospermic cases, the results are often disappointing and a glass wool filtration using the SpermFertil columns or a Nycodenz gradient would appear to be the method of choice for such samples.

Experimental studies on human sperm physiology often require very large numbers of spermatozoa and the ultimate clinical applicability of such studies will be dependent upon being able to obtain sufficient numbers of spermatozoa. This is important, not only for donor samples, but also for the ejaculates of patients undergoing infertility investigations.

Therefore, the goal of any sperm separation procedure is to retrieve a maximum of viable sperm whose biological functions are maintained by means of the separation technique. This is mandatory not only for treatment cycles in assisted reproduction, but also for the assessment of spermatozoa functions which should be performed in the diagnostic work-up of male infertility.

Intrauterine insemination (IUI)

Depending upon the patient and the required final yield, the preparation method should be carefully chosen. For example, IUI requires some 5 million motile spermatozoa in a 100–500 μL volume for insemination, whereas IVF or GIFT requires only 50 000 to 100 000 motile spermatozoa per oocyte (although one may need larger numbers in male factor cases to improve the likelihood of successful fertilization)[72].

If no male factor is present for intrauterine insemination, the whole semen sample is diluted 1:3 to 1:5 of Ham's F-10 or equivalent medium, for example T9, plus 10% inactivated serum (or 10 mg/mL HIV-controlled human serum albumin) and centrifuged at 300–400***g*** for 10 min; the supernatant is discarded. The pellet is washed once more with 2 mL of Ham's F-10 or equivalent plus 10% serum. The final pellet is overlaid with 0.6 mL of Ham's F-10 plus 10% serum and incubated for 1 h at 37°C to allow sperm to swim up. Then 0.4 to 0.5 mL of the top layer is aspirated; the count, motility and forward progression are noted and used for insemination. A morphology slide of the swim-up sample is prepared for later evaluation.

In cases of male factor subfertility, even for retrograde ejaculation samples, a method which is gentle to spermatozoa should be chosen. Depending on the semen characteristics, MiniPercoll, glass wool filtration or Nycodenz gradients can be selected. At the Department of Dermatology and Andrology, Justus-Liebig-University, Giessen, Germany, glass wool filtration with SpermFertil columns is normally used. Motility of spermatozoa can be improved by a short stimulation (5–10 min) by means of 1 mg/mL pentoxifylline which is added to the semen. In addition, pentoxifylline scavenges excess reactive oxygen species[40] which have been found to be significantly higher in men with oligozoospermia[53]. Then semen is filtered through the glass wool, washed with HEPES-buffered medium supplemented with 10% inactivated material serum, the pellet is resuspended in 500 μL fresh medium and is inseminated subsequently.

In cases with retrograde ejaculation, patients are requested to urinate with a small residue of urine remaining in the bladder before collection, then to masturbate and urinate into a plastic jar containing pre-warmed medium supplemented with 10% inactivated maternal serum (or 10 mg/mL HIV-controlled human serum albumin) and 2 mg/mL pentoxifylline. This mixture is centrifuged at 300***g*** for 10 min, the pellet resuspended in 2 mL fresh medium without pentoxifylline, and subsequently passed through glass wool columns. The filtrate is centrifuged and the pellet is once again resuspended for insemination in 500 μL fresh medium. Because of a higher yield following sperm preparation we use the MiniPercoll in cases of a volume less than 1 mL.

In vitro fertilization (IVF) and gamete intrafallopian tube transfer (GIFT)

In the wash procedure for IVF and GIFT, 1 mL of semen is washed twice with 2 mL of Ham's F-10 plus 10% serum and centrifuged at 300–400***g*** for 10 min. The final sperm pellet is overlaid with 1 mL of Ham's F-10 plus 10% serum. The spermatozoa are allowed to swim up for 30 min at 37°C in an incubator with 5% CO_2 in air. The top layer containing the swim-up sperm is aspirated and investigated for concentration, motility and forward progression; a slide is made for morphology. A count for the determination of the final swim-up sperm concentration is performed, and the appropriate volume is added to the ova to obtain the recommended number of sperm per ovum.

For GIFT, the resultant swim-up samples are diluted to a sperm concentration of 4×10^6/mL and 20×10^6/mL to achieve a final count of 100 000 and 500 000 sperm in normal males (>14% morphologically normal sperm) and in teratozoospermic males (<14% morphologically normal sperm), respectively.

We have found that when we use sperm preparations as described, we obtain improved semen samples. The resulting swim-up samples contain a high proportion of motile sperm (80% to 100%), with improved forward progression and free of any foreign cells or debris. Sperm survival is usually very good, up to 72 h. We have also found an increased percentage of morphologically normal sperm in the swim-up samples[13].

Antisperm antibodies

Our studies have shown that washed, swim-up sperm from men with antisperm antibodies do not differ from unwashed samples in terms of sperm-bound antibodies. Swim-up procedures are exactly the same as for IUI preparation, antibodies are detected with the immunobead test (IBT) and sperm cervical mucus contact (SCMC) test before and after sperm separation. However, the semen parameters – morphology, forward progression, and motility – are all improved by the wash and swim-up procedures.

Our results suggest that patients can achieve pregnancy despite antisperm antibodies[55]. Improvement in sperm parameters[55], minimizing the distance between sperm and ova, and bypassing the cervical mucus may be reasons for the relatively high pregnancy rate (see Chapter 30).

Choosing an appropriate sperm preparation method should take into account not only the relative simplicity and rapidity of a method, for reasons of laboratory efficiency, but should also consider the quality of the semen samples to be processed and the absolute yield that will be required. One must remember that an individual man's response to a given preparation method, in terms of the motile sperm yield, will not necessarily be constant over time. Furthermore, there may well be substantial interindividual variability in the method providing optimum yield even for samples of apparently similar semen quality.

IDENTIFICATION AND SEPARATION OF X- AND Y-BEARING SPERM

The sex of one's offspring has remained important both historically and culturally. The Egyptians (2000 BC) defined the role of the testis in reproduction, while the Greeks defined women as the nurturers of the eggs and men as the source of genetic characteristics. The general sex preference is for the firstborn to be male with the second child being a female. Prospective parents have been pressured for centuries by these social and personal issues to attempt to modify the sex selection process. According to the standard meiotic model in which equivalent numbers of X- and Y-bearing sperm are produced, the primary X:Y chromosome ratio is 1:1, which is in contrast with the secondary sex ratio of 106 males:100 females[56]. Information for sex determination is carried in mammalian sperm, and so most sex control schemes have concentrated on semen manipulations. The ability to ensure a male or female offspring by artificial insemination using purified X- and Y-bearing sperm would offer chances for healthy children to every woman heterozygous for harmful X-linked hereditary disorders. Any method influencing the sex ratio of agriculturally important animals would also have a major impact on the genetic improvement of animals and should produce substantial economic benefits. Several physical, biochemical and immunological methods of semen treatment have been investigated in various laboratories trying to alter the sex ratio of the offspring, but the results remain controversial at best. To some extent, the lack of progress might have been due to the lack of appropriate methods to monitor the success of sperm sex separation techniques.

Identification of X- and/or Y-bearing sperm

This section deals with different techniques employed for identification of X- and/or Y-bearing sperm. Apart from helping in determining the sex of the offspring, methods used for monitoring the proportion of X- and Y-chromosome-bearing sperm are F-body analysis[57], cytogenetic analysis of penetrated hamster oocytes[58] and fluorescence-aided cell sorting (FACS)[58]. More recently, *in situ* hybridization with X- and/or Y-chromosome-specific probes[60] and polymerase chain reaction (PCR)[61] became relevant approaches for the identification of X- and Y-bearing sperm.

Quinacrine mustard staining

Until 1969, there was no standard technique known of differentiating the X- from the Y-bearing spermatozoa. It was then discovered that the distal part of the long arm of the Y chromosome could be stained with quinacrine hydrochloride[62]. Quinacrine intercalates and binds to the minor groove of the double helix DNA. Quinacrine contains a terminal mustard configuration in the side chain and alkylating groups of the mustard variety have a well known affinity for the N-7 atom of guanine[63]. It was found that quinacrine mustard staining of metaphase chromosome preparations reveals a bright fluorescent spot on the long arm of the Y chromosome[63]. The fluorescent spot (F-body) can also be detected in sperm and it is assumed that these fluorescent spots represent Y-bearing spermatozoa[57]. A fixed, air-dried preparation of a few drops of semen on a glass slide can be used for F-body determination. The Y-chromosome can be stained with an aqueous solution of quinacrine hydrochloride followed by fluorescence examination. Barlow and Vosa[57] reported that 45.1% of human spermatozoa had a fluorescent body in their heads. In a study with 20 patients[64] we found the mean percentage Y-bearing sperm to be 45.85% ± 6.51 (± SD). Another study[65] found the percentage of Y-bearing sperm, according to the F-body count, in 18 untreated semen samples to be 52%. Controversy, however, exists regarding the reliability of the quinacrine mustard staining method as a sperm sex assay because some fluorescent spots may also represent normal polymorphic regions of certain autosomes. Increases and decreases in the length of the Y-chromosome also directly reflect similar changes in fluorescent pattern. Normal males have been described possessing very short Y-chromosomes that lacked an intensely fluorescent portion[66]. Since the incidence of spermatozoa with F-body was almost always less than 50% and those showing two or more F-bodies was relatively high, it was suspected that not all Y-sperm exhibited a F-body, and that some spermatozoa with F-body-like regions were not Y-bearing sperm[67]. Furthermore, since the counting of F-bodies is to a great extent viewer dependent[67] and the fluorescent viewing time per microscopic field is limited to 40 s, we concluded that the F-body count does not reflect reliably the percentage of Y-bearing sperm in a given semen sample. In a comparative study with a DNA-probe and quinacrine mustard it was finally concluded that the latter staining technique is not suitable for evaluation of methods that claim to separate X- and Y-bearing sperm[68].

Karyotype analysis of human sperm

Karyotype analysis of human sperm after fusion with denuded hamster oocytes offers an alternative for the verification of results of sperm separation techniques[58]. The use of hamster eggs as 'reactivating vehicles' for human sperm nuclei was first described by Yanagimachi *et al.*[70]. Rudak[58] obtained the first human sperm chromosome preparations after culturing zona-free hamster oocytes penetrated by human spermatozoa[71]. One of the major sites of species specificity in mammals is the zona pellucida[70], and most species retain their strong species specificity even after the removal of the zona pellucida. The golden hamster is unique in this aspect and when the zona pellucida is removed, most of the species specificity is lost. After penetration by human sperm, both male and female gametes organize their pronuclei in such a way that individual chromosomes may be visualized.

We obtained sperm chromosome complements using Martin's technique[72] with slight modifications. Briefly, the semen sample was washed with Biggers–Whitten–Whittingham (BWW) and incubated at 37°C for 5–7 h in BWW or, alternatively, kept at 4°C in Test yolk buffer overnight, to induce capacitation. The oviducts of super-ovulated hamsters were dissected and the oocytes were freed from the cumulus mass enzymatically with hyaluronidase. The zona pellucida was removed by trypsin, thus allowing cross-species fertilization. The hamster oocytes and human sperm were coincubated until 50% of the oocytes were fertilized (determined by squash mounts), or after a 3-h coincubation period. The oocytes were then transferred to Ham's F-10 media overnight (12–13 h) followed by a 6–8-h incubation with colcemid to arrest the chromosomes at metaphase. The oocytes were fixed onto slides using Tarkowski's method[73]. Giemsa staining was used to examine the chromosomes.

A total of 3187 historical control karyotypes were reviewed by Brandriff[74] and an overall sex chromosome ratio (X:Y) of 50.2:49.8 was found. These results certainly suggest that the initial ratio of X- to Y-bearing sperm present in the ejaculate in 50/50, as expected on theoretical grounds. We found[75] that sperm capacitated better in Test yolk buffer compared to BWW medium. Sperm capacitated in Test yolk buffer yielded several sperm chromosome complements with varying degrees of quality. The success of the technique greatly depends on specific precautions during oocyte handling and chromosome fixation. First, it is important to check the hamster oocytes for fertilization since this is the first opportunity to determine the success of the technique. Secondly, the number of usable chromosome spreads is impaired by (1) multiple penetrations, (2) oocyte loss (burst) during the process of chromosome fixation and (3) inadequate spreading[72]. Thirdly, oocyte handling should be restricted to a minimum in order to prevent parthenogenesis.

In contrast to the F-body scoring in which a random sampling of the spermatozoa is guaranteed the issue of sample bias is raised with the hamster ovum penetration technique, as only sperm with fertilizing capacity penetrate zona-free eggs and are being analyzed. The hamster ovum penetration technique is time consuming, it is technically difficult and provides data on only a small number of sperm cells, thereby limiting the usefulness of this method.

From the experience gained in our laboratory the success of the experiment depended greatly on the time taken for manipulations. The hamster ovum penetration technique, however, offers interesting research possibilities in the direct analysis of the chromosome constitution of human spermatozoa. This area of research includes, among others, the group of infertile patients with <15% normal sperm morphology, capable of ovum penetration, and especially cases of gamete micromanipulation therapy for those patients with low penetration capabilities.

Flow cytometry

Apart from sperm chromosomal character as measured by karyotyping and chromosome specific probes, the measurement of DNA mass is one of the most scientifically valid methods for differentiating between X- and Y-chromosome-bearing sperm. The human Y chromosome is smaller than the X chromosome and it has been reported to differ by 3% of DNA content[76,77]. However, no evidence existed that could demonstrate that the sex chromosome constitution of a sperm presented a specific shape or any particular morphological characteristics. Recently, however, Cul[78] showed for the first time that human X sperm are indeed statistically larger and longer than Y sperm. They determined the sex of 233 non-motile sperm, which were individually selected for direct photography before PCR amplification. They magnified photographs of individual sperm a further 30× and directly measured them. Statistical analysis showed that the length, perimeter and area of heads, the length of the neck and tail in X-bearing sperm are significantly larger than those of Y-bearing sperm.

Separation of X and Y sperm using a method based on differences in total DNA (weight) requires a technique with exceptionally high resolution ability. Differentiation of sperm cells can be accomplished by flow cytometry, as it permits separation of cells after measurement of their relative DNA content, based on the fluorescence emission intensity after vital staining of cells with a DNA specific fluorochrome.

According to Johnson[77], sperm samples were washed and sperm nuclei prepared by sonication to break the tail from the head. Sperm nuclei and fresh, viable spermatozoa were stained by adding a vital fluorochrome, bisbenzimide. Samples were flow-analyzed and sorted at room temperature.

The flow cytometer/cell sorter was specifically modified for the analysis of spermatozoa for DNA content and for their flow sorting capabilities. Briefly, the forward angle light scatter detector was replaced with a fluorescence detector and the standard cylindrical sample injection tip was slanted to produce a ribbon-shaped core stream. These adaptations are required if one is to control the orientation of the spermatozoa to the laser beam and measure the fluorescence from the properly orientated spermatozoa allowing detection of small differences in DNA content between X- and Y-bearing sperm[77].

The fluorescence signal collected by the detector is highly proportional to sperm DNA content. Two peaks, representing X- and Y-bearing sperm, were found in unmanipulated sperm that were ~2.8% apart in terms of DNA content. This flow cytometric determination[77] of human spermatozoal DNA content difference agrees with the value reported by Sumner[76], determined on the basis of dry mass differences of X- and Y-bearing sperm.

Johnson[77] illustrated the usefulness of DNA content as a marker by which viable human X- and Y-bearing sperm can be identified and separated. Although small differences such as 3% in DNA content require that the resolving capability of the instrumentation be pressed to its basic (inherent) cutoff point, flow cytometry promises unlimited applications in the identification and separation of X- and Y-bearing sperm.

Polymerase chain reaction

The polymerase chain reaction (PCR) is a powerful technique for selectively amplifying DNA or RNA sequences. It is so sensitive that a single DNA molecule may be amplified to produce microgram amounts of DNA which may be visualized on agarose gels. The technique requires a pair of oligonucleotide primer sequences which flank the region of interest, which are complementary to the opposite strand of the target DNA. The basis of the technique is a thermal cycle consisting of three stages:

(1) Denaturation – the target molecule is heat denatured to produce single stranded template molecules.

(2) Annealing – the primers which are in molar excess to the template molecule competitively anneal to the complementary target DNA.

(3) Extension – the thermostatic enzyme Taq polymerase initiates the synthesis of new strands using target sequences as template.

This cycle is repeated for 20–30 rounds, resulting in a theoretical doubling of the target sequence with each cycle.

We have used PCR amplification, with a common pseudoautosomal primer and X- and Y-specific primers, on human blood DNA from 20 subjects (male and female). We correctly sexed 19 of the 20 blood samples finding the primers suitable for distinguishing between human male and female DNA (unpublished results). Handyside *et al.*[79] have reported the accurate sexing of preimplantation embryos from single cells biopsied at the eight-cell stage using PCR to amplify a repeated sequence specific for the Y chromosome. Using this technique pregnancies have been established and female births have resulted following transfer of embryos identified as females[80].

The analysis of the genotype of single sperm at the DNA level (the gene coding for the low density lipoprotein receptor) by PCR was accomplished by Li[82]. After purification from seminal plasma, individual sperm were drawn into a fine plastic needle under microscopic observation and delivered to a tube for lysis and amplification.

Lobel[61] established the primary sex ratio of unselected sperm. Sperm DNA from whole semen was isolated and purified. PCR amplification and quantitation of X and Y chromosome sequences was performed. The mean primary sex ratio of unmanipulated sperm in 98 samples investigated with quantitative PCR was 1:1, with an average Y chromosome content of 50.3%. Another study[78] individually amplified 233 sperm and found that 48.8% were Y-bearing sperm and 51.2% were X-bearing sperm.

There are several factors affecting the success of PCR, e.g. temperatures and incubation times, primers, magnesium ion concentration, deoxyribonucleotide triphosphates, enzyme, buffer and target DNA. For instance, we managed independently to amplify and detect the X- and Y-chromosomal fragments of lymphocyte DNA; however, as soon as the X and Y primers were added together in the PCR cocktail, for simultaneous amplification of the X- and Y-chromosmal fragments, only the X-fragments were detected on the agarose gel. A possible explanation for the repeated amplification failure of the Y-chromosome fragment could lie in the critical importance of target DNA length. It could be explained that due to the relative smaller length of the X-specific fragment (450 bp) compared to the Y-specific fragment (830 bp), annealing to the complementary sequence and extension of the annealed primer resulted in more rapid amplification of the X-specific segment. To optimize the simultaneous amplification of different primers one should choose target DNA sequences of similar length. Although the basis of this technique is fundamentally the same for general applications, unfortunately no single protocol is appropriate to all situations. Ideally, the precise conditions of the reaction should be adjusted and optimized for each combination of template and primers.

One of the great advantages of PCR is the incredible sensitivity of the technique. It also has a negative side to it: the risk of contamination. Contamination can be from two sources – either foreign DNA entering the reaction or previously amplified DNA carried over in solutions and equipment. However, by simultaneous scoring of X and Y chromosome targets[61], the relative abundance of the two chromosomes is directly measured with increased precision, accuracy and speed.

An alternative to the use of PCR is *in situ* hybridization of X and/or Y chromosome specific probes to fixed nuclei.

In situ *hybridization*

The application of X- and/or Y-specific DNA probes is an alternative method for monitoring the proportion of X- and Y-bearing sperm following separation efforts. By the process of *in situ* hybridization, specific nucleic acid sequences are traced in morphologically preserved chromosomal cells[83]. *In situ* hybridization involves labelling of a specific nucleic acid probe, denaturation of target material, *in situ* hybridization of the probe to the target DNA and finally detection. Fluorescent *in situ* hybridization (FISH)[84] with an X- or Y-chromosome specific DNA probe reveals a highly specific fluorescent spot in sperm nuclei.

Joseph *et al.*[85] used isotopic cRNA–DNA *in situ* hybridization with a Y-chromosome specific probe to identify human Y-bearing spermatozoa obtained from human testicular biopsies. They found 48.3% Y-bearing sperm. West *et al.*[60] first reported the successful identification of human Y-bearing sperm, from ejaculated semen, by *in situ* hybridization with tritiated DNA. They followed a pretreatment regimen designed to decondense the sperm head to allow the DNA probe access to the chromatin.

The success of the *in situ* hybridization technique depends on the efficient decondensation of the sperm heads to allow access of the probe to sperm chromatin. Sperm heads could be decondensed in the presence of an anionic detergent solution (SDS) containing dithiothreitol to break the disulfide bonds.

A decondensed, fixed and air-dried preparation of a few drops of semen on a glass slide can be used for FISH. In our laboratory the Y-centromere specific DNA probe DYZ3 (Wolfe *et al.*[86]: ATCC) was labeled with digoxigenin (Boehringer Mannheim, Randburg, South Africa) by nick translation. Sperm preparations, lymphocyte preparations (obtained using standard cytogenetic techniques) and DNA probe were simultaneously denatured in a solution of 60% formamide, 2×SSC, 50 mM sodium phosphate at 80°C for 3 min. Hybridization of probe to target DNA occurred at 37°C overnight in a humid chamber. The digoxigenin labeled probe was detected with fluorescein-conjugated sheep antidigoxigenin (200 μg/mL stock solution) as described by the Boerhaave's Course for *in situ* hybridization[87]. Cells were counterstained with propidium iodide (PI). The FITC and PI were viewed under a fluorescence microscope.

Using the probe DYZ3, we found the sperm sex ratio of 20 untreated semen samples (2100 spermatozoa scored) to be 50.3% Y:49.7% X[88]. West[60] found 46.7% labeled spermatozoa among 3900 scored. Han[89] found that single FISH with an X-chromosome specific probe hybridized to 48.2% among 6460 sperm nuclei scored. Using double FISH, Han[90], using X- and Y-chromosome specific probes, found that the overall proportions of X- and Y-bearing sperm in ejaculates is 47.9% and 47.2%, respectively. Simultaneous detection of X- and Y-bearing sperm rules out any doubt that may occur as to whether the non-fluorescent cells are nullisomic or have failed to hybridize. Correlation between single sex chromosome and double sex chromosome FISH is, however, very high, indicating that FISH with one sex chromosome probe may be used with equal confidence.

In conclusion, the different identification techniques applied to differentiate between X- and Y-bearing sperm vary from less reliable to extremely reliable. However, these techniques all convey the same basic message, namely that the sperm sex ratio outcome of native semen is close to the expected 1:1 distribution. The aim of any sperm sex separation technique is thus to successfully separate X- from Y-bearing sperm in such a way that will significantly change the expected 1:1 ratio.

XY sperm separation techniques

This section deals with attempts aimed to successfully separate X- from Y-bearing sperm. Eight scientific hypotheses for producing the desired sex of offspring by separation of X- and Y-bearing sperm were reviewed by Gledhill[91]. These hypotheses are based on physical characteristics of sperm, and differences in size, shape, density and surface charge. Others are based on the presence of H-Y antigen on all Y-chromosome bearing cells, flow fractionation, Sephadex gel filtration, albumin centrifugation and the most significant method to date, namely flow cytometry. The following discussion will focus mainly on the latter three topics.

Sephadex gel filtration

Gel filtration with Sephadex relies on the separation of large molecules from smaller ones. This is accomplished by the pore size of the Sephadex gel which permits diffusion of smaller molecules into the three-dimensional network of the gel, whereas larger molecules are excluded from the gel matrix. Ultimately, larger molecules will move through the gel column at a more rapid rate, thus effecting separation based on molecular size. Theoretically, smaller Y-bearing sperm should be trapped within the network of the Sephadex gel, while the larger X-bearing sperm would pass through the column more rapidly, effecting separation into X- and Y-bearing sperm.

Steeno *et al.*[92] originally claimed an enrichment of 95% X-chromosome-bearing sperm using Sephadex gel filtration. Sephadex G50 fine powder was suspended in a solution to swell overnight. A glass column was filled with Sephadex, semen was added on the column and filtration was performed with a specific solution at room temperature. After the void volume, the fractions rich in motile sperm were collected in 1 mL aliquot fractions, in separate tubes. Nine to 15 tubes were collected after filtration and approximately 35% of the original number of spermatozoa were recovered.

Corson *et al.*[93] reported 73% females born after therapeutic donor insemination of 19 women with Sephadex-treated sperm. Twelve of the 19 women conceived with an overall result of seven daughters, two sons and one set of mixed twins. Since clomiphene citrate was administered to some of the patients, different hormonal levels might have contributed to the change in sex ratio.

Using a modified version of Steeno *et al.*'s[92] Sephadex gel filtration, Beckett *et al.*[94] tested the effectiveness of the latter separation technique by direct sperm chromosome and DNA analysis. However, no consistent enrichment for X-chromosome-bearing sperm was demonstrated according to any of the testing methods employed and nor was a significant difference detected in sex ratio between untreated and Sephadex-treated sperm. These results question the utility of the Sephadex sperm separation technique for female sex selection.

Albumin gradient centrifugation

One of the best known and successfully applied X- and Y-bearing sperm separation techniques has been described by Ericsson and colleagues[95–97]. Ericsson and co-workers[95] first reported the enrichment of Y-bearing human sperm fraction after layering semen over liquid albumin gradient columns. It was reported that approximately 85% of the sperm migrating to the lowest part of the column were Y-bearing sperm. This observation was based on differential staining obtained with the quinacrine mustard staining method[57] (previously discussed), and was later confirmed by male:female birth ratio[96,97]. Some reports agree with Ericsson's human Y-sperm enrichment[93], while others contradict his results[74].

We conducted an *in situ* hybridization study[88] that evaluated the enrichment of Y-bearing sperm, as proposed by the Ericsson's albumin gradient separation (modified protocol 3)[96], on 20 semen samples. Ejaculates were diluted, centrifuged and the pellet resuspended in medium after which a small aliquot of the sample was removed to serve as the control specimen. The remainder of the sample was divided into 0.5 mL aliquots and layered over a 10% solution of human serum albumin (HSA) in glass columns for 45 min. The initial sperm layer was removed and the albumin centrifuged for 10 min. Sperm pellets were resuspended in Tyrode's salt solution and layered over a two-layer HSA column consisting of a 12.5% layer over a 20% layer. The sperm layer was removed after 30 min and the 12.5% layer after another 30 min. The 20% HSA (test sample) and control sample were centrifuged and each pellet was resuspended in BWW.

Manipulated and unmanipulated sperm fractions were treated for nucleus chromatin decondensation, fixed and a few drops put onto glass slides followed by air drying. Each fraction was probed for the presence of Y-bearing sperm using FISH with the probe DYZ3.

There was a statistically significant increase in the mean percentage of Y-bearing sperm after albumin separation, compared to the percentage of Y-bearing sperm before separation. The global sex ratio before separation was 50.3% Y: 49.7% X and after albumin separation, 53.4% Y: 46.6% X.

Using the human sperm–hamster egg system, Gledhill *et al.*[91] found no significant increase in sex ratio of albumin processed spermatozoa compared to unprocessed control samples. Brandriff *et al.*[74] also reported that they could not confirm the Y enrichment of spermatozoa after the albumin density procedure. They found that the sex ratio (Y:X) after separation (42.8%:57.2%) was not significantly different to that of unprocessed spermatozoa (50.2%:49.8%)[74]. Ueda *et al.*[98] found a slight, but significant, increase in the percentage of Y-bearing sperm.

We found a slight but statistically significant increase in the mean percentage of Y-bearing sperm after albumin treatment. Although the result is statistically significant, the question remains whether the 3 percentage-point increase in Y-bearing sperm is of any clinical significance. This is in conflict with the live-born data of Ericsson[96] from women artificially inseminated with albumin isolated sperm. From 1034 births after intrauterine insemination with albumin-processed sperm 749 (72%) were male. However, the degree of enrichment was only slight in our hands and the clinical relevance uncertain. A randomized controlled clinical study should help to clarify the above laboratory results.

Flow cytometric cell sorting

Once the small differences in DNA content between individual X- and Y-bearing sperm were identified by flow cytometry as previously described, it was possible to separate the X- from Y-bearing sperm. The specially modified sorting system allows the generation of a fluorescent signal from spermatozoa stained with Hoechst[77]. Spermatozoa were sorted directly onto standard microscope slides according to fluorescence intensity detected (emitted) from stained spermatozoa. These two separated sperm populations were then probed for the presence of the X or Y chromosome by FISH.

Flow cytometric sorting for the enrichment of X- and Y-bearing sperm populations showed 82.2% and 75.5% positive signals, respectively, after probing with FISH. Statistical correlation indicated a significant difference from the theoretical human sex ratio. Moreover, sorted X- and Y-bearing sperm were found to maintain their viability for several hours after sorting and no significant deleterious effect was evident due to the fluorescent staining[77]. All animal offspring born after flow cytometric separation proved morphologically and functionally normal[99].

Human spermatozoa are not easily sorted or analyzed for DNA content by this method for three reasons. First, the head morphology of the human spermatozoon is more angular than the paddle shape of spermatozoa of domestic animals. The sorting process relies on orientating the flattest side of the spermatozoon to the laser beam, so that variation in fluorescent signal can be minimized and separation achieved[58]. Fluorescence emitted from the edge of the spermatozoon is much brighter than fluorescence emitted from its larger flat surface. This fluorescence heterogeneity is maximal when it is detected at a right angle to the incident excitation source. Secondly, human spermatozoa are more polymorphic and have greater heterogeneity of chromatin composition than animal spermatozoa. Thirdly, small differences such as 3% in DNA content require that the resolving capability of the instrumentation be pressed to its basic (inherent) cutoff point[58].

However, Johnson *et al.*[77] illustrated the usefulness of DNA content as a marker by which viable human X- and Y-bearing sperm can be identified and separated. Their results demonstrate that the human sperm sex ratio can be significantly shifted to favor the selection of female-producing (X) sperm or male-producing (Y) sperm when spermatozoa are flow cytometrically sorted on the basis of DNA content. Flow cytometry and cell sorting for the purpose of XY sperm separation is a very promising procedure with multiple potential clinical applications.

Clinical applications

The medical community has desired to have available the technology of effective sex preselection to improve therapeutic alternatives in cases of X-linked genetic diseases. Approximately 200 X-linked recessive disorders have been documented. Of these diseases muscular dystrophy, the Fragile X Syndrome, hemophilia, Lesch–Nyhan Syndrome, Hunter's Syndrome, Fabry Disease and Testicular Feminization Syndrome are some of the more common examples. An accurate sex preselection technique would replace the current therapeutic approach of prenatal and preimplantation genetic diagnosis for X-linked recessive diseases. Selective abortion of the affected sex biopsy and sex selection would be replaced by medical intervention before implantation by means of artificial insemination with a purified X-bearing sperm population.

With the improvements of IVF, less spermatozoa are required to fertilize a single ovum. This tendency is of immense value for those patients with low penetration capabilities where gamete micromanipulation therapy (intracytoplasmic microinjection of whole spermatozoa or sperm heads from the separated sperm population) should be utilized. The successful use of sorted sperm microinjection in several species has been demonstrated[100]. All animal offspring born after flow cytometric separation proved morphologically and functionally normal[99].

Apart from sex selection used when the prospective mother carries an X-linked disease, data indicated that allowing sex selection by desire would not greatly disturb the existing sex proportions, and would not alter, in any sensible way, our social structure[101]. It has always been proclaimed that all children should be desired and, therefore, in those families where the sex of children is a problem a child of the desired sex would be a wanted child.

References

1. Mortimer, D. (1989). Sperm transport in the human female reproductive tract. In Finn, C. A. (ed.) *Oxford Reviews of Reproductive Biology*, Vol. 5, p. 30. (Oxford: Oxford University Press)
2. Mortimer, D. (1990). Semen analysis and sperm washing techniques. In Gagnon, C. (ed.) *Control of Sperm Motility: Biological Clinical Aspects*, pp. 263–84. (Boca Raton: CRC Press)
3. Franken, D. R., Oehninger, S. C., Burkman, L. I., Coddington, C. C., Kruger, T. F., Rosenwaks, Z., Acosta, A. A. and Hodgen, G. D. (1989). The hemizona assay (HZA): a predictor of human sperm

fertilization potential in *in vitro* fertilization (IVF) treatment. *J.* In Vitro *Fertil. Embryo Transf.*, **6**, 44–9
4. Henkel, R., Müller, C., Miska, W., Gips, H. and Schill, W.-B. (1993). Determination of the acrosome reaction in human spermatozoa is predictive of fertilization *in vitro. Hum. Reprod.*, **8**, 2128–32
5. Edwards, R. G., Bavister, B. D. and Steptoe, P. C. (1969). Early stages of fertilization *in vitro* of human oocytes matured *in vitro. Nature*, **221**, 632–5
6. Edwards, R. G., Steptoe, P. C. and Purdy, J. M. (1980). Establishing full-term human pregnancies using cleaving embryos grown *in vitro. Br. J. Obstet. Gynaecol.*, **87**, 737–56
7. Purdy, J. M. (1982). Methods for fertilization and embryo culture *in vitro*. In Edwards, R. G. and Purdy, J. M. (eds.) *Human Conception* In Vitro, pp. 135–48. (London: Academic Press)
8. Trounson, A. O., Leeton, J. F., Wood, C., Webb, J. and Kovacs, G. (1980). The investigation of idiopathic infertility by *in vitro* fertilization. *Fertil. Steril.*, **34**, 431–8
9. Mahadevan, M. M., Trounson, A. O. and Leeton, J. F. (1983). The relationship of tubal blockage, infertility of unknown cause, suspected male infertility, and endometriosis to success of *in vitro* fertilization and embryo transfer. *Fertil. Steril.*, **40**, 755–62
10. Yates, C. A. and de Kretser, D. M. (1987). Male-factor infertility and *in vitro* fertilization. *J.* In Vitro *Fertil. Embryo Transf.*, **4**, 141–7
11. Aitken, R. J. and Clarkson, J. S. (1988). Significance of reactive oxygen species and antioxidants in defining the efficacy of sperm preparation techniques. *J. Androl.*, **9**, 367–76
12. Tea, N. T., Jondet, M. and Scholler, R. (1984). A migration–gravity sedimentation method for collecting motile spermatozoa from human semen. In Harrison, R. F., Bonnar, J. and Thompson, W. (eds.) In Vitro *Fertilization and Embryo Transfer in Early Pregnancy*, p. 117. (Lancaster: MTP Press)
13. Menkveld, R., Stander, F. S. H., Kotze, T. J. vW., Kruger, T. F. and van Zyl, J. A. (1990). The evaluation of morphological characteristics of human spermatozoa according to stricter criteria. *Hum. Reprod.*, **5**, 586–92
14. Huszar, G., Willetts, M. and Corrales, M. (1990). Hyaluronic acid (Sperm Select) improves retention of sperm motility and velocity in normozoospermic and oligozoospermic specimens. *Fertil. Steril.*, **54**, 1127–34
15. Wikland, M., Wik, O., Steen, Y., Qvist, K., Söderlund, B. and Janson, P. O. (1987). A self-migration method for preparation of sperm for *in vitro* fertilization. *Hum. Reprod.*, **2**, 191–5
16. Harrison, R. A. P. (1976). A highly efficient method for washing mammalian spermatozoa. *J. Reprod. Fertil.*, **48**, 347
17. Bolton, V. N. and Braude, P. R. (1984). Preparation of human spermatozoa for *in vitro* fertilization by isopycnic centrifugation on self-generating density gradients. *Arch. Androl.*, **13**, 167
18. Pousette, A., Akerlöf, E., Rosenborg, L. and Fredricsson, B. (1986). Increase in progressive motility and improved morphology of human spermatozoa following their migration through Percoll gradients. *Int. J. Androl.*, **9**, 1
19. Dravland, J. E. and Mortimer, D. (1985). A simple discontinuous Percoll gradient procedure for washing human spermatozoa. *IRCS Med. Sci.*, **13**, 16
20. Arcidiacono, A., Walt, H., Campana, A. and Balerna, M. (1983). The use of Percoll gradients for the preparation of subpopulations of human spermatozoa. *Int. J. Androl.*, **6**, 433
21. Gellert-Mortimer, S. T., Clarke, G. N., Baker, H. W. G., Hyne, R. V. and Johnston, W. I. H. (1988). Evaluation of Nycodenz and Percoll density gradients for the selection of motile human spermatozoa. *Fertil. Steril.*, **49**, 335–41
22. Mortimer, D., Curtis, E. F. and Dravland, J. E. (1986). The use of strontium-substituted media for capacitating human spermatozoa: an improved sperm preparation method for the zona-free hamster penetration test. *Fertil. Steril.*, **46**, 97
23. Laws-King, A., Trounson, A., Sathananthan, H. and Kola, I. (1987). Fertilization of human oocytes by microinjection of a single spermatozoon under the zona pellucida. *Fertil. Steril.*, **48**, 637
24. Suarez, S. S., Wolf, D. P. and Meizel, S. (1986). Induction of the acrosome reaction in human spermatozoa by a fraction of human follicular fluid. *Gamete Res.*, **14**, 107–21
25. Mortimer, S. T. and Mortimer, D. (1988). Percoll selection of human spermatozoa is dependent upon motility not concentration. *J. Reprod. Fertil.* Abstr. Ser., **1**, 65
26. Bisson, J. P. and David, G. (1975). Anomalies morphologiques du spermatozoide humain. II. Étude ultrastructurale. *J. Gynecol. Obstet. Biol. Reprod.*, **4** (Suppl. 1), 37
27. Tanphaichitr, N., Millette, C. F., Agulnick, A. and Fitzgerald, L. M. (1988). Egg-penetration ability and structural properties of human sperm prepared by Percoll-gradient centrifugation. *Gamete Res.*, **20**, 67–81
28. Bolton, V. N., Warren, R. E. and Braude, P. R. (1986). Removal of bacterial contaminants from semen for *in vitro* fertilization or artificial insemination by the use of buoyant density centrifugation. *Fertil. Steril.*, **46**, 1128
29. Pardo, M., Barri, P. N., Bancells, N., Coroleu, B., Buxederas, C., Pomerol, J. M., Jr. and Sabater, J. (1988). Spermatozoa selection in discontinuous Percoll gradients for use in artificial insemination. *Fertil. Steril.*, **49**, 505–9
30. Ord, T., Patrizio, P., Marello, E., Balmaceda, J. P. and Asch, R. H. (1990). Mini-Percoll: a new method of semen preparation for IVF in severe male factor infertility. *Hum. Reprod.*, **5**, 987–9
31. Serafini, P., Blank, W., Tran, C., Mansourian, M.,

Tan, T. and Batzofin, J. (1990). Enhanced penetration of zona-free hamster ova by sperm prepared by Nycodenz and Percoll gradient centrifugation. *Fertil. Steril.*, **53**, 551–5
32. Paulson, J. D. and Polakoski, K. L. (1977). A glass wool column procedure for removing extraneous material from the human ejaculate. *Fertil. Steril.*, **28**, 178–81
33. Sherman, J. K., Paulson, J. D. and Lui, K. C. (1981). Effect of glass wool filtration on ultrastructure of human spermatozoa. *Fertil. Steril.*, **36**, 643
34. Van der Ven, H. H., Jeyendren, R. S., Al-Hasani, S., Tünnerhoff, A., Hoebbel, K., Diedrich, K., Krebs, D. and Perez-Pelaez, M. (1988). Glass wool filtration of human semen: relation to swim-up procedure and outcome of IVF. *Hum. Reprod.*, **3**, 85–8
35. Rhemrev, J., Jeyendran, R. S., Vermeiden, J. P. W. and Zaneveld, L. J. D. (1989). Human sperm selection by glass wool filtration and two-layer, discontinuous Percoll gradient centrifugation. *Fertil. Steril.*, **51**, 685–90
36. Henkel, R., Franken, D. R., Schill, W.-B. and Lombard, C. J. (1994). The selective capacity of glass wool filtration for normal chromatin condensed human spermatozoa: A therapeutic modality for male factor cases? *Int. J. Androl.*, submitted
37. Rana, N., Jeyendran, R. S., Holmgren, W. J., Rotman, C. and Zaneveld, L. J. D. (1989). Glass wool-filtered spermatozoa and their oocyte penetrating capacity. *J.* In Vitro *Fertil. Embryo Transf.*, **6**, 280–4
38. Aitken, R. J. and Clarkson, J. S. (1987). Cellular basis of defective sperm function and its association with the genesis of reactive oxygen species by human spermatozoa. *J. Reprod. Fertil.*, **81**, 459–69
39. Mortimer, D. (1991). Sperm preparation techniques and iatrogenic failures of *in-vitro* fertilization. *Hum. Reprod.*, **6**, 173–6
40. Gavella, M. and Lipovac, V. (1992). Pentoxifylline-mediated reduction of superoxide anion production by human spermatozoa. *Andrologia*, **24**, 37–9
41. Lui, C. W., Mrsny, R. J. and Meizel, S. (1979). Procedures for obtaining high percentages of viable *in vitro* capacitated hamster sperm. *Gamete Res.*, **2**, 207
42. Daya, S., Gwatkin, R. B. L. and Bissessar, H. (1987). Separation of motile human spermatozoa by means of a glass bead column. *Gamete Res.*, **17**, 375
43. Sofikitis, N., Toda, T., Miyagawa, I., Terakawa, N., Iino, A. and Zavos, P. M. (1993). Morphometric parameters of human spermatozoa recovered via the sperm prep filtration column. In Vitro *International Congress of Andrology*, Tokyo, Miniposter, p. 145
44. Chijioke, P. C., Crocker, P. R., Gilliam, M., Owens, M. D. and Pearson, R. M. (1988). Importance of filter structure for the trans-membrane migration studies of sperm motility. *Hum. Reprod.*, **3**, 241
45. Raoof, N. T., Pearson, R. M. and Turner, P. (1987). A modified trans-membrane migration method for measuring the effect of drugs on sperm motility. *Br. J. Clin. Pharmacol.*, **24**, 319
46. Agarwal, A., Manglona, A. and Loughlin, K. R. (1991). Filtration of spermatozoa through L4 membrane: a new method. *Fertil. Steril.*, **56**, 1162–5
47. Ikemoto, I., Fanning, L., Loughlin, K. R. and Agarwal, A. (1993). Human sperm acrosin levels: Comparison of Kennedy and Accu-Sperm methods. In Vitro *International Congress of Andrology*, Tokyo, Miniposter, p. 1
48. Laughlin, K. R., Ikemoto, I., Fanning, L. and Agarwal, A. (1993). Levels of reactive oxygen species before and after sperm processing: Comparison of swim-up and L4 filtration methods. In Vitro *International Congress of Andrology*, Tokyo, Miniposter, p. 245
49. Forman, R., Guillett-Rosso, F., Fari, A., Volante, M., Frydman, R. and Testart, J. (1987). Importance of semen preparation in avoidance of reduced *in vitro* fertilization results attributable to bacteria. *Fertil. Steril.*, **47**, 527
50. Wong, P. C., Balmaceda, J. P., Blanco, J. D., Gibbs, R. S. and Asch, R. H. (1986). Sperm washing and swim-up technique using antibiotics removes microbes from human semen. *Fertil. Steril.*, **45**, 97
51. Sun, L-S., Gastaldi, C., Peterson, E. M., de la Maza, L. M. and Stone, S. C. (1987). Comparison of techniques for the selection of bacteria-free sperm preparations. *Fertil. Steril.*, **48**, 659
52. World Health Organization. (1987). *WHO Laboratory Manual for the Examination of Human Semen and Semen–Cervical Mucus Interaction*, 2nd edn, p. 67. (London: Cambridge University Press)
53. Aitken, R. J., Clarkson, J. S., Hargreave, T. B., Irvine, D. S. and Wu, F. C. W. (1989). Analysis of the relationship between defective sperm function and the generation of reactive oxygen species in cases of oligozoospermia. *J. Androl.*, **10**, 214–20
55. Mortimer, D. (1985). The male factor in infertility. Part I. Semen analysis. In *Current Problems in Obstetrics, Gynaecology and Fertility*, Vol. VIII, No. 7, p. 87. (Chicago: Year Book Medical Publishers)
56. Zarutski, P. W., Muller, C. H., Magone, M. and Soules, M. R. (1989). The clinical relevance of sex selection techniques. *Fertil. Steril.*, **52**, 891–905
57. Barlow, P. and Vosa, C. G. (1970). The Y chromosome in human spermatozoa. *Nature*, **226**, 961–2
58. Rudak, E., Jacobs, P. A. and Yanagimachi, R. (1978). Direct analysis of the chromosome constitution of human spermatozoa. *Nature*, **274**, 911–3
59. Johnson, L. A. and Pinkel, D. (1986). Modification of a laser-based flow cytometer for high resolution DNA analysis of mammalian spermatozoa. *Cytometry*, **7**, 268–73
60. West, J. D., West, K. M. and Aitken, R. J. (1989). Detection of Y-bearing spermatozoa by DNA–DNA *in situ* hybridization. *Mol. Reprod. Dev.*, **1**, 201–7
61. Lobel, S. M., Pomponio, R. J. and Mutter, G. L.

(1993). The sex ratio of normal and manipulated human sperm quantitated by the polymerase chain reaction. *Fertil. Steril.*, **59**, 387–92

62. Caspersson, T., Zech, L., Modest, E. J., Foley, G. E., Wagh, U. and Simonsson, E. (1969). DNA-binding fluorochromes for the study of the organization of the metaphase nucleus. *Exp. Cell Res.*, **58**, 141–52
63. Pearson, P. (1972). The use of new staining techniques for human chromosome identification. *J. Med. Genet.*, **9**, 264
64. Claassens, O. E., Stander, F. S. H., Kruger, T. F., Menkveld, R. and Lombard, C. J. (1989). Does the wash-up and swim-up method of semen preparation play a role in sex selection? *Andrology*, **23**, 23–6
65. Quinlivan, W. L. G., Preciado, K., Long, T. L. and Sullivan, H. (1982). Separation of human X and Y spermatozoa by albumin gradient and Sephadex chromatography. *Fertil. Steril.*, **37**, 104–7
66. Boaonkar, D. S. and Hollander, D. H. (1971). Quinacrine fluorescence of the Y chromosome. *Nature*, **230**, 52
67. Beatty, R. A. (1977). F-bodies as chromosome markers in mature human sperm heads. *Cytogenet. Cell Genet.*, **18**, 33–49
68. Roberts, A. M. and Goodall, H. (1976). Y chromosome visibility in quinacrine-stained human spermatozoa. *Nature*, **262**, 493–4
69. Van Kooij, R. J. and Van Oost, B. A. (1992). Determination of sex ratio of spermatozoa with a deoxyribonucleic acid-probe and quinacrine staining: a comparison. *Fertil. Steril.*, **58**, 384–6
70. Yanagimachi, R., Yanagimachi, H. and Rogers, B. J. (1976). The use of zona-free animal ova as a test-system for the assessment of the fertilizing capacity of human spermatozoa. *Biol. Reprod.*, **15**, 471–6
71. Yanagimachi, R. (1984). Zona-free hamster eggs: their use in assessing fertilization capacity and examining chromosomes of human spermatozoa. *Gamete Res.*, **10**, 187–232
72. Martin, R. H. (1983). A detailed method for obtaining preparations of human sperm chromosomes. *Cytogenet. Cell Genet.*, **35**, 252–6
73. Tarkowski, A. K. (1966). An air-drying method for chromosome preparations from mouse eggs. *Cytogenetics*, **5**, 394–400
74. Brandriff, B. F., Gordon, L. A., Haendel, S., Singer, S., Moore, D. H. and Gledhill, B. L. (1986). Sex chromosome ratios determined by karyotypic analysis in albumin-isolated human sperm. *Fertil. Steril.*, **46**, 678–85
75. Claasens, O. E., Franken, D. R., Menkveld, R. and Kruger, T. F. (1992). The use of hamster ova as reactivating vehicles to obtain human sperm chromosomes. *Med. Tech. S. Africa*, **6**, 32–5
76. Sumner, A. T. and Robinson, J. A. (1976). A difference in dry mass between the heads of X- and Y-bearing sperm. *J. Reprod. Fertil.*, **48**, 9–15
77. Johnson, L. A., Welch, G. R., Keyvanfar, K., Dorfman, A., Fugger, E. F. and Schulman, J. D. (1993). Gender preselection in humans? Flow cytometric separation of X and Y spermatozoa for the prevention of X-linked diseases. *Hum. Reprod.*, **8**, 1733–9
78. Cul, K. and Matthews, C. D. (1993). X larger than Y. *Nature*, **366**, 117–8
79. Handyside, A. H., Pattinson, K. K., Penketh, R. J., Delhanty, J. D., Winston, R. M. and Tuddenham, E. G. (1989). Biopsy of human preimplantation embryos and sexing by DNA amplification. *Lancet*, **1**, 347–9
80. Handyside, A. H., Kontogianni, E. H., Hardy, K. and Winston, R. M. (1990). Pregnancies from biopsied human preimplantation embryos sexed by Y-specific DNA amplification. *Nature*, **344**, 768–70
82. Li, H., Gyllensten, U. B., Cui, X., Saiki, R. K., Erlich, H. A. and Arnheim, N. (1988). Amplification and analysis of DNA sequences in single human sperm and diploid cells. *Nature*, **335**, 414–7
83. John, H., Bimstiel, M. and Jones, K. (1969). RNA/DNA hybrids at the cytological level. *Nature*, **223**, 582–7
84. Raap, A. K., Van de Rijke, F. M., Dirks, R. W., Sol, C. J., Boom, R. and Van der Ploeg, M. (1991). Bicolor fluorescence *in situ* hybridization to intron and exon mRNA sequences. *Exp. Cell Res.*, **197**, 319–22
85. Joseph, A. M., Gosden, J. R. and Chandley, A. C. (1984). Estimation of aneuploidy levels in human spermatozoa using chromosome specific probes and *in situ* hybridization. *Hum. Genet.*, **66**, 234–8
86. Wolfe, J., Darling, S. M., Erickson, R. P., Craig, I. W., Buckle, V. J., Rygby, P. W., Willard, H. F. and Goodfellow, P. N. (1985). Isolation and characterization of an alphoid centromeric repeat family from the Y chromosome. *J. Mol. Biol.*, **182**, 277–485
87. Raap, A. K. (1992). *In Situ Hybridization, Boerhaave Committee for Postgraduate Medical Education*, pp. 1–23. (Leiden: Leiden University)
88. Claassens, O. E., Oosthuizen, C. J. J., Brusnicky, J., Franken, D. R. and Kruger, T. F. (1995). Fluorescent *in situ* hybridization (FISH) evaluation of human Y-bearing spermatozoa separated by albumin density gradients. *Fertil. Steril.*, **63**, 417–18
89. Han, T. L., Webb, G. C., Flaherty, S. P., Correll, A., Matthews, C. D. and Ford, J. (1992). Detection of chromosome 17- and X-bearing human spermatozoa using fluorescence *in situ* hybridization. *Mol. Reprod. Dev.*, **33**, 189–94
90. Han, T. L., Ford, J. H., Webb, G. C., Flaherty, S. P., Correll, A. and Matthews, C. D. (1993). Simultaneous detection of X- and Y-bearing human sperm by double fluorescence *in situ* hybridization. *Mol. Reprod. Dev.*, **34**, 308–13
91. Gledhill, B. L. (1988). Selection and separation of X- and Y-chromosome-bearing sperm. *Gamete Res.*, **20**, 377–95

92. Steeno, O., Adimoelja, A. and Steeno, J. (1975). Separation of X and Y bearing human spermatozoa with the Sephadex gel-filtration method. *Andrology*, **7**, 95–7
93. Corson, S. L., Batzer, F. R., Alexander, N. J., Schlaff, S. and Otis, C. (1984). Sex selection by sperm separation and insemination. *Fertil. Steril.*, **42**, 756–60
94. Beckett, T. A., Martin, R. H. and Hoar, D. I. (1989). Assessment of the sephadex technique for selection of X-bearing human sperm by analysis of sperm chromosomes, deoxyribonucleic acid and Y-bodies. *Fertil. Steril.*, **52**, 829–35
95. Ericsson, R. J., Langevin, C. N. and Nishino, M. (1973). Isolation of fractions rich in human Y sperm. *Nature*, **246**, 421–4
96. Beernick, F. J., Dmowski, W. P. and Ericsson, R. J. (1993). Sex preselection through albumin separation of sperm. *Fertil. Steril.*, **59**, 382–6
97. Ericsson, S. A. and Ericsson, R. J. (1992). Couples with exclusively female offspring have an increased probability of a male child after using male sex preselection. *Hum. Reprod.*, **7**, 372–3
98. Ueda, K. and Yanagimachi, R. (1987). Sperm chromosome analysis as a new system to test human X- and Y-sperm separation. *Gamete Res.*, **17**, 221–8
99. Johnson, L. A. (1991). Sex preselection in swine: altered sex ratios in offspring following surgical insemination of flow sorted X- and Y-bearing sperm. *Reprod. Dom. Anim.*, **26**, 309–14
100. Johnson, L. A. and Clarke, R. N. (1988). Flow sorting of X- and Y-sorted bull, boar, and ram sperm microinjected into hamster oocytes. *Gamete Res.*, **21**, 335–43
101. Egozcue, J. (1993). Sex selection: why not? *Hum. Reprod.*, **8**, 1777

Prediction of sperm fertilizing potential 23

T. F. Kruger, D. R. Franken, R. R. Henkel and S. Oehninger

INTRODUCTION

The currently reported high incidence of male factor infertility mandates a complete andrological consultation and basic semen evaluation in all male partners of couples consulting for infertility. Clinicians and research scientists are still confronted with the question of whether a given laboratory test or a battery of tests can predict the outcome in assisted reproduction. No simple solution to these problems is available and there is no wide consensus on the value of the different tests available in clinical practice today.

BASIC SEMEN ANALYSIS

As far as routine evaluation of male infertility is concerned, the basic semen analysis is still the cornerstone of laboratory evaluation of the male.

Physical examination of semen, e.g. coagulation, liquefaction and viscosity, are important and gross abnormalities when present should be detected and carefully reported by the Andrology Laboratory regardless of the quality of other semen parameters. Semen processing using different separation techniques is often hampered by physical abnormalities[1].

Semen volume, unless extremely low, seldom represents a problem for assisted reproduction (normal >2.0 mL). pH should be checked routinely because its value may indicate the presence of chronic or acute infections that can impair fertilization *in vitro* or *in vivo* (normal pH = 7.2–8.0)[1].

The basic semen analysis will be considered normal for *in vivo* fertilization according to World Health Organization's (WHO) latest manual[2], when a concentration of >20 million/mL, percentage of motile sperm >50% (categories a and b) and normal sperm morphology >30% are found[2]. The morphology threshold for assisted reproduction according to the Tygerberg and Norfolk groups is at the level of 14% normal forms if strict criteria are used[3–5].

We consider a bacteriological as well as immunological screening essential parts of the initial semen analysis evaluation.

Influence of motility on fertilization *in vitro*

In a report by Acosta *et al.*[6] from the Jones Institute, it was noted that even a very low percentage of motile spermatozoa (10%) in a given sample did not have a significant negative influence on fertilization and pregnancy rates. They divided their patients into three groups: those with motility between 10% and 20% (group 1), 21% to 30% (group 2), and 31% to 40% (group 3). The fertilization rate was 68% for group 1, 72% for group 2 and 73% for group 3 with a pregnancy rate per embryo transfer of 42.9% (group 1), 32.5% (group 2), and 24.4% (group 3). There were no significant differences between the groups. However, it is possible that motility values <10% may represent a problem in *in vitro* fertilization (IVF).

Sperm concentration

The number of sperm is evaluated in terms of both sperm density and recoverable sperm. This is very important in handling patients for assisted reproduction. If the sperm density is <20 million/mL, the specimen is considered abnormal[2]. However, in assisted reproduction patients with severe oligozoospermia can still do well in terms of fertilization and pregnancy outcome if enough sperm can be obtained with separation techniques. In a prospective study performed at our own institution, no impact could be found on pregnancy outcome using, for example, the concentration/ml in the initial sample as a yardstick (Table 1)[7].

The number of recoverable sperm is determined by the swim-up procedure. A minimum figure

Table 1 The effect of different semen parameters on pregnancy rate. Reproduced from Kruger *et al.* 1993[7] with permission of the Hemisphere Publishing Corporation

Parameter	*Ongoing pregnancies (%)*
Sperm morphology (%)	
0.0–4.0	14*
5.0–14.0	21*
Insemination semen volume in oviduct	
0.01–0.09	20*
0.1–0.19	14*
0.2–0.9	19*
Seminal sperm concentration/mL	
3.0–10.0	17*
11.0–19.0	8*
>20.0	22*
Swim-up concentration	
0.1–4.9	18*
5.0–9.9	11*
>10.0	30*

* No significant difference

compatible for fertilization seemed to be 1.5 million total motile sperm assuming that the other parameters are normal[6]. In our own gamete intrafallopian transfer (GIFT) program, it is possible to achieve a good pregnancy rate if only 500 000 sperm/mL are recovered[5,7].

Spermatozoon morphology

In our experience, morphological characteristics appear to be the best predictors for fertilization. Strict criteria should be employed during the morphological examination of spermatozoa. Based on previous publications, this gives the best predictive ability[3–5].

The normal spermatozoon should have a single sperm head with a well-defined acrosome comprising between 40% and 70% of the sperm head area, and a perfectly smooth oval head, or one that tapers slightly at the level of the postacrosomal region. The head length should be 4–5 μm and the width 2.5–3 μm when Papanicolaou staining is utilized. When the DiffQuik stain is used, the length should be 5–6 μm and the width 2.5–3.5 μm[8]. (WHO 1992 with a stricter approach towards morphology criteria gives measurements for Papanicolaou of 4–5.5 μm [length]×2.5–3.5 μm [width].) No abnormalities in the neck, midpiece or tail should be present. The midpiece should be slender, axially attached and <1 μm wide, and its length should be approximately 1.5 times the head length. No cytoplasmic droplet greater than half the area of the sperm head should be present. The tail should be uniform, slightly thinner than the midpiece, uncoiled and approximately 45 μm long. Trivial variations in head morphology should be considered normal, but borderline normal heads are classified in a subgroup called slightly abnormal.

The 14% threshold for normal forms

When these strict criteria for normality are utilized in patients undergoing IVF, patients with fewer than 14% normal morphological forms were found to have a decreased fertilization rate according to previous publications (Table 2)[2,6]. Furthermore, in this same group of patients, two subgroups could be identified. The first appeared to have a good prognosis in terms of fertilizing ability although the percentage of eggs fertilized was lower than normal. This group was said to demonstrate the good prognostic pattern, or G pattern (lower fertilization potential than the normal group if only 100 000 sperm/mL/egg are used to fertilize the oocytes) (Table 2).

The second group in which fertilization was observed, exhibited a poor prognostic pattern, or P pattern (Table 3).

These morphological patterns have been found to be consistent and interpretation of the slides reproducible among technicians. In patients with 0–4% normal sperm morphology, classified as the P pattern, fertilization rates per oocyte were found to be 7.6% compared to the fertilization rate of 63.9% in the G pattern group ($P<0.0001$)[4].

Recently, independent researchers from various international centers looking at the role of sperm morphology in assisted reproduction have confirmed these results[9–13]. It was also observed in studies by Enginsu[10,13] that the predictive ability of strict criteria was significantly better compared to the WHO 1987 approach[10].

In a prospective study of patients in our GIFT program, we have also observed a significant difference in pregnancy rate when utilizing the 14% threshold of normal sperm morphology. A significantly lower pregnancy rate was observed in the group of patients with <14% normal morphology compared to those individuals in whom normal morphological forms comprised >14% of the

Table 2 Sperm morphology as a predictor of human IVF. Reproduced from Acosta (1988)[6] with permission of B. C. Dekko Inc.

	Group 1 (n=25) *Normal forms <14%*	*Group 2* (n=71) *Normal forms >14%*
Fertilization rate (% per oocyte)	49.4	88.3*
MI–MII	0=28%	0=1.4%
	<50%=36%	<50%=11.2%
	>50%=36%	>50%=87.4%
Pregnancies	3	24
Pregnancy rate/laparoscopy	12%	34.8%
Ongoing	4%	18.3%$^+$
Pregnancy rate/transfer	16%	34.3%
Ongoing	5%	18.5%$^+$

*P<0.0001; $^+$no significant difference

Table 3 Prognostic patterns of sperm morphology in human IVF. Reproduced from Kruger *et al.* (1988)[4] with permission of the American Society for Reproductive Medicine

	Fertilization in P pattern group (n=13)	*Fertilization in G pattern group* (n=32)
Normal forms (%)±SD	1.8±2.4	7.7±3.3
Concentration (million/mL) ±SD	63.3±42.8	83.3±57.8 (NS)
Motility (%)±SD	45.6±13.2	55.3±18.6 (NS)
Fertilization rate (%) per oocyte	7.6	63.9*
Embryos (%)±SD per patient	0.4	2.6*

SD=standard deviation; NS = not significant; *P<0.0001

specimen. In this study 423 cycles were analyzed prospectively, and the ongoing pregnancy rate in the group with abnormal sperm morphology (<14% normal forms) was 12%; meanwhile, an ongoing pregnancy rate of 23% was recorded in those couples in whom the male was found to have adequate sperm morphology (P<0.01)[5].

Two factors can be taken into consideration when handling a patient with low morphology to improve prognosis in assisted reproduction: (1) fertilization rate can be improved by simply increasing the insemination concentration/mL/egg from 100 000 sperm to at least 500 000 sperm[5,9]; and (2) to carefully consider the maturation stage of the oocyte. Patients with metaphase II oocytes will do better with IVF[14] and have an improved pregnancy rate in GIFT[5].

NEW DEVELOPMENTS IN THE FIELD OF SPERM MORPHOLOGY

In recent studies, sperm morphology was evaluated using computerized sperm analyzers. Four recent studies examined the value of the computerized system[15–18]. Wang[15,16] concluded that no benefit could be found in the system she had tested above the manual method. Davis[17], however, found the evaluation of the Motion Analysis System valuable. The studies by Wang and Davis looked at comparative analysis between manual and computerized systems on a cell by cell basis. In a recent study by our own group, we looked at the correlation between sperm morphology (normal forms, strict criteria) using slide by slide evaluation between manual and computerized systems (FERTECH). A good correlation was observed between the two methods[18]. The computer evaluation was also compared with the manual evaluation in a clinical study using fertilization as an endpoint. The computerized system identified the <14% of normal forms very well and showed a significant difference in fertilization rate in the groups with <14% and >14% normal forms (Figures 1,2). This difference was even more pronounced when a group of patients with <10% normal forms was considered (Figures

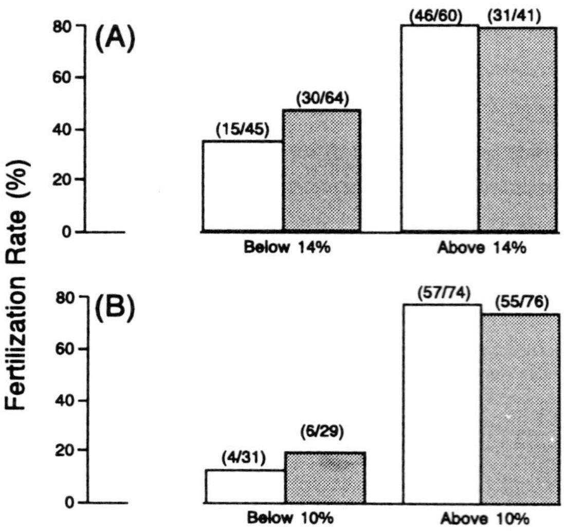

Figure 1 Tygerberg study. (A) Comparison of the ability of the manually recorded method and FERTECH (computer program) to predict IVF results. A threshold of 14% normal sperm forms was used to divide the two groups of patients. Numbers of oocytes fertilized/inseminated are provided in parenthesis. (B) Comparison of the ability of the manually recorded method and FERTCH to predict IVF results. A threshold of 10% normal sperm forms was used to divide the two groups of patients. □, Manual; ■, FERTECH. Reproduced from Kruger *et al.*[18] with permission of the American Society for Reproductive Medicine

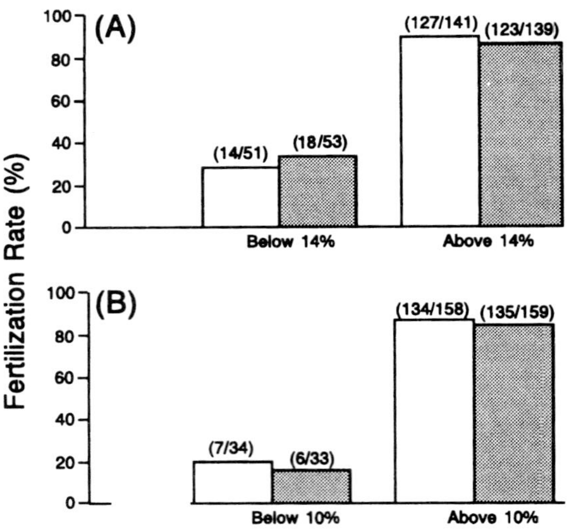

Figure 2 Norfolk study. (A) Comparison of the ability of the manually recorded method and FERTECH to predict IVF results. A threshold of 14% normal sperm forms was used to divide the two groups of patients. (B) Comparison of the ability of the manually recorded method and FERTECH to predict IVF results. A threshold of 10% normal sperm forms was used to divide the two groups of patients. □, Manual; ■, FERTECH. Reproduced from Kruger *et al.*[18] with permission of the American Society for Reproductive Medicine

1,2). It was concluded that this new development holds promise for clinical practice[18].

In a recent, still unpublished, study we evaluated the IVOS system readings against the human readings (experienced worker) in a slide by slide evaluation. Thirty slides were compared in each group. The Kappa statistical evaluation was used and man-versus-computer (IVOS) was in the same category as man-versus-man looking at percentage normal morphology per slide (Kappa, respectively, 0.73 and 0.58; both in the good agreement group).

When the Spearman correlation coefficient was applied to the same set of data, Kappa was 0.88 in the man-versus-man and 0.85 man-versus-IVOS experiments.

The repeatability per cell for the IVOS system showed a Kappa value of 0.83 (excellent category). This new development, fast enough for day to day use, holds promise in routine andrology laboratories as well as in clinical practice in assisted reproduction.

Bacteriological screening

Routine bacteriological screening includes cultures for *Neisseria gonorrhea*, *Ureaplasma urealyticum* and other mycoplasma strains, and *Chlamydia trachomatis* detected by the monoclonal antibody immunofluorescence technique in the urethral smear. In men with a history of chronic urogenital infectious disease or a white cell count in semen of >1 million leukocytes/mL, regular bacteriological investigation should also be performed. In general, a micro-organism count of >3000 Gram-negative pathogens/mL of semen or >10 000 Gram-positive non-pathogenic bacteria/mL of 1:2 diluted seminal plasma should be considered significant[6].

Immunological factors

In our institution, we use the mixed agglutination reaction test to screen for sperm antibodies in semen. If a value of more than 10% is obtained, we consider this test positive and confirm it with a

Table 4 Outcome of IVF in the Norfolk group. Reproduced from Acosta *et al.* (1994)[21] with permission of the American Society for Reproductive Medicine

	Fert. rate (%)	*Total preg rate (%)*	*Term preg. rate*		*Abort. rate*	
			Cycle (%)	*Transf. (%)*	*Cycle (%)*	*Transf. (%)*
Study group (29 patients, 38 cycles)	41.9	21.0	23.5	13.1	14.7	37.5
G pattern (21 patients, 29 cycles)	52.2	24.1	25.0	13.8	14.3	42.8
P pattern (8 patients, 9 cycles)	18.5	11.1	16.7	11.1	16.7	0.0
Control group (23 patients, 23 cycles)	77.9	65.2	60.0	52.2	48.0	40.0
G pattern (16 patients, 16 cycles)	82.8	81.2	72.2	68.7	61.1	30.8
P pattern (7 patients, 7 cycles)	67.8	28.6	28.6	14.3	14.3	100.0

Fert. = fertility; preg. = pregnancy; Transf. = transfer; Abort. = abortion

direct immunobead test on the semen. In a study performed at our institution[19], we found a good correlation doing sperm antibodies in serum and in semen, thus supporting the use of the mixed agglutination reaction (MAR) test as a screening procedure to detect sperm autoantibodies.

When antibodies are detected, we tend to offer assisted reproduction techniques to these patients if there are no other abnormalities present, one reason being that we find the best pregnancy result with GIFT[20]. There was a significantly lower pregnancy rate within the same patients if only intrauterine insemination was performed compared to the GIFT outcome (3% pregnancy per cycle, compared to a 16% pregnancy rate per cycle, respectively).

In a recent study performed at the Jones Institute and Tygerberg Hospital, it was shown that low normal sperm morphology is playing a detrimental role in the fertilization process both in the control group and in the antibody positive group. One can clearly note the influence on fertilization and pregnancy outcome in the different morphology groups, as well as between the antibody positive and control groups (Tables 4, 5) (see Chapters 13, 27 and 28)[21].

Spermatozoa separation methods

Sperm separation is essential in assisted reproductive procedures to remove spermatozoa from the seminal plasma, thus eliminating anticapacitation factors in the seminal plasma, and to obtain a highly motile sperm fraction with increased normal forms. In our program, we use Ham's F-10 media plus maternal serum for preparation of semen in a double wash and swim-up procedure[3]. Other methods of separation include layering and swim-up, albumin gradient separation, glass-wool separation, glass bead column separation and Percoll separation[22]. Recently, a new method of semen preparation by MiniPercoll has been reported that was shown to be particularly beneficial in patients with severe oligozoospermia[23]. It was also used successfully in cases in which epididymal sperm was aspirated to be used in IVF. It is the authors' opinion that each male patient must be approached as an individual. The assisted reproduction laboratory must have different separation techniques available for oligozoospermic and asthenozoospermic patients. Some patients will do better using the swim-up technique and deliver sufficient sperm for

Table 5 Outcome of GIFT in the Tygerberg group. Reproduced with permission from Acosta *et al.* (1994)[21] with permission of the American Society of Reproductive Medicine

	Fert. rate (%)	*Total preg. rate (%)*	*Term preg. rate transf. (%)*	*Abort. rate transf. (%)*
Study group (54 patients, 89 cycles)	27.1	28.1	16.9	33.3
N (>14% normal) (26 patients, 49 cycles)	33.9	36.7	22.4	28.0
G pattern (25 patients, 35 cycles)	19.1	20.0	11.4	23.1
P pattern (3 patients, 5 cycles)	0	0	0	0
Control group (89 patients, 89 cycles)	62.9	43.8	32.6	23.2
N (>14% normal) (49 patients, 49 cycles)	70.6	51.0	36.7	38.9
G pattern (35 patients, 35 cycles)	52.3	37.1	28.6	42.9
P pattern (5 patients, 5 cycles)	42.8	20.0	20.0	0

Fert. = fertility; preg. = pregnancy; Abort. = abortion; transf. = transfer

assisted reproduction. On the other hand, other patients would need support to obtain a sufficient number of motile sperm, i.e. using the glass-wool technique or other separation techniques with or without pentoxifylline. In a patient with asthenozoospermia the days of abstinence can be important and often, one day or less of abstinence can improve the motility of sperm in the sample.

Testing of sperm function

Despite progress in IVF and other assisted reproduction techniques, the diagnosis and treatment of male factor infertility is still a major challenge for reproductive biologists as well as clinicians in reproductive medicine. Since evaluation of sperm function test results prior to any male factor treatment seems to be mandatory, the diagnostic work-up and the success in male infertility have recently incorporated more sophisticated diagnostic methods for evaluation of sperm quality. Some of these assays determine biochemical parameters which have been found to be important for sperm function. Most of them, however, determine the biological functions of spermatozoa and consequently the capability to fertilize an oocyte.

Biochemical assays

Creatine kinase

Recently, a cellular marker of sperm quality, creatine kinase, has been found to be a key enzyme in the synthesis of energy transport factors. Higher levels seem to indicate a defect in sperm cytoplasmic extrusions[24]. Motile sperm fractions from oligozoospermic samples enriched by the swim-up method were found to have lower creatine kinase levels than the original samples. Furthermore, when IVF was performed in oligozoospermic men, the group that proved to be fertile could be predicted on the basis of their sperm creatine kinase activity. However, more work is necessary to make this observation valuable for routine clinical use.

Recently, we have found that mature sperm selectively bind to the zona pellucida using immunocytochemistry for creatine kinase[25]. Spermatozoa with immature creatine kinase-staining patterns seem to be deficient in oocyte recognition and binding. This corroborates the report of Menkveld *et al.*[26], that morphologically superior sperm have a higher binding capacity than abnormally shaped sperm forms. Furthermore, a good relationship has been found between the sperm biochemical parameters of creatine kinase concentration, lipid peroxidation and abnormal sperm morphology[27].

Bioassays of sperm–oocyte interaction

Acrosin activity

Acrosin (EC 3.4.21.10), a trypsin-like serine proteinase which is exclusively found within the acrosome of mammalian spermatozoa[28,29], is associated with zona pellucida binding and zona pellucida penetration of spermatozoa[30–33]. Human spermatozoa that are almost devoid of acrosin fail to fertilize an egg, even if they are motile and possess an intact plasma membrane[34–38]. Considering the important function of acrosin for the fertilization process, several techniques have been described in the past to assess human sperm acrosin activity[39–42]. However, there are still uncertainties regarding the value of acrosin as a sole predictor of fertilization[43]. More work is needed in this field.

Two different assays quoted from the literature are evaluated in IVF programs: one spectrophotometric assay, using BAPNA as a substrate[44], and another based on lysis of a gelatine layer which is evaluated in our unit[45]. Using a cutoff point of 10 μm for the halo diameter and 60% for the halo formation rate in the gelatinolytic assay, our data indicated that men whose spermatozoa show these parameters in the low range are infertile with high probability (Table 6). Using that gelatinolytic assay, we found relatively low sensitivity besides high specificity (Table 6). This clearly supports the hypothesis that functional parameters of spermatozoa are more or less independent from each other. To reach the main goal of reproductive events, i.e. successful fertilization of oocytes by spermatozoa, each of these specific spermatozoal functions must be optimal. If one parameter is suboptimal, fertilization is affected.

Table 6 Statistical calculations of predictive values for cutoff values of halo diameter (10 μm) and halo formation rate (60%) for the gelatinolytic assay to predict fertilizing capacity of spermatozoa from different patients. Reproduced from Henkel *et al.* (1995)[45] with permission of J. B. Lippincott

	Halo diameter (10 μm)	*Halo formation rate (60%)*
Specificity (%)	98.7	92.0
Sensitivity (%)	25.7	37.1
Positive predictive value (%)	90.0	68.4
Negative predictive value (%)	74.0	75.8

Hypo-osmotic swelling test

The hypo-osmotic swelling (HOS) test is a measure of sperm membrane integrity and has been proposed as a predictor of IVF success[46]. Some investigations, however, have not found significant correlations between the results of the HOS test and the fertilizing ability of sperm *in vitro*[47,48].

Acrosome reaction

Apart from motility, membrane integrity, ability to bind to the zona pellucida, acrosin activity and membrane fusion abilities, the acrosome reaction is of essential importance for fertilization. The acrosome is a membrane-bound organelle which appears during spermatogenesis as a product of the Golgi complex. Acrosomal membranes underlying the plasma membrane are referred to as outer acrosomal membranes, those overlying the nuclear membrane as inner acrosomal membranes. The acrosome reaction is an exocytotic process involving fusion of sperm plasma membrane and outer acrosomal membrane. Only acrosome-reacted spermatozoa can penetrate the zona pellucida[49]. Patients showing aberrations of the acrosome are subfertile[37].

Data recently obtained by us[50] support the hypothesis by Tesarik[51] that higher levels of acrosome-reacted spermatozoa are required for fertilization, which will occur under physiological induction of the acrosome reaction. This means that the spontaneous acrosome reaction of capacitated spermatozoa, induced by random formation of clusters of the ZP3 receptors in the sperm membrane[52] and reported to be 4–10%[53,54], is not sufficient for fertil-

Table 7 Statistical calculations of predictive values for cutoff values of the inducibility of the acrosome reaction (AR) (difference between test value of AR after low-temperature induction and the spontaneous AR) (7.5%) and the percentage of acrosome-reacted spermatozoa after induction of acrosome reaction by means of low temperature to predict the fertilizing capacity of spermatozoa from different patients. Reproduced from Henkel *et al.* (1993)[50] with permission of IRL Press Ltd

	Inducibility (7.5%)	*Percentage of acrosome-reacted sperm (13.0%)*
Specificity (%)	50.0	21.7
Sensitivity (%)	86.0	98.0
Positive predictive value (%)	63.1	83.3
Negative predictive value (%)	78.2	73.5

ization of oocytes. This is in accordance with a recent report by Henkel *et al.*[50], that the percentage of acrosome-reacted spermatozoa should exceed 13% after induction of acrosome reaction in a diagnostic system using low temperature to induce acrosome reaction (Table 7). Consequently, an increased number of acrosome-reacted spermatozoa (more than those occurring during spontaneous acrosome reaction) is a prerequisite for fertilization. Nevertheless, the percentage of acrosome-reacted spermatozoa after induction of the acrosome reaction (AR) by means of low temperature in patients showing good fertilization is not significantly different from that in patients showing poor fertilization[50]. In contrast, the inducibility of the acrosome reaction, i.e. the difference between spontaneous acrosome reaction and the percentage of acrosome-reacted spermatozoa after induction, shows highly significant correlation. Inducibility of acrosome reaction should be at least 7.5% to be assessed as normal. Normal acrosome reaction and/or normal inducibility of the acrosome reaction indicate good fertilizing capacity of spermatozoa (Table 7).

Sperm penetration assay

The zona-free hamster ovum–sperm penetration assay (SPA) is often used as a prognostic test to assess male fertility *in vitro* as well as to measure the improvement of sperm function after therapy. This

Table 8 Sperm morphology as a predictor of the sperm penetration assay (SPA). Reproduced from Kruger *et al.* (1988)[56] with permission of Blackwell Science Ltd

	70 patients, sperm concentration >10×10⁶/mL motility >30%	
	Group 1a (n=*41*) *Normal forms <14%* *(teratozoospermia)*	*Group 1b* (n=*29*) *Normal forms >14%* *(normospermia)*
SPA<10%	35 (85.4%)	4 (13.8%)*
SPA>10%	6 (14.6%)	25 (86.2%)*

*P<0.0001, in comparison with group 1a

heterologous bioassay evaluates the ability of the proportion of acrosome-reacted sperm in a given sperm population and its ability to fuse with the oolemma and decondense within zona-free hamster eggs. Originally proposed as a test for assessing the fertilizing capacity of human spermatozoa, the SPA reflects specifically the ability of sperm samples to undergo the acrosome reaction[1].

The existence of a correlation between SPA and conventional semen parameters has been examined by numerous authors, yet no consensus has been attained, mainly because of the varied experimental conditions and assessment criteria used by different laboratories. Most early investigators found no correlation between SPA and the traditional semen parameters, sperm density, motility or morphology. In contrast, Rogers *et al.*[55] reported a correlation with motility and morphology, but found the latter to be more important. A prospective study of the SPA at Norfolk evaluated 70 patients with a normal sperm concentration (exceeding 20×10^6/mL), a normal motile sperm fraction (>30%) and varied levels of sperm morphology, ranging from 1% to 39% normal forms. Biggers–Whitten–Whittingham (BWW) medium was utilized for incubation, with 3% bovine serum albumin (BSA) as the protein source during a short (6-h) incubation protocol. A statistical significant relationship was noted between the percentage of sperm with normal forms (>14%) and the penetration rate in the SPA (P=0.001) (Table 8)[56,57].

Furthermore, the outcome of the SPA was correlated with IVF retrospectively in 84 patients. Thirty-eight patients had an SPA of <10%; no fertilization *in vitro* was demonstrated in 13 patients (34.2%), whereas successful fertilization was noted in 25 (65.8%). Forty-six couples had an SPA exceeding 10%; fertilization occurred in 38 (82.6%) and no fertilization in 8 (17.4%). Based on these results, it was concluded that SPA appeared to have a positive predictive value for IVF when it was normal, but was less reliable when egg penetration was <10%. This relatively poor predictability of fertilization by means of SPA might be attributed to the fact that this bioassay is still not really evaluated. According to all previous protocols, acrosome reaction has to be induced before coincubation of human sperm with zona-free hamster oocytes. However, no attention is paid to the percentage of acrosome-reacted spermatozoa (high percentage or low percentage). Thus, one does not know whether low binding and/or penetration results from a poorly induced acrosome reaction or from an impaired binding of sperm to the oolemma. Moreover, there is no agreement about the cutoff value. Apart from the large-scaled procedure for performance of SPA, after comparing the new criteria of sperm morphology and our SPA standards, and taking the mentioned disadvantages into consideration, morphology seems to be a better predictor of IVF outcome and a more useful adjunct for counseling patients.

Hemizona assay

Tight binding of human spermatozoa to the human zona pellucida is a critical event in gamete interaction leading to fertilization. This binding step may provide unique information predictive of sperm's ultimate fertilizing potential. However, due to species specificity human spermatozoa will bind firmly only to human zona pellucida. In view of this, the feasibility of tight human sperm binding to the zona pellucida of non-living human oocytes was first examined by Overstreet and Hembree[58]. Sperm binding and zona penetration were tested using oocytes recovered from *post mortem* ovarian tissue and, later, from ovaries removed from surgical indications. This study, however, did not investigate the kinetics of zona binding or the specific relationship between the binding event and male fertility.

Burkman and colleagues developed a new sperm function assay based on the relative binding of patient versus control spermatozoa to the matching halves of a bisected human oocyte[59]. This hemizona assay (HZA) assesses tight binding of sperm to the outer surface of the zona hemisphere. A threshold of 30% for the hemizona assay index (HZI) was established with the better prognosis in IVF for those sperm samples with an index >30%. In a prospective, blinded study, we investigated the relationship between sperm binding to the hemizona and IVF success. The positive predictive value of this test was 85%, and negative predictive value was 70%[60].

This functional test holds promise as an adjustment to the basic semen analysis to counsel patients prior to an assisted reproduction procedure.

It is interesting to note that most of the spermatozoa bound to the hemizona were morphologically normal[26], and 80% acrosome-reacted. The zona glycoproteins from salt-stored human zona pellucida retained not only the capability for tight binding, but also the ability to induce acrosome reaction. The ZP3 complex thus serves both as a sperm receptor and a trigger for the acrosome reaction (see Chapter 20).

Additional investigations

Acridine orange test

The acridine orange (AO) test has recently been introduced as an indicator of the DNA status of human spermatozoa. Tejada *et al.*[61] introduced a simplified method for fixation and denaturing sperm DNA. Specimens with high percentages of denatured sperm heads were associated with decreased fertility, whereas specimens with high numbers of sperm heads showing a distinct green fluorescence were indicative of normal semen samples containing a high percentage of sperm with normal DNA content.

The results of the AO test were compared with human sperm morphology and fertilization *in vitro*[14]. Seventy-six patients from the IVF and GIFT programs were randomly selected for the study. All patients underwent routine semen analysis, sperm DNA evaluation and standard IVF procedures. The results indicated a moderate positive correlation (r=0.38, P=0.0006) between the AO test results and normal sperm morphology. Patients with an AO test value exceeding 24% had significantly higher oocyte fertilization rates than did patients with lower values: results for metaphase I were 74% versus 51% (P=0.0008) and, in metaphase II oocytes, 88% versus 60% (P=0.0001).

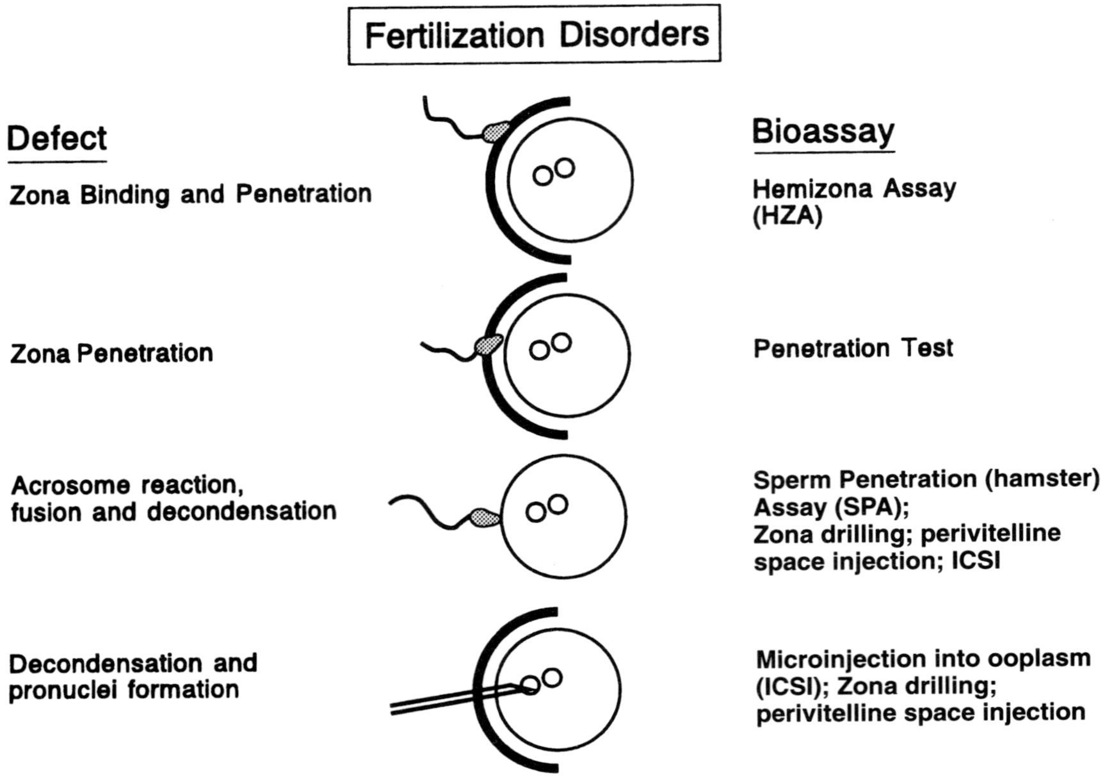

Figure 3 Sequential analysis of specific sperm defects in cases of recurrent failed fertilization. Reproduced from Oehninger *et al.*[65] with permission of Mosby – Year Book Inc.

We concluded from this study that, although there is a good predictive value in the AO test, sperm morphology is still the best predictor and easier to do on a day to day basis.

Chromatin condensation

Another parameter of spermatozoal function which has been shown to be predictive of fertilization *in vitro* is the chromatin condensation[62]. Normally, during spermatogenesis, the histones in late spermatids are replaced by protamines. The ratio of replacement can be determined by means of aniline blue staining[63], because acid aniline blue binds to the very basic residues of histones. If this replacement is not performed properly sperm will stain blue, indicating immaturity of nuclei and, consequently, probability of successful fertilization will decrease. According to Liu and Baker[64], poor fertilization in patients with normal sperm morphology might be caused by poor zona binding or poor nuclear maturity. Recently, it was demonstrated that the percentage of mature nuclei can be enriched by means of glass wool filtration[65].

Sequential analysis

It was proposed by Oehninger *et al.*[66] that, by combining the two bioassays, the HZA, a zona penetration assay, and the heterologous SPA, it might be possible to evaluate tight sperm–oocyte binding, zona penetration, sperm oocyte fusion and sperm head decondensation in sequence (Figure 3). This is an interesting concept that may refine our ability to diagnose male factor infertility. It is postulated that if an abnormality in a specific step of the binding–fertilization chain could be identified, the information gained could then be used in selecting optimal therapy for a specific patient. This may even be of value in identifying patients with the best prognoses for intracytoplasmic sperm injection and vice versa.

Sperm receptors

Sperm receptors, i.e. wheat germ agglutinin receptors, on the sperm head is an interesting development in the field of diagnostic andrology[67]. Gabriel indicated a correlation between wheat germ agglutinin receptors at the equatorial region with semen parameters and, specifically, morphology (Table 9). Potentially, this observation can be of clinical value as well as part of the parameters evaluated in sequential analysis (see Chapter 24, 25).

Oxygen species

This aspect of semen evaluation and its clinical relevance will be covered by Aitken in Chapter 21 of this textbook.

CONCLUSION

The aim of this chapter is to highlight some of the exciting new developments in diagnostic andrology with emphasis on the latest ones in the field of sperm morphology. The concept of sequential diagnosis in this field seems to be important and can possibly prove to be of practical help in the future to decide on a specific treatment with assisted reproduction or assisted fertilization.

Table 9 Percentage wheat germ agglutinin receptor localization on human sperm membrane domains in P, G pattern and normal semen samples (mean ± SD). Reproduced with permission from Gabriel *et al.*[66] with permission of Blackwell Wissenschafts Verlag

	Patient group		
Analysis % morphology	*P pattern 0–4*	*G pattern 5–14*	*Normal >14*
Acrosomal	6.46 ± 14	33.06 ± 21	32.91 ± 21
Equatorial	20.15 ± 9[al]	36.15 ± 19[b]	34.5 ± 2[c]
Post acrosome	93.54 ± 5	87.7 ± 19	91.83 ± 10
Neck	20.92 ± 13	19.18 ± 13	18.92 ± 12
Midpiece	2.85 ± 5	1.56 ± 2	1.0 ± 2
Tail	3.4 ± 7	7.5 ± 12	5.33 ± 10

[a] versus [b] = $P<0.05$; [a] versus [c] = $P<0.05$

References

1. Menkveld, R. and Kruger, T. F. (1990). Laboratory procedures: review and background. In Acosta, A. A., Swanson, R. J., Ackerman, S. B., Kruger, T. F., Van Zyl, J. A. and Menkveld, R. (eds.) *Human Spermatozoa in Assisted Reproduction*, pp. 68–94. (Baltimore: Williams and Wilkins)
2. World Health Organization (1992). *World Health Organization Manual for the Examination of Human Semen and Sperm–Cervical Mucus Interaction*. (London: Cambridge University Press)
3. Kruger, T. F., Menkveld, R., Stander, F. S. H., Lombard, C. J., Van der Merwe, J. P., Van Zyl, J. A. and Smith, K. (1986). Sperm morphologic features as a prognostic factor in *in vitro* fertilization. *Fertil. Steril.*, **46**, 1118–23
4. Kruger, T. F., Acosta, A. A., Simmons, K. F., Swanson, R. J., Matta, J. F. and Oehninger, S. (1988). Predictive value of abnormal sperm morphology in *in vitro* fertilization. *Fertil. Steril.*, **49**, 112–17
5. Van der Merwe, J. P., Kruger, T. F., Swart, Y. and Lombard, C. J. (1992). The role of oocyte maturity in the treatment of infertility because of teratozoospermia and normozoospermia with gamete intrafallopian transfer. *Fertil. Steril.*, **58**, 581–6
6. Acosta, A. A., Kruger, T. F., Swanson, R. J. and Ackerman, S. (1988). *In vitro* fertilization in male infertility. In Garcia, C.-R., Mastroianni, L. Jr. and Dublin, L. (eds.) *Current Therapy of Infertility – 3*, pp. 233–9. (Philadelphia: B.C. Decker Inc.)
7. Kruger, T. F., Franken, D. R., Stander, F., Swart, Y. and Van der Merwe, J. P. (1993). Effect of semen characteristics on pregnancy rate in a gamete intrafallopian transfer program. *Arch. Androl.*, **31**, 127–31
8. Kruger, T. F., Ackerman, S. B., Simmons, K. F., Swanson, R. J., Brugo, S. S. and Acosta, A. A. (1987). A quick reliable staining technique for human sperm morphology. *Arch. Androl.*, **18**, 275–7
9. Oehninger, S., Acosta, A. A., Morshedi, M., Veeck, L. L., Swanson, R. J., Simmons, K. and Rosenwaks, Z. (1988). Corrective measures in pregnancy outcome in *in vitro* fertilization in patients with severe sperm morphology abnormalities. *Fertil. Steril.*, **50**, 283–7
10. Enginsu, M. E., Dumoulin, J. C. M., Pieters, M. H. E. C., Bras, M., Evers, J. L. H. and Geraedts, J. P. M. (1991). Evaluation of human sperm morphology using strict criteria after Diff-Quik staining: correlation of morphology with fertilization *in vitro*. *Hum. Reprod.*, **6**, 854–8
11. Liu, D. Y. and Baker, H. W. G. (1988). The proportion of human sperm with poor morphology but normal intact acrosomes detected with *Pisum sativum* agglutinin correlates with fertilization *in vitro*. *Fertil. Steril.*, **50**, 288–93

12. Hinting, A., Comhaire, F., Vermeulen, L., Dhont, M., Vermeulen, A. and Vanderkerckhove, D. (1990). Value of sperm characteristics and the result of *in vitro* fertilization for predicting the outcome of assisted reproduction. *Int. J. Androl.*, **13**, 59–64
13. Enginsu, M. E., Dumoulin, J. C. M., Pieters, M. H. E. C., Evers, J. L. H. and Geraedts, J. P. M. (1993). Predictive value of morphologically normal sperm concentration in the medium for *in-vitro* fertilization. *Int. J. Androl.*, **16**, 113–20
14. Claassens, O. E., Menkveld, R., Franken, D. R., Pretorius, E., Swart, Y., Lombard, C. J. and Kruger, T. F. (1992). The acridine orange test: determining the relationship between sperm morphology and fertilization *in vitro*. *Hum. Reprod.*, **7**, 242–7
15. Wang, C., Leung, A., Tsoi, W., Leung, J., Ng, V. and Lee, V. (1991). Computer-assisted assessment of human sperm morphology: comparison with visual assessment. *Fertil. Steril.*, **55**, 983–8
16. Wang, C., Leung, A., Tsoi, W-L., Leung, J., Ng, V. and Lee, K-F. (1991). Computer-assisted assessment of human sperm morphology: usefulness in predicting fertilizing capacity of human spermatozoa. *Fertil. Steril.*, **55**, 989–93
17. Davis, R. O., Bain, D. E., Siemers, R. J., Thal, D. M., Andrew, J. B. and Gravance, C. G. (1992). Accuracy and precision of the CellForm-Human* automated sperm morphometry instrument. *Fertil. Steril.*, **58**, 763–9
18. Kruger, T. F., Du Toit, T. C., Franken, D. R., Acosta, A. A., Oehninger, S. C., Menkveld, R. and Lombard, C. J. (1993). A new computerized method of reading sperm morphology (strict criteria) is as efficient as technician reading. *Fertil. Steril.*, **59**, 202–9
19. Windt, M-L., Menkveld, R., Kruger, T. F., Van der Merwe, J. P. and Van Zyl, J. A. (1989). Effect of sperm washing and swim-up on antibodies bound to sperm membrane: use of immunobead/sperm cervical mucus contact tests. *Arch. Androl.*, **22**, 55–9
20. Van der Merwe, J. P., Kruger, T. F., Windt, M-L., Hulme, V. A. and Menkveld, R. (1990). Treatment of male sperm autoimmunity by using the gamete intrafallopian transfer procedure with washed spermatozoa. *Fertil. Steril.*, **53**, 682–7
21. Acosta, A. A., Van der Merwe, J. P., Doncel, G., Kruger, T. F., Sayilgan, A., Franken, D. R. and Kolm, P. (1994). Fertilization efficiency of morphologically abnormal spermatozoa in assisted reproduction is further impaired by antisperm antibodies of the male partner's sperm. *Fertil. Steril.*, **62**, 826–33.
22. Oehninger, S. and Hodgen, G. D. (1991). How to evaluate human spermatozoa for assisted reproduction In DeCherney, A. (ed.) *Assisted Reproduction Reviews*, pp. 15–27. (Baltimore: Williams and Wilkins)
23. Ord, T., Patrizio, P., Marello, E., Balmaceda, J. P. and Asch, R. H. (1990). A new method of semen preparation for IVF in severe male factor infertility – Minipercoll. *Presented at the 46th Annual Meeting of the American Fertility Society*, October, Washington, DC
24. Huszar, G., Vigue, L. and Corrales, M. (1990). Sperm creatine kinase activity in fertile and infertile oligospermic men. *J. Androl.*, **11**, 40–6
25. Huszar, G., Vigue, L. and Oehninger, S. (1994). Creatine kinase immunocytochemistry of human sperm–hemizona complexes: Selective binding of sperm with mature creatine kinase-staining pattern. *Fertil. Steril.*, **61**, 136–42
26. Menkveld, R., Franken, D. R., Kruger, T. F., Oehninger, S. and Hodgen, G. D. (1991). Sperm selection capacity of the human zona pellucida. *Mol. Reprod. Dev.*, **30**, 346–52
27. Huszar, G. and Vigue, L. (1994). Correlation between the rate of lipid peroxidation and cellular maturity as measured by creatine kinase activity in human spermatozoa. *J. Androl.*, **15**, 71–7
28. Hedrick, J. L., Urch, U. A. and Hardy, D. M. (1988). The structure-function properties of the sperm enzyme acrosin. In Shoemaker, S., Sonnet, P. and Whitaker, J. (eds.) *Enzymes in Agricultural Biotechnology*, pp. 55–73. (Washington, DC: ACS Books)
29. Zaneveld, L. J. D. and De Jonge, C. J. (1991). Mammalian sperm acrosomal enzymes and the acrosome reaction. In Dunbar, B. S. and O'Rand, M. G. (eds.) *A Comparative Overview of Mammalian Fertilization*, pp. 63–79. (New York: Plenum Press)
30. Rogers, B. J. and Bentwood, B. (1982). Capacitation, acrosome reaction and fertilization. In Zaneveld, L. J. D. and Chatterton, R. T. (eds). *Biochemistry of Mammalian Reproduction*, p. 203. (New York: John Wiley)
31. Polakoski, K. L. K. and Siegel, M. S. (1986). The proacrosin–acrosin system. In Paulson, J. D., Negro-Vilar, A., Lucena, E. and Martini, L. (eds.). *Andrology, Male Fertility and Sterility*, pp. 359–75. (Orlando: Academic Press)
32. Töpfer-Petersen, E. and Henschen, A. (1987). Acrosin shows zona and fucose binding, novel properties for a serin proteinase. *FEBS Lett.*, **226**, 38–42
33. Tesarik, J., Drahorad, J. and Peknicova, J. (1988). Subcellular immunochemical localization of acrosin in human spermatozoa during the acrosome reaction and zona pellucida penetration. *Fertil. Steril.*, **50**, 133–41
34. Mohsenian, M., Syner, F. N. and Moghissi, K. S. (1982). A study of sperm acrosin in patients with unexplained infertility. *Fertil. Steril.*, **37**, 223–9
35. Goodpasture, J. C., Zavos, P. M., Cohen, M. R. and Zaneveld, L. J. D. (1982). Relationship of human sperm acrosin and proacrosin to semen parameters. I. Comparison between symptomatic men of infertile couples and asymptomatic men, and between different split ejaculate fractions. *J. Androl.*, **3**, 151–6
36. Schill, W.-B. (1974). Quantitative determination of acrosin activity in human spermatozoa. *Fertil. Steril.*, **25**, 703–12
37. Schill, W.-B., Töpfer-Petersen, E. and Heissler, E. (1988). The sperm acrosome: functional and clinical aspects. *Hum. Reprod.*, **3**, 139–45

38. Schill, W.-B. (1991). Some disturbances of acrosomal development and function in human spermatozoa. *Hum. Reprod.*, **6**, 969–78
39. Schill, W.-B., Feifel, M., Fritz, H. and Hammerstein, J. (1981). Inhibitors of acrosomal proteinase as antifertility agents. A problem of acrosomal membrane permeability. *Int. J. Androl.*, **4**, 25–38
40. Welker, B., Bernstein, G. S., Dietrich, K., Nakamura, R. M. and Krebs, D. (1988). Acrosomal proteinase activity of human spermatozoa and relation of results to semen quality. *Hum. Reprod.*, **3**, 75–80
41. Kennedy, W. P., Kaminski, J. M., Van der Ven, H. H., Jeyendran, R. S., Reid, D. S., Blackwell, J., Bielfeld, P. and Zaneveld, L. J. D. (1989). A simple, clinical assay to evaluate the acrosin activity of human spermatozoa. *J. Androl.*, **10**, 221–31
42. Schill, W.-B. (1990). Determination of active, non-zymogen acrosin, proacrosin and total acrosin in different andrological patients. *Arch. Dermatol. Res.*, **282**, 335–42
43. Liu, D. Y. and Baker, H. W. G. (1990). Relationships between human sperm acrosin, acrosomes, morphology and fertilization *in vitro*. *Hum. Reprod.*, **5**, 298–303
44. Tummon, I. S., Yuzpe, A. A., Daniel, S. A. J. and Deutsch, A. (1991). Total acrosin activity correlates with fertility potential after fertilization *in vitro*. *Fertil. Steril.*, **56**, 933–8
45. Henkel, R., Müller, C., Miska, W., Schill, W.-B., Kleinstein, J. and Gips, H. (1995). Acrosin activity of human spermatozoa by means of a gelatinolytic technique. A method useful for IVF. *J. Androl.*, **16**, 272–7
46. Jeyendran, R. S., van der Ven, H. H., Perez-Pelaez, M., Crabo, B. G. and Zaneveld, L. J. D. (1984). Development of an assay to assess the functional integrity of the human sperm membrane and its relationship to other semen characteristics. *J. Reprod. Fertil.*, **70**, 219–28
47. Sjöblom, P. and Coccia, E. (1989). On the diagnostic value of the hypoosmotic sperm swelling test in an *in vitro* fertilization (IVF) program. *J.* In Vitro *Fertil. Embryo Transf.*, **6**, 41–3
48. Coetzee, K., Kruger, T. F., Menkveld, R., Lombard, C. J. and Swanson, R. J. (1989). Hypoosmotic swelling test in the prediction of male fertility. *Arch. Androl.*, **23**, 131–8
49. Koehler, J. K., De Curtis, I., Stechener, M. A. and Smith, D. (1982). Interaction of human sperm with zona free hamster eggs. A freeze fracture study. *Gamete Res.*, **6**, 371–86
50. Henkel, R., Müller, C., Miska, W., Gips, H. and Schill, W.-B. (1993). Determination of the acrosome reaction in human spermatozoa is predictive of fertilization *in vitro*. *Hum. Reprod.*, **8**, 2128–32
51. Tesarik, J. (1989). Appropriate timing of the acrosome reaction is a major requirement for the fertilizing spermatozoon. *Hum. Reprod.*, **4**, 957–61
52. Leyton, L., Bunch, D., Le Guen, P., Selub, M. and Saling, P. (1990). Regulation of acrosomal exocytosis by sperm binding to the zona pellucida. In *Gamete Interaction: Prospects for Immunocontraception*, p. 225. (Wiley-Liss Inc.)
53. Plachot, M., Mandelbaum, J. and Junca, A. M. (1984). Acrosome reaction of human sperm used for *in vitro* fertilization. *Fertil. Steril.*, **42**, 418–23
54. Cummins, J. M., Pember, S. M., Jequier, A. M., Yovich, J. L. and Hartmann, P. E. (1991). A test of the human sperm acrosome reaction following ionophore challenge. Relationship to fertility and other seminal parameters. *J. Androl.*, **12**, 98–103
55. Rogers, B. J., Bentwood, B. J., Van Campen, H., Helmbrecht, G., Soderdahl, D. and Hale, R. W. (1983). Sperm morphology assessment as an indicator of human fertilizing capacity. *J. Androl.*, **4**, 119
56. Kruger, T. F., Swanson, R. J., Hamilton, M., Simmons, K. F., Acosta, A. A., Matta, J. F., Oehninger, S. and Morshedi, M. (1988). Abnormal sperm morphology and other semen parameters related to the outcome of the hamster oocyte human sperm penetration assay. *Int. J. Androl.*, **11**, 107–13
57. Kruger, T. F. and Franken, D. R. (1993). Evaluation of male-factor infertility. In Behrman, S. J., Patton, G. W. Jr. and Holtz, G. (eds.) *Progress in Infertility*, pp. 113–21. (Boston: Little, Brown and Company)
58. Overstreet, J. W. and Hembree, W. E. (1976). Penetration of the zona pellucida of non-living human oocytes by human spermatozoa *in vitro*. *Fertil. Steril.*, **27**, 815–31
59. Burkman, L. J., Coddington, C. C., Franken, D. R., Kruger, T. F., Rosenwaks, Z. and Hodgen, G. D. (1988). The hemizona assay (HZA): development of a diagnostic test for the binding of human spermatozoa to the human hemizona pellucida to predict fertilization potential. *Fertil. Steril.*, **49**, 688–97
60. Franken, D. R., Kruger, T. F., Oehninger, S. C., Coddington, C. C., Lombard, C. J., Smith, K. and Hodgen, G. D. (1993). The ability of the hemizona assay to predict human fertilization in different and consecutive *in-vitro* fertilization cycles. *Hum. Reprod.* **8**, 1240–44
61. Tejada, R. I., Mitchell, J. C., Norman, A., Marik, J. J. and Friedman, S. (1984). A test for the practical evaluation of male fertility by acridine orange (AO) fluorescence. *Fertil. Steril.*, **42**, 87–91
62. Auger, J., Mesbah, M., Huber, C. and Dadoune, J. P. (1990). Aniline blue staining as a marker of sperm chromatin defects associated with different semen characteristics between proven fertile and suspected infertile men. *Int. J. Androl.*, **13**, 452–62
63. Terquem, A. and Dadoune, J. P. (1983). Aniline blue staining of human spermatozoon chromatin. Evaluation of nuclear maturation. In Andro, J. (ed.). *The Sperm Cell*, pp. 249–52. (The Hague: Martinus Nijhoff Publishers)
64. Liu, D. Y. and Baker, H. W. G. (1992). Sperm nuclear chromatin normality: relationship with sperm mor-

phology, sperm-zona pellucida binding, and fertilization rates. *Fertil. Steril.*, **58**, 1178–84

65. Henkel, R., Franken, D. R., Schill, W. B. and Lombard, C. J. (1994). The selective capacity of glass wool filtration for the separation of human spermatozoa with condensed chromatin: A possible therapeutic modality for male factor cases? *Int. J. Androl.*, in press
66. Oehninger, S. C., Acosta, A. A., Veeck, L. L., Brzyski, R., Kruger, T. F., Muasher, S. J. and Hodgen, G. C. (1991). Recurrent failure of *in vitro* fertilization: Role of the hemizona assay in the sequential diagnosis of specific sperm–oocyte defects. *Am. J. Obstet. Gynecol.*, **164**, 1210–5
67. Gabriel, L. K., Franken, D. R., Van der Horst, G., Kruger, T. F. and Oehninger, S. C. (1994). Wheat germ agglutinin receptors on human sperm membranes and sperm morphology. *Andrologia*, **26**, 5–8

New frontiers in male factor diagnosis 1: sperm membrane moieties 24

L. K. Gabriel

INTRODUCTION

Standard semen analysis including sperm concentration, motility and sperm morphology is widely used as a functional indicator of male fertility. However, the results do not provide precise diagnostic or prognostic information for human fertility *in vivo* or *in vitro*[1,2]. Because standard semen analyses have limited clinical value for predicting fertility, many other tests of human sperm function have been developed. Among these are assessment of normal sperm morphology[3,4] (strict criteria), computer-assisted motility evaluation, hypo-osmotic swelling[5], tests for sperm nuclear maturity[6], acrosin activity[7], hamster zona-free oocyte penetration[8] and human sperm–zona binding[9]. Although these tests provide additional valuable information that may improve the prediction of fertility, there is no single test of sperm function that will predict fertility accurately. Fertility failure can only be predicted in cases where there is an absolute disorder affecting all sperm, such as azoospermia or total absence of morphologically normal forms (e.g. globozoospermia).

Prospective studies to relate semen analysis results to fertility are difficult to perform in humans due to financial, social and ethical reasons. Liu *et al.*[6] demonstrated the use of *in vitro* fertilization (IVF) results to investigate the potential value of sperm function tests. In a study of several putative tests of human sperm function only normal sperm morphology, sperm insemination concentration and vitality were found to show a significant positive correlation with IVF rates.

To date, there appears to be no sperm assay to assess human sperm surface receptors that correlates significantly with fecundity or fertilization rates in IVF. Immunofluorescence tests using polyclonal or monoclonal antibodies and lectins have been employed to assess acrosomal status and the dynamics of the acrosome reaction[10,11] Fenichel *et al.*[12] reported that impaired acrosomal status (assessed using a mouse monoclonal antibody and fluorescein isothiocyanate (FITC)-conjugated rabbit anti-mouse immunoglobulin) may be associated with low fertilization rates (<50%) in humans. In a similar study, acrosome loss (FITC concanavalin A staining of the inner acrosomal membrane) correlated with an increase in IVF of zona-free human eggs ($r = +0.98$)[9]. This and similar studies demonstrated the potential use of lectins as molecular probes of cell membrane dynamics and transformations.

LECTINS AS MOLECULAR PROBES

Lectins have been isolated from a wide variety of plants and animals, ranging from legumes to horseshoe crabs. The general property of lectins is that of agglutinating cells through their cell surface oligosaccharide determinants. Because of the carbohydrate binding specificities of lectins, some of these agglutinins have proven to be quite useful for clinical blood typing and structural studies of blood group substances[13], in analysis of the surface structure of normal and tumor cells[14], for specific isolation of glycoproteins[15] and for many other reasons[16]. At present, enormous interest centers on probing the nature and distribution of membrane-bound, carbohydrate-containing structures by using lectins of defined specificity[17]. The past decade has seen the extension of lectin studies to a large number of specialized cell types, with the male gamete receiving its just share of attention[18].

LECTIN–CELL INTERACTIONS

Numerous articles and reviews have appeared in recent years that provide detailed information about lectin biochemistry and interactions of lectins with cell surfaces and specific saccharides[14,19]. A general picture has emerged regarding interactions of lectins with cell surfaces. Although many exceptions exist, it appears that many lectin receptor sites are more mobile in the membranes of tumor cells and embryonic cells than in a variety of untransformed cell lines. Lectins induce a clustering or capping of receptor sites in the membranes of tumor (transformed) or embryonic cells but not in the membranes of many normal (non-transformed) cell lines[14]. Numbers of exposed cell surface lectin receptor sites may vary among cell types[19] or at different stages in the cell cycle[20]. In general, the difference between heterogeneous populations of transformed and embryonic cells versus non-transformed cells appears to be a mobility of receptor sites rather than in numbers of surface sites[14].

If we consider the maturation and capacitation processes in mammalian spermatozoa to entail 'transformation' processes, involving the various cell surface changes and physiologcal processes that occur during this complex cascade of events, it seems feasible to equate sperm surface lectin receptor activity through capacitation, in terms of receptor mobility and exposure (unmasking) of lectin receptor sites.

Mammalian spermatozoan membranes have increasingly become the subject of experimental studies, particularly in the field of spermatogenesis[16,17,21,22]. Much of the work has focused on surface receptors involved in mutual adhesion of spermatogonia during spermatogenesis. Since glycoproteins have been implicated in intercellular adhesion and information transfer during differentiation[16,21], it is not surprising that researchers have devoted much attention to the development of various techniques to investigate the intricate distributions, identities and biological functions of these important membrane components.

LECTINS IN SPERMATOLOGY

Methodology

Lectins from a wide variety of sources are now commercially available in purified form. In many cases, lectins coupled to fluorescent or electron optical markers can also be purchased and utilized with a minimum of further purification.

Studies of male gametes using lectins generally fall into two categories depending on the assay method employed to detect sperm–lectin interactions. The first of these involves simple agglutination determinations whereby the extent of the sperm agglutination can be estimated in the light microscope using an arbitrary scale[23–34]. An indirect measure of agglutination or, more precisely, lectin binding sites, can be obtained, by radio-iodination of the agglutinins and scintillation counting of the treated sperm populations[33]. Although very useful in providing average numbers of lectin binding sites per cell, this and similar methods provide no information about the distribution of binding sites over the surface of the spermatozoon.

Most of the studies involving sperm–lectin interactions have utilized fluorescent or ultrastructural markers attached to the agglutinins. Such studies have the obvious advantage of providing direct evidence of the location of lectin binding sites over the surface of the sperm and changes in such distributions during physiological or experimental transformations.

It is possible to use either fixed or living sperm for such localization studies. In our experience, living sperm label in a rather variable fashion, possibly due to lectin-induced redistribution, membrane damage due to cytotoxic effects or a combination of factors. Although aldehyde-fixed sperm probably have a reduced affinity for most lectins, the distribution obtained after labeling is probably more representative of the native state. It would be advantageous to combine morphological observations with some of the more quantitative methods mentioned above; however, financial and practical implications do not permit such combined experimental protocols in most laboratories.

The use of lectins in studying the surface changes associated with capacitation of spermatozoa has been a useful adjunct to other structural and physiological approaches in attempts to elucidate a mechanism for the capacitation process. A wide variety of lectins, having various specificities, have been shown to undergo a similar loss of binding activity over the acrosomal surface during capacitation and prior to the occurrence of the acrosome reaction. The observations that many of these lectins behave in a similar fashion on sperm from several species suggest that the alteration of substances on the sperm surface during capacitation is rather indiscriminate in terms of the kinds of molecules (primarily glycoproteins) that are removed, unmasked or rearranged, but not in terms of the location at which such processes take place (primarily over the acrosomal and equatorial regions).

The fact that spermatozoa from even a single species (e.g. man) are receptive to a wide variety of lectins, demonstrates the highly intricate and complex membrane organization of this specialized cell type. The search for molecules on the surface of mammalian spermatozoa that are responsible for the binding of sperm to the zona pellucida has led to the identification of a number of different surface proteins. To isolate and identify the single most specific sperm surface component that is most instrumental in the preparation of spermatozoa (capacitation and the acrosome reaction) for interaction with the oocyte and/or sperm–zona pellucida binding, will be like searching for the proverbial 'needle in a hay-stack'.

Sperm–lectin interactions – clinical value

The biological and biochemical properties of lectins have afforded much weight to their employment as membrane probes to examine the role of cell surface components of various cell types, in morphogenesis and other biological events[35,36]. Lectin-induced agglutination studies and fluorescence techniques have been widely employed in the identification and localization of membrane glycoprotein and glycolipid moieties of human spermatozoa[37–41]. Attention has been focused on the alterations of sperm surface receptors (oligosaccharides) during the germinal differentiation pathway, epididymal transit and capacitation[39,42,43]. Such subtle maturational alterations of membrane constituents and the masking and unmasking of membrane receptors are apparently of prime importance in the determination of sperm fertilizing ability and, hence, male fertility *per se*[44].

Wheat germ agglutinin (WGA) has been reported to show important interactions with human sperm surfaces in this regard[37,43] and WGA receptor deficiency has been implicated as a possible underlying cause of male infertility in humans[22,45]. More recent studies have demonstrated the relationship between WGA receptor abundance and localization on human spermatozoa and sperm morphology (evaluated by strict criteria)[46].

The percentage of morphologically normal spermatozoa, a direct product of spermatogenesis and sperm maturation processes, represents an important criterion for male fertility, if one accepts that normal morphology is a requisite in the process of fertilization. In studies where evaluation of sperm morphology has been done by strict criteria[47], this parameter is highlighted among other semen parameters as a predictor of sperm fertilizing capacity in *in vitro* fertilization (IVF)[3]. Although the mechanisms of sperm–zona penetration are not fully understood an initial cell-to-cell binding, which may involve certain receptor–ligand events, adequate motility patterns and enzymatic mechanisms, is probably required. Subtle disorders in any of these mechanisms may thus contribute to impaired zona penetration.

Analysis of WGA (mean±SD) receptor localization on spermatozoa categorized according to strict criteria into P pattern, G pattern and normal forms, showed a significant difference ($P<0.05$) in the percentage of equatorial staining of the P patterns (20.15±9.54) when compared to the G patterns (36.12±19.25) and the normal forms (34.50±20.23). There were no significant differences in the percentages of WGA staining in the acrosomal, post-acrosomal, neck, intermediate segment and tail regions (Table 1).

Furthermore, fluorescence intensity assessment (indicative of receptor abundance) of the P patterns showed a higher frequency of low intensity ratings (44% 1-rating, 22% 4-rating) when compared to the G (15% 1-rating, 32.5% 4-rating) and normal (22% 1-rating, 50% 4-rating) patterns (Figure 1).

Sperm morphology has been significantly and positively correlated with fertilization rates in IVF. The importance of sperm morphology as recorded by strict criteria, has been demonstrated to be a powerful predictive indicator in human fertilization[3,47]. Since fertilization involves a number of molecular interactions between gametes, it is important to examine the possibilities for the establishment of molecular assays for gamete defects.

Table 1 Percentage WGA receptor localization on human sperm membrane domains among different morphological groups

Analysis	*Group*		
	P pattern	*G pattern*	*Normal*
Morphology %	0–4	5–14	>14
	2.10±0.94	8.95±2.49	20.13±4.14
Acrosomal	46.46±14.22[a]	33.06±21.77[b]	32.92±21.25[c]
Equatorial	20.15±9.54[d]	36.12±19.25[e]	34.50±20.22[f]
Post acrosomal	93.54±5.73	87.70±19.72	91.83±10.80
Neck	20.92±13.59	19.18±13.67	18.92±12.63
Midpiece	2.85±5.77	1.56±2.49	1.08±2.27
Tail	3.46±7.59	7.50±12.36	5.33±10.56

Values are means ± standard deviation. [a] versus [b]: NS, $P=0.06$; [a] versus [c]: NS, $P=0.07$; [b] versus [c]: NS, $P=0.98$; [d] versus [e]: $P<0.05$; [d] versus [f]; $P<0.05$

The molecular modifications of the sperm surface plasma membrane, demonstrated in part by changes in the lectin affinity to the specific morphological zones of the sperm membranes (Figure 2), are reported to be essential to the subsequent rearrangement of intrinsic membrane proteins, creating 'high-fluidity' areas which may represent the presumed sites for sperm binding to the zona pellucida and the acrosome reaction, which are prerequisite to fertilization.

In this respect, deficiencies in sperm maturational events will be reflected in defective spermatozoa by a deviation from the expected lectin-binding patterns. Significantly lower WGA binding to the equatorial region in the P patterns when compared to the G pattern and normal forms, reported here, may represent this deviation. WGA receptors in the equatorial region of human spermatozoa play important roles during sperm–egg recognition and zona binding[37]. A decrease in the number of sperm carrying these binding receptors at the fertilization site may thus negatively affect the fertilization potential of the spermatozoa *per se*. A significant impairment of sperm binding under hemizona assay (HZA) con-

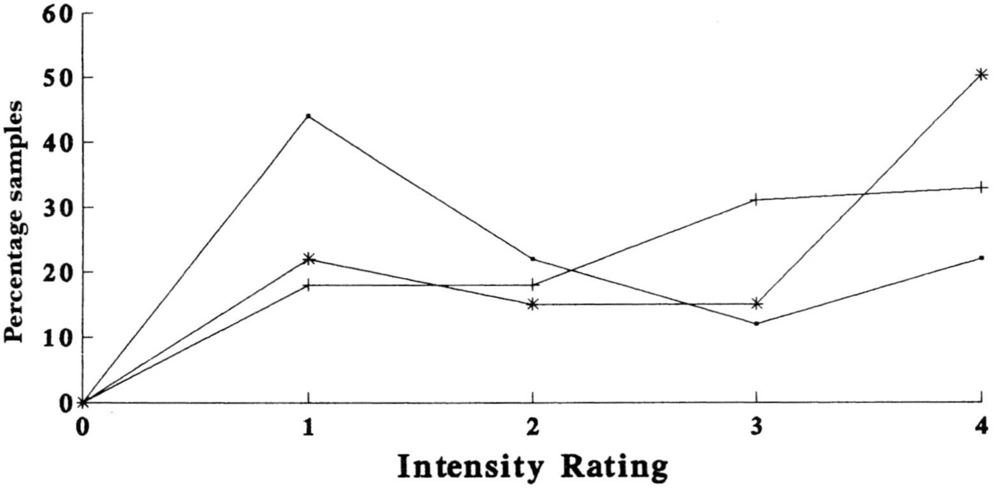

Figure 1 Relative frequencies of intensity values for human spermatozoa categorized into three morphological groups (i.e. P patterns, G patterns and normal forms). Rating scale: 0=absent, 1=very weak, 2=weak, 3=good, 4=very good. ■, P patterns; +, G patterns; *, normal patterns. Reproduced from Gabriel *et al.* (1994)[46] with permission of Blackwell Wissenschafts Verlag

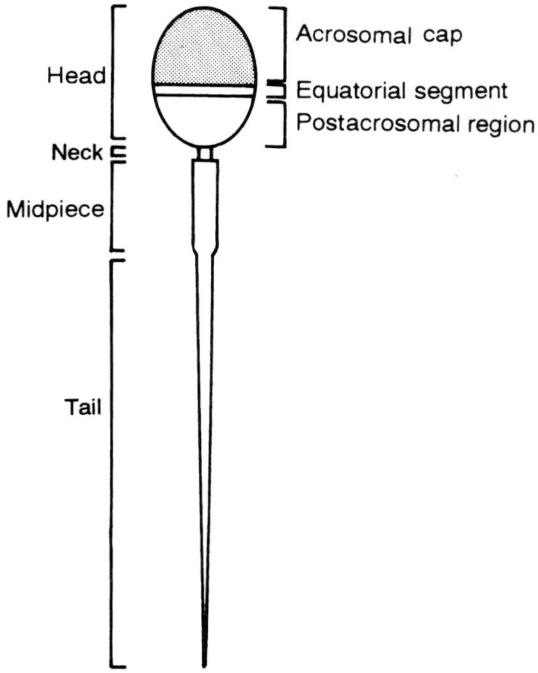

Figure 2 Sperm membrane regions for the evaluation of WGA receptor localization. Reproduced from Gabriel *et al.* (1994)[48] with permission of Hemisphere Publishing Corporation

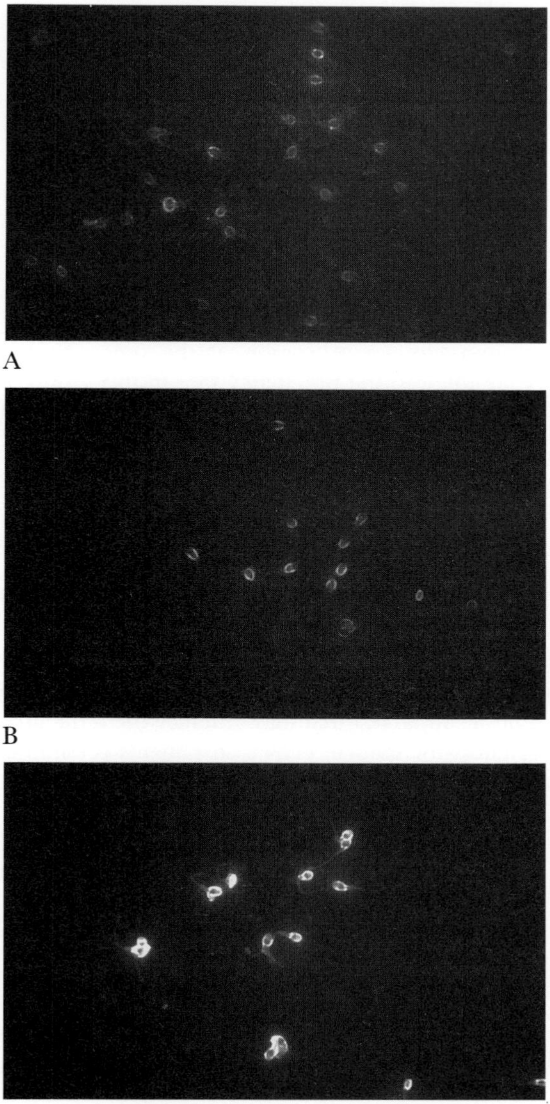

A

B

C

Figure 3 Photomicrographs showing receptor intensity differences among (A) P patterns; (B) G patterns; and (C) normal forms

ditions has been reported in semen specimens that were classified as P patterns[49]. Also, previous studies have shown a positive correlation between the percentage normal morphology and the number of tightly bound sperm during HZA[50,51]. Franken *et al.*[49] reported an increase in the number of zona-bound sperm in severely teratozoospermic patients after increasing the sperm concentration and therefore, the number of morphologically normal forms during HZA. Since receptor localization appears to be closely related to sperm morphology, the increase in sperm concentration and percentage of sperm with normal morphology may result in an increase in the percentage of sperm carrying the receptors at the binding/fertilization site.

Also, the normal WGA receptor intensity is an important consideration with regard to sperm maturity and fertilizing ability. Assessment of fluorescence intensity, indicative of WGA receptor abundance, showed distinct differences in the relative frequencies of values in the 0–4 rating scale, given in each of the three morphology groups (Figures 1 and 3). An increase in the number of morphologically normal sperm may, therefore, also represent an increase in the number of sperm with adequate binding-receptor intensity. Therefore, abnormalities of WGA receptor, both in quantity and/or localization, evident in teratozoospermia, may be one cause of poor HZA indices and failed *in vitro* fertilization.

This might be an important factor in the explanation of those P patterns where good *in vitro* fertilization rates occurred, as well as in cases of unexplained infertility where normal forms show a poor prognosis in IVF. We refer here to the few P patterns that showed normal WGA receptor localization and intensity, as well as the normal forms which display primarily normal WGA receptor localization, but extremely low intensity. In the P pattern group, however, the fertilization rate can be increased (up to 62%)[52] when increasing the insemination concentration at the time of IVF. None the less, the pregnancy rate in this group of patients remains quite low despite having achieved a major improvement in the fertilization sites. This suggests that the potential for establishment of a pregnancy by these sperm populations is clearly impaired, indicating that the morphological aberrations may be markers for other functional defects. This further emphasizes the requirement for clinical analyses to steer toward the incorporation of assays on a more molecular level of sperm assessment.

The technique employed in this study[46] represents a simple test that may enhance the sequential diagnosis of gamete defects in patients presenting with severe teratozoospermia and couples with recurrent failure of fertilization *in vitro*.

An independent study examined the correlation between human sperm WGA receptor activity and fertilization rate in IVF, with calculations of the predictive values of the 'WGA assay'[53]. When the total number of metaphase II oocytes involved in this study was divided into the number of oocytes that fertilized and those that were unfertilized, it was found that 68 of 107 fertilized oocytes were inseminated with sperm with WGA acrosomal staining of >35%. Similarly, 35 of 56 unfertilized oocytes were inseminated with spermatozoa with WGA acrosomal staining of <35% (Table 2). The calculated positive predictive value of the WGA assay with these results was 76%.

However, comparison of results of the percentage FITC–WGA staining of the insemination spermatozoa and the fertilization rates revealed an interesting pattern of correspondence. Values of FITC–WGA acrosomal region staining <35% in 15 of 27 patients showed corresponding *in vitro* fertilization rates of <50% (group 1) compared to FITC–WGA acrosomal region staining of >35% with corresponding fertilization rates ⩾50% (group 2) in 10 of 27 patients (Table 3, Figure 4 A,B), giving a positive predictive value of 90.9%.

Table 2 Linear discriminant analysis of the number of oocytes fertilized using 35% WGA acrosomal staining as the minimum cutoff for successful fertilization prediction

WGA acrosomal staining	*Number of oocytes*		
	Fertilized	*Unfertilized*	*Total*
>35%	68	21	89
<35%	39	35	74
Total	107	56	163

χ^2=10.06 (d.f. 1), P<0.01; sensitivity: 68/107=64%; specificity: 35/56=63%; positive predictive value: 68/89=76%; negative predictive value: 35/74=47%; overall predictive value: 103/163=63%

Table 3 Two-by-two contingency table determined with 35% FITC–WGA acrosomal staining as minimum value versus *in vitro* fertilization outcome

Acrosomal staining	In vitro *fertilization group*		*Total*
	*Total fertilization rate**		*Frequency*
>35%	10	1	11
<35%	1	15	16
Total frequency	11	16	27

*The total fertilization rate ⩾50%, <50% is in spite of corrective measures. χ^2=19.361 (d.f. 1), P<0.001; positive predictive value=90.90%; negative predictive value=93.75%

Comparison between FITC–WGA staining of group 1 versus group 2 sperm samples showed that the mean values in percentage staining of the acrosomal region were 30.92±18.53 and 62.70±21.70 (P<0.01), respectively (Table 4). Analysis of the percentage change in FITC–WGA staining in each of the sperm morphological zones, following sperm processing for IVF insemination in groups 1 and 2, revealed significant differences (P<0.01) in the acrosomal (13.76±8.92 and 34.36±17.38) and equatorial (10.25±6.69 and 20.16±9.46) regions (Table 4).

Correlation between the percentage of FITC–WGA staining and fertilization rates in the combined group (groups 1 and 2) showed a highly significant positive correlation with acrosomal region staining (r=0.73, P=0.0001). In the examination of the percentage change of the FITC–WGA staining,

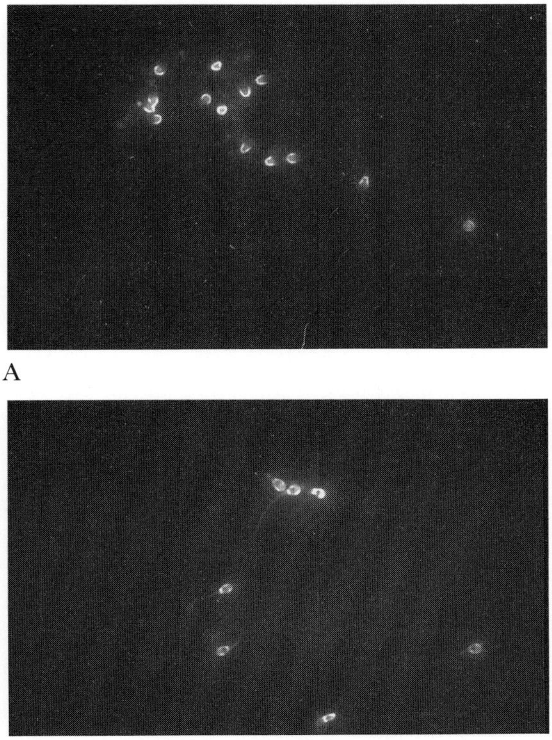

A

B

Figure 4 FITC-WGA staining patterns observed (A) in sample with fertilization rate <50%. No acrosomal staining observed in this field; (B) in sample with fertilization rate ⩾50%. Acrosomal staining evident. Reproduced from Gabriel *et al.* (1995)[52] with permission of the American Society for Reproductive Medicine

acrosomal (r=0.51, P=0.01) and equatorial (r=0.53, P=0.01) staining correlated significantly with IVF rates (Table 5).

When the individual correlations between the percentage of FITC–WGA staining of the different morphological zones of the insemination sperm were considered, only acrosomal and equatorial staining correlated significantly (r=0.46, P<0.05) (Table 6).

The development of successful *in vitro* fertilization (IVF) systems has permitted more accurate evaluation of gamete interactions. The examination of sperm populations used in IVF has contributed much to the establishment of more precise criteria for fertility. The ability to mimic capacitation conditions *in vitro* has enabled the study of the membrane alterations that occur.

Table 4 Percentage and percentage change[§*] FITC–WGA staining of human spermatozoa in groups with <50% and ⩾50% total fertilization rate of preovulatory oocytes

Morphological zone	*%FITC–WGA staining (% change in FITC–WGA staining following swim-up)* in vitro *fertilization groups*	
	Group 1 *<50%*	*Group 2* *⩾50%*
Acrosomal	30.92±18.53[a] (13.76±8.92)[c]	62.70±21.70[b] (34.36±17.38)[d]
Equatorial	34.83±18.15 (10.25±6.69)[e]	42.60±19.87 (20.16±9.46)[f]
Post-acrosomal	91.92±8.89 (3.79±3.37)	93.20±7.49 (4.31±3.69)
Neck	16.50±15.22 (22.38±15.49)	12.20±5.49 (23.59±29.82)
Midpiece	0.33±0.65 (0.00±0.00)	0.90±1.59 (2.78±9.62)
Tail	2.50±4.72 (6.42±12.97)	3.60±4.37 (9.05±16.05)

Values are means±SD; [§*]values in parenthesis [a,b], P<0.01; [c,d], P<0.01; [e,f], P<0.01

Table 5 Correlation[a] between *in vitro* fertilization rates and percentage and percentage change[b] FITC–WGA staining of human sperm

	Sperm morphological zones					
	A	*E*	*PA*	*N*	*MP*	*T*
IVF	0.73**	0.23	–0.10	–0.12	0.26	0.13
Rate	(0.0001)	(0.31)	(0.65)	(0.61)	(0.24)	(0.56)
	0.51*	0.53*	0.34	–0.19	0.29	–0.19
	(0.01)	(0.01)	(0.12)	(0.40)	(0.20)	(0.39)

[a] Correlation coefficient (significance level); [b] coefficient underlined; **significant (P<0.001); *significant (P<0.05). A=acrosomal; E=equatorial; PA=post-acrosomal; N=neck; MP=midpiece; T=tail

It would appear, from this study, that a minimum of 35% FITC–WGA acrosomal staining in a sample is necessary for good (⩾50%) IVF. The 64% positive predictive value of the WGA assay, calculated when the total fertilization of oocytes was considered, does not represent a convincing figure for the application of the assay as the prognosis for fertilization of a specific number of oocytes. The data suggest that the assay may, however, be used as a possible indicator of functional aberrations of oocytes. Of the oocytes inseminated with sperm exhibiting >35% WGA acrosomal staining, 23.6% remained unfertilized

Table 6 Multivariate correlation[a] between percentage FITC–WGA staining of individual sperm zones[b]. Reproduced from Gabriel *et al.* (1995)[52] with permission of the American Society for Reproductive Medicine

Zones	*A*	*E*	*PA*	*N*	*MP*
E	0.46*				
	(0.03)				
PA	–034	0.64*			
	(0.12)	(0.001)			
N	–0.14	–0.16	0.32		
	(0.55)	(0.48)	(1.14)		
MP	0.21	–0.12	0.10	0.06	
	(0.36)	(0.96)	(0.65)	(0.80)	
T	0.02	0.29	–0.24	–0.04	0.45
	(0.93)	(0.20)	(0.28)	(0.85)	(0.06)

[a] Correlation coefficient (significance level); [b] A=acrosomal; E=equatorial; PA=post-acrosomal; N=neck; MP=midpiece; T=tail; * significant ($P<0.05$)

(Table 2). This could be a reflection of defective oocytes if no other male factor is diagnosed.

Using the 50% minimum cutoff value for IVF total fertilization rate[54] and the 35% lower limit for WGA acrosomal staining, the calculated positive predictive value of the WGA assay increases to 90% (Table 3). This implies that the assay may hold much potential as a possible prognostic indicator for IVF. By determining the WGA activity over the acrosomal region of the spermatozoa and using the 35% cutoff value, patients may possibly be grouped into a good prognosis or a poor prognosis pattern for IVF, provided that all other semen parameters are within the normal range.

When the two fertilization rate groups (i.e. <50% and ≥50%) were compared for FITC–WGA activity, staining of the acrosomal region was significantly greater ($P<0.01$) in the ≥50% fertilization rate group (62.70±21.70) than in the <50% fertilization rate group (30.92±18.53). Also, the percentage of changes in acrosomal (13.76±8.92 and 34.36±17.38) and equatorial (10.25±6.69 and 20.16±9.46) region staining, following swim-up separation were significantly different ($P<0.01$).

The fact that staining occurs in suspension would suggest that this represents staining of the plasma membrane[6] and may therefore be related to the unmasking of sperm surface receptors during capacitation. If this is the case, the results suggest an impairment in the mechanisms for removal of decapacitation factors in the <50% fertilization rate group when compared to the ≥50% group. Alternatively, the <50% IVF rate group could inherently possess a larger percentage of spermatozoa that are devoid of these membrane constituents at the acrosomal region, thus rendering these spermatozoa unable to fertilize. The actual localization of these WGA receptors, however, should be verified by ultrastructural examination of the sperm vestments using colloidal gold- or ferritin-labeled WGA and transmission electronmicroscopy.

The question may also be raised as to whether FITC–WGA staining of the acrosomal and equatorial regions are indicative of the dynamics of the acrosome reaction. This being true, the percentage increase in acrosomal and percentage decrease in equatorial region staining would represent the exposure of the inner acrosomal membrane and modification of the equatorial region which are apparently essential for fertilization[10,11]. The significant positive correlation ($r=0.46$, $P<0.05$) between the percentage of FITC–WGA acrosomal and equatorial region staining demonstrates the close interaction between these membrane domains. Spermatozoa that are not stained by FITC–WGA in the acrosomal region may thus demonstrate an impairment in the initiation of the acrosome reaction by these sperm or they may have acrosome reacted beyond the exposure of the inner acrosomal membrane. These sperm will thus be unable to fertilize since the acrosome reaction at the oocyte zona surface is a requisite in the fertilization process. Elucidation of such assumptions may, however, be achieved by comparative studies with *in vitro*-induced acrosome reaction using calcium ionophore (A23187) and sperm in IVF insemination medium.

The results of this study[53] indicate a significant positive correlation ($r=0.73$, $P=0.0001$) between FITC–WGA staining of the acrosomal region of human spermatozoa and fertilization recorded *in vitro*. This would imply that the WGA receptors in the acrosomal region of human spermatozoa play a vital role in the fertilization process. Samples that do not conform to the observed correlation may indicate other functional defects. Samples should, therefore, be assessed in relation to other semen parameters. Since no single parameter, in isolation, may determine fertility, the use of multivariate correlation both intra- and interassay is reiterated. The WGA assay may be included among and in conjunction with other semen parameters as a possible prognostic indicator of fertilization success *in vitro*. Thus, it would appear that there is a close relationship between WGA receptors on human sperm and sperm morphology as well as sperm–egg fusion. WGA receptor deficiency (both in quantity and/or localization) may be one underlying cause of male infertility and could be considered as 'sperm membrane molecular disease'.

References

1. Bostofte, E., Serup, J. and Rebbe, H. (1982). Relation between sperm count and semen volume, and pregnancies obtained during a twenty-year follow-up period. *Int. J. Androl.*, **5**, 267–75
2. Jeulin, C., Feneux, D., Serres, C., Jouannet, P., Guillet-Rosso, F., Belaisch-Allart, J., Frydman, R. and Testart, J. (1986). Sperm factors related to failure of human *in vitro* fertilization. *J. Reprod. Fertil.*, **76**, 735–44
3. Kruger, T. F., Acosta, A., Simmons, K. F., Swanson, R. J., Matta, J. F. and Oehninger, S. (1988). Predictive value of abnormal sperm morphology in *in vitro* fertilization. *Fertil. Steril.*, **49**, 112–17
4. Menkveld, R., Stander, F. S. H., Kotze, T. J., Kruger, T. F. and Van Zyl, J. A. (1990). The evaluation of morphological characteristics of human spermatozoa according to stricter criteria. *Hum. Reprod.*, **5**, 586–92
5. Van der Ven, H. H., Jeyendran, R. S., Al-Hasani, S., Perez-Palaez, M., Diedrich, K. and Zaneveld, L. J. D. (1986). Correlation between human sperm swelling in hypoosmotic medium (hypoosmotic swelling test) and *in vitro* fertilization. *J. Androl.*, **7**, 190–6
6. Liu, D. Y., Du Plessis, Y. P., Nayudu, P. L., Johnston, W. I. H. and Baker, H. W. G. (1988). The use of *in vitro* fertilization to evaluate putative tests of human sperm function. *Fertil. Steril.*, **49**, 272–7
7. Goodpasture, J. C., Zavos, P. M., Cohen, M. R. and Zaneveld, L. J. D. (1981). Effects of various conditions of semen storage on the acrosin system of human spermatozoa. *J. Reprod. Fertil.*, **63**, 397–405
8. Yanagimachi, R., Yanagimachi, H. and Rogers, B. J. (1986). The use of zona-free animal ova as a test system for the fertilizing capacity of human spermatozoa. *Biol. Reprod.*, **15**, 471–6
9. Franken, D. R., Acosta, A. A., Kruger, T. F., Lombard, C., Oehninger, S. and Hodgen, G. D. (1993). The hemizona assay: Its role in identifying male factor infertility in assisted reproduction. *Fertil. Steril.*, **59**, 1075–80
10. Holden, C. A. and Trounson, A. O. (1991). Staining of the inner acrosomal membrane of human spermatozoa with concanavalin A as an indicator of potential egg penetration ability. *Fertil. Steril.*, **56**, 967–74
11. Kallajoki, M., Virtanen, I. and Suominen, J. (1986). The fate of acrosomal staining during the acrosomal reaction of human spermatozoa as revealed by a monoclonal antibody and PNA-lectin. *Int. J. Androl.*, **9**, 181–94
12. Fenichel, P., Donzeau, M., Farahifar, D., Basteris, B., Ayraud, N. and Hsi, B.-L. (1991). Dynamics of human sperm acrosome reaction: relation with *in vitro* fertilization. *Fertil. Steril.*, **55**, 994–9
13. Badel, P. and Brilliantine, L. (1969). Agglutination of spermatozoa of clams and of human A, B and O blood groups by phytoagglutinins. *Proc. Cos. Expl. Biol. Med.*, **130**, 621–3
14. Nicolson, G. L. (1974). The interactions of lectins with animal cell surfaces. *Int. Rev. Cytol.*, **39**, 89–190
15. Lotan, R. and Nicolson, G. L. (1979). Purification of cell membrane glycoproteins by lectin affinity chromatography. *Biochim. Biophys. Acta*, **559**, 329–766
16. Brown, J. C. and Hunt, R. C. (1978). Lectins. *Int. Rev. Cytol.*, **52**, 277–349
17. Grant, G. W. M. and Peters, M. W. (1984). Lectin-membrane interactions. Information from model systems. *Biochim. Biophys. Acta*, **779**, 403–22
18. Koehler, J. K. (1978). The mammalian sperm surface: studies with specific labelling techniques. *Int. Rev. Cytol.*, **54**, 73–108
19. Sharon, N. and Lis, H. (1974). Use of lectins for the study of membranes. In Korn, E. D. (ed.) *Methods in Membrane Biology*, Vol. 3, pp. 147–99 (New York: Academic Press)
20. Noonan, K. D. and Burger, M. M. (1973). Binding of (3H) concanavalin A to normal and transformed cells. *J. Biol. Chem.*, **248**, 4286–92
21. Boyd, W. C. (1954). In Neurath, H. and Bailey, K. (eds.) *The Proteins*, Vol. 2, Part B, pp. 755–839. (New York: Academic Press)
22. Fei, W. Y. and Hao, X. W. (1990). Wheat germ agglutinin (WGA) receptor on human sperm membrane and male infertility. *Arch. Androl.*, **24**, 97a
23. Kashiwabara, T., Tanaka, R. and Matsumoto, T. (1965). Tail-to-tail agglomeration of bull spermatozoa by phytoagglutinins present in soy beans. *Nature*, **207**, 831–2
24. Kinsey, W. H. and Koehler, J. K. (1976). Fine structural localization of Concanavalin A binding sites on hamster spermatozoa. *J. Supramol. Struct.*, **5**, 185–9

25. Kinsey, W. H. and Koehler, J. K. (1978). Cell surface changes associated with *in vitro* capacitation of hamster sperm. *J. Ultrastruct. Res.*, **64**, 1–13
26. Koehler, J. K. (1976). Changes in antigenic site distribution on rabbit spermatozoa after incubation in capacitating media. *Biol. Reprod.*, **15**, 444–56
27. Koehler, J. K. and Gaddum-Rosse, P. (1975). Media induced alterations of membrane associated particles of the guinea pig sperm tail. *J. Ultrastruct. Res.*, **51**, 106–18
28. Koehler, J. K. and Sato, K. (1978). Changes in lectin labelling pattern of mouse spermatozoa accompanying capacitation and the acrosome reaction. (Abstr.) *J. Cell. Biol.*, **79**, 165
29. Kopecny, V. (1979). Acrosome labelling in mammalian spermatozoa. *Ann. Biol. Anim. Biochem. Biophys.*, **19**, 695–701
30. Lewin, L. M., Weissenberg, R., Sobel, J. S., Marcus, Z. and Nebel, L. (1979). Differences in Con A-FITC binding to rat spermatozoa during epididymal maturation and capacitation. *Arch. Androl.*, **2**, 279–81
31. Millette, C. F. (1977). Distribution and mobility of lectin binding sites on mammalian spermatozoa. In Edindin, M. and Johnson, M. H. (eds.) *Immunobiology of Gametes*, pp. 51–71. (Cambridge: Cambridge University Press)
32. Nicolson, G. L. (1978). Ultrastructural localization of lectin receptors. In Koehler, J. K. (ed.) *Advanced Techniques in Biological Electron Microscopy*, Vol. II, pp. 1–38. (Heidelberg: Springer Verlag)
33. Nicolson, G. L., Lacorbiere, M. and Yanagimachi, R. (1972). Quantitative determination of plant agglutinin membrane sites on mammalian spermatozoa. *Proc. Soc. Exp. Biol. Med.*, **141**, 661–3
34. Nicolson, G. L. and Yanagimachi, R. (1972). Terminal saccharides on sperm plasma membranes. Identification by specific agglutinins. *Science*, **177**, 276–9
35. Koehler, J. K. (1981). Lectins as probes of the spermatozoan surface. *Arch. Androl.*, **6**, 197–217
36. Thoss, K. and Roth, J. (1975). The use of fluoresceine isothiocyanate labelled lectins for the immunohistochemical demonstration of saccharides. *Exp. Path. Bd.*, **11**, 155–61
37. Cerezo, J. M. S., Beuno, M. I., Skowronski, B. and Cerezo, A. S. (1982). Immunohistochemical localization of Concanavalin A and wheat germ lectin receptors in the normal human spermatozoa. *Am. J. Reprod. Immunol.*, **2**, 246–9
38. Cerezo, J. M. S., Levit, L., Nardone, P. and Cerezo, A. S. (1989). Sperm peroxidases and their possible role as glycoprotein-containing Con A and Wheat germ lectin receptors. *Am. J. Reprod. Immunol.*, **20**, 13–16
39. Cross, N. L. and Overstreet, J. W. (1987). Glycoconjugates of the human sperm surface: Distributions and alterations that accompany capacitation *in vitro*. *Gamete Res.*, **16**, 23–5
40. Kallojoki, M., Malmi, R., Virtanen, I. and Suominen, J. (1985). Glycoconjugates of human sperm surface. A study with fluorescent lectins and *Lens culinaris* agglutination affinity chromatography. *Cell. Biol. Int. Rep.*, **9**, 151–64
41. Wollina, U., Schreiber, G., Zollmann, C., Hipler, C. and Gunther, E. (1989). Lectin binding sites in normal human testis. *Andrologia*, **21**, 127–30
42. Lee, M. C. and Damjonov, I. (1985). Lectin binding sites on human sperm and spermatogenic cells. *Anat. Rec.*, **212**, 282–7
43. Singer, S. L., Lambert, H., Cross, N. L. and Overstreet, J. W. (1985). Alteration of the human sperm surface during *in vitro* capacitation as assessed by lectin-induced agglutination. *Gamete Res.*, **12**, 291–9
44. Myles, D. G. and Primakoff, P. (1991). Sperm proteins that serve as receptors for the zona pellucida and their post-testicular modification. *Ann. N.Y. Acad. Sci.*, **637**, 486–93
45. Zhixing, P. and Yifei, W. (1990). Quantification and localization of wheat germ agglutinin receptor on human sperm membrane and male fertility and infertility (Abstr). *Arch. Androl.*, **24**, 103
46. Gabriel, L. K., Franken, D. R., Van Der Horst, G., Kruger, T. F. and Oehninger, S. C. (1994). Wheat germ agglutinin receptors on human sperm membranes and sperm morphology. *Andrologia*, **26**, 5–8
47. Kruger, T. F., Menkveld, R., Stander, F. S. H., Lombard, C. J., Van Der Merwe, J. P., Van Zyl, J. A. and Smith, K. (1986). Sperm morphologic features as a prognostic factor in *in vitro* fertilization. *Fertil. Steril.*, **46**, 1118–23
48. Gabriel, L. K., Franken, D. R., Van der Horst, G. and Kruger T. F. (1994) Localization of wheat germ agglutinin lectin receptors on human sperm by fluorescence microscopy: utilization of different fixatives. *Arch. Androl.*, **33**, 77–85
49. Franken, D. R., Kruger, T. F., Menkveld, R., Oehninger, S., Coddington, C. C. and Hodgen, G. D. (1990). Hemizona assay and teratozoospermia: increasing sperm insemination concentrations to enhance zona pellucida binding. *Fertil. Steril.*, **54**, 497–503
50. Franken, D. R., Oehninger, S., Burkman, L. J., Coddington, C. C., Kruger, T. F., Rosenwaks, Z., Acosta, A. A. and Hodgen, G. D. (1989). The hemizona assay (HZA): a predictor of human sperm fertilizing potential in *in vitro* fertilization (IVF) treatment. *J.* In Vitro *Fertil. Embryo Transf.*, **6**, 44–50
51. Oehninger, S., Coddington, C. C., Scott, R., Franken, D. R., Burkman, L. J., Acosta, A. A. and Hodgen, G. D. (1989). Hemizona assay (HZA): assessment of sperm dysfunction and prediction of *in vitro* fertilization outcome. *Fertil. Steril.*, **51**, 665–70
52. Oehninger, S. C., Acosta, A. A., Morshedi, M., Veeck, L., Swanson, R. J., Simmons, K. and Rosenwaks, Z. (1988). Corrective measures and preg-

nancy outcome in *in vitro* fertilization outcome in patients with severe sperm morphology abnormalities. *Fertil. Steril.*, **50**, 283–7

53. Gabriel, L. K., Franken, D. R., Van Der Horst, G. and Kruger, T. F. (1995). FITC-wheat germ agglutinin staining of human spermatozoa and fertilization *in vitro. Fertil. Steril.*, **63**, 894–901

54. Franken, D. R., Acosta, A. A., Kruger, T. F., Lombard, C., Oehninger, S. and Hodgen, G. D. (1993). The hemizona assay: its role in determining male factor infertility in assisted reproduction. *Fertil. Steril.*, **59**, 1075–80

New frontiers in male factor diagnosis 2: current trends and future prospects

25

G. F. Doncel

INTRODUCTION

The last 20 years have seen an explosion in the amount of information in reproductive biology. Spermatogenesis and its end-product, the spermatozoon, did not escape this phenomenon[1]. However, despite all this frenetic activity, the striking reality is that there has been virtually no advance in the clinical treatment of male infertility. Where advances have occurred, they have affected relatively few patients[2].

About 75% of patients seen for male infertility have semen quality ranging from normal to severe oligozoospermia[3]. Other factors may be present in these patients, such as varicoceles, subclinical inflammation of the accessory sex organs, poor general health, stress or heat exposure, but altering these factors generally has no dramatic or continuing beneficial effect[4]. The clinician attempting to deal with male infertility is constantly reminded of the lack of detailed understanding of the pathophysiology of spermatogenesis and spermiogenesis defects which appear to underlie the disorders observed in the majority of patients.

Male infertility is associated with alterations in the number or the quality of spermatozoa; however, these defects are not a disease entity in their own right, but probably the end result of an array of multiple interacting factors which may have their main effects during sperm production and differentiation.

The variability that occurs in semen quality from day to day in an individual is controversial and very poorly understood. Besides the laboratory errors, there appears to be true biological variations that are of marked degree[5]. Some pathological disorders of the semen, such as oligo- or asthenozoospermia, can also be transient. More interestingly, even the fertilizing potential of a sample with otherwise normal semen parameters may vary.

Fertilization rates are governed by multiple factors linked to both sperm and eggs. Unfortunately, with the current battery of tests to study sperm quality, we are unable to accurately predict the fertilization chances of a couple undergoing assisted reproduction or to advise them to avoid the trial. Even worse, if a sperm alteration is detected, we fail to describe the defective molecular mechanism and therefore, a rational therapy cannot be attempted.

Several studies have clearly demonstrated that standard semen parameters such as sperm concentration, motility and gross morphology have limited clinical value in predicting both natural and assisted fertilization[6–8]. Since the basic semen analysis does not appropriately address sperm function, numerous assays have been developed with this purpose.

Computer-assisted motion analysis, hyperosmotic swelling test (HOST), acrosomal and nuclear maturity assessments, hamster-egg penetration test (HEPT), and zona binding penetration assays are part of today's armamentarium (see previous chapters).

Although primarily intended as a therapy, *in vitro* fertilization (IVF) represents the ultimate assay to evaluate sperm–oocyte interactions and a significantly valuable endpoint. Therefore, almost all of the above-mentioned sperm functional tests have been correlated with fertilization rates *in vitro*, and their predictive values determined. It is important to note, however, that work-ups for the initial screening of a presumptive clinical male factor patient and a male factor patient being studied for IVF are substantially different. Tests with good prognostic value in one situation may not be so useful in the other.

Current sperm functional assays attempt to determine potential alterations on the sperm capacity to undergo some of the biological processes involved in fertilization.

However, using logistic regression analysis, a powerful statistical tool to correlate the binary probability of a given event (fertilization) to occur or not, and multiple potentially causative variables, only strict morphology, acrosomal status, mean linearity (one of the computerized motion parameters) and binding to the zona pellucida, were significantly related to fertilization rates *in vitro*[9]. But even these assays are not able to predict fertilization in all cases, nor are they free from technical pitfalls. For instance, zona-binding tests utilize human oocytes which are largely unavailable, at least in the amount needed to allow the assays to become part of routine sperm evaluation. Strict morphology is technically simple and possesses a good correlation with IVF rates; however, it requires well-trained technicians to be performed and the subjectivity involved makes inter-laboratory standardization very difficult. Assessment of acrosome status may provide additional information, particularly in men with high proportions of spermatozoa with abnormal morphology. Nevertheless, in the way it is usually performed, it fails to examine acrosome reaction inducibility and, with that, a dynamic process that plays a crucial role in fertilization.

Keeping in mind that it is very unlikely that a single test would be able to predict sperm fertilizing ability with total accuracy, several are the evaluation trends that can be anticipated for the near future. We will attempt to briefly outline some of the potential applications of recent findings in the areas of capacitation and sperm plasma membrane, sperm zona receptors, signal-transduction mechanisms, motility regulation, mitochondrial and genomic DNA, post-fusion events and, lastly, analysis of fertility data.

SPERM CAPACITATION AND PLASMA MEMBRANE

Capacitation encompasses the processes that transform the morphologically complete, but non-functional male gamete into a fertilizing sperm cell, giving it the capacity to penetrate the zona pellucida and fuse with the oocyte itself.

Assessing the ability of human spermatozoa to undergo capacitation is particularly difficult because of the absence of unequivocal morphological correlates, because individuals vary markedly in the rate at which spermatozoa capacitate, and because capacitation within any one population of sperm is strongly asynchronous both *in vivo* and *in vitro*[10,11].

However, since capacitation is a prerequisite for sperm to undergo hyperactivated motility, acrosome reaction and ultimately, fertilization, it would be very important to verify its characteristics before any treatment modality is recommended for an infertile patient. The individual variability noted earlier[10] may imply that different semen samples may require different incubation times and media to achieve full capacitation in enough spermatozoa.

Several lines of evidence[12] suggest that mammalian plasma membranes are a heterogenous mosaic of at least two kinds of microdomains: (1) gel-like areas where molecular motion is very slow; and (2) liquid crystal-like microdomains in which molecules move relatively freely.

Cholesterol has previously been demonstrated to limit protein insertion into phospholipid bilayers, to restrict lateral mobility of functional receptors, and to modulate the activity of membrane proteins[13,14]. Cholesterol concentration is preferentially reduced within the plasma membrane domain overlying the acrosomal cap during capacitating incubations[15]. Further, Hoshi *et al.*[16] found that, in normozoospermic men, a lower cholesterol/phospholipid ratio of fresh sampled spermatozoa is correlated with a shorter incubation time required to achieve a positive sperm penetration assay. It is thus apparent that loss or reduction of plasma membrane cholesterol constitutes an important step in the capacitation of human spermatozoa.

It has been reported that normozoospermic men who do not fertilize human eggs *in vitro* constitute an identifiable class of occult male factor infertility. In a recent report[17], the abnormal fertilization potential of a group of these men could be correlated with elevated sperm membrane cholesterol content, decreased spontaneous acrosome reaction rates and sperm inability to express surface receptors.

The integrity of the plasma membrane is an obvious parameter for assessment because it is crucially involved in sperm–egg interactions and it is an essential requirement for general cell function. The use of fluorescent probes to assess membrane integrity in mammalian spermatozoa has already been reported[18]. Propidium iodide, which binds to and stains cellular DNA, is impermeable to the plasma membrane and therefore can only enter and stain damaged (permeable) cells. Carboxyfluorescein diacetate, on the other hand, is permeant, but is de-esterified inside the cell by non-specific esterases; the resultant free carboxyfluorescein is fluorescent and impermeant and builds up in the cytoplasm of intact cells, causing them to fluoresce green throughout. New probes are currently being assessed in human sperm. Lectin-coated beads which recognize intracellular molecules are also being explored[20]. In this case, the need for a cytofluorometer or a fluorescence microscope could be avoided.

There is a growing body of evidence to indicate that a significant factor in the etiology of male infertility involves a loss of sperm function as a consequence of oxidative stress[21]. This stress originates from the excessive generation of reactive oxygen species by the spermatozoa and results in the peroxidation of unsaturated fatty acids in the sperm plasma membrane. It is possible that reactive oxygen species originating from infiltrating leukocytes could also stress the sperm, although protective properties of seminal plasma would render this unlikely *in vivo*. Whatever the source of the reactive oxygen species, the lipid peroxides generated thereby exhibit powerful negative correlations with the movement characteristics of the spermatozoa and their capacity for sperm–oocyte fusion.

New chemiluminescent techniques used to detect production of reactive oxygen species have incorporated horseradish peroxidase to focus on hydrogen peroxide generation[22] and luminol analogues to increase the efficiency of the luminescent reaction[23].

The measurement of lipid peroxidation, especially of pre-existing lipid peroxides[24], can be taken to give an indication of the degree of oxidative stress experienced by a sperm population during its life history. In this respect, lipid peroxidation may be a more informative and ultimately more useful diagnostic tool than the analysis of the generation of reactive oxygen species *per se*. Prospective studies are currently underway to establish this point.

ZONA-BINDING SPERM RECEPTORS

A variety of proteins from mammalian spermatozoa have been implicated as possible zona binding receptors which would function in the adherence of the sperm plasma membrane to the zona pellucida of the oocyte. Since sperm samples displaying normal semen parameters can fail fertilization, one of the potential pathogenetic defects may be an abnormal expression of sperm–zona-binding receptors. Several candidates have been postulated as zona binding glycoproteins; however, the precise nature of these receptors in mammalian sperm remains yet to be determined[25].

Concerning the human sperm, several authors have utilized labeled lectins in order to identify the expression of surface glycoproteins with potential zona-receptor activity. Encouraging results have been obtained and are reviewed later in this chapter.

Recently, two carbohydrate-binding sites have been correlated with the fertilization potential of human spermatozoa. The mannose ligand-binding capacity of a sperm population was microscopically assessed after reaction with a mannosylated fluorescein-conjugated bovine serum albumin[26,27]. The unlabeled probe specifically blocked human sperm–zona binding in a concentration-dependent manner[28]. Recognition between the probe and the mannose-binding sites appeared to be calcium-dependent.

The incidence of sperm expressing mannose–ligand receptors increased during an incubation under capacitating conditions and the fluorescent patterns on the sperm-head changed after the acrosome reaction[27,28]. However, the precise location of these receptors on the sperm has not yet been determined and, therefore, the sperm-head fluorescent patterns that represent receptor surface expression are still a matter of controversy. In our opinion, the mannose staining should be combined with a positive identification of membrane integrity, e.g. Hoechst 33258 or hypo-osmotic swelling test. In a recent study by Benoff and co-workers[17], of 338 human semen specimens with normal profiles, 10 failed to fertilize *in vitro*. Six of these occult male factors were distinguished from controls (good fertilization) by their failure to show time-dependent increases in the percentage of spermatozoa exhibiting head-directed mannose–ligand activity, by the loss or apparent increase in membrane cholesterol and by the absence of spontaneous and/or mannose-induced acrosome exocytosis.

Abnormal expression of mannose–ligand receptors has also been reported in a group of men with varicocele[29] and in patients who were under medication with calcium-channel blockers such as nifedipine[30].

Another fluorescein-conjugated neoglycoprotein, similar to the one described above but containing fucose residues instead of mannose, was shown to label a small subpopulation of normal human spermatozoa[31]. The neoglycoprotein binding was competitively inhibited by solubilized human zona pellucida giving physiological relevance to such sperm binding sites. The fluorescent patterns were located at the acrosomal area of the acrosome-intact sperm, increasing their incidence with time of exposure to capacitating conditions.

Although these probes are easy to use, inexpensive and commercially available, the fact that they recognize a sugar that can be in more than one glycoprotein may dilute their specificity to identify a particular zona binding receptor. Because of this, we have studied monoclonal antibodies directed against putative zona-binding sperm proteins.

Sperm surface β-1,4-galactosyltransferase (GalTase) is a well-characterized protein that has been suggested to mediate fertilization in mice[32]. It specifically recognizes those oligosaccharides on ZP_3 that possess sperm-binding activity, but do not interact with other zona pellucida glycoproteins[33]. We have demonstrated[34] that an anti-bovine GalTase polyclonal IgG and a monoclonal IgM directed against human GalTase were able to specifically inhibit human sperm–zona binding. Neither of the antibodies altered sperm motion parameters nor induced the acrosome reaction during the incubation period. Immunofluorescent localization of GalTase on live human spermatozoa revealed a faint patchy pattern at the head level.

Using a Western-blot technique, GalTase has been immunodetected in a 'high density' subpopulation of human spermatozoa[35]. Interestingly, a population of men whose sperm demonstrated an inability to penetrate zona-free hamster eggs showed a reduced level of enzyme activity. Analysis of DNA from those individuals identified a mutated allelic variant for the GalTase gene[36].

Mouse sperm contain a major phosphotyrosine-containing protein of M_r 95 000 which has been implicated as a sperm membrane receptor for the egg zona pellucida glycoprotein ZP_3[37]. A similar antigen has been described in human sperm, and antibodies against it proved to inhibit sperm–zona interaction[34,38,39]. This antigen represents another interesting candidate to be assessed in sperm samples of infertile men.

As described above, several probes have been employed to detect putative zona-binding receptors in the human sperm. However, not knowing the precise nature of the receptor(s), the best possible biomarker would be a recombinant human ZP_3. The bulk of evidence in different mammalian species points to this protein as the main zona pellucida ligand involved in sperm–zona primary binding. Human ZP_3 genomic sequence(s) has been reported[40,41] and cloning and expression are under way. Once a physiologically active product is obtained, three lines of applications in male factor diagnosis can be envisioned. First, ZP_3 linked to silica beads or fluorochromes could be used to characterize the expression of ZP_3-binding receptors in spermatozoa from infertile men. This would provide evidence to understand the *in vitro* fertilization failure observed in some sperm samples displaying classical semen parameters within normal range. However, presence does not suffice and ZP_3 would represent a way to assess function of the receptor through signal-transduction endpoints such as the acrosome reaction. Lastly, zona-binding assays correlate very well with fertilization potential and are highly predictive for the *in vitro* fertilization outcome (Chapter 20). However, scarcity of human eggs is a difficult obstacle to overcome. If the human ZP_3 were incorporated successfully in the mouse genome the transgenic animal, expressing a mouse zona pellucida with a human ZP_3, could provide a much-needed source of oocytes to assess sperm function[42].

SPERM SIGNAL-TRANSDUCTION MECHANISMS AND ACROSOME REACTION

The acrosome reaction is essential for mammalian fertilization because it is required for sperm penetration through the zona and for oolemma fusion[43,44]. Morphologically abnormal acrosomes, as well as altered acrosome reaction kinetics, have been correlated with poor *in vitro* fertilization rates[45,46]. However, data on the molecular defects underlying these deficiencies have not been reported.

It is increasingly evident that the acrosome reaction can be initiated after activation of membrane receptors, ultimately leading to protein phosphorylation and/or increase in intracellular calcium ions[47]. Three signal transduction pathways have so far been identified that can result in protein phosphorylation and acrosome reaction: (1) the adenylate cyclase, cAMP, protein kinase A pathway; (2) the phospholipase C, diacylglycerol, protein kinase C pathway; and (3) the guanylate cyclase, cGMP, protein kinase G pathway. An acrosome reaction induced by isolated human zonae pellucida appears to involve all three[48]. Tyrosine phosphorylation, another important mechanism of signal transduction, has been described on sperm-head proteins and associated with zona pellucida stimulation[39]. Phosphotyrosine-containing proteins localized at the equatorial segment of human sperm seem to be involved in sperm–zona binding since their specific blockage by means of monoclonal antibodies significantly impaired this interaction[49].

It has recently been shown that spermatozoa from oligozoospermic[50] and teratozoospermic[51] patients have a reduced capacity to increase intracellular calcium after progesterone stimulation. This demonstrates an inability to initiate the cascade of transductional events that lead to acrosome reaction, possibly explaining, at least in part, the decreased fertilizing capacity of these patients.

Evaluation of receptor-induced production of second messengers could provide the information needed for a more rational approach to the *in vitro* therapy of acrosome-reaction deficiencies. For example, if a low cAMP content were determined after proper sperm stimulation, *in vitro* treatment of the sperm sample with a phosphodiesterase inhibitor such as pentoxifylline would be in order.

It is important to remark that spontaneous acrosome reactions bear no relation to fertility and therefore induced reactions should be those added to the existing semen analysis. Currently, the techniques most used to assess acrosome reaction inducibility employ a calcium ionophore[52] or human follicular fluid[53]. Induced reactions have been shown to be significantly reduced in subfertile men and their assessment to have a good predictive value for fertility.

Innovations in this area are focused on stimulation of the reaction and methods of detection of acrosomal status. Concerning the stimuli, here again, in the near future, a recombinant human ZP_3 would be the best option. However, separate stimulation of each of the different transduction pathways by specific agents could reveal the precise defect underlying the acrosome reaction deficiency.

In regard to the methodology, new probes (lectins or monoclonal antibodies) targeting outer and inner acrosomal membranes and acrosomal contents are being tried, alone or in combination, to better define the stages of the acrosome reaction[54]. Although monoclonal antibody-coated beads have been used in combination with inverted phase-contrast microscopy[55], flow cytometric or fluorescence microscopic capabilities may soon be an integral part of the image analyzers currently used for motility and morphology assessments.

SPERM MOTILITY

Evaluation of sperm movement characteristics has become notoriously more detailed with the introduction of computer-assisted motion analyzers (Chapter 7). Multiple motion parameters, as well as hyperactivated motility, can be sorted out and precisely measured in an objective manner. Correlations with *in vitro* fertilization rates have been extensively reported.

Improved software with advantages, such as continuous tracking in real time, operator-overriding capacity and very low sample density analysis, is now being marketed.

Although the computer-aided systems have become more and more descriptive, little information has been produced in terms of the pathophysiological mechanisms underlying the sperm motility disorders. Ultrastructural studies have revealed absence of dynein arms and other flagellar abnormalities in some asthenozoospermic semen; however, the overall incidence of these anomalies within the infertile population is considerably low[56].

Using an immunofluorescent technique and specific monoclonal antibodies, we have studied the tyrosine-phosphorylation of tail proteins in normo- and asthenozoospermic sperm samples[57]. Tail phosphotyrosine-containing proteins increase during capacitation, being present in 70% of the spermatozoa from normal samples. Asthenozoospermic samples (<30% motility), however, show an inability to respond to capacitating conditions with an increase in motility parameters and phosphorylation values. After 6 h incubation, both hyperactivated motility and tail tyrosine-phosphorylation are significantly lower than in normal samples. Both defects appear to be concomitantly reversed by *in vitro* treatment of the spermatozoa with pentoxifylline.

Sperm motility alterations may also be caused by mitochondrial dysfunctions. Fluorochromes, such as rhodamine 123, have been used to compare mitochondrial membrane potential with sperm motility[58] and to evaluate simultaneously sperm mitochondrial activity and motion parameters with the aid of image analyzers[59]. The relationship between aerobic ATP and sperm motility has also been established[60].

SPERM MITOCHONDRIAL AND GENOMIC DNA

During recent years, a number of mitochondrial DNA mutations that cause human disease have been identified[61]. These are associated with a broad spectrum of clinical manifestations. The molecular and biochemical characterizations of mitochondrial DNA diseases have provided new insights into the nature of human degenerative disorders and spontaneous body aging, and have raised the possibility that deleterious mitochondrial DNA mutations may be much more common than previously thought.

Changes appearing in unexplained spermatogenic failure are strikingly similar to those seen in spontaneous body aging and it has been suggested that the same mechanisms may be underlying both phenomena[62]. Two important molecular mechanisms are now thought to be associated with general body aging. These are tissue damage due to release of toxic-free radicals and reactive oxygen species, and defects in oxidative phosphorylation. Both of these factors are seen in unexplained male infertility. They may in turn be related to inherited or acquired mutations in the mitochondrial DNA of the germ cell line and/or associated testicular support cells. In fact, it has been reported[63] that a patient suffering an encephalomyopathy known to be caused by a mitochondrial DNA disease showed a marked asthenozoospermia associated with ultrastructurally and functionally abnormal sperm mitochondria. Sperm mitochondrial DNA evaluations are currently being performed in our laboratory and others in order to provide evidence to support or reject the hypothetical association between mitochondrial DNA anomalies and sperm dysfunctions.

Screening of sperm genomic DNA is currently more advanced than its mitochondrial counterpart. Chromosomal abnormalities have been observed in about 50% of all spontaneous abortions in humans. The great majority of these anomalies comprise numerical rather than structural chromosome aberrations[64]. Whereas, in human live-borns, only numerical sex chromosome aberrations and trisomy 13, 18, and 21 are found, aneuploidy has been described for almost every chromosome complement in spontaneous abortions. Since human oocytes are difficult to obtain and are available only in small numbers, limited data on them exist so far[65]. Sperm cells, on the other hand, are easy to obtain in large numbers.

In the late 1970s a method was described that permitted a direct analysis of sperm chromosome complements after *in vitro* fertilization of hamster eggs with human sperm[66]. This technique is suitable to detect both numerical as well as structural chromosome aberrations[67,68]. However, the method is time-consuming, and only limited number of spermatozoa per donor are available for analysis. Non-radioactive *in situ* hybridization with chromosome-specific DNA probes offers a good alternative for determining numerical chromosomal aberrations. This method has recently been applied to the detection of aneuploidy of several chromosomes from sperm nuclei[69–71]. Our group has just reported the use of this technique in the screening of infertile male patients (Chapter 26)[72].

Genetic screening of the haploid complement of spermatozoa, as well as the dipiloid complement of the male and female partners of an infertile couple, will be an important requisite in the diagnostic evaluation of patients undergoing assisted reproduction. There has been an increasing number of human diseases associated with mutated allelic variants of normal genes. The pathogenetic mechanisms directly or indirectly linking genes and diseases are now becoming clear. However, the potential association between these abnormal genes and the fertilization capability of the carrier's gametes has not been established for the most part.

In this respect, the recent demonstration that congenital absence of the vas deferens (CAVD) is a mild form of cystic fibrosis (CF)[73], almost exclusively involving the genital tract, has prompted a research group to investigate the association between CF genotype mutations and *in vitro* performance of epididymal sperm (Chapter 32)[74]. Sixty-three patients with CAVD undergoing microsurgical epididymal sperm aspiration and *in vitro* fertilization were evaluated. A total of 12 mutations in the CF transmembrane regulator gene, representing around 90% of the total known CF mutations, were screened on DNA extracted from peripheral lymphocytes and amplified by the polymerase chain reaction. The difference in fertilization rates between patients testing positive for CF mutations and those whose screening was negative was highly significant. Moreover, those patients bearing the most common and lethal of the CF mutations, ΔF508, as the only detectable, showed the poorest fertilization rate. Such poor outcome was repeated with several attempts. Therefore, the association between CF-mutated genotype and sperm intrinsic defects, e.g. alteration of chloride channels, is a clear possibility.

This example and the almost complete ignorance on the genetic background of human diseases should remind us of the potential for iatrogenically increasing the transmission of pathological genetic characters. Assisted fertilization techniques, such as intracytoplasmic sperm injection (ICSI) that bypasses all natural sperm selection barriers, should therefore be executed with caution.

SPERM–EGG POST-FUSION EVENTS

The intracytoplasmic injection of human spermatozoa into eggs now seems to be the most beneficial approach to obtain fertilization and live births in cases of severe male infertility[75,76].

Egg activation and the events that it implicates are a key step for the success of such type of assisted fertilization. Physiologically, this process is triggered by fusion of the sperm and egg plasma membranes and a number of theories have been put forth to account for the mechanism by which this phenomenon occurs. Egg activation could be naturally initiated by: (1) the introduction of a soluble factor from the sperm into the egg cytoplasm; (2) the fusion of the sperm and egg membranes solely; and/or (3) the interaction of a sperm component with a specific egg plasma membrane receptor.

In ICSI, the injection of a spermatozoon into the ooplasm seems to be a sufficient stimulus to activate the oocyte, without the requisite of a membrane fusion. However, the intracellular signals mediating the egg activation, as well as the sperm contribution to it, have not yet been elucidated clearly.[77]

Sperm evaluations that can provide information to predict ICSI outcomes will have to wait until knowledge on biochemical mechanisms controlling the early events of human egg activation is accumulated.

FERTILITY DATA ANALYSIS

Revising the preceding chapters and the topics we have discussed above, it becomes clear that prediction of male fertility on the basis of a sole sperm assay is an unattainable goal. Furthermore, prediction of a couple's fertility potential should take into consideration sperm and oocyte biological variables, technical conditions and epidemiological factors, altogether making analysis of fertility data a complex and unique problem.

Statistical methods in reproductive medicine have been borrowed from other medical fields and do not properly address the special challenges of fertility data analysis. New mathematical models and statistical methods have been designed for this purpose[78,79]. An artificial neural network, a computational algorithm inspired by the biological structure of the neuron, was 'trained' to predict whether or not any ovum would fertilize from variables including number of cases that the micromanipulator had performed, site of the IVF laboratory, number of ova injected, average number of sperm injected, egg quality, semen analysis and sperm penetration assay results. The system predicted if any fertilization occurred 100% correctly in a test set that the neural network had not previously encountered[79].

Although complex in nature, the spreading of powerful personal computers and user-friendly software will soon make these analytical methods applicable in routine laboratory and clinical fertility evaluation.

CONCLUSIONS

The need for a better prediction of the fertilization potential of human spermatozoa has resulted in the incorporation of new tests to the screening armamentarium applied to infertile couples today. These tests assess several sperm functions involved in the process of fertilization. However, in spite of the battery of assays currently available, accurate prediction of fertilization and pregnancy rates for a couple undergoing assisted reproduction remains an elusive goal.

Owing to the basic research done in sperm biology, a new wave of sperm tests is under way. In contrast to those presently existing, these tests point to the assessment of molecular structures or mechanisms underlying sperm fertilization events. Evaluation of capacitation and molecular structure of sperm plasma membranes, putative zona-binding receptors, signal-transduction mechanisms, acrosome reaction inducibility, and sperm motion regulation are just a few of these tests.

Along this line of molecular characterization of sperm defects, probably the most innovative trend is the evaluation of sperm mitochondrial and genomic DNA. The association between human genetic disorders and sperm fertilizing ability presents a very interesting hypothesis yet to be proved.

Since accurate prediction of fertility does not appear feasible by employing only one or two tests, new computerized statistical methods that can process multiple variables and 'learn' from the outcome of the cases are going to spread rapidly once user-friendly software becomes available.

With the advent of highly successful microassisted fertilization techniques, there have been colleagues claiming that sperm evaluation, and even basic and applied research on human spermatozoa, will no longer be necessary or relevant. This chapter owes most of its content to the basic knowledge on sperm physiology acquired in recent years. Therefore, it seems appropriate to finish by stating that decreasing our interest in understanding the causes of male infertility will lead to a regrettable delay in the acquisition of scientific knowledge in this area, ultimately and unfortunately impeding the future development of better therapeutic modalities for the infertile couple.

References

1. Bacetti, B. (ed.) (1991). *Comparative Spermatology 20 Years After*, p. 75. (New York: Serono Symposia Publications, Raven Press)
2. Baker, H. W. B. (1993). Treatment of male infertility – what does the future hold? *Int. J. Androl.*, **16**, 343–8
3. Baker, H. W. G., Burger, H. G., de Kretser, D. M. and Hudson, B. (1986). Relative incidence of etiologic disorders in male infertility. In Santen, R. J. and Swerdloff, R. S. (eds.) *Male Reproductive Dysfunction: Diagnosis and Management of Hypogonadism, Infertility and Impotence*, pp. 341–72. (New York: Marcel Dekker Inc.)
4. Baker, H. G. W. (1986). Requirements for controlled therapeutic trials in male infertility. *Clin. Reprod. Fertil.*, **4**, 13–25
5. World Health Organization. (1992). *WHO Laboratory Manual for the Examination of Human Semen and Semen–Cervical Mucus Interaction*, 3rd edn. (Cambridge: Cambridge University Press)
6. Polansky, F. F. and Lamb, E. J. (1988). Do the results of semen analysis predict future fertility? A survival analysis. *Fertil. Steril.*, **49**, 1059–65
7. Mahadevan, M. M. and Trounson, A. O. (1984). The influence of seminal characteristics on the success rate of human *in vitro* fertilization. *Fertil. Steril.*, **42**, 400–5
8. Dunphy, B., Neal, N. L. and Cooke, I. D. (1989). The clinical value of conventional semen analysis. *Fertil. Steril.*, **51**, 324–9
9. Liu, D. Y. and Baker, H. W. G. (1992). Test of human sperm function and fertilization *in vitro*. *Fertil. Steril.*, **58**, 465–83
10. Perrault, S. D. and Rogers, B. J. (1982). Capacitation pattern of human spermatozoa. *Fertil. Steril.*, **38**, 258–60
11. Bedford, J. M. (1983). Significance of the need for sperm capacitation before fertilization in eutherian mammals. *Biol. Reprod.*, **28**, 108–20
12. Benoff, S., Cooper, G. W., Hurley, I., Mandel, F. S. and Rosenfeld, D. L. (1993). Antisperm antibody

binding to human sperm inhibits capacitation induced changes in the levels of plasma membrane sterols. *Am. J. Reprod. Infertil.*, **30**, 113–30
13. Muller, C. P. and Krueger, G. R. F. (1986). Modulation of membrane proteins by vertical phase separation and membrane lipid fluidity. Basis for a new approach to tumor immunotherapy. *Anticancer Res.*, **6**, 1181–94
14. Yeagle, P. L. (1985). Cholesterol and the cell membrane. *Biochim. Biophys. Acta*, **822**, 267–87
15. Tesarik, J. and Flechon, J. E. (1986). Distribution of sterols and anionic lipids in human sperm plasma membrane: Effects of *in vitro* capacitation. *J. Ultrastruct. Mol. Struct. Res.*, **97**, 227–37
16. Hoshi, K., Aita, T., Yanagida, K., Yoshimatsu, N. and Sato, A. (1990). Variation in the cholesterol/phospholipid ratio in human spermatozoa and its relationship with capacitation. *Hum. Reprod.*, **5**, 71–4
17. Benoff, S., Hurley, I., Cooper, G. W., Mandel, F. S., Hershlag, A., Scholl, G. M. and Rosenfeld, D. L. (1993). Fertilization potential *in vitro* is correlated with head-specific mannose–ligand receptor expression, acrosome status and membrane cholesterol content. *Hum. Reprod.*, **8**, 2155–66
18. Garner, D. L., Pinkel, D., Johnson, L. A. and Pace, M. M. (1986). Assessment of spermatozoal function using dual fluorescent staining and flow cytometric analyses. *Biol. Reprod.*, **34**, 127–38
19. Harrison, R. A. P. and Vickers, S. E. (1990). Use of fluorescent probes to assess membrane integrity in mammalian spermatozoa. *J. Reprod. Fertil.*, **88**, 343–52
20. Kohn, F. M., Mack, S. R., Anderson, R. A. and Zaneveld, L. J. D. (1994). Detection of human spermatozoa with absent anterior head membranes by lectin coated beads. *J. Androl.* Jan/Feb (Suppl.), Abstr., p. 45
21. Aitken, R. J. (1994). A free radical theory of male infertility. *Reprod. Fertil. Dev.*, **6**, 19–24
22. Aitken, R. J., Buckingham, D. W. and West, K. M. (1992). Reactive oxygen species and human spermatozoa; analysis of the cellular mechanisms involved in luminol and lucigenin-dependent chemiluminescence. *J. Cell Physiol.*, **151**, 446–77
23. Aitken, R. J. and Buckingham, D. (1992). Enhanced detection of reactive oxygen produced by human spermatozoa with 7-dimethylamino-naphthalin-1, 2-decarbonic acid hydrazide. *Int. J. Androl.*, **15**, 211–19
24. Aitken, R. J., Harkins, D. and Buckingham, D. (1993). Relationship between iron-catalyzed lipid peroxidation potential and human sperm function. *J. Reprod. Fertil.*, **98**, 257–65
25. Sailing, P. M. (1989). Mammalian sperm interaction with extracellular matrices of the egg. *Oxf. Rev. Reprod. Biol.*, **2**, 339–88
26. Tesarik, J., Mendoza, C. and Carreras, A. (1991). Expression of D-mannose binding sites on human spermatozoa: comparison of fertile donors and infertile patients. *Fertil. Steril.*, **56**, 113–18
27. Benoff, S., Cooper, G. W., Hurley, I., Napolitano, B., Rosenfeld, D. L., Scholl, G. M. and Hershlag, A. (1993). Human sperm fertilizing potential *in vitro* is correlated with differential expression of a head-specific mannose–ligand receptor. *Fertil. Steril.*, **59**, 854–62
28. Chen, J. S., Doncel, G. F., Alvarez, C. and Acosta, A. A. (1995). Expression of mannose-binding sites on human spermatozoa and their role in sperm–zona pellucida binding. *J. Androl.*, **16**, 55–63
29. Benoff, S., Cooper, G. W., Hurley, I. R., Barcia, M. and Gilbert, B. R. (1994). Varicocele legation affects sperm mannose lectin expression and acrosome status. *J. Androl.*, Jan/Feb (suppl.), Abstr., 54
30. Benoff, S., Cooper, G. W., Hurley, I., Rosenfeld, D. L., Hershlag, A. and Scholl, G. M. (1993). The effect of calcium ion channel blockers on sperm fertilization potential. *Am. Fertil. Soc.*, Abstr., **2**, 1
31. Tesarik, J., Mendoza, C., Ramirez, J. P. and Moos, J. (1993). Solubilized human zona pellucida competes with a fucosylated meoglycoprotein for binding sites on the human sperm surface. *Fertil. Steril.*, **60**, 344–50
32. Shur, B. D. and Neely, C. A. (1988). Plasma membrane association, purification, and partial characterization of mouse sperm β1,4-galactosyltransferase. *J. Biol. Chem.*, **263**, 17706–14
33. Miller, D. J., Macek, M. B. and Shur, B. D. (1992). Complementarity between sperm surface β-1,4-galactosyltransferase and egg-coat ZP3 mediates sperm–egg binding. *Nature*, **357**, 589–93
34. Doncel, G. F., Valerio, E., Alvarez, C. and Acosta, A. A. (1993). In search of biomarkers for zona receptors in human sperm. *J. Androl.*, **14**, 1 (suppl.), Abstr., 27
35. Sullivan, R., Ross, P. and Berube, B. (1989). Immunodetectable galactosyltransferase is associated only with human spermatozoa of high buoyant density. *Biochem. Biophys. Res. Commun.*, **162**, 184–8
36. Humphreys-Beher, M. G. and Blackwell, R. E. (1989). Identification of a deoxyribonucleic acid allelic variant for β1-4 galactosyltransferase expression associated with male sperm binding/penetration infertility. *Am. J. Obstet. Gynecol.*, **160**, 1160–5
37. Leyton, L. and Saling, P. (1989). 95 kd sperm proteins bind ZP3 and serve as tyrosine kinase substrates in response to zona binding. *Cell*, **57**, 1123–30
38. Moore, H. D. M., Hartman, T. D., Bye, A. P., Lutjen, P., DeWitt, M. and Trounson, A. O. (1987). Monoclonal antibody against sperm antigen M_r 95,000 inhibits attachment of human spermatozoa to the zona pellucida. *J. Reprod. Immunol.*, **11**, 157–66
39. Naz, R. K., Ahmad, K. and Kumar, R. (1991). Role of membrane phosphotyrosine proteins in human spermatozoal function. *J. Cell Sci.*, **99**, 157–65
40. Chamberlin, M. E. and Dean, J. (1990). Human homolog of the mouse sperm receptor. *Proc. Natl Acad. Sci. USA*, **87**, 6014–18

41. Van Duin, M., Polman, J. E. M., Verkoelen, C. E. H., Bunschoten, H., Meyerink, J. H., Olive, W. and Aitken, R. J. (1993). Cloning and characterization of the human sperm receptor ligand ZP3: evidence for a second polymorphic allele with a different frequency in the Caucasian and Japanese populations. *Genomics*, **14**, 1064–70
42. Dean, J. (1992). Biology of mammalian fertilization: role of the zona pellucida. *J. Clin. Invest.*, **89**, 1055–9
43. Yanagimachi, R. (1981). Mechanisms of fertilization in mammals. In Mastroianni, L. and Biggers, J. D. (eds.) *Fertilization and Embryonic Development* In Vitro, p. 81. (New York: Plenum Press)
44. Talbot, P. (1985). Sperm penetration through oocyte investments in mammals. *Am. J. Anat.*, **174**, 331–46
45. Liu, D. Y. and Baker, H. W. G. (1988). The proportion of human sperm with poor morphology but normal intact acrosomes detected with *Pisum sativum* agglutinin correlates with fertilization *in vitro*. *Fertil. Steril.*, **50**, 288–93
46. Takahashi, K., Wetzels, A. M. M., Goverde, H. J. M., Bastiaans, B. A., Janssen, H. J. and Rolland, R. (1992). The kinetics of the acrosome reaction of human spermatozoa and its correlation with *in vitro* fertilization. *Fertil. Steril.*, **57**, 889–94
47. Zaneveld, L. J. D., Anderson, R. A., Mach, S. R. and De Jonge, C. J. (1993). Mechanism and control of the human sperm acrosome reaction. *Hum. Reprod.*, **8**, 2006–8
48. Bielfeld, P., Faridi, A., Zaneveld, L. J. D. and De Jonge, C. J. (1994). The zona-pellucida-induced acrosome reaction of human spermatozoa is mediated by protein kinases. *Fertil. Steril.*, **61**, 536–41
49. Doncel, G. F., Alvarez, C., Chen, J. S. and Acosta, A. A. (1993). Phosphotyrosine containing proteins in human sperm: immunolocalization and role in sperm–zona binding. *Am. Fertil. Soc.*, Abstr., **85**, 41
50. Falsetti, C., Baldi, E., Krausz, C., Casano, R., Failli, P. and Forti, G. (1993). Decreased responsiveness to progesterone of spermatozoa in oligozoospermic patients. *J. Androl.*, **14**, 17–22
51. Oehninger, S., Blackmore, P., Morshedi, M., Sueldo, C., Acosta, A. A. and Alexander, N. (1994). Defective calcium influx and acrosome reaction (spontaneous and progesterone-induced) in spermatozoa of infertile men with severe teratozoospermia. *Fertil. Steril.*, **61**, 349–54
52. Cummins, J. M., Pember, S. M., Jequier, A. M., Yovich, J. L. and Hartmann, P. E. (1991). A test of the human sperm acrosome reaction following ionophore challenge. Relationship to fertility and other seminal parameters. *J. Androl.*, **12**, 98–103
53. Calvo, L., Vantman, D., Banks, S. M., Tezon, J., Koukoulis, G. N., Dennison, L. and Sherins, R. J. (1989). Follicular fluid-induced acrosome reaction distinguishes a subgroup of men with unexplained infertility not identified by semen analysis. *Fertil. Steril.*, **52**, 1048–54
54. Aitken, R. J. and Brindle, J. P. (1993). Analysis of the ability of three probes targeting the outer acrosomal membrane or acrosomal contents to detect the acrosome reaction in human spermatozoa. *Hum. Reprod.*, **8**, 1663–9
55. Ohashi, K., Saji, F., Kato, M., Okabe, M., Mimura, T. and Tanizawa, O. (1992). Evaluation of acrosomal status using MH61-beads test and its clinical application. *Fertil. Steril.*, **58**, 803–8
56. Marmor, D. and Grob-Menendez, F. (1991). Male infertility due to asthenozoospermia and flagellar anomaly: detection in routine semen analysis. *Int. J. Androl.*, **14**, 108–16
57. Yunes, R., Doncel, G. F. and Acosta, A. A. (1994). Tyrosine phosphorylation of sperm-tail proteins and hyperactivated motility in normozoospermic and asthenozoospermic human sperm samples. In *Proceedings of 50th Annual Meeting of the American Fertility Society*, San Antonio, Texas, November, p. 53 (abstr. 5)
58. Auger, J., Ronot, X. and Dadoune, J. P. (1989). Human sperm mitochondrial function related to motility: a flow and image cytometric assessment. *J. Androl.*, **10**, 439–48
59. Evenson, D. P., Darzynkiewicz, Z. and Melamed, M. R. (1982). Simultaneous measurement by flow cytometry of sperm cell viability and mitochondrial potential related to cell motility. *J. Histochem. Cytochem.*, **30**, 279–80
60. Mitchell, J. A., Nelson, L. and Hafez, E. S. E. (1976). Motility of spermatozoa. In Hafez, E. S. E. (ed.), *Human Semen and Fertility Regulation in Men*, pp. 83–106. (Saint Louis: C. V. Mosby Co)
61. Wallace, D. C. (1992). Diseases of the mitochondrial DNA. *Ann. Rev. Biochem.*, **61**, 1175–212
62. Cummins, J. M., Jequier, A. M. and Kan, R. (1994). Molecular biology of human male infertility: links with aging, mitochondrial genetics and oxidative stress? *Mol. Reprod. Dev.*, **37**, 345–62
63. Folgero, T., Bertheussen, K., Lindal, S., Torbergsen, T. and Oian, P. (1993). Mitochondrial disease and reduced sperm motility. *Hum. Reprod.*, **8**, 1863–8
64. Hassold, T., Chen, N., Funkhouser, J., Jooss, T., Manuel, B., Matsura, J., Matsuyama, A., Wilson, C., Yamane, J. A. and Jacobs, P. A. (1980). A cytogenetic study of 1000 spontaneous abortions. *Ann. Hum. Genet.*, **44**, 154–64
65. Martin, R. H., Ko, E. and Rademaker, A. (1991). Distribution of aneuploidy in human gametes: comparison between human sperm and oocytes. *Am. J. Med. Genet.*, **39**, 321–31
66. Rudak, E., Jacobs, P. A. and Yanagimachi, R. (1978). Direct analysis of the chromosome constitution of human spermatozoa. *Nature*, **274**, 911–13
67. Martin, R. H. (1983). A detailed method for obtaining preparations of human sperm chromosomes. *Cytogenet. Cell Genet.*, **35**, 253–6
68. Genesca, A., Benet, J., Caballin, M. R., Miro, R., Germa, J. R. and Egozcue, J. (1990). Significance of

structural chromosome aberrations in human sperm: analysis of induced aberrations. *Hum. Genet.*, **85**, 495–9
69. Han, T. L., Ford, J. H., Webb, G. C. and Flaherty, S. P. (1993). Simultaneous detection of X- and Y-bearing human sperm by double fluorescence *in situ* hybridization. *Mol. Reprod. Dev.*, **34**, 308–13
70. Holmes, J. M. and Martin, R. H. (1993). Aneuploidy detection in human sperm nuclei using fluoresence *in situ* hybridization. *Hum. Genet.*, **91**, 20–4
71. Guttenbach, M., Schakowski, R. and Schmid, M. (1994). Incidence of chromosome 3, 7, 10, 11, 17 and X disomy in mature human sperm nuclei as determined by nonradioactive *in situ* hybridization. *Hum. Genet.*, **93**, 7–12
72. Pang, M. G., Zackowski, J. L., Ryu, B. Y., Moon, S. Y., Acosta, A. A. and Kearns, W. G. (1994). Aneuploidy detection for chromosomes 1, X and Y by fluorescence *in situ* hybridization in human sperm from oligo-astheno-teratozoospermic patients. *Am. Soc. Hum. Genet.*, abstr.
73. Anguiano, A., Oates, R. H., Amos, J. A., Dean, M., Gerrard, B., Stewart, C., Maher, T. A., White, M. B. and Milunsky, A. (1992). Congenital bilateral absence of the vas deferens: A primarily genital form of cystic fibrosis. *J. Am. Med. Assoc.*, **67**, 1794–7
74. Patrizio, P., Ord, T., Silber, J. and Asch, R. H. (1993). Cystic fibrosis mutations impair the fertilization rate of epididymal sperm from men with congenital absence of the vas deferens. *Hum. Reprod.*, **8**, 1259–63
75. Palermo, G., Joris, H., Devroey, P. and Van Steirteghem, A. C. (1992). Pregnancies after intracytoplasmic injection of a single spermatozoon into an oocyte. *Lancet*, **340**, 17–18
76. Van Steirteghem, A. C., Nagy, Z., Joris, H., Liu, J., Staessen, C., Smitz, J., Wisanto, A. and Devroey, P. (1993). High fertilization and implantation rates after intracytoplasmic sperm injection. *Hum. Reprod.*, **8**, 1061–6
77. Van Steirteghem, A. C. (1993). Intracytoplasmic sperm injections (ICSI) and human fertilization: does calcium hold the key to success? *Hum. Reprod.*, **8**, 988–9
78. Katz, D. F. and Paveri Fontana, S. L. (1994). Model relationships between sperm biomarkers, fertility and its perturbations. (Abstr.) *J. Androl.*, Jan/Feb (Suppl.), **28**
79. Niederberger, C. S., Stockton, J., Lipshultz, L. I. and Lamb, D. J. (1993). A neural network to analyze fertility data and predict gamete micromanipulation success. *Am. Fertil. Soc.*, **231**, 186 (abstr.)

Chromosomes of human spermatocytes, sperm and the male pronucleus 26

W. G. Kearns, S. F. Hoegerman, M. G. Pang and J. L. Zackowski

INTRODUCTION

In the past, it has been difficult to predict fertility from *in vitro* measures of sperm quality[1]. The development of experimental techniques to predict sperm function is complicated by the fact that many interacting biological processes are required for normal sperm function *in vivo*. For example, sperm with damaged acrosomes but normal motility probably lack fertilizing capacity *in vivo*[2]. Additional parameters such as surface charge, chromosome complement, surface adhesiveness or the expression of specific membrane receptors might also affect sperm transport and *in vivo* fertilization. The elucidation of the biological, including the genetic, processes required for normal sperm function *in vivo* is a prerequisite for the full understanding of the ontogeny of male infertility.

MEIOTIC CHROMOSOME STUDIES IN MALES

In an extensive and early study, Skakkebaek *et al.*[3] (1973) reported on the meiotic chromosomes of 18 controls and 74 infertile men. They reported on the frequency of numerical chromosome aberrations, chiasma frequency, the presence of unpaired homologous chromosomes and the occurrence of polyploidy. All subjects had normal somatic karyotypes. Normal controls ranging in age from 19 to 39 years had sperm counts greater than 60×10^6/mL and sperm of good motility with <50% morphologically abnormal cells. The infertile men ranged in age from 23 to 51 years and were classified as infertile by the authors on the basis of aspermia, severely impaired fertility, poor sperm motility, and/or abnormal sperm morphology. Testicular material was obtained and orcein stained meiotic chromosome preparations were analyzed from each individual. Meiotic cells were scored for the relative frequency of cells in the first meiotic division (MI) and in the second meiotic division (MII), chiasma frequency at MI, non-pairing of both autosomes and sex chromosomes at MI and polyploidy. Structural chromosome abnormalities were not evaluated.

Skakkebaek *et al.*[3] questioned whether decreased sperm production in the infertile men was due to inhibition before MI, between MI and MII, or following MII. Their results showed that the mean ratio of MII to MI cells was 0.9 in controls and 0.5 in the infertile males. The lower value in the latter group indicates that, in these men, many cells failed to progress from MI to MII. Therefore, the patients' infertility was, at least in part, a consequence of the failure of primary spermatocytes to divide to form secondary spermatocytes. Twelve of the 18 infertile males whose spermatogenesis progressed to MII had MII/MI ratios below that of the lowest control.

An additional three infertile males showed complete inhibition of spermatogenesis between MI and MII. These data were supportive of previous work[4–6] showing six of 53 infertile males with an arrest of spermatogenesis between these stages.

Their data also showed that the relative frequency of spermatogonial metaphases was higher in infertile men (19.7%) versus normal controls (9.4%). Skakkebaek *et al.*[3] suggested that the absolute number of spermatogonia may be the same in both groups. The elevated frequency seen in the infertile subjects may have resulted from the reduction in their number of spermatocytes.

Skakkebaek *et al.*[3] found an average of 51.2 and 48.7 chiasmata per cell for normal controls and infertile males, respectively. The difference was not significant. However, significantly greater variability in chiasma frequency did occur within the infertile male population with 10 of 17 infertile patients having chiasma frequencies lower than the lowest of the six normal controls.

Skakkebaek *et al.*[3] evaluated pairing of sex chromosomes and autosomes at MI. The failure of the X and Y chromosomes to be paired, seen in 15% of 1159 cells, was the most common finding noted. Their data showed only a few small autosomes separated in a rare cell; no significant differences existed between infertile patients and normal control donors. Unpaired homologous chromosomes at MI could lead to non-disjunction and the production of aneuploid sperm. Such abnormalities could give rise to zygotes showing, for example, 47,XXY (Klinefelter's syndrome), 45,X (Turner's syndrome) and 47,XY,+21 (Down's syndrome).

Polyploidy was observed in 4.8% of spermatogonial (mitotic) metaphases and in 1.3% of MI metaphases in both infertile and control subjects. There was a significant difference in the frequency of polyploidy at MII in the two populations. At MII, polyploidy was seen in 3.6% of control and 10.6% of patient metaphases. Polyploidy seen at any of these stages results from either the abnormal occurrence of two rounds of DNA synthesis (endoreduplication) or from an abortive nuclear division. These abnormalities, along with failure of secondary spermatocytes to complete the second meiotic division (an abnormality which could not be scored by the technique used by Skakkebaek *et al.*[3]), will potentially produce diploid sperm.

By this time, polyploid cells had been found in mice and other mammalian species[7] and were believed to result from cell fusion or endoreduplication[8]. In addition, diploid spermatozoa had been found in animals and men[8–12]. The finding of increased polyploidy at MII by Skakkebaek *et al.*[3] demonstrated that failure of a meiotic division may also generate polyploidy and that polyploidy generated in this way occurs at elevated frequencies in infertile males.

Several studies published from the mid-1970s to the mid-1980s demonstrated that the incidence of meiotic chromosome abnormalities in infertile males was much higher than in fertile males[13]. The collective results of Chandley *et al.*[14] in 1976, Ferguson-Smith[15], Hendry *et al.*[16], Mićić *et al.*[17] in 1981 and Koulischer *et al.*[18] in 1982 indicated that an average frequency of 8.9% (98/1101) of infertile males had elevated frequencies of meiotic abnormalities, especially meiotic arrest and desynapsis (the failure of homologous chromosomes that have synapsed normally during pachynema to remain paired during diplonema; desynapsis is usually the result of a failure of chiasma formation). Individual studies showed frequencies that ranged from 1.44% to 17%. Koulischer *et al.*[18] suggested that this wide range was primarily due to different interpretations of what should be scored as a meiotic abnormality. They held that one should not include anomalies such as separation of the sex chromosomes at MI as a meiotic abnormality.

In 1983, Egozcue *et al.*[19] performed meiotic studies on spermatocytes from testicular biopsies or semen samples from 1100 infertile and sterile males attending fertility clinics. 'Meiotic arrest', probably corresponding to the decreased MII/MI ratio reported by Skakkebaek *et al.*[3], was the most common anomaly noted. This was followed in frequency by the absence of germ cells and then by desynapsis. Somatic abnormalities, which included Robertsonian translocations, reciprocal translocations, inversions, a deletion, a mosaic 45,X/46,XY karyotype, a mosaic 46,XY/47,XXY karyotype and a 47,XYY karyotype, were seen in 1.9% of the subjects. The authors presented the results of semen analysis in 55 patients with meiotic and/or somatic abnormalities. Only two of the 55 were normozoospermic. Oligo-astheno-teratozoospermia and oligo-asthenozoospermia were found in 14 cases each. Asthenozoospermia was found in seven cases, followed by oligozoospermia in five, azoospermia in four, cryptozoospermia in four, astheno-teratozoospermia in two, oligo-teratozoospermia in two, and polyastheno-teratozoospermia in one patient.

CHROMOSOME ANALYSIS OF SPERMATOZOA AND THE MALE PRONUCLEUS

In order to assess the value of estimating the ploidy of sperm cells by the size of the sperm head, Carothers and Beatty[20] (1975) first classified sperm heads as being small, medium or large based upon subjective size evaluation of Feulgen stained preparations and then correlated these subjective determinations with photometric determinations of ploidy based on light absorption by the Feulgen stained DNA. Their data on rabbits showed that haploid or diploid sperm, as determined by the Feulgen–DNA absorption assay, were always classified as being small or large in size, respectively. In humans, however, no consistent relationship was noted between sperm head size and ploidy. While all small sperm heads were determined to be haploid by the Feulgen–DNA assay, haploidy was also the most common finding for both the medium and large nuclei. Based on the Feulgen–DNA absorption assay of 5554 spermatozoa from two normal controls; 99.3% were haploid, 0.56% were diploid and 0.07% had higher ploidy levels. These data closely resemble those of Sumner *et al.*[12] (1971), who evaluated 1670 spermatozoa from four patients of an infertility clinic by fluorescence and DNA content analysis. Sumner *et al.*[12] reported 98.98% of sperm as haploid, 0.96% diploid and 0.06% tetraploid. Considering the small number of subjects in both of these studies, it remains unclear as to whether infertile males, relative to normal fertile donors, showed a significant increase in either their absolute number or percentage of diploid sperm.

Numerical and structural chromosome abnormalities play an important role in the etiology of prenatal wastage. Approximately 8% of all human concepti surviving long enough to produce clinically recognized pregnancies have a chromosome aberration in either structure or number. It is estimated that approximately 50% of all first trimester abortions are chromosomally abnormal[21]. Most numerical chromosome abnormalities arise *de novo* due to an error in chromosome disjunction during meiosis in a parent or as a result of a disjunctional error in mitotic divisions in the zygote. In contrast, most major structural abnormalities (e.g. translocations and inversions) are transmitted to offspring from a carrier parent; the remainder arise *de novo*.

The frequency of *de novo* chromosome abnormalities in sperm is only partially known. Prior to the mid-1970s the inspection of sperm chromosomes proved impossible because, in the course of spermatogenesis, sperm chromatin becomes highly compacted and does not become visible again until the first cleavage division of the newly formed zygote. In 1976, Yanagimachi *et al.*[22] developed a technique for the *in vitro* fertilization of zona-free golden hamster eggs with capacitated human sperm which then decondensed within the ooplasm. Using this technique, Rudak *et al.*[23] (1978) established a system in which human sperm were fused with Syrian hamster eggs which then proceeded through the initial stages of development. The human sperm heads decondensed and the human chromatin formed metaphase chromosomes in preparation for first cleavage. This allowed the first extended cytogenetic observation of countable human sperm chromosomes in which numerical as well as structural abnormalities could be identified. From 1978 until 1992, many investigators used the human–hamster fusion technique to analyze the chromosome constitution of approximately 20 000 sperm. The results of Rudak *et al.*[23], Sele *et al.*[24], Brandriff *et al.*[25,35], Jenderny and Rohrborn[26], Kamiguchi and Mikamo[27], Martin *et al.*[28–30], Estop *et al.*[31], Rosenbush and Sterzik[32], Benet *et al.*[33] and Tateno[34] are summarized in Table 1.

The data summarize chromosome analyses for hypohaploidy, per cent aneuploidy, conservative estimate of aneuploidy and frequency of structural abnormalities. Hypohaploidy refers to cells containing one or more fewer chromosomes than the normal haploid number; hyperhaploidy refers to cells containing more chromosomes than the normal haploid number, per cent aneuploidy is the sum of the per cent hypohaploid plus the per cent hyperhaploid. The conservative estimate of aneuploidy is defined as twice the percentage of hyperhaploidy.

Twelve studies reported per cent hypohaploidy, per cent hyperhaploidy, per cent aneuploidy and per cent structural abnormalities; 9 of 13 also reported the X:Y sex chromosome ratio. One group reported on per cent aneuploidy and per cent structural abnormalities. Overall, the investigators showed a mean per cent hypohaploidy of 2.75%, a mean per cent hyperhaploidy of 1%, a mean per cent aneuploidy of 3.69%, a mean per cent of pronuclei with structural abnormalities of 8.44% and an X:Y sex chromosome ratio of 52:48.

The findings of Martin *et al.*[28–30] and Brandriff *et al.*[25,35] will be reviewed in detail to illustrate the values of such studies. In 1983, Martin *et al.*[29] reported on the karyotypes of 1000 human male pronuclei from 33 normal donors using the human–hamster fusion technique. Donors ranged in age from 22 to 50 years with no history of chemotherapy, radiation treatments or infertility.

Table 1 Summary of sperm chromosome abnormalities in sperm from normal men using hamster technique

Study	*No. of karyotypes*	*% Hypo-haploid*	*% Hyper-haploid*	*% Aneuploid*	*Conservative estimate of aneuploidy (%)*	*% Structural abnormalities*	*Sex ratio (X : Y)*
Rudak *et al.*, 1978[23]	60	3.3	1.7	5.0	3.3	1.7	57.0 : 43.0
Martin *et al.* 1982[28]	240	2.1	5.4	7.5	10.8	1.7	59.6 : 40.4
Martin *et al.* 1983[29]	1000	2.7	2.4	5.2	4.8	3.3	53.9 : 46.1
Brandriff *et al.* 1984[35]	909	1.0	0.6	1.5	1.2	6.5	—
Brandriff *et al.*, 1985[25]	2468	0.9	0.7	1.7	1.5	7.7	50.1 : 49.9
Sele *et al.* 1985[24]	70	7.1	5.7	12.9	11.4	1.4	—
Kamiguchi and Mikamo, 1986[27]	1091	0.5	0.5	1.0	1.0	13.0	53.0 : 47.0
Jenderny and Rohrborn, 1987[26]	129	0.8	0.8	1.6	1.6	3.9	51.9 : 48.1
Martin *et al.* 1991[30]	5629	3.5	0.6	4.2	1.2	9.4	—
Estop *et al.* 1991[31]	555	6.3	2.0	8.3	4.0	3.6	54.5 : 45.5
Rosenbusch and Sterzik, 1991[32]	413	1.0	1.0	2.0	2.0	7.0	49.2 : 50.8
Benet *et al.*, 1992[33]	505	9.1	2.0	4.0	4.0	6.9	50.4 : 49.6
Tateno *et al.* 1992[34]	519	—	—	0.8	—	18.9	—
Mean (weighted)		2.75	1.00	3.69	2.0	8.44	52.0 : 48.0

Twenty-one were of proven fertility while 12 had no confirmed children. Sixty-five per cent of the chromosome spreads were successfully karyotyped using Q-banding; in the remaining cells, chromosomes were placed in groups using routine Giesma staining. The total frequency of abnormalities was 8.5%. Fifty-two were aneuploid (24 were hyperhaploid, 27 were hypohaploid and one had double aneuploidy) and 33 showed structural chromosome abnormalities. The 24 hyperhaploid sperm complements included 17 with one extra chromosome and seven with more than one extra chromosome. Eighteen of the 27 hypohaploid complements were missing one chromosome and nine were missing more than one chromosome. The percentage of X-bearing sperm was 53.9%, whereas the percentage of sperm with one Y chromosome was 46.1%. Structural chromosome abnormalities included 2.2% chromosome breaks, 0.2% chromosome gaps, 0.2% fragments, 0.1% deletions, 0.4% dicentrics or quadriradials and 0.2% reciprocal translocations.

Aneuploidy was seen in all chromosome groups and Martin *et al.*[29] suggested that all chromosomes may be equally susceptible to non-disjunction. Numerical chromosome abnormalities were more common than structural aberrations. The frequency of abnormalities was not uniform across all donors; two males of unproven fertility had 33% of the total structural aberrations identified. The frequency of aneuploidy was higher in the human chromosome complement than in the hamster chromosome complement. The numbers of hyperhaploid to hypohaploid complements (24 and 27, respectively) were close to the predicted 1:1 ratio expected if all aneuploidy results from meiotic non-disjunction and there is no differential selection against the resulting hypo- and hyperhaploid gametes. Martin *et al.*[29] did not select donors based upon their ability to fertilize hamster eggs. Consequently, the number of sperm complements analyzed per donor varied between four and 134. Martin *et al.*[29] stated that, with this range, they could not adequately assess the variation in the frequency of chromosome aberrations between donors.

In 1984, Brandriff *et al.*[35] compared the frequencies of structural and numerical chromosome aberrations in 909 karyotypes from four healthy donors. They reported frequencies of structural abnormalities of 1.3, 4.8, 9 and 10.4%. The frequencies of aneuploidy were 1.3, 1.4, 1.4 and 1.9% in these four donors. For three donors, the frequencies of structural abnormalities were significantly higher in their sperm than in their peripheral blood lymphocytes. Sex chromosome frequencies did not significantly differ from the expected 1:1 ratio.

In 1985, Brandriff *et al.*[25] analyzed the chromosomal constitution of an additional 2468 male pronuclei. Healthy donors ($n=11$) ranging in age from 21 to 49 years participated in the study and, as in previous studies, donor-to-donor variation in the ability of their sperm to fuse with hamster eggs was noted. Variations in fusion rate necessitated repeat samples from donors. Numerical as well as structural abnormalities were scored. Of the 2468 karyotpyes analyzed, 7.7% had structural abnormalities and 1.7% were aneuploid. Aneuploidy included 0.9% hypohaploid and 0.7% hyperhaploid. The sex chromosome frequencies were 50.1% for X and 49.9% for the Y chromosome.

The human–hamster technique is difficult, time consuming and expensive. Sperm from some males produce a high mitotic index of metaphase chromosomes, whereas other males' sperm yield few metaphase chromosome spreads, possibly indicating genetic variability in the ability of human sperm to fertilize hamster eggs *in vitro*.

Large numbers of suitably primed golden hamsters are needed to provide the eggs and the ability to produce metaphase chromosome preparations of suitable quality is problematic. Chromosomes may be clumped or too widely spread. The chromosomes are somewhat resistant to banding with results usually inferior to those of high resolution banding techniques applied to typical somatic cells. Furthermore, it is possible that structural or numerical chromosome abnormalities may be induced by the culture system or harvest procedure[36], or that some sperm may be selected for or against by the *in vitro* fertilization system[35]. Approximately 20 000 sperm have been analyzed to date using this technique. As aneuploidy in human sperm is rare, precise quantification of aneuploidy rates is not feasible using the human–hamster technique[37].

Fluorescent *in situ* hybridization (FISH) is a powerful tool which permits the direct visualization of specific chromosomes or chromosome regions[38,39]. Using DNA probes specific for a particular chromosome, FISH provides a rapid, alternative technique for the detection of aneuploidy and polyploidy in human sperm. Two types of non-radioactive hybridization method exist, direct and indirect. In the direct method, the detectable reporter molecule (fluorochrome) is bound directly to the nucleic acid probe so that formed hybrids can be visualized immediately using a fluorescent microscope. The indirect method uses hapten-labeled probes with subsequent signal detection by affinity cytochemistry. Recently, the availability of microscopes equipped with double or triple band pass filter sets has permitted the simultaneous detection of two or more differentially labeled probes by FISH.

The successful application of the FISH technique to mammalian spermatozoa depends primarily upon the efficiency of probe penetration following decondensation of the sperm nucleus. The chromatin of mammalian sperm is packaged in a condensed and inactive state. The histones found in somatic nuclei are replaced by sperm-specific protamines during late spermatogenesis. Intermolecular disulfide bonds form between adjacent protamines during epididymal maturation and maintain the tightly packaged state of chromatin. This tight packaging of the DNA–protamine complex in the human sperm nucleus makes it difficult for DNA probes to access target chromatin. Thus, sperm nucleus decondensation must precede the successful application of FISH.

Since 1984, at least 14 studies using FISH on sperm chromosomes from normal men have been reported. The results of Joseph *et al.*[40], Guttenbach and Schmidt[41,47], Pieters *et al.*[42], Coonen *et al.*[50], Han *et al.*[51,54], Holmes and Martin[53], Robbins *et al.*[55], Bischoff *et al.*[43], Guttenbach *et al.*[44,45], Miharu *et al.*[46] and Pang *et al.*[56] are summarized in Table 2.

Disomy frequencies for chromosomes 1, 3, 4, 6, 7, 8, 10, 11, 12, 15, 16, 17, 18, X and Y have been reported in sperm from normal donors. Seven investigators have reported on the disomy frequency for chromosome 1; mean=0.37% (range 0.06% to 0.8%). In comparison, only one group has reported on the disomy frequency (0.2%) for chromosome 15. Seven investigators reported on the disomy frequency of the X chromosome; mean=0.24% (range 0.03% to 0.38%), whereas eight investigators reported on the disomy frequency for the Y chromosome; mean=0.13% (range=0.0% to 0.27%). Representative studies are now discussed in detail.

In an early attempt to analyze the chromosome complements in human sperm, Joseph *et al.*[40] (1984) used ^{3}H-labelled satellite DNA probes to detect aneuploidy for chromosomes 1 and Y, but noted that the sperm heads were too condensed for precise signal detection. The disomy frequencies for chromosomes 1 and Y were 0.35% and 0.18%, respectively.

Guttenbach and Schmid[47] (1990) performed non-radioactive *in situ* hybridization on sperm nuclei from eight normal donors using a biotin-labeled Y chromosome-specific satellite DNA probe. The sperm nuclei were not chemically pretreated to disrupt disulfide bonds, but were

Table 2 Sperm from normal men showing two signals for specific chromosomes using FISH technique

Study	*Chromosome*														
	1	*3*	*4*	*6*	*7*	*8*	*10*	*11*	*12*	*15*	*16*	*17*	*18*	*X*	*Y*
Joseph *et al.* 1984[40]*	0.35														0.18
Guttenbach and Schmid, 1990[47]															0.27
Pieters *et al.* 1990[42]	0.80														0.00
Coonen *et al.* 1991[50]	0.67														
Guttenbach and Schmid, 1991[41]	0.41														
Han *et al.*, 1992[51]												0.33		0.29	
Holmes and Martin, 1993[53]	0.06								0.04					0.03	
Han *et al.*, 1993[54]														0.28	0.21
Robbins *et al.*, 1993[55]	0.14														0.06
Bischoff *et al.*, 1994[43]		0.34	0.24	0.08	0.05	0.11	0.10		0.31	0.20	0.39	0.10		0.38	0.09
Guttenbach *et al.*, 1994[45]		0.31			0.31		0.32	0.34				0.31		0.34	
Guttenbach *et al.*, 1994[44]													0.36		
Miharu *et al.* 1994[46]	0.14										0.17			0.13	0.08
Pang *et al.*, 1995[56]					0.28			0.13	0.05				0.08	0.20	0.15
Mean (unweighted)	0.37	0.03	0.24	0.08	0.21	0.11	0.26	0.24	0.13	0.20	0.28	0.25	0.22	0.24	0.13

*Used ^{3}H-labeled DNA

prepared for FISH by incubation in Hanks's balanced salt solution. Guttenbach and Schmid[47] did not decondense the sperm head chemically because they felt the sperm decondensed during the DNA denaturation process. They reported 49.4% Y-bearing sperm and assumed the remainder to be X-bearing (50.3%). The frequency of disomy for the Y chromosome was 0.27%, which exceeds the observed frequency of XYY live births of 0.1%. They speculated that either 24,YY sperm have a reduced fertilizing capacity or that chance led to the discrepancy. An alternative explanation is that some of the YY-bearing sperm were diploid as a consequence of non-reduction of chromosome number, specifically failure of MII. Hybridization with only one probe cannot distinguish between disomy due to non-disjunction or diploidy due to non-reduction. The ability of Guttenbach and Schmid[47] to successfully identify the presence of a Y chromosome without chemical decondensation, and the observation of the expected 1:1 ratio, suggests that some sperm nucleus decondensation did indeed occur, possibly during denaturation.

Studies have shown that partially decondensed human sperm nuclei contain a complex network of chromatin fibers[48] and Wyrobek *et al.*[49] (1990) analyzed and discussed the importance of sperm nuclei decondensation in order for successful probe hybridization to take place. Sperm nuclei from three normal donors were decondensed with lithium diiodosalicylate (LIS) and then analyzed by FISH for the presence of a Y chromosome. The decondensed sperm nuclei showed the presence of one Y chromosome in 50.1% of the nuclei examined. Their results of 50% of human sperm carrying a Y chromosome are consistent with data reported by others using the human–hamster fusion technique and support the hypothesis that X and Y-bearing human gametes are produced in equal numbers.

Coonen *et al.*[50] (1991) decondensed sperm nuclei using dithiothreitol (DTT) treatments of variable duration and analyzed sperm from 32 normal healthy men by FISH for the presence of chromosome 1. They reported that chromosome 1-specific signals were observed in 40–90% of the analyzed sperm and hypothesized that this variation was due to maturational heterogeneity of the sperm present in the ejaculate. Alternatively, variability in signal detection may have resulted from the variable duration of DTT treatment (i.e. variations in denaturation). They reported that 0.67% (range 0.2–1.3%) of successfully hybridized sperm had two copies of chromosome 1. This frequency represents the sum of cells disomic for chromosome 1 and diploid cells.

Han *et al.*[51] (1992) used single-probe FISH to analyze decondensed sperm nuclei for chromosomes 17 and X. Thirteen healthy donors were studied. Sperm nuclei decondensation was by a modification of the method of West *et al.*[52] using 6 mM EDTA and 2 mM DTT. Han *et al.*[51] distinguished between diploid and disomic sperm based upon the size of the sperm head; sperm nuclei of normal size with two hybridization signals were scored as disomic, whereas large nuclei with two hybridization signals were classified as diploid. Hybridization signals for chromosome 17 were detected in 96.1% of sperm nuclei analyzed; 95.4% were haploid (range 89.8–99.3%), 0.33% disomic (range 0.16–0.54%) and 0.37% diploid (range 0.0–0.89%). The hybridization results for the X chromosome showed 48.2% of sperm nuclei with positive signals; 47.7% haploid (range 43.4–50.4%), 0.29% disomic (range 0.18–0.4%) and 0.2% diploid (range 0.0–0.55%).

Holmes and Martin[53] (1993) also evaluated FISH for its ability to detect aneuploidy successfully in human sperm. Repetitive DNA sequences specific for chromosomes 1, 12 and X were used separately as probes and decondensed sperm nuclei were used as target DNA. Decondensation protocols used cetyltrimethylammonium bromide and DTT. A total of 10 524 sperm was analyzed for chromosome 1, 10 263 sperm nuclei were scored for chromosome 12 and 7003 sperm were analyzed for the X chromosome. Hybridization efficiency was >98%. Reported disomy frequencies were 0.06% for chromosome 1, 0.04% for chromosome 12 and 0.03% for the X chromosome. Holmes and Martin[53] compared their frequencies using the FISH technique to published data using the human–hamster fusion protocol and found no significant differences.

Using simultaneous two-probe, two-color FISH, Han *et al.*[54] (1993) studied the sex chromosome constitution of sperm nuclei obtained from 12 normal donors ranging in age from 20 to 45 years. Diploid and disomic sperm were distinguished as described above. Ninety-six per cent of 12 636 decondensed sperm nuclei showed fluorescent labeling. Forty-seven per cent were X and 46.8% were Y; 0.28% were disomic XX, and 0.18% were diploid XX; 0.21% were disomic YY and 0.17% were diploid YY. The frequency of XY-bearing sperm was 0.83%. When compared to male pronucleus karyotyping data, these FISH sex chromosome aneuploidy rates are much higher.

Robbins *et al.*[55] used FISH to evaluate aneuploidy for chromosomes 1 and Y in sperm from three healthy men whose sperm had been previously studied using the human–hamster fusion technique. Frequencies of sperm disomic for chromosome 1 were 0.14% and for chromosome Y were 0.056%. These frequencies were not significantly different from the frequencies of hyperhaploidy seen using the human–hamster technique. However, the frequencies of disomy for chromosomes 1 and Y in one donor were approximately 2.5× higher than in the other two donors. Such donor-to-donor variation has been observed with the human–hamster sperm karyotyping technique[30].

Oligo-astheno-teratozoospermic patients (n=9) of an *in vitro* fertilization program as well as normal controls (n=4) were studied by Pang *et al.*[56] (1995). Four of the nine patients previously had their sperm utilized for intracytoplasmic sperm injection (ICSI). Sperm nuclei decondensation was accomplished using a modification of the method of West *et al.*[52] using 6 mM EDTA and 2 mM DTT. Simultaneous two-probe, two-color FISH was performed using probe sets for either chromosomes 7 and 18, 11 and 12 or X and Y, scoring 1000 sperm for each probe set. For autosomes, two-probe, two-color FISH enables one to successfully differentiate disomy due to non-disjunction or diploidy due to non-reduction.

A sperm cell was scored as disomic for a particular chromosome if it showed two signals for that chromosome, but not for the other simultaneously probed chromosome. The absence of signal for a single chromosome was scored as nullisomy for that chromosome. Cells were scored as diploid if there were two signals for both probed autosomes (Figure 1). Sperm showing signal for neither chromosome of a probe set were not scored, as this outcome may have been an artifact resulting from inadequate decondensation of the cell's nucleus.

The mean sum of the frequencies of sperm with disomy for any of the four tested autosomes was 0.53% (range 0.0–1.1%) for the controls and 5.5% (range 1.5–9.5%) for the patients. The corresponding data for autosomal nullisomy were 0.45% (range 0.0–0.7%) for fertile controls and 9.2% (range 1.0–18.1%) for the oligo-astheno-teratozoospermic

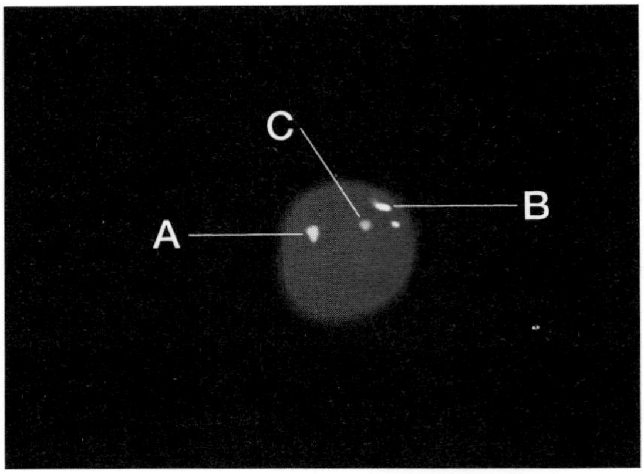

Figure 1 Decondensed sperm head from an oligo-astheno-teratozoospermic patient analyzed by FISH using direct labeled satellite DNA probes for chromosomes 7 and 18. If the figure was in colour chromosome 7 would be green (A), chromosome 18 would be red (B) and the sperm nucleus counterstained with DAPI would be blue (C). This sperm head was classified as diploid

patients. From these data, it was calculated that the average frequency of aneuploidy, expressed on a per chromosome basis, was 0.25% for controls and 3.7% for patients. Under the assumption that all 22 autosomes disjoin at the same frequency as the four tested autosomes, and that non-disjunctional events occur independently, Pang *et al.*[56] calculated that, in non-polyploid sperm, the total frequencies of autosomal aneuploidy would have been approximately 5.3% for controls and 56.1% for the oligo-astheno-teratozoospermic patients.

The frequencies of non-disjunctional gain or loss of sex chromosomes could not be established when using an X and Y pooled probe set. Cells with two sex chromosomes could be diploid due to failure of a meiotic division or disomic due to non-disjunction.

As determined from analyses using the autosomal probes, proven fertile donors showed a frequency of diploidy of <0.1% (range 0.0–0.1%), while patients' frequencies ranged between 0.3% and 9.8% with a mean of 2.1%. For the oligo-astheno-teratozoospermic patient with 9.8% diploid sperm, Pang *et al.*[56] identified the type of error which occurred primarily. Of the 1000 sperm analyzed for the X and Y chromosomes, 14.6% had two signals; of these, 11.1% were XY, 2.4% were XX and 1.1% were YY. Based upon the high frequency of diploidy found using autosomal probes, it was concluded that most of the cells with two sex chromosomes must be diploid. The distribution of sex chromosome types indicates that there was a failure of the first meiotic division in the majority of diploid sperm cells. This was deduced from the meiotic behavior of the sex bivalent. If the first division is abortive, the sex bivalent and all autosomal bivalents will not disjoin and the resulting sperm will have both an X and a Y chromosome, as well as two of every autosome. On the other hand, if a normal first meiotic division is followed by an abortive second division, the two chromatids of all chromosomes, including the single X or Y chromosome, do not separate and the sperm will have either two Xs or two Ys.

The data of Pang *et al.*[56] show a significant increase ($P<0.05$) in the frequencies of diploidy, autosomal disomy, autosomal nullisomy, sex chromosome number and total abnormalities from oligo-astheno-teratozoospermic patients versus proven fertile donors. The data suggest that meiotic errors occur at highly elevated frequencies in oligo-astheno-teratozoospermic patients. Such errors may be causally related to the patients' decreased fertility.

It is clear that FISH can be a rapid, reliable method for numerical chromosome evaluation of decondensed human sperm nuclei. The procedure is easily learned, shows a high efficiency of hybridization, permits the rapid scoring of thousands of sperm nuclei and is very sensitive. Sperm nuclei decondensation, probe labeling, hybridization conditions and immunocytochemistry are parameters which require optimization for enhanced signal detection by FISH. Successful FISH requires high efficiency rates of hybridization while not destroying sub-populations of sperm nuclei. Overall comparisons for disomy frequencies between FISH and sperm karyotyping show fair consistency between the two techniques. However, investigator-to-investigator variability exists for FISH results on disomy frequencies studying fertile donors. This variability may have resulted from different degrees of sperm nuclei decondensation, yielding variable probe access for FISH. Additional factors, such as variation in signal scoring criteria, fluorescence microscope configuration, as well as DNA cross-hybridization and donor-to-donor variation may have contributed to this chromosome frequency variability.

CONCLUSIONS

Tremendous progress has been made over the past quarter-century studying the cytogenetics of male gametogenesis and the resulting gamete. Cytogeneticists have moved from studying spermatogenesis itself, which sheds light on the nature of meiotic errors, to the study of the chromosomes of successful sperm cells; that is, those cells which succeed in fertilizing hamster ova. Studies merging molecular techniques and conventional cytogenetics are now beginning to bridge the gap between what we have learned about the meiotic process in males and what we know of the mitotic chromosomes of zygotes.

The results of meiotic studies of spermatogenesis and FISH studies of sperm are consistent with one another. Taken collectively, the meiotic studies have shown that failure of primary spermatocytes to progress from MI to MII is common in infertile males. Although there is currently sparse FISH data from infertile males, the data of Pang *et al.*[56] suggest that, in at least some cases, frequencies of diploidy will be found to be elevated. It is probable that most diploid sperm have an XY sex chromosome constitution. Diploid XY sperm results from a failed first meiotic division (as frequently observed in the meiotic studies), followed by an essentially normal second meiotic division.

Meiotic studies also revealed that infertile males may have a small decline in their average chiasma frequency. Some infertile men show a marked reduction in chiasma frequency and desynapsis. Decreased chiasma frequency could result in premature disjunction of bivalents (desynapsis). In turn, this would increase aneuploidy as the resulting univalents may migrate randomly to one pole or the other during anaphase of MI. The limited FISH data of Pang *et al.*[56] on sperm from oligo-asthenoteratozoospermic patients suggest increased frequencies of aneuploidy in such males.

It is difficult to relate the results of sperm studies utilizing FISH to the studies of the male pronucleus chromosomes. The human sperm–hamster egg fusion technique data summarized were on sperm from normal men and can only assess the cytogenetic status of sperm capable of successful fertilization. FISH, on the other hand, assesses all sperm. If aneuploidy has no effect on the fertilizing capacity of human sperm (i.e. human sperm–hamster egg), and if the calculation of the mean aneuploidy rate for controls given by Pang *et al.*[56] is correct, then there is fair agreement between these studies. Using unweighted means, the average frequencies of nullisomy plus disomy in the studies of male pronuclei given in Table 1 was 3.7%. Pang *et al.*[56] estimated the overall frequency of autosomal nullisomy plus disomy in sperm from normal donors to be 5.3%.

In order to assess the role that chromosome complement plays in normal and abnormal fertility, additional molecular cytogenetic studies must be done on sperm samples both from men with normal fertility and from men with abnormal semen. Care should be taken to fully characterize each patient's clinical picture so that data on subjects with identical presentations can be pooled later. Correlations of meiotic cytology and FISH studies on sperm from the same individuals may also prove highly informative.

Molecular cytogenetic studies on sperm will have clinical utility. For example, the delineation of subpopulations of infertile men based upon the cytogenetic quality of their sperm could identify both appropriate and inappropriate candidates for procedures such as intracytoplasmic sperm injection.

References

1. Bavister, B. D. (1990). Tests of sperm fertilizing ability. In Asch, R. H., Balmaceda, J. P. and Johnston, I. (eds.) *Gamete Physiology* pp. 77–105. (Norwell, MA: Serono Symposia)
2. Saacke, R. G. and White, I. G. (1972). Semen quality tests and their relationship to fertility. In *Proceedings of the 4th Technical Conference on Artificial Insemination and Reproduction*, Chicago, IL, pp. 22–27
3. Skakkebaek, N. E., Bryant, J. I. and Philip, J. (1973). Studies on meiotic chromosomes in infertile men and controls with normal karyotypes. *J. Reprod. Fertil.*, **35**, 23–36
4. McIlree, M. L., Price, W. H., Court Brown, W. M.,

Tulloch, W. S., Newsam, J. E. and MacLean, N. (1966). Chromosome studies on testicular cells from 50 subfertile men. *Lancet*, **ii**, 69–71

5. Hultèn, M., Eliasson, R. and Tillinger, K. G. (1970). Low chiasma count and other meiotic irregularities in two infertile, 46,XY men with spermatogenic arrest. *Hereditas*, **65**, 285–90
6. Pearson, P. L., Ellis, J. D. and Evans, H. J. (1970). A gross reduction in chiasma formation during meiotic prophase and a defective DNA repair mechanism associated with a case of human male infertility. *Cytogenetics*, **9**, 460–7
7. Hultèn, M., Karlman, A., Lindsten, J. and Tiepolo, L. (1970). Aneuploidy and polyploidy in germline cells of the chinese hamster. *Hereditas*, **65**, 197–202
8. Beatty, R. A. (1961). Genetics of gametes. V. The frequency distribution of the head length of rabbit spermatozoa, and search for dimorphism. *Proc. Roy. Soc. Edinb.* (B), **68**, 72–82
9. Gledhill, R. L. (1964). Quantitative ultramicrospectrophotometry of presumed diploid spermatozoa. *Fifth Int. Congr. Anim. Reprod. & A. I.*, **3**, 489
10. Salisbury, G. W. and Baker, F. N. (1966). Frequency of occurrence of diploid bovine spermatozoa. *J. Reprod. Fertil.*, **11**, 477–80
11. Sumner, A. T. (1971). Frequency of polyploid spermatozoa in man. *Nature*, **231**, 49
12. Sumner, A. T., Robinson, J. A. and Evans, H. J. (1971). Distinguishing between XY and YY bearing human spermatozoa by fluorescence and DNA content. *Nature – New Biol.*, **229**, 231–3
13. Zuffardi, O. and Tiepolo, L. (1982). Frequencies and types of chromosome abnormalities associated with human male infertility. In Crosignani, P. G. and Rubin, B. L. (eds.) *Genetic Control of Gamete Production and Function*, pp. 261–73. (New York: Academic Press)
14. Chandley, A. C., Maclean, N., Edmond, P., Fletcher, J. and Watson, G. S. (1976). Cytogenetics and infertility in man. II. Testicular histology and meiosis. *Ann. Hum. Genet.*, **40**, 165–76
15. Ferguson-Smith, M. A. (1976). Meiosis in the human male. In Pearson, P. L. and Lewis, K. R. (eds.) *Chromosomes Today, Vol. 5*, pp. 33–41. (New York: Wiley)
16. Hendry, W. E., Polani, P. E., Pugh, R. C., Sommerville, J. F. and Wallace, D. M. (1976) 200 infertile males: correlation of chromosomes, histological, endocrine, and clinical studies. *Br. J. Urol.*, **47**, 899–908
17. Mićić, S., Mićić, M., Ilić, V. (1981). Histological and meiotic evaluation of infertile men. *Andrologia*, **13**, 499–503
18. Koulischer, L., Schoysman, R., Gillerot, Y. and Derby, J. M. (1982). Meiotic chromosome studies in human male infertility. In Crosignani, P. G. and Rubin, B. L. (eds.). *Genetic Control of Gamete Production and Function*, pp. 239–60. (New York: Academic Press)
19. Egozcue, J., Templado, C., Vidal, F., Navarro, J., Morer-Fargas, F. and Marina, S. (1983). Meiotic studies in a series of 1100 infertile and sterile males. *Hum. Genet.*, **65**, 185–8
20. Carothers, A. D. and Beatty, R. A. (1975). The recognition and incidence of haploid and polyploid spermatozoa in man, rabbit, and mouse. *J. Reprod. Fertil.*, **44**, 487–500
21. Hassold, T. J., Matsuyama, A., Newlands, I. M., Matsuurg, J. S., Jacobs, P. A., Manuel, B. and Tsuei, J. (1978). A cytogenetic survey of spontaneous abortions in Hawaii. *Ann. Hum. Genet.*, **41**, 443–54
22. Yanagimachi, R., Yanagimachi, H. and Rogers, B. J. (1976). The use of zona-free animal ova as a test-system for the assessment of the fertilizing capacity of human spermatozoa. *Biol. Reprod.*, **15**, 471–6
23. Rudak, E., Jacobs, P. A. and Yanagimachi, R. (1978). The chromosome constitution of human spermatozoa: A method of direct chromosome analysis. *Nature*, **274**, 911–13
24. Sele, B., Pellestor, F., Jalbert, P. and Estrade, C. (1985). Analyze cytogenetique des pronucleus a partir du modele de fecondation interspecifique homme hamster. *Ann. Genet.*, **28**, 81–85
25. Brandriff, B., Gordon, L., Ashworth, L., Watchmaker, G., Moore, D. II, Wyrobek, A. J. and Carrano, A. V. (1985). Chromosomes of human sperm: variability among normal individuals. *Hum. Genet.*, **70**, 18–24
26. Jenderny, J. and Rohrborn, G. (1987). Chromosome analysis of human sperm. First results with a modified method. *Hum. Genet.*, **76**, 385–8
27. Kamiguchi, Y. and Mikamo, K. (1986). An improved, efficient method for analyzing human sperm chromosomes using zona-free hamster ova. *Am. J. Hum. Genet.*, **38**, 724–40
28. Martin, R. H., Lin, C. C., Balkan, W. Burns, K. (1982). Direct chromosomal analysis of human spermatozoa: preliminary results from 18 normal men. *Am. J. Hum. Genet.*, **34**, 459–68
29. Martin, R. H., Balkan, W., Burns, K., Rademaker, A. W., Lin, C. C. and Rudd, N. L. (1983). The chromosome constitution of 1000 human spermatozoa. *Hum. Genet.*, **63**, 305–9
30. Martin, R. H., Ko, E. and Rademaker, A. (1991). Distribution of aneuploidy in human gametes: comparison between human sperm and oocytes. *Am. J. Med. Genet.*, **39**, 321–31
31. Estop, A. M., Cieply, K., Vankirk, V., Munne, S. and Garver, K. (1991). Cytogenetic studies in human sperm. *Hum. Genet.*, **87**, 447–51
32. Rosenbusch, B. and Sterzik, K. (1991). Sperm chromosomes and habitual abortion. *Fertil. Steril.*, **56**, 370–2
33. Benet, J., Genesca, A., Navarro, J., Egozcue, J. and Templado, C. (1992). Cytogenetic studies in motile sperm from normal men. *Hum. Genet.*, **89**, 176–80
34. Tateno, H., Kamiguchi, Y. and Mikamo, K. (1992). A freezing and thawing method of hamster oocytes designed for both the penetration test and chromo-

some assay of human spermatozoa. *Mol. Reprod. Dev.*, **33**, 202–9
35. Brandriff, B., Gordon, L., Ashworth, L., Watchmaker, G. and Wyrobek, A. (1984). Chromosomal abnormalities in human sperm: comparisons among four healthy men. *Hum. Genet.*, **66**, 193–201
36. Genesca, A., Benet, J., Caballin, M. R., Germa, J. R. and Egozcue, J. (1990). Significance of structural chromosome aberrations in human sperm: analysis of induced aberrations. *Hum. Genet.*, **85**, 495–9
37. Martin, R. H. and Rademaker, A. W. (1990). The frequency of aneuploidy among individual chromosomes in 6821 human sperm chromosome complements. *Cytogenet. Cell Genet.*, **53**, 103–7
38. Kearns, W. G. and Pearson, P. L. (1994). Fluorescent *in situ* hybridization using chromosome-specific DNA libraries. In Choo, K. H. A. and Totowa, N. J. (eds.) *Methods in Molecular Biology*, pp. 15–22. (Tutowa, N. J.: Humana Press)
39. Kearns, W. G. and Pearson, P. L. (1994). Detection of chromosomal aberrations in metaphase and interphase cells in prenatal and postnatal studies. In Choo, K. H. A. and Totowa, N. J. (eds.) *Methods in Molecular Biology*, pp. 459–76. (Humana Press)
40. Joseph, A. M., Gosden, J. R. and Chandley, A. C. (1984). Estimation of aneuploidy levels in human spermatozoa using chromosome specific probes and *in situ* hybridization. *Hum. Genet.*, **66**, 234–8
41. Guttenbach, M. and Schmid, M. (1991) Non-isotopic detection of chromosome 1 in human meiosis and demonstration of disomic sperm. *Hum. Genet.*, **87**, 261–5
42. Pieters, M. H. E. C., Geraedts, J. P. M., Meyer, H., Dumoulin, J. C. M., Evers, J. L. H., Jongbloed, R. J. E., Nederlof, P. M. and van der Flier, S. (1990). Human gametes and zygotes studied by nonradioactive *in situ* hybridization. *Cytogenet. Cell Genet.*, **53**, 15–19
43. Bischoff, F. Z., Nguyen, D. D., Burt, K. J. and Shaffer, L. G. (1994). Estimates of aneuploidy using multicolor fluorescence *in situ* hybridization on human sperm. *Cytogenet. Cell Genet.*, **66**, 237–43
44. Guttenbach, M., Schakowski, R. and Schmid, M. (1994). Incidence of chromosome 18 disomy in human sperm nuclei as detected by nonisotopic *in situ* hybridization. *Hum. Genet.*, **93**, 421–42
45. Guttenbach, M., Schakowski, R. and Schmid, M. (1994). Incidence of chromosome 3, 7, 10, 11, 17 and X disomy in mature human sperm nuclei as determined by nonradioactive *in situ* hybridization. *Hum. Genet*, **93**, 7–12
46. Miharu, N., Best, R. G. and Young, R. (1994). Numerical chromosome abnormalities in spermatozoa of fertile and infertile men detected by fluorescence *in situ* hybridization. *Hum. Genet.*, **93**, 502–6
47. Guttenbach, M. and Schmid, M. (1990). Determination of Y chromosome aneuploidy in human sperm nuclei by nonradioactive *in situ* hybridization. *Am. J. Hum. Genet.*, **46**, 553–8
48. Evenson, D. P., Witkins, S. S., deHarven, E. and Bendich, A. (1978). Ultrastructure of partially decondensed spermatozoal chromatin. *J. Ultrastructure Res.*, **63**, 178–87
49. Wyrobek, A. J., Alhborn, T., Balhorn, R., Stanker, L. and Pinkel, D. (1990). Fluorescence *in situ* hybridization to Y chromosomes in decondensed human sperm nuclei. *Mol. Reprod. Dev.*, **27**, 200–8
50. Coonen, E., Pieters, M. H. E. C., Dumoulin, J. C. M., Meyer, H., Evers, J. L. H., Ramaekers, F. C. S. and Geraedts, J. P. M. (1991). Nonisotopic *in situ* hybridization as a method for nondisjunction studies in human spermatozoa. *Mol. Reprod. Dev.*, **28**, 18–22
51. Han, T. L., Webb, G. C., Flaherty, S. P., Correll, A., Matthews, C. D. and Ford, J. H. (1992). Detection of chromosome 17- and X-bearing human spermatozoa using fluorescence *in situ* hybridization. *Mol. Reprod. Dev.*, **33**, 189–94
52. West, J. D., West, K. M. and Aitken, R. J. (1989). Detection of Y-bearing spermatozoa by DNA-DNA *in situ* hybridization. *Mol. Reprod. Dev.*, **12**, 201–7
53. Holmes, J. M. and Martin, R. H. (1993). Aneuploidy detection in human sperm nuclei using fluorescence *in situ* hybridization. *Hum. Genet.*, **91**, 20–4
54. Han, T. L., Ford, J. H., Webb, G. C., Flaherty, S. P., Correll, A. and Matthews, C. D. (1993). Simultaneous detection of X- and Y-bearing human sperm by double fluorescence *in situ* hybridization. *Mol. Reprod. Dev.*, **34**, 308–13
55. Robbins, W. A., Seagraves, R., Pinkel, D. and Wyrobek, A. J. (1993). Detection of aneuploid human sperm by fluorescence *in situ* hybridization: evidence for a donor difference in frequency of sperm disomic for chromosomes 1 and Y. *Am. J. Hum. Genet.*, **52**, 799–807
56. Pang, M. G., Zackowski, J. L., Hoegerman, S. F., Moon, S. Y., Cuticchia, A. J., Acosta, A. A. and Kearns, W. G. (1995). Detection by fluorescence *in situ* hybridization of chromosomes 7, 11, 12, 18, X, and Y abnormalities in sperm from oligo-astheno-teratozoospermic patients of an *in vitro* fertilization program. In *Proceedings IXth World Congress on* In Vitro *Fertilization and Assisted Reproduction*, Vienna, Austria, April 3–7

Section 3

Male factor treatment

Assisted reproduction 1: *in vitro* fertilization

27

A. A. Acosta

INTRODUCTION

The technological breakthrough of intracytoplasmic sperm injection (ICSI) has dramatically changed the approach to diagnosis and treatment of the male factor by assisted reproductive methods. Nevertheless, it is our responsibility in the future to try to improve results in assisted reproduction in such a way that fewer and fewer cases need to resort to assisted fertilization; having obtained identical results, we also need to try to find a battery of diagnostic tests to select which cases should be allocated to assisted fertilization and which cases can be treated by assisted reproduction.

The need for unification of definitions and testings of the male factor when assisted reproduction is going to be used for treatment has already been discussed in Chapter 5. It is imperative, in my view, that when assisted reproduction is used one of the main questions that should be answered by that procedure, which therefore becomes not only a therapeutic method but also a diagnostic test, is whether fertilization can occur and, if it occurs, whether it can be considered normal (similar to the normal gamete population) or abnormal by the standards of the laboratory performing the procedure. If at the end of that trial the question has not been answered, we have wasted a unique opportunity to evaluate and quantify the fertilizing potential of the sperm.

We will not refer in this chapter to the simpler and most common modalities of assisted reproduction, namely insemination in any one of its many variants; they have been addressed in other sections of this book (see Chapters 29 and 30), but we will devote the discussion to the higher complexity methods (*in vitro* fertilization and embryo transfer [IVF–ET], gamete intrafallopian transfer [GIFT] and zygote intrafallopian transfer [ZIFT]). Assisted fertilization will be dealt with in Chapter 31.

The problem of low or absent fertilization in the male factor when clearly established and demonstrated can be treated by: (1) systemic medical treatment to improve sperm quality; (2) sperm manipulation in the laboratory to enhance fertilizing ability; (3) the use of assisted fertilization when the other methods fail. These therapeutic approaches may improve the low fertilization rates but seldom, if ever, will the rates reach the fertilization efficiency of normal gametes. In spite of all the literature published on the subject of fertilization prediction, the most useful tools seem to be the morphology pattern[1], the hemizona assay[2] and the evaluation of acrosome reaction by any one of the methods proposed[3]. Nevertheless, when it comes to predicting whether a specific sperm sample will fertilize normally or abnormally (low fertilization rate) there is no clear, useful tool to separate these two categories. Therefore, *in vitro* fertilization becomes the final test of sperm efficiency for the male factor and has to be utilized as such.

The clinical male factor, as previously defined (see Chapter 5), is usually treated empirically by medical means (gonadotropins, androgens, antiandrogens or aromatase inhibitors) or by surgery, according to the etiological factors presumably involved, trying to improve the sperm quality to achieve a pregnancy naturally. The male factor in assisted reproduction can also be treated empirically, not with the idea of normalizing sperm characteristics but trying to improve them, or trying to stabilize the quality of the sperm in patients providing very different samples at different times; this will allow the embryology laboratory to work with a better specimen. The intractable severe male factor leaves no option but assisted fertilization (micromanipulation).

The possibility of a male factor in assisted reproduction can be suspected when the sperm density is <20 million sperm/mL (or $<20\times10^6$ sperm /mL), when the sperm total progressive motility is <30%, the sperm normal morphology is <14% and there is a total recovered sperm motile fraction after swim-up of $<5\times10^6$. It becomes severe and, therefore, fertilization could be predicted to be low or not to occur at all when the sperm morphology is <4% (poor prognosis pattern)[4], which is a common denominator to all these patients, and/or sperm density is $<5\times10^6$ sperm/mL, and/or motility is <10%, and/or the total motile fraction recovered after swim-up is $<1.5–1\times10^6$, and/or the hemizona index is <36%, which may indicate no fertilization in 75% of the cases.

The same semen evaluation methodologies indicated for the clinical male factor can be used for evaluation of semen in assisted reproduction, namely basic semen analysis, bacteriological and immunological investigation, characteristics of sperm recovered after using some of the separation procedures previously described and tests of sperm functions, such as acrosine activity, adenosine triphosphate, and creatinine kinase content, sperm cervical mucus penetration assay, hyperosmotic swelling test, acrosome reaction test, hamster-zona free penetration assay and hemizona assay. In spite of all these investigations, the definitive test is certainly *in vitro* fertilization in a well established laboratory. Most of these aspects of semen evaluation have been already reviewed in Section 2 of this book.

BASIC SEMEN ANALYSIS

The general requirements for semen collection have already been described (Chapter 6). The general characteristics of semen (coagulation, liquefaction and viscosity), if grossly abnormal, should be reported to the embryology laboratory to alert them of possible difficulties in semen processing.

Volume, unless it is extremely low, should not represent a problem for the embryology laboratory to work with.

In the Norfolk experience, when the sperm density in the original specimen drops below 20 million/mL, a clear effect on fertilization rate can be seen, with a drop of fertilization to around 60% but no impact in pregnancy rate; when it reaches <10 million/mL, fertilization rate drops below 50% and pregnancy rate is impaired; below 5 million/mL, there is a further drop to 30% and the term pregnancy rate is also decreased. Sperm density below one million represents a very severe male problem and fertilization is most unlikely. Unfortunately sperm density, as any one of the other parameters, cannot be judged as an isolated factor as it is usually combined with abnormalities of motility and morphology, which makes overall evaluation more difficult.

Sperm motility has a secondary role in the IVF results, and even samples with slightly <10% progressive motility still are able to fertilize as long as the other parameters are acceptable. Nevertheless, specimens with <10% progressive motility should be considered as severe male factor in assisted reproduction, mainly when abnormalities are present in the other diagnostic criteria.

Patients with poor sperm density and motility should be treated empirically to try to improve these characteristics, and provide the embryology laboratory with a better specimen. A similar approach can be taken with patients who deliver sperm samples with extremely variable parameters; systemic treatment can stabilize the count and motility in some of these cases.

Automated sperm assessment

The introduction of automated assessment of the sperm by computer-assisted sperm analysis (CASA), allows determination of several different characteristics of sperm motility that cannot be evaluated manually. A pattern of motility, including mean velocity, mean linearity, fertility index, curvilinear velocity and amplitude of lateral head displacement, introduced a kinematic approach to the sperm motility evaluation that may help in prediction of fertilization. Barlow *et al.*[5] reviewed the correlation of fertilizing ability of the sperm with several different parameters evaluated by manual and computer-assisted methods, both in fresh semen and after swim-up preparations, and found a significant correlation between sperm concentration, motility, velocity, vitality and normal morphology in both types of specimens. They propose a predictive function to calculate the potential fertilization rate for a patient using the post-swim-up motility and the normal sperm morphology in the fresh sample. There are several computer systems on the market that allow investigation of these parameters.

Evaluation of hyperactivated motility

Evaluation of hyperactivated motility can also be added to the prediction armamentarium; this type of motility is one of several expressions of sperm capacitation. It was described originally in laboratory animals (hamsters) by Yanagimachi and there are current efforts being made to define similar changes in the human sperm[6–9]. It can be evaluated by high speed videomicrography with slow motion analysis, or by standard videomicrography with time exposure analysis. Several patterns of hyperactivation have been identified: circling, high curvature, thrashing, helical and star-spin[7]. Three criteria have been proposed to automatically determine hyperactivated motility[7]: linearity $\leqslant 65$, velocity $\geqslant 100$ μm and head displacement $\geqslant 7.5$ μm. Wang *et al.*[10] investigated this type of motility in fresh and post-swim-up specimens, as well as 24 h after incubation. Hyperactivated motility reached a peak at 1 h and plateaued at 3 h, and they could not find a correlation between the presence of hyperactivated motility and the results of sperm penetration assay in the hamster system. In the abnormal samples, the incidence of hyperactivated motility and the percentage with star-spin at 3 h was significantly lower. The authors believe that hyperactivated motility may be useful as an early indicator of capacitation abnormalities in human spermatozoa that are not measured by sperm penetration assay (SPA). Murad *et al.*[11] concluded that the expression of hyperactivated motility requires interdependent changes at the axonemal and cytosolic levels, and determined that the highest percentage of hyperactivation was induced by decomplemented fetal cord serum in the medium.

We are still in need of a simplified method of evaluation of hyperactivated motility and a clear demonstration of a correlation with the fertilization ability of the sperm in order to be able to incorporate this criterion into the clinical arena. The complicated and expensive equipment needed, the difficulties in studying a large number of sperm by this method, the discrepancies in the descriptions and interpretation of the sperm hyperactivated patterns in the human being, the change in pattern of motility in the same sperm with time, the lack of sufficient studies showing a positive correlation between this type of sperm motility and fertilization *in vitro*, or fertilizability *in vivo* and the small number of sperm detected in the hyperactivated state in some reports indicate that this method will not be available in the clinical evaluation of sperm parameters for quite some time.

Modifying agents

Agents modifying conditions of sperm to induce better motility and hyperactivated motility have been tried in the human *in vitro* system. One of these agents is the steroid-rich fraction of human follicular fluid[12], due to the presence of progesterone and 17-hydroxyprogesterone which stimulate calcium flux[13] and, therefore, improve motility. When calcium ionophore is used the number of hyperactivated sperm is significantly reduced[14], and the presence of cumulus oophorus or solubilized cumulus intercellular matrix induces a linear high velocity motility different from the hyperactivated one which is reduced[15].

Other agents have also been used to improve the ability of the sperm to move adequately. Imoedemhe *et al.*[16], looking at normal human spermatozoa after being exposed to different concentrations of caffeine, were able to demonstrate a significant improvement in the various motility parameters in a dose-dependent manner, but that did not lead to an improvement in the fertilization rates; high concentrations adversely affected the fertilization rate, and embryonic development was also retarded. The authors do not recommend, for the time being, the use of this stimulant in assisted reproduction programs. The same authors[17] have used 2-deoxyadenosine for the same purposes in asthenospermic males. The sperm motility pattern was significantly improved, as well as the number of sperm recovered; the fertilization rate(s) was also enhanced with a higher number of embryos being replaced. The pregnancy rate was comparable to the historic pregnancy rates for the group, so they do not believe that 2-deoxyadenosine has an adverse effect on embryonic development, although they have not been able to assess actual pre-embryos. Lacham[18], using the mouse model, demonstrated that 2-deoxyadenosine produced significant embryonic arrest between the two and four-cell stage. In the human, 2-deoxyadenosine induced 80% blockage. Pentoxifylline showed a similar effect, but that was not statistically significant.

Adenosine is a very potent blocker of the G-1 or G-2 phase of the cell cycle. Pentoxifylline, on the other hand, seems to have the advantage of reducing production of superoxide anions by human spermatozoa[19]. Chao *et al.*[20] have also used human follicular fluid to stimulate sperm motility and velocity; the amplitude increase of motility peaked at 12 h, the amplitude increase of curvilinear velocity also peaks at 12 h after sperm washing in phosphate buffered saline. They believe that there is a non-dialyzable and heat-stable factor with a molecular weight of around 50 000 in human follicular fluid that improved and maintained the motility and velocity of washed human sperm.

Morphology

The last crucial parameter to be investigated in semen analysis is morphology, using either the WHO[21], Düsseldorf guidelines[22] or the strict criteria for head and neck normality, as proposed by the University of Stellenbosch and modified by Norfolk, which allows better reproducibility, predictability of fertilization and/or pregnancy outcome[23]. A high number of sperm morphological abnormalities seem to be characteristic of men and sperm selected by cervical mucus screening after ejaculation in the vagina, recovered from the peritoneal cavity or attached to the surface of the zona pellucida in the hemizona assay shows morphological characteristics that are normal, and the population's morphology is more homogeneous. The characteristics of these populations can be used to determine the criteria for normal morphology.

The morphology classification utilized in our laboratory (strict criteria) is a modification of the methods of MacLeod[24] and Eliasson[25], taking into account the total morphological characteristics of the sperm. Normal ideal spermatozoa according to strict criteria should have a head with a small oval configuration, a well-defined acrosome comprising between 40% and 70% of the sperm-head area, a perfectly small oval head, or one that tapers slightly at the level of the post-acrosomal region. The head length should be 3–5 μm, and the width 2–3 μm when Papanicolaou staining is used and 5–6 μm in length, and 3–4 μm in width when the Diff-Quik[26] staining is utilized. No abnormalities in the neck, midpiece or tail should be present. The midpiece should be slender, axially attached, and <1 μm in width, and the length should be approximately 1.5 times the head length. No cytoplasmic droplets larger than half the area of the sperm head should be present. The tail should be uniform, slightly thinner than the midpiece, uncoiled, and approximately 45 μm in length. Trivial variations in head morphology may still be considered normal, but borderline normal heads are classified in a different category as slightly abnormal forms.

Acrosomal abnormalities could be classified as secondary when the changes in the sperm membranes are determined by external factors, or when there is loss of acrosome content due to damage or aging and, in some of these cases, these abnormalities may be reversible. The term 'primary acrosomal abnormalities' is used when the changes occur during development and differentiation of the spermatozoa, and may be caused by abnormal formation, distribution or attachment of the acrosome. Head abnormalities that may be considered major may affect size, shape and the presence of vacuoles. Elongated or tapered heads may be due to environmental factors or stress. Minor head abnormalities are of unknown significance.

Midpiece anomalies involve mitochondria, centrioles, microtubular formation and/or retention of abnormally large cytoplasmic droplets. This type of abnormality may occur in an isolated fashion, or may be present simultaneously with both head and tail defects. Tail abnormalities are characterized by various degrees of coiling within an intact plasma membrane, duplication, angulations and so forth.

Using these criteria, a population with normal fertilization rates in IVF shows more than 14% normal forms; figures below 14% indicate progressive deterioration of sperm morphology and, consequently, of function. Two subgroups have been identified within this abnormal group: patients who have between 5% and 14% normal forms are considered to have a good prognosis pattern (G pattern) and patients with 4% or less normal forms are considered to have a poor prognosis pattern (P pattern) and show the worst performance in IVF[1]. This type of evaluation should be carried out in at least 200 sperm cells per slide.

The normal male population having >14% normal sperm forms has a morphology index (summation of normal forms plus slightly abnormal forms) >40%; patients with a P pattern have a morphology index well below 30%; and the G pattern subgroup constitutes an intermediate category whose prognosis is more difficult to establish, and is perhaps between that of the other two groups; its morphology index is 30–40%. When a discrepancy is found between the percentage abnormal morphology and the morphology index, the former seems to be a more reliable parameter for prediction.

The G pattern has to be judged according to its characteristics. All those that are very close to the P pattern should be considered as having a poor prognosis; those that are close to the normal pattern should be considered as having a much better function.

Performance of each sperm group and subgroup is clearly different in IVF[6]. When insemination is performed utilizing the regular 50 000 to 100 000 sperm/mL/egg in 3 mL, as is done in our laboratory, patients with normal sperm morphology had a fertilization rate of 88.3%. Meanwhile, patients with normal forms <14% showed a fertilization rate of 49.5%. The pregnancy rate per retrieval or per transfer was also significantly lower in this group. Patients with a G pattern, on the other hand, had a fertilization rate of 63.9%, and patients with a P pattern showed only 7.6% fertilization capacity[1].

The fertilization decrease in the P pattern can be solved partially by a 5–10 times increase in the number of sperm used at insemination (500 000–1 000 000 sperm/mL/egg). When these corrective measures are used the fertilization rate improves to 63.6% and up to 89.8%, as demonstrated in the original work[27]. The miscarriage rate may be high; therefore, the ongoing term pregnancy rates per cycle and per transfer are much lower. In a more recent evaluation of a larger number of patients in Norfolk (1988–89)[6], in terms of fertilization rate of preovulatory oocytes in 381 cycles performed using sperm of normal characteristics with a concentration at insemination of $120.6 \pm 26.5 \times 10^5$ ($x \pm SD$) sperm/mL/egg, a fertilization rate of 92.6%, with a subsequent total pregnancy rate per cycle and per transfer of 26.1% and 28.0% was achieved, respectively, and term ongoing pregnancy rates of 17.3 and 18.5% were obtained. In the P pattern group using $1.3 \pm 0.1 \times 10^6$ sperm/mL/egg as sperm concentration at insemination, the fertilization rate was 55.6%, the total pregnancy rates per cycle and per transfer were 17.1 and 23.2%, and the term/ongoing pregnancy rates per cycle and per transfer were 7.8% and 10.7%, respectively, in a total of 76 cycles examined. Meanwhile, in the G pattern subgroup a total fertilization rate, using $6.4 \pm 0.5 \times 10^5$ sperm concentration at insemination, the fertilization rate was quite satisfactory (85.2%), the total pregnancy rates per cycle and per transfer were 22.4% and 24.0%, respectively, but the term/ongoing pregnancy rates per cycle and per transfer decreased to 11.2 and 12.0%, respectively. The abortion rate in the normal sperm population group was 34%, in the G pattern it was 50%, and in the P pattern 53%. These figures seem to indicate a severe impairment of results in terms of IVF when abnormal sperm is used with both the G pattern and P pattern, although the P pattern continues to show the poorest outcome. A report of the results in the male factor treatment by assisted reproduction should accordingly be done as term pregnancy rate by cycle of aspiration in order to express the real efficiency of the sperm in establishing term pregnancies.

On the other other hand, as in any biological system, there are exceptions to these rules, and patients with a P pattern of morphology, but excellent sperm density and motility, may behave in a completely different fashion, and even spontaneous pregnancies are possible in this category.

This information obtained in the human IVF system can be confirmed in the heterologous hamster SPA and in the homologous hemizona assay, as will be seen later in this chapter. We propose therefore that, using these criteria for morphology diagnosis, severely dysmorphic sperm will perform poorly and therefore the prognosis for that patient is not even close to the prognosis in patients with normal sperm populations. Similar results were obtained by Enginsu *et al.*[28], who also found the strict criteria much more useful in predicting fertilization than the hypo-osmotic swelling test (HOST) and morphology evaluated by WHO criteria.

Effects of stress on performance

In spite of all the efforts to determine the sperm fertilizing ability by the close scrutiny of each one of the parameters, there is something else that cannot be assessed properly by them. If the sperm is put under stress by laboratory procedures it can be demonstrated that the performance is worse than could be predicted by studying the fresh sample. For instance, if a sperm separation procedure is performed using a swim-up technique, this seems to give an overall evaluation of the effect of each and every abnormality found in the specimen in the final quality and potential efficiency of the sperm. Early in the Norfolk program it was determined that when using the double-wash, double-swim-up technique, $<1.5\times10^6$ total motile sperm were recovered from the specimen, and results of fertilization were greatly decreased[29]. Re-investigation of this matter during the years 1988–89 revealed very few exceptions, even when insemination in a microtiter dish was performed. When the motility before and after swim-up was compared in 73 cases, 41.1% improvement was obtained with highly significant differences between motility before and after swim-up[30]. One should remember that the selection of the highly motile fraction is achieved after losing a high proportion of sperm that will never be available for utilization in the actual process of insemination, unless the pellet is resuspended and utilized. Only 10–30% of the motile sperm present are recovered by this procedure. Similar considerations could be made for morphological characteristics of the sperm recovered[30]. A significant increase is obtained in the percentage of the normal forms and morphology index in the post-swim-up specimen at the expense of losing a tremendous amount of sperm. In terms of separation of the motile sperm fraction for therapeutic purposes at the time of *in vitro* fertilization insemination, different methodological procedures can be utilized. In the very poor specimens with borderline parameters (severe male factor in assisted reproduction by Norfolk criteria) simple washing by dilution and centrifugation can be utilized. Sperm washing techniques do not remove dead sperm cells, which according to results in the zona-free hamster eggs decrease and impair the process of sperm fusion with the hamster oocytes[31]. The regular swim-up procedure in those cases will diminish substantially the number of sperm available and, therefore, the chances of fertilization. Unfortunately, damage to the sperm mainly in abnormal samples have been reported with this technique, either due to the centrifugation process itself, or to oxidative stress (hydrogen peroxide generation), which impairs lipid quality at the sperm membrane level[32].

These mechanisms of oxidative stress (lipid peroxidation) are due probably to the sedimentation of the sperm, together with other cellular and particulate matters, although spermatozoa themselves, mainly when they are abnormal, produce oxidation substances that can stimulate lipid peroxidation and modify the membranes. Aitken[33] has utilized 7-dimethyl-amino-naphthalin-1,2-dicarbolic acid hydrazide, a luminol analog, in combination with horseradish peroxidase to enhance the detection of reactive oxygen species produced by human spermatozoa. DeLamirande and Gagnon[34], using Percoll separated spermatozoa treated with hydrogen peroxide, or the combination of xanthine and xanthine oxidase, noticed a progressive decrease leading to complete arrest in sperm flagellar beat frequency; partial recovery can be obtained if the sperm is demembranated in a medium containing magnesium adenosine triphosphate; the recovery is transient. The most damaging effect came from hydrogen peroxide, but oxygen and hydroxy radicals also played a role. ATP depletion, according to those authors[34], induced by reactive oxygen species generation, was responsible for the effects observed in the sperm. Kobayashi *et al.*[35] have used superoxide dismutase to try to interfere with lipid peroxidation in human spermatozoa that causes loss of motility, and tried to inhibit this lipid peroxidation by using the enzyme. Addition of exogenous superoxide dismutase to the sperm suspension significantly decreased the loss of motility and the increase of malondialdehyde concentration in spermatozoa, suggesting the possibility of using this agent to improve the situation.

Other less popular migration procedures are the migration into albumin or into an intraviscous hyaluronate layer.

Separation procedures

Another way to recover a more efficient sperm motile fraction is to use gradient or column separation procedures. The best known one utilizes silicone particles coated with polyvinyl pyrrolidone (Percoll) in continuous or discontinuous gradients. This avoids the oxidation stress referred to previously and allows recovery of a similar or higher proportion of sperm cells than the swim-up. Furthermore, it seems to favor capacitation and membrane fusion.

A trial was made in the Norfolk program to compare the effect of the swim-up separation in patients with G and P patterns of morphology[36]. The only difference found in the fresh specimens before processing was a significantly less mean velocity in the P pattern; after swim-up, percentage motility was also significantly lower in that group, and the velocity and linearity were decreased, although that did not reach statistical significance. As a final result, a recovery rate of 42.0±4% (x±SD) in the G pattern group, versus 19±2.8% (x±SD) recovery rate in the P-pattern group was observed. This seemed to indicate that, although minor differences can be found in terms of motility, a more significant difference is seen after swim-up in terms of total motile recovery fraction and recovery rate.

TEST OF SPERMATOZOAL FUNCTION

Adenosine triphosphate and creatinine kinase system in the sperm

Since the recognition that a semen sample is composed of a heterogeneous sperm population, the shortcomings of the basic semen analysis were apparent, one being the inability of that test to be of accurate diagnostic and prognostic value in assisted reproduction. New approaches based on biochemical and molecular markers of sperm function have been pursued. However, no single evaluation has been developed yet to predict the sperm fertilizing ability.

Many sperm functions are energy-requiring processes, and the evaluation of biochemical markers of sperm energy metabolism seems to be a logical approach. Among them, the determination of sperm ATP content and the activity of phosphocreatine kinase (CK) and sperm-specific lactate dehydrogenase (LDH-C4, LDH-X) are typical examples. The most commonly accepted viewpoint is that sperm cells are able to synthesize the energy source (ATP) needed, by utilizing a variety of exogenous substrates such as glucose, fructose, pyruvate and lactate. This is accomplished via the glycolytic pathway or the oxidative phosphorylation in sperm mitochondria. Ivanov *et al.*[37], more than 45 years ago, suggested that the ATP thus formed diffuses in sperm flagellum and is used by the sperm to maintain its important energy-requiring functions. In several recent investigations it has been suggested that ATP alone may not be the only factor involved in the subcellular biochemical energy accumulation of the sperm[38–41]. Saks *et al.*[42], in their studies of cardiac muscle cells, reported that although ATP utilization occurs in muscular contractions the use of ATP cannot be detected. The implication is that the ATP pool is kept at a constant level at the expense of another energy source. Another energy supply at the sperm level is the phosphocreatine (creatine phosphate) system. ATP produced is converted to phosphocreatine in mitochondria, giving rise to ADP for further ATP synthesis. Phosphocreatine diffuses out from the site of production to the sites of utilization, where it can be dephosphorylated to produce ATP. Under normal conditions, this mechanism allows the immediate energy source, ATP, to be kept at an adequate level while the reserve source, phosphocreatine, is synthesized, transferred, accumulated and utilized as needed.

Several investigators have reported the existence of a similar mechanism in the sperm[39,40,43]. It is believed that via this 'shuttle system', ATP is transferred from the site of synthesis to the sites of utilization, namely the sperm membranes and the dynein arms of the flagellum.

The enzyme responsible for the reversible conversion of ATP to phosphocreatine is ATP:creatine *N*-phosphotransferase (creatine kinase, CK). Since the equilibrium constant for the conversion is low and the ATP production from phosphocreatine is kinetically favorable, there must be different types of CK to direct this reversible reaction toward the desired direction. In mitochondria, a mitochondrial type of CK converts ATP to phosphocreatine, and at the site of utilization, another CK subtype catalyzes the reverse reaction. In the sea urchin the CK of the sperm head is in the conventional range of 40 kDa, whereas the flagellar type has been identified to be 145 kDa[44,45]. Specific inhibition of CK by low levels of 1-fluoro-2,4 dinitrobenzene attenuates flagellar beating, indicating that the energy shuttle involves CK, and that it is essential for normal flagellar motion. CK was reported to be associated with the flagellar axonemes, and may bind directly to polarize flagellar microtubules[45,46]. There are three CK subtypes (isoenzymes) identified in humans: CK-MM, CK-MB and CK-BB. With high voltage electrophoresis, these isoenzymes can further be subdivided to six isoforms as they exist in the body. Isoforms of CK-MM and CK-BB have been detected in human sperm, and are believed to be involved in the proposed phosphocreatine shuttle system.

LDH, on the other hand, found in many organs, has five major isoenzymes. A sixth isoenzyme, LDH-C4 (LDH-X), is found specifically in ejaculated sperm[47,48]. Its gene locus is on chromosome 11 and first appears in primary spermatocytes. Since it is unique to sperm, autoimmunity against it may occur spontaneously, or can be stimulated to try to develop a contraceptive method[49]. LDH catalyzes interconversion of lactate and pyruvate, two important energy substrates for sperm. Its evaluation may be useful in some instances. Location of these isoenzymes has been reported to be in the sperm cytosol as well as in mitochondrial matrix.

The relative value of ATP, CK or LDH-C4 determinations in assisted reproduction has been reported by several investigators. Calamera *et al.*[50] and Comhaire *et al.*[51,52] found a close relationship between sperm ATP content, its motility and its fertilizing potential in a therapeutic insemination program. Our own limited study of samples used for IVF showed a good negative correlation ($P<0.001$) between sperm ATP in the swim-up sample and the pregnancy outcome. Swim-up samples with ATP levels below 40 pmol/10^6 sperm showed no pregnancies[53]. Chan *et al.*[54] determined ATP levels in whole semen and found no correlation with penetration in the hamster zona-free oocyte system. Methodological differences may very well be the reason for such discrepancies. There have been several reports of close association between the sperm total CK content, and the rate CK-MM/CK-BB plus CK-MM in samples used in assisted reproduction with the fertilization rate[55,56]. It has also been reported that oligozoospermic patients have much higher total CK per sperm and much lower CK-MM than normozoospermic patients[57]. Higher total CK values have been correlated with a higher incidence of the presence of sperm cells with cytoplasmic droplets in oligozoospermic samples. The presence of higher CK-MM as compared to CK-BB is an indication of sperm maturity.

The role of LDH-C4 evaluation in assisted reproduction has not been investigated fully. Simultaneous determination of ATP, CK and LDH-C4 perhaps will be of value diagnostically and prognostically. Since the process of sperm and egg interaction and fertilization is very complex, it is probable that problems can emerge at different steps of that process and, therefore, no single test, biochemical parameter or marker can be accurate in all patients.

The World Health Organization (WHO) designed a prospective study to evaluate sperm characteristics and adenosine triphosphate content to try to predict the occurrence of pregnancy in infertile couples. Neither the common sperm parameters nor ATP content were good predictors[45].

The levels of ATP have been reported lower in patients with good motility, both in terms of mean sperm ATP concentration and ATP concentration per living spermatozoon, the implication being that highly motile spermatozoa consume ATP more than sperm with impaired motility[58]. DeLamirande and Gagnon[34] have proposed that reactive oxygen species induce ATP depletion on the sperm, leading mainly to loss of sperm motility due to axonemal damage induced by the depletion of ATP. All these studies, although very significant in understanding sperm physiology and some aspects of sperm pathophysiology, do not allow us to propose ATP determination as a routine test in evaluating the sperm.

RESULTS

In general, the results obtained in *in vitro* fertilization when abnormal semen is used are not as satisfactory as the results obtained with normal gametes, even when fertilization occurs. The number of papers covering this subject published recently is scanty. Patients should be aware of those results before entering the program and certainly they should know what results are obtained in the particular center they are applying to. The first results from the Norfolk experience were published in 1985 and 1986[29,59,60].

Hirsch *et al.*[60] reviewed 83 cycles of IVF-ET in which a male factor was the sole cause for the couple's infertility, or was one of the factors in multifactorial infertility. The male factor was defined as a sperm density of $<20\times10^6$ sperm/mL, motility <60%, forward progression <2, and/or an abnormal sperm morphology feature >40%, and a score of fewer than two sperm penetrations per hamster egg, as determined by the sperm penetration assay. Clomiphene citrate and hMG were used for ovarian stimulation, sperm concentration varying between 0.5 and -1×10^6 motile sperm/mL of media were used at insemination, and in severely oligospermic specimens more than one oocyte was placed in a dish. The cumulus mass was mechanically removed. The overall fertilization rate was 70% and an average of 2.6 embryos per patient were transferred. The fertilization rate for non-male factors was 85% for mature oocytes; with a sperm density <20 million/mL, the fertilization was impaired and when it dropped to <10 million/mL, for the most part the fertilization rate dropped below 30%. Thirty per cent motility seemed to be the most useful threshold. No significant relationship with morphology was found. Two penetrations per hamster ova in the SPA seemed to be a useful threshold to determine normal fertilization versus low fertilization. The pregnancy rate per cycle in the male factor population was 20%, while in the non-male factor population it was 10%. Therefore, this is one of the few reports in which the male factor pregnancy rate is better than the non-male factor pregnancy rate. A second paper by the same authors[61] states once again that IVF in the male factor is 'rewarded with a pregnancy rate that is not statistically different from that for the overall IVF population'. They obtained a pregnancy rate of 20% without specification of the type of pregnancy rate that was being reported. Hinting[62] reported a significantly reduced fertilization rate when the spermatozoa presented abnormal morphology with or without poor motility and a low sperm concentration. The pregnancy rate with abnormal semen seems to decrease with GIFT, but not with IVF-ET. Enginsu *et al.*[63], reporting on the male factor in *in vitro* fertilization outcome, demonstrated that the only semen parameter of clinical significance was sperm morphology using strict criteria. The pregnancy rates cannot be compared because there are few pregnancies in most of the categories.

The Norfolk results have already been given in this chapter.

References

1. Kruger, T. F., Acosta, A. A., Simmons, K. F., Swanson, R. J., Matta, J. F. and Oehninger, S. (1988). Predictive value of abnormal sperm morphology in *in vitro* fertilization. *Fertil Steril.*, **49**, 112–7
2. Franken, D. R., Acosta, A. A., Kruger, T. F., Lombard, C. J., Oehninger, S. and Hodgen, G. D. (1993). The hemizona assay: its role in identifying male factor infertility in assisted reproduction. *Fertil Steril.*, **59**, 1075–80
3. Henkel, R., Muller, C., Miscka, W., Gips, H. and Schill, W. B. (1993). Determination of the acrosome reaction in human spermatozoa is predictive of fertilization *in vitro*. *Hum. Reprod.*, **8**, 2128–32
4. Acosta, A. A. (1992). Male factor in assisted reproduction. Presented at the 17th Annual Meeting of American Society of Andrology. *Infertil. Reprod. Med. Clin. North Am.*, **3**, 487–503
5. Barlow, P., Delvigne, A., Van-Dromme, J., Van-Hoeck, J., Vandenbosch, K. and Leroy, F. (1991). Predictive value of classical and automated sperm analysis for *in-vitro* fertilization. *Hum. Reprod.*, **6**, 1119–24
6. Burkman, L. J. (1984). Characterization of hyperactivated motility by human spermatozoa during capacitation: comparison of fertile and oligozoospermic sperm populations. *Arch. Androl.*, **13**, 153–65
7. Burkman, L. J. (1991). Discrimination between non-hyperactivated and classical hyperactivated motility patterns in human spermatozoa using computerized analysis. *Fertil. Steril.*, **55**, 363–71
8. Mortimer, D., Courtot, A. M., Giorangrandi, Y., Jeulin, C. and David, G. (1984). Human sperm motility after injection and incubation in synthetic media. *Gamete Res.*, **9**, 131–44
9. Wothe, D. D., Charbonneau, H. and Shapiro, B. M. (1990). The phosphocreatine shuttle of sea urchin sperm: flagellar creatine kinase resulted from a gene triplication. *Proc. Natl Acad. Sci. USA.*, **87**, 5203–7
10. Wang, C., Leung, A., Tsoi, W. L., Leung, J., Ng, V., Lee, K. F., Chan, S. Y. (1991). Evaluation of human sperm hyperactivated motility and its relationship with the zona-free hamster oocyte sperm penetration assay. *J. Androl.*, **12**, 253–7
11. Murad, C., deLamirande, E. and Gagnon, C. (1992).

Hyperactivated motility is coupled with interdependent modifications at axonemal and cytosolic levels in human spermatozoa. *J. Androl.*, **13**, 323–31

12. Mbizvo, M. T., Burkman, L. J. and Alexander, N. J. (1990). Human follicular fluid stimulates hyperactivated motility in human sperm. *Fertil. Steril.*, **54**, 708–12
13. Blackmore, P. F., Beebe, S. J., Danforth, D. R. and Alexander, N. (1990). Progesterone and 17-α-hydroxyprogesterone: Novel stimulators of calcium. *J. Biol. Chem.*, **265**, 1376–80
14. Grunert, J.-H., De Geyter, C. and Nieschlag, E. (1990). Objective identification of hyperactivated human spermatozoa by computerized sperm motion analysis with the Hamilton–Thorne sperm motility analyzer. *Hum. Reprod.*, **5**, 593–9
15. Tesarik, J., Mendoza Oltras, C. and Testart, J. (1990). Effect of the human cumulus oophorus on movement characteristics of human capacitated spermatozoa. *J. Reprod. Fertil.*, **88**, 665–75
16. Imoedemhe, D. A., Sique, A. B., Pacpaco, E. L. and Olazo, A. B. (1992). The effect of caffeine on the ability of spermatozoa to fertilize mature human oocytes. *J. Assist. Reprod. Genet.*, **9**, 155–60
17. Imoedemhe, D. A., Sique, A. B., Pacpaco, E. A. and Olazo, A. B. (1992). Successful use of the sperm motility enhancer 2-deoxyadenosine in previously failed human *in vitro* fertilization. *J. Assist. Reprod. Genet.*, **9**, 53–6
18. Lacham, O. (1992). Immobilized sperm motility stimulation and embryo development. *Advances in Assisted Reproductive Technology for the Infertile Male, Serono International Clinical Meeting*, Adelaide, Australia, 30 November–1 December
19. Gavella, M. and Liporac, V. (1992). Pentoxifylline-mediated reduction of superoxide anion production by human spermatozoa. *Andrologia*, **24**, 37–9
20. Chao, H. T., Ng, H. T., Tsai, K. L., Hong, C. Y. and Wei, Y. H. (1992). Human follicular fluid stimulates motility and velocity of washed human sperm *in vitro*. *Andrologia*, **24**, 47–51
21. World Health Organization. (1992). *WHO Laboratory Manual for the Examination of Human Semen and Sperm–Cervical Mucus Interaction*, 3rd edn. (Cambridge: Cambridge University Press)
22. Hofmann, N. and Haider, S. G. (1985). Neue Ergebnisse Morphologischer Diagnostik der Spermatogenesestorungen. *Gynäkologe*, **18**, 70–80
23. Kruger, T. F., Menkveld, R., Stander, F. S. H., Lombard, C. J., Van der Merwe, J. P., van Zyl, J. A. and Smith, K. (1986). Sperm morphologic features as a prognostic factor in *in vitro* fertilization. *Fertil. Steril.*, **46**, 1118–23
24. MacLeod, J. and Gold, R. Z. (1951). The male factor in fertility and infertility. IV. Sperm morphology in fertile and infertile marriage. *Fertil. Steril.*, **2**, 394–414
25. Eliasson, R. (1971). Standards for investigation of human semen. *Andrologia*, **3**, 49
26. Kruger, T. F., Ackerman, S. B., Simmons, K. F., Swanson, R. J., Brugo, S. S. and Acosta, A. A. (1987). A quick reliable staining technique for human sperm morphology. *Arch. Androl.*, **18**, 275–7
27. Oehninger, S., Acosta, A. A., Morshedi, M., Veeck, L., Swanson, R. J., Simmons, K. and Rosenwaks, Z. (1988). Corrective measures and pregnancy outcome in *in vitro* fertilization patients with severe sperm morphology abnormalities. *Fertil. Steril.*, **50**, 283–7
28. Enginsu, M. E., Dumoulin, J. C., Pieters, M. H., Bergers, M., Evers, J. L. and Geraedts, J. P. (1992). Comparison between the hypo-osmotic swelling test and morphology evaluation using strict criteria in predicting *in vitro* fertilization (IVF). *J. Assist. Reprod. Genet.*, **9**, 259–64
29. van Uem, J. F., Acosta, A. A., Swanson, R. J., Mayer, J., Ackerman, S., Burkman, L. J., Veeck, L., McDowell, J. S., Bernardus, R. and Jones, H. W. Jr. (1985). Male factor evaluation in IVF: Norfolk experience. *Fertil. Steril.*, **44**, 375–83
30. Acosta, A. A., Oehninger, S., Morshedi, M., Swanson, R. J., Scott, R., Irianni, F. (1989). Assisted reproduction in the diagnosis and treatment of the male factor. *Obstet. Gynecol. Surv.*, **44**, 1–18
31. Rana, N., Jeyendran, R. J., Holmgren, W. J., Rotman, C. and Zaneveld, L. J. D. (1989). Glass wool-filtered spermatozoa and their oocyte penetrating capacity. *J.* In Vitro *Fertil. Embryo Transf.*, **6**, 280–4
32. Aitken, J. (1991). Molecular basis of sperm improvement *in vitro*. *Proceedings of the Seventh World Congress of In Vitro Fertilization and Medically Assisted Procreation*, Paris, France, 30 June–3 July
33. Aitken, R. J. and Buckingham, D. (1992). Enhanced detection of reactive oxygen species produced by human spermatozoa with 7-dimethyl amino-naphthalin-1,2-dicarbonic acid hydrazide. *Int. J. Androl.*, **15**, 211–9
34. DeLamirande, E. and Gagnon, C. (1992). Reactive oxygen species and human spermatozoa. II. Depletion of adenosine triphosphate plays an important role in the inhibition of sperm motility. *J. Androl.*, **13**, 379–86
35. Kobayashi, T., Miyazaki, T., Natori, M. and Nozawa, S. (1991). Protective role of superoxide dismutase in human sperm motility: superoxide dismutase activity and lipid peroxide in human seminal plasma and spermatozoa. *Hum. Reprod.*, **6**, 987–91
36. Oehninger, S., Acosta, R., Morshedi, M., Philput, C., Swanson, R. J. and Acosta, A. A. (1990). Relationship between morphology and motion characteristics of human spermatozoa in semen and in swim-up fractions. *J. Androl.*, **11**, 446–52
37. Ivanov, I. I., Kassavina, B. S. and Fomenko, L. D. (1946). Adenosine triphosphate in mammalian spermatozoa. *Nature*, **158**, 624–9
38. Dadoune, J. P., Mayaux, M. J. and Guihard-Moscato, M. L. (1988). Correlation between defects in chromatin condensation of human spermatozoa stained

by aniline blue and semen characteristics. *Andrologia*, **20**, 211–17

39. Sherman, J. K. (1990). Cryopreservation of human semen. In Kee, B. A. and Webster, B. W. (eds.) *Handbook of the Laboratory Diagnosis and Treatment of Infertility*, Chapter 13, pp. 224–59. (Boca Raton: CRC Press)
40. Smith, K. D. and Steinberger, E. (1973). Survival of spermatozoa in a human sperm bank. *J. Am. Med. Assoc.*, **223**, 774–7
41. Vincenzo, T. (1980). Artificial insemination and semen banks in Italy. In David, G. and Price, W. S. (eds.) *Human Artificial Insemination and Semen Preservation*, pp. 51–6. (New York: Plenum Press)
42. Saks, V. A., Rosenshtraukh, L. V., Smirnov, V. N. and Chazov, E. I. (1978). Role of creatine kinase in cellular function and metabolism. *Can. J. Physiol. Pharmacol.*, **65**, 691–6
43. Jouannet, P., Frydman, R., Van Steirteghem, A., Wolf, J. P., Czyglik, F. and Van Den/Abbeel, E. (1990). Cryopreservation and infertility. In Seibel, M. M. (ed.) *Infertility, A Comprehensive Text*, Chapter 37, pp. 525–38. (Norwalk: Appleton & Lange)
44. Tombes, R. M. and Shapiro, B. M. (1987). Enzyme termini of a phosphocreatine shuttle. Purification and characterization of two creatine kinase isoenzymes from sea urchin sperm. *J. Biol. Chem.*, **262**, 1–9
45. World Health Organization. (1992). Adenosine triphosphate in semen and other sperm characteristics: Their relevance for fertility prediction in men with normal sperm concentration. *Fertil. Steril.*, **57**, 877–81
46. Tombes, R. M. and Shapiro, B. M. (1985). Metabolic channeling: A phosphorylcreatine shuttle to mediate high energy phosphate transport between mitochondrion and tail. *Cell*, **41**, 325–34
47. Blanco, A. and Zimkhim, W. H. (1963). Lactate dehydrogenase in human testes. *Science*, **139**, 601–2
48. Goldberg, E. (1963). Lactic and malic dehydrogenases in human spermatozoa. *Science*, **139**, 602–3
49. Evrev, T. I. (1975). Auto antigenicity of LDH-X isoenzymes. In Markert, C. L. (ed.) *Isoenzymes: Physiological Function*, Vol. II, pp. 129–41. (New York: Academic Press)
50. Calamera, J. C., Brugo, S. and Vilar, O. (1982). Relation between motility and adenosine triphosphate (ATP) in human spermatozoa. *Andrologia*, **14**, 239–41
51. Comhaire, F. and Thiery, M. (1985). Methods of improvement of the success rate of artificial insemination with donor semen. *Int. J. Androl.*, **9**, 14–20
52. Comhaire, F., Vermeulen, L., Ghedira, K., Mas, J., Irvine, S. and Callipolitis, G. (1983). Adenosine triphosphate in human semen – a quantitative estimate of fertilizing potential. *Fertil. Steril.*, **40**, 500–4
53. Morshedi, M. (1989). Andrological methods of predicting the pregnancy outcome of an IVF program. Doctoral thesis, Eastern Virginia Medical School/Old Dominion University, pp. 148–56
54. Chan, S. Y. W. and Wang, C. (1987). Correlation between semen adenosine triphosphate and sperm fertilizing capacity. *Fertil. Steril.*, **47**, 717–19
55. Huszar, G., Corrales, M. and Vigue, L. (1988). Correlation between sperm creatine phosphokinase activity and sperm concentrations in normospermic and oligospermic men. *Gamete Res.*, **19**, 67–75
56. Huszar, G. and Vigue, L. (1987). Serial sperm CPK measurements in oligospermic and normospermic patients. *Poster #79, presented at the 5th World Congress on* In Vitro *Fertilization and Embryo Transfer*, Program supplement, April 5–10, p. 56
57. Huszar, G. and Vigue, L. (1990). Spermatogenesis-related changes in the synthesis of the creatine kinase B-type and M-type isoforms in human spermatozoa. *Mol. Reprod. Dev.*, **25**, 258–62
58. Gottlieb, C., Svanborg, K. and Bjdgeman, M. (1991). Adenosine triphosphate (ATP) in human spermatozoa. *Andrologia*, **23**, 421–5
59. Acosta, A. A., Chillik, C. F., Brugo, S., Ackerman, S., Swanson, R. J., Pleban, P., Yuan J. and Haque, D. (1986). *In vitro* fertilization and the male factor. *Urology*, **28**, 1–9
60. Hirsch, I., Gibbons, W. E., Lipshultz, L. I., Rossavik, K. K., Young, R. L., Poindexter, A. N., Dodson, M. G. and Findley, W. E. (1986). *In vitro* fertilization in couples with male factor infertility. *Fertil. Steril.*, **45**, 659–64
61. Gibbons, W. (1987). *In vitro* fertilization as therapy for male factor infertility. *Urol. Clin. North Am.*, **14**, 563–7
62. Hinting, A., Comhaire, F., Vermeulen, L., Dhont, M., Vermeulen, A. and Vandekerckhove, D. (1990). Possibilities and limitations of techniques of assisted reproduction for the treatment of male infertility. *Hum. Reprod.*, **5**, 544–8
63. Enginsu, M. E., Pieters, M. H., Dumoulin, J. C., Evers, J. L. and Geraedts, J. P. (1992). Male factor as determinant of *in vitro* fertilization outcome. *Hum. Reprod.*, **7**, 1136–40

Assisted reproduction 2: gamete intrafallopian transfer

28

J. P. Van der Merwe and T. F. Kruger

INTRODUCTION

The birth of the first baby after *in vitro* fertilization and embryo transfer (IVF-ET) marked the beginning of a new era in human reproductive medicine[1]. This treatment modality provided the possibility of a child to many infertile couples for whom very limited or no treatment alternative existed. An alternative technique for the treatment of infertile couples when the spouse has at least one patent Fallopian tube was described by Asch[2]. This technique involved the laparoscopic placement of both sperm and oocytes into the Fallopian tube, the normal site of human fertilization[3]. GIFT has since also been used in the treatment of male infertility. Some authors have reported relatively good results, provided that a sufficient number of motile spermatozoa were transferred[4], while others found very poor pregnancy rates in cases with abnormal sperm parameters[5]. Very little is reported on the outcome of GIFT as a treatment for male factor applying the strict criteria as a measure of normality of the spermatozoa[6].

The fertilization potential of the spermatozoa and oocytes cannot be determined in GIFT unless the patient conceives. In order to make sure that fertilization has taken place, a combination of *in vitro* fertilization with subsequent zygote intrafallopian transfer (ZIFT)[7] or tubal embryo stage transfer (TEST), embryo intrafallopian transfer was introduced[8]. This technique comprises two invasive procedures, namely oocyte retrieval and tubal embryo transfer.

In this chapter, we will concentrate on the influence of the different semen parameters on the outcome of the GIFT procedure with emphasis on sperm morphology.

NORMAL SPERM MORPHOLOGY

The role of sperm morphology in assisted reproduction (IVF) was questioned by different authors. Wiedemann *et al.*[9] have shown that the andrological factor becomes relevant in GIFT when patients present with <30% morphologically normal spermatozoa, and/or <30% motility, and/or sperm density of $<10\times10^6$/mL (according to WHO classification criteria).

The Tygerberg Unit recently performed a retrospective study in order to determine the effect of sperm morphology according to the strict criteria[6] in a GIFT program. The outcome of 1952 consecutive GIFT cycles was analyzed with patients classified in three categories according to the percentage of morphologically normal spermatozoa based on previous publications[6] (0% to 4%, or P pattern; 5% to 14%, or G pattern; >14%, or normal pattern).

A couple is considered for infertility work-up after failure to achieve a pregnancy over 2 years of unprotected intercourse. Patients who have at least one patent Fallopian tube on hysterosalpingogram and laparoscopy are considered for GIFT when more conventional and simpler treatments have failed. Patients with the following diagnosis or combination of factors are accepted for the GIFT program: unexplained infertility, male factor, endometriosis (mild to severe), cervical factor, immunological factor, pelvic adhesions that interfered with oocyte pick-up during normal ovulation and unsuccessful donor insemination.

In order to maximize the recovery of fertilizable oocytes, all patients undergo controlled ovarian hyperstimulation[10,11].

The husband was required to produce a semen sample 1 h before laparoscopy was performed. The semen was prepared by either washing and swim-up[12] or glass wool separation[13]. The latter was performed in patients with a sperm concentration of $<5\times10^6$ spermatozoa/mL.

Oocyte retrieval was performed by laparoscopy[13]. Aspirated oocytes were placed in individual culture dishes containing Ham's F-10 medium with 50% maternal serum in a CO_2 in air incubator (Forma Scientific 3157). Three or four oocytes were replaced per patient undergoing GIFT treatment.

Oocyte handling and influence on pregnancy outcome

In the event of males with a P pattern[14] or women over 40 years of age, more oocytes may be transferred to increase the chances of fertilization and pregnancy. Whenever possible, only metaphase II (MII) oocytes[15] were selected to enhance the chances of pregnancy[16]. In a previous study it was shown that, by increasing the number of metaphase II oocytes, the chances of a pregnancy were increased[16]. Of the 537 GIFT treatment cycles that were prospectively analyzed by the Tygerberg unit, 423 cycles yielded four or more oocytes. Patients were divided into two groups according to sperm morphology: those with <14% normal forms and those with >14% normal morphology (as judged by strict criteria). These two groups were further divided into five subcategories depending upon the number of metaphase II oocytes transferred: category 1 received four MI oocytes back; category 2, three MIs and one MII; category 3, two MIs and two MIIs. Category 4 received one MI and three MIIs, and category 5 received four MIIs. The extreme or pure categories were those with four MI oocytes back (category 1) and those with four MIIs back (category 5).

In the group with <14% normal forms (category I; four MI oocytes replaced), three pregnancies resulted from 33 cycles (9.09%); and in category V, four MII oocytes replaced, the pregnancy rate was 15% (14/95) per cycle. In the group with >14% normal forms, in category I, the pregnancy rate was 16% (3/19) per cycle; and in category V, the pregnancy rate was 33% (20/61) per cycle. In the group with >14% normal forms there was a significant improvement in pregnancy rate (P=0.04) in category V. Furthermore, the effect of morphology on pregnancy outcome (<14% normal forms versus >14% normal forms) is significant (P=0.0161) (12% versus 23% ongoing pregnancies).

Increasing motile sperm concentration in the fallopian tube to improve pregnancy rate

In the Tygerberg unit, the transfer catheter is loaded as follows: first, 25 μL of medium containing 100 000 sperm, as was traditionally done for normal semen parameters[3]; in cases with a normal morphology of <14%, 500 000 sperm or more are loaded and transferred. Oehninger[17] has shown that the *in vitro* fertilization rate can be improved by increasing the insemination concentration/mL/egg from 100 000 to at least 500 000. Matson *et al.*[4] investigated the usefulness of GIFT in treating oligospermic couples. The number of spermatozoa that were insemianted was increased from 100 000 to 325 000 (the minimum number associated with pregnancy). Khan *et al.*[12] found that pregnancy rates were no different if the number of inseminated spermatozoa was reduced from 100 000 to 2500. However, the strict criteria for morphological evaluation of spermatozoa were not applied in both studies, which in our opinion must be taken into consideration.

Results of 1952 GIFT cases of different morphology categories

From 1952 consecutive cycles analyzed, 59 were omitted mainly because adjustments were made to the protocol, i.e. GIFT was done as well as replacement of embryos, or the morphology slides of the semen on the day of the procedure were not adequate to assess.

In Table 1, the outcome of 1893 consecutive cycles were classified into groups A, B and C according to the morphologically normal spermatozoa. Group A (P pattern morphology)[18] was compared with group B (G pattern morphology)[8] and group C (normal morphology >14%).

The pregnancy rate of 28.3% in group B (G pattern) was significantly better than the 20.4% in group A (P pattern patients: P=0.0087; OR [odds ratio] =1.54; 95% CI, 1.11–2.13) (Table 1). In both groups, 500 000 spermatozoa per Fallopian tube were used. During the second stage of the study, no

Table 1 The outcome of 1893 consecutive cycles classified according to the morphology of spermatozoa

Group	*% Normal morphology*	*Cycles*	*Total pregnancy rate (%)*	*Ongoing pregnancy rate (%)*
A	0–4	313	64 (20.4)[a]	47 (15)[d]
B	5–14	830	235 (28.3)[b]	152 (18.3)[e]
C	>15	750	257 (34.3)[c]	175 (23.3)[f]

[a] versus [b] $P=0.008$; [b] versus [c] $P=0.01$; [d] versus [e] not significant; [e] versus [f] $P=0.007$

more than three oocytes were returned in group B patients in order to reduce the chances of multiple pregnancies. Four oocytes were returned in group A patients if four or more oocytes were retrieved. The pregnancy rate of 34.3% in patients in group C was also significantly better than the 28.3% pregnancy rate in group B ($P=0.013$; OR = 1.32, 106–1.64). In group C (patients with morphology >14%), 100 000 spermatozoa were replaced. Early pregnancy loss was 32.7% and the ectopic pregnancy rate was 3.7%.

The 175 ongoing pregnancies in 750 cycles (23.3%) in group C (>14% normal forms) was significantly better than the 152 (18.3%) ongoing pregnancies from 830 cycles in group B (G pattern) ($P=0.07$; OR = 1.36, 1.06–1.75) (5–14% normal forms). The ongoing pregnancy rate of 18.3% in group B (normal morphology 5–14%) was not significantly higher than the 15% in group A (normal morphology 0–4%). This was due to a high percentage of early pregnancy losses in group B. This increase in the pregnancy rate in the various morphology groups was previously published in IVF[6] and GIFT[15] programs where it was shown that the morphology applying strict criteria has an effect on the fertilization and pregnancy rates. It was also shown by Guzick *et al.*[19] that sperm morphology has a strong association with pregnancy, although strict criteria were not used.

SEMINAL SPERM CONCENTRATION

The seminal sperm concentration/mL does not seem to affect the pregnancy rate[9,19,20]. Kruger *et al.*[20] have shown that the pregnancy rate of a semen concentration of between 3 and 10 million

Table 2 The effect of different semen parameters on pregnancy rate. Reproduced from Kruger *et al.* (1993)[20] with permission of the Hemisphere Publishing Corporation

Parameter	*Ongoing pregnancies (%)*
Sperm morphology (%)	
0–4	14*
5–14	21*
Insemination semen volume in oviduct/mL	
0.01–0.09	20*
0.1–0.19	14*
0.2–0.9	19*
Seminal sperm concentration/mL	
3–10	17*
11–19	8*
>20	22*
Swim-up concentration/mL	
0.1–4.9	18*
5–9.9	11*
>10	30*

*No significant difference

sperm/mL did not differ significantly with the pregnancy rate with a sperm concentration of >20 million/mL. This study, therefore, agrees with the finding of Wiedemann *et al.*[9], that isolated oligozoospermia is not an important cause for infertility, especially in assisted reproduction. Kruger *et al.*[20] pointed out that, in patients with morphology <14% normal forms, at least 500 000 motile sperm must be retrieved to achieve success (Table 2).

Rodrigues-Rigau *et al.*[21] found an association between sperm counts and pregnancy rates without mentioning the effect of morphology of the spermatozoa as a factor on pregnancy outcome.

SPERM MOTILITY

Guzick *et al.*[19] found a pregnancy rate that was significantly higher if the motility was >30% compared to a motility of ≤20%. Other workers[21] found no significant relationship between percentage motility or velocity and clinical or chemical pregnancy rates in GIFT. It was found that linearity (motility efficiency index), an index of directional motility, correlated strongly with clinical and chemical pregnancy rates, as well as with the overall incidence of positive hCG[19]. A strong correlation to clinical pregnancy rate was observed with total motile sperm count. Men with decreased total motile sperm counts show not only diminished

Table 3 Outcome of GIFT in the Tygerberg group in patients with positive antisperm antibodies on the sperm. Reproduced from Acosta *et al.* (1994)[24] with permission of the American Society for Reproductive Medicine

	Fert. rate (%)	*Total preg. rate transfer (%)*	*Term preg. rate transfer (%)*	*Abortion rate (%)*
Study group (54 patients, 89 cycles)	27.1[e]	28.1[a]	16.9[c]	33.3
N (>14% normal) (26 patients, 49 cycles)	33.9	36.7	22.4	28.0
G pattern (25 patients, 35 cycles)	19.1	20.0	11.4	23.1
P pattern (3 patients, 5 cycles)	0	0	0	0
Control group (89 patients, 89 cycles)	62.9[f]	43.8[b]	32.6[d]	23.2
N (>14% normal) (49 patients, 49 cycles)	70.6	51.0	36.7	38.9
G pattern (35 patients, 35 cycles)	52.3	37.1	28.6	42.9
P pattern (5 patients, 5 cycles)	42.8	20.0	20.0	0

Fert. = fertility; preg. = pregnancy; [a] versus [b] $P=0.0288$; [c] versus [d] $P=0.0150$; [e] versus [f] $P<0.0001$

incidence of pregnancy in their partners, but also a dramatic increase in the incidence of early pregnancy wastage[19].

IMMUNOLOGICAL INFERTILITY

The problem of standardizing diagnostic procedures and lack of good means of treatment for sperm antibodies in either or both partners were causes of inadequate identification of this infertility problem.

The MAR test[22] was used to screen all the males for the presence of antibodies. If the test showed >10% binding of motile sperm, the direct immunobead test was done[23]. The semen specimen was considered positive if >20% of the sperm showed binding to the immunobeads.

A matched controlled retrospective review to investigate the influence of antisperm antibodies on the sperm surface on the outcome of GIFT was done[24]. Fifty-four GIFT cycles were done in these patients. These couples were matched with controls with negative antisperm antibodies, by wives' stimulation protocol and baseline semen analysis. Study and control groups were divided according to sperm morphology pattern in normal, good and poor prognosis subgroups for comparison.

The pregnancy and fertilization rates of supernumerary preovulatory oocytes were taken as outcome measures (Table 3).

The fertilization rate in the study group was significantly lower (27.1%) than in the control group (62.9%). Total and term pregnancy rates in the study group (28.1% and 16.9%) were also significantly lower when compared with their control counterparts (43.8%). The abortion rate in the study group was 33% ± 9.4% and 23.2% abortions were recorded in the control group (not significant) (Table 3).

The presence of antisperm antibodies on the sperm surface clearly impairs the outcome of the GIFT treatment of these patients. This is also

Table 4 Review of published prospective, randomized studies with concurrent controls comparing IVF and uterine embryo transfer with GIFT or ZIFT (including transfer of embryos). No significant differences in pregnancy or implantation rates were found for any of the studies. Reproduced from Abyholm and Tanbo (1993)[29] with permission of Rapid Science Publishing

Author	*Indications*	*Pregnancy rate (%)*			*Implantation rate (%)*		
		IVF-ET	*GIFT*	*ZIFT*	*IVF-ET*	*GIFT*	*ZIFT*
Leeton *et al.*	Unexplained infertility	20	19				
Tanbo *et al.*	Unexplained infertility/ endometriosis/male infertility	46	26	38	16	7	10
Amso *et al.*	Unexplained infertility/ endometriosis/male infertility	17		29	9		16
Balmaceda *et al.*	Ovum donation	55		58	17		21
Ron-El *et al.*	Unexplained infertility/ male infertility	38		38	19		15
Tournaye *et al.*	Male infertility	22		27	10		12

shown in the impaired fertilization rate of supernumerary oocytes where the influence of morphology can clearly be seen (Table 3). Retrieval of at least 500 000 motile spermatozoa for GIFT is, however, important to warrant success[25]. The GIFT procedure appears to be a safe and effective treatment modality for male immunological infertility; as previously stated by us, assisted reproduction has an important place in the treatment of these patients[25]. The use of corticosteroids must be limited only to those cases where not enough motile spermatozoa (>500 000/mL) can be obtained for GIFT.

ZIFT AND TRANSTUBAL PROCEDURES

Some authors are of the opinion that the ZIFT procedure seems to make more sense because the clinician is assured that fertilization has taken place, which is not the case with the GIFT procedure[26]. Diedrich[27] described the transvaginal sonographic oocyte retrieval, IVF and ET into the Fallopian tube transvaginally as a treatment of male infertility.

Higher pregnancy rates are reported following ZIFT or tubal embryo transfer than after GIFT. Amso and Shaw[28] reviewed the different publications and found that many of these reports are either non-randomized studies or retrospective analyses, have no clearly defined inclusion criteria, have no controls or use only historical controls, or suffer from a combination of the above faults. The few prospective randomized studies performed generally fail to show a higher pregnancy rate with ZIFT or GIFT compared with IVF-ET (Table 4)[29]. We propose GIFT as a good assisted reproductive method for the treatment of male infertility with especially satisfactory results in the low morphology groups in spite of potentially low fertilization results *in vitro* (Table 5)[20].

Table 5 Fertilization rate of oocytes in patients with normal morphology 0–14% and >14%. Reproduced from Kruger *et al.* (1993)[20] with permission of the Hemisphere Publishing Corporation

Sperm morphology (%)	*Fertilization rate (%)*
0–4	18[a]
5–14	39[b]
>14	73[c]

[a] versus [b] P=0.0005; [a] versus [c] P=0.0001; [b] versus [c] P=0.0001

In an article by Grow *et al.*[30] it is interesting to note that in their P pattern group, the ongoing pregnancy rate is 14% versus 26.5% in the patients with higher morphology (Table 6). Comparable GIFT pregnancy rates are reported from the Tygerberg group (15% versus 23.3%) where the same morphology criteria are used (Table 1).

In light of the current literature, it is therefore our opinion that different units must follow the method of treatment with which they feel comfortable. We favor the GIFT method of treatment because it is easy to perform and treatment is completed in one session. Usually, the whole procedure takes less than 25 min. As in IVF, excess embryos can be frozen for future use. More prospective randomized controlled studies are, however, needed on the role of IVF, ZIFT and GIFT on male factor infertility.

Table 6 Patient characteristics and results in a Tygerberg retrospective cohort study

Characteristic	*P pattern*	*Controls*
No. of cycles	172	172
Age of wife*	35.5±3.9	35.4±3.8
Peak estradiol*	982±653	968±603
Preovulatory eggs per retrieval	8.3±6.2	79.9±6.1
Fertilization rate (%)	80.8 (1076/1332)	91.3 (1224/1340)**
High grade transfer (%)	65 (98/150)	66 (110/166)
No. of embryos transferred per transfer*	3.6±1.1	3.7±1.0
Implantation rate (%)*	7.4 (40/538)	11.9 (70/590)***
Miscarriage rate (%)*	30 (9/30)	23 (13/57)
Ongoing pregnancy per transfer (%)	14 (21/150)	26.5 (44/166)****

* Values are mean±SD; ** P<0.0001, controls versus P pattern; *** P<0.02, controls versus P pattern; **** P<0.01, controls versus P pattern

References

1. Steptoe, P. C. and Edwards, R. C. (1978). Birth after reimplantation of a human embryo. *Lancet*, **2**, 366
2. Asch, R. H., Ellsworth, L. R., Balmaceda, J. P. and Wang, P. C. (1984). Pregnancy following translaparoscopic gamete intrafallopian transfer (GIFT). *Lancet*, **2**, 1034–5
3. Asch, R. H., Balmaceda, J. P., Ellsworth, L. R. and Wang, P. C. (1985). Gamete intrafallopian transfer (GIFT): a new treatment for infertility. *Int. J. Fertil.*, **30**, 41–5
4. Matson, P. L., Blackledge, D. G., Richardson, P. A., Turner, S. R., Yovich, J. M. and Yovich, J. L. (1987). The role of gamete intrafallopian transfer (GIFT) in the treatment of oligospermic infertility. *Fertil. Steril.*, **48**, 608–12
5. Guastella, G., Cefalu, E., Ciriminna, R., Comparetto, G., Gullo, D., Palermo, R., Salerno, P., Amodeo, G. and Cittadini, E. (1986). One year's experience with the GIFT method. *Acta Eur. Fertil.*, **17**, 93–7
6. Kruger, T. F., Menkveld, R., Stander, F. S. H., Lombard, C. J., Van der Merwe, J. P., Van Zyl, J. A. and Smith, K. A. (1986). Sperm morphologic features as a prognostic factor in *in vitro* fertilization. *Fertil. Steril.*, **46**, 1118–23
7. Devroey, P., Braeckmans, P. and Smitz, I. (1986). Pregnancy after translaparoscopic zygote-intrafallopian transfer in a patient with sperm antibodies. *Lancet*, **1**, 1329
8. Balmaceda, J. P., Gestaldi, C., Remohi, J., Borrero, C., Ord, T. and Asch, R. H. (1988). Tubal embryo transfer as a treatment of infertility due to male factor. *Fertil. Steril.*, **50**, 476–9
9. Wildemann, R., Noss, U. and Hepp, H. (1989). Gamete intra-Fallopian transfer in male sub-fertility. *Hum. Reprod.*, **4**, 408–11
10. Kruger, T. F., Van der Merwe, J. P., Stander, F. S. H., Menkveld, R., Van den Heever, A. D., Kopper, K., Odendaal, H. J., Van Zyl, J. A. and De Villier, J. N. (1986). Results of the *in vitro* fertilization programme at Tygerberg Hospital: phases II and III. *S. Afr. Med. J.*, **69**, 297–300
11. Van der Merwe, J. P., Kruger, T. F., Lombard, C. J. and Muller, L. M. (1987). Ovulation induction for *in vitro* fertilization in Tygerberg Hospital. *S. Afr. Med. J.*, **71**, 515–17
12. Glass, R. H. and Ericson, R. J. (1978). Intrauterine insemination of isolated motile sperm. *Fertil. Steril.*, **29**, 535–8
13. Paulson, J. D., Polakoski, K. and Leto, S. (1979). Further characterization of glass wool column filtration of human semen. *Fertil. Steril.*, **32**, 125–6
14. Kruger, T. F., Acosta, A. A., Simmons, K. F., Swanson, R. J., Matta, I. F. and Oehninger, S. (1988). Predictive value of abnormal sperm morphology in *in vitro* fertilization. *Fertil. Steril.*, **49**, 112–17
15. Veeck, L. L. and Maloney, M. (1986). Insemination and fertilization. In Jones, H. W. Jr., Jones, G. S., Hodgen, G. D. and Rosenwaks, Z. (eds.) In Vitro *Fertilization – Norfolk*, pp. 168, 82. (Baltimore: Williams and Wilkins)
16. Van der Merwe, J. P., Kruger, T. F., Swart, Y. and Lombard, C. J. (1992). The role of oocyte maturity in the treatment of infertility because of teratozoospermia and normozoospermia with gamete intrafallopian transfer. *Fertil. Steril.*, **58**, 581–6
17. Oehninger, S., Acosta, A. A., Morshedi, M., Veeck, L., Swanson, R. J., Simmons, K. and Rosenwaks, Z. (1988). Corrective measures and pregnancy outcome in *in vitro* fertilization in patients with severe morphology abnormalities. *Fertil. Steril.*, **50**, 283–7
18. Khan, I., Camus, M., Staessen, C., Wisanto, A.,

Devroey, P. and Van Steirteghem, A. C. (1988). Success rate in gamete intrafallopian transfer using low and high concentrations of washed spermatozoa. *Fertil. Steril.*, **50**, 922–7

19. Guzick, D. S., Balmaceda, J. P., Ord, T. and Asch, R. H. (1989). The importance of egg and sperm factors in predicting the likelihood of pregnancy from gamete intrafallopian transfer. *Fertil. Steril.*, **52**, 795–800
20. Kruger, T. F., Franken, D. R., Stander, F. S. H., Swart, Y. and Van der Merwe, J. P. (1993). Effect of semen characteristics on pregnancy rate in a gamete intrafallopian transfer program. *Arch. Androl.*, **31**, 127–31
21. Rodriguez-Rigau, R. J., Ayala, D., Grurert, G. M., Woodward, R. M., Lotze, E. C., Feste, J. R., Gibbons, W., Smith, K. D. and Steinberger, E. (1989). Relationship between the results of sperm analysis and GIFT. *J. Androl.*, **10**, 139–44
22. Henry, W. F., Stredonska, J. and Lake, R. A. (1982). Mixed erythrocyte spermatozoa antiglobulin reaction (MAR) test for IgA and sperm antibodies in subfertile males. *Fertil. Steril.*, **37**, 108–12
23. Clarke, G. N., Stojandoff, A. and Cauchi, M. N. (1982). Immunoglobulin class of sperm-bound antibodies in semen. *Proceedings of the Fifth International Symposium on Immunology of Reproduction*, May, Bulgaria
24. Acosta, A. A., van der Merwe, J. P., Doncel, G., Kruger, T. F., Sayilgan, A., Franken, D. R. and Kolm, P. (1994). Fertilization efficiency of morphologically abnormal spermatozoa in assisted reproduction is further impaired by antisperm antibodies on the male partner's sperm. *Fertil. Steril.*, **62**, 826–33
25. Van der Merwe, J. P., Kruger, T. F., Windt, M.-L., Hulme, V. A. and Menkveld, R. (1990). Treatment of male sperm autoimmunity by using the gamete intrafallopian transfer procedure with washed spermatozoa. *Fertil. Steril.*, **53**, 682–7
26. Bayer, S. R., Lee, M. A., Robert McInnes, D. and Cardone, V. R. S. (1993). *In vitro* fertilization and male factor infertility: a critical review and update. *Ass. Reprod. Rev.*, **3**, 244–54
27. Diedrich, K., Bauer, O., Werner, A., Van der Ven, H., Al-Hasani, D. and Krebs, D. (1991). Transvaginal intratubal embryo transfer: a new treatment of male infertility. *Hum. Reprod.*, **6**, 672–5
28. Amso, N. N. and Shaw, R. W. (1993). A critical appraisal of assisted reproduction techniques. *Hum. Reprod.*, **8**, 168–74
29. Abyholm, T. and Tanbo, T. (1993). GIFT, ZIFT, and related techniques. *Curr. Opin. Obstet. Gynecol.*, **5**, 615–22
30. Grow, D. R., Oehninger, S., Seltman, H. J., Toner, J. P., Swanson, R. J., Kruger, T. F. and Muasher, S. J. (1994). Sperm morphology as diagnosed by strict criteria: probing the impact of teratozoospermia on fertilization rate and pregnancy outcome in a large *in vitro* fertilization population. *Fertil. Steril.*, **62**, 559–67

Artificial insemination 1: using a donor's sperm

29

M. Morshedi

HISTORY

With lessons learned from new assisted reproductive techniques such as *in vitro* fertilization (IVF), we have been able to improve the outcome of therapeutic insemination. Realistically, the process of therapeutic insemination is carried out in almost all *in vitro* and *in vivo* assisted reproductive techniques. However, therapeutic insemination mainly refers to such *in vivo* techniques as intravaginal, cervical, uterine, tubal and peritoneal inseminations.

The term 'artificial insemination' was initially used in animal husbandry as a science of breeding. It was, and is, also used for humans. Because of the negative connotation associated with the term 'artificial', replacement with a more descriptive and appropriate term, therapeutic insemination, has been suggested[1]. In this chapter, therapeutic donor insemination (TDI) and artificial insemination by donor (AID) will be used interchangeably and will refer to the exclusive use of cryopreserved semen unless otherwise stated.

Recent advances in the field of reproduction have brought us a multitude of assisted reproductive techniques. Strategy for the management of infertility, however, remains complex. It often requires a compromise between the diagnostic methods, their efficacy and complexity, and the choices of treatment with their own risks, costs and efficacy. In almost all instances of infertility management, therapeutic insemination combined with sperm manipulation techniques is one of the first options practised. It has been one of the oldest methods of assisted reproduction and often the most cost-efficient procedure.

The first known report of artificial insemination was hypothetical, dating back to approximately 222 AD. A Talmudic document entails an academic debate between a Rabbi and one of his students on the accidental insemination of a female by semen previously deposited in the bathwater in which she bathed. Because the woman unknowingly became pregnant, said the Rabbi, she could not be at fault[1]. The same reasoning has also been used by young females in some strict societies, even in the twentieth century.

The first alleged report of artificial insemination dating back to 1322 had, unfortunately, a destructive objective. It relates to the classic Arabic tale of how an enemy secretly inseminated a pure strain of very valuable Arabic mares with the semen from inferior stallions[1].

The first documented case of artificial insemination in humans goes back to early 1790. The Englishman John Hunter, one of the pioneers of modern cryobiology, advised a London cloth merchant who had hypospadias to inject his 'seminal fluid' with a prewarmed syringe into his wife's vagina. A pregnancy was achieved, although it is unclear whether or not Hunter did the insemination[1]. In 1838, Girault[2] of France treated a woman with a 'long cervix' and a 'narrow ostium' with the husband's semen blown into her uterus through a hollow tube. He later treated nine additional patients similarly and seven conceived.

The first artificial insemination using the husband sample (AIH) in the United States was performed in 1866 by Dr J. Marion Sims of the Women's Hospital in New York City[2]. He performed 55 intracervical (ICI) and intrauterine (IUI) inseminations using normal semen samples obtained from the vagina after intercourse. Only one pregnancy ensued, but the success rate might have been higher had Sims not mistakenly believed that ovulation occurred during menstruation.

The first reported TDI was performed in 1884, but it was not reported until 25 years later by the donor himself. The procedure was performed by Dr William

Pancoast of Jefferson Medical College in Philadelphia to treat a case of 'postgonococcal azoospermia'. The insemination apparently came about as a result of the jokes made by some medical students, one of whom, the best-looking member of the class, became the semen donor. An IUI was performed without the knowledge of the couple. When a pregnancy resulted the husband was informed of the actual happening. Fortunately he was pleased with the outcome, but he asked that his wife not be told[2].

The credit for TDI practice, however, goes to Dr Robert Dickinson of New York City who began the practice in the early 1890s. He, one of his students, Dr Sophia Kleegman, and Dr Margaret Jackson, of England, made great contributions to the acceptance of the procedure as a lawful, legitimate, practical and somewhat acceptable way of overcoming childlessness[2]. Nevertheless, some religious authorities still regard TDI as a form of non-coital reproduction and consider it unacceptable. Islam forbids it, Roman Catholic Holy Office rejects it and Orthodox Jews, Lutherans and most Anglican churches oppose it. From 1930 on, Dr Kleegman and others used both TDI and artificial insemination by husband (AIH) routinely in their practices. Dr Kleegman performed TDI on four couples between 1930 and 1934, on 10 couples from 1935 to 1939 and 181 couples between 1945 and 1959. Inseminations were timed based on basal body temperature (BBT), and many of them were ICIs and some IUIs using whole semen. Few cases of complications, such as 'trichomonal vaginalis' and 'streptococcic pelvic infections', were reported. In one of her reports in 1954[1], Dr Kleegman gave a cumulative pregnancy rate of 68% after one to six treatment cycles of TDI. It is interesting to note that some of the couples requesting TDI were denied the procedure because they did not meet the 'required standards and emotional adjustments'[1]. In a survey conducted in 1941 it was reported that 5164 of 7642 (67.6%) infertility specialists used TDI in their practices[1]. The Office of Technology Assessment conducted a survey and reported annual births of 30 000–60 000 from TDI in the United States[3].

INDICATIONS

As one of the unique methods of assisted reproduction, TDI has been the subject of major emotional, legal and religious issues often not associated with any other procedures. Although infertility of the husband is the prime indication for TDI, many other applications can also be listed (Table 1). However, advances in reproductive technology have given patients hope that some of the indications for TDI may be treatable without the aid of TDI. Methods of sperm microaspiration from the epididymis and testis, sperm microinjection, advances in understanding the organic basis of ejaculatory dysfunctions, preimplantation genetic diagnosis, gene therapy and cryopreservation of spermatozoa and haploid cell lines in cancer patients may eventually help couples overcome their infertility without submitting to TDI.

Table 1 Indications for TDI

Continue to be practised	*May become obsolete*
Azoospermia	Oligo-astheno-teratozoospermia
Single female	Genetic disorders
	Chemotherapy
	Ejaculatory defects
	Sexual dysfunction
	Repeated failed fertilization
	Vasectomy, immunological infertility

PSYCHOLOGICAL AND LEGAL ASPECTS OF TDI

Infertility may not appear to be a disease in the minds of the public. However, it is generally perceived by many couples who experience it as an enormous emotional burden. Since infertility has traditionally been considered to be more female-related, the crisis becomes even more disturbing when it is related to the male. Even if some couples have a slight chance of spontaneous conception after prolonged exposure, stress from the emotional aspect of infertility and the prospect of TDI may further delay such success. In a psychological analysis of patients considering TDI, it was reported that the psychologist's rating of the couples was predictive of pregnancy rates. Those rated as 'excellent candidates' gave a cumulative pregnancy rate of 59%, those rated as 'acceptable candidates' gave a 41% rate, and those considered 'psychologically at risk' gave a 14% pregnancy rate[4]. Evidence for the development of stress-related secondary anovulation and luteal phase defects in some patients has been reported[5]. Batzer *et al.*[6] presented several studies related to the association between stress and anovulation in TDI patients.

Dealing with anxiety

Tradition plays a major role in associating infertility with sexual inadequacy, failure and lack of fulfillment. To most, the presence of a child completes the family structure, fulfills our dreams of the future and gives us a sense of wholeness. We have been raised with societal expectations that there are only two options available for having children: one, to get married; the other, to adopt. Adoption may be seen by some couples as confirmation of their infertility, but the unconventional (natural) appearance of TDI prevents them from thinking that way. Lack of knowledge about TDI brings about anxiety when it is suggested as an option. Both healthcare professional and the patients themselves must bear the burden of dealing with the emotional factors associated with TDI. Knowledge brings understanding and comfort. Emotional factors of TDI can be dealt with successfully if they are understood and if both the healthcare providers and the patients have the necessary endurance to explore all of its aspects. Couples dealing with their infertility perceive themselves as being different and deviant. They must be given time to recover from the shock that overwhelms many men, and it is wise not to accept the couples too soon after the husband's sterility has been ascertained. We must provide them with the information that, unlike natural procreation where partners choose each other without any medical considerations, TDI is medically controlled in an attempt to minimize the risks. They need help to understand that TDI could provide them with bonding to the child from the outset of pregnancy and that it is more comparable with the natural decision to 'bear children, not to rear them'. All facets must be discussed with the couples when TDI is suggested. These include methods of donor selection and screening, cryopreservation of samples and the advantages and disadvantages of cryopreservation, methods of selection of donors for the couples and their role and control in the selection process, costs, success rate and the legal issues related to TDI and the resulting births. They must be told that they can discontinue TDI anytime they wish. The possibility of disappointment must also be discussed. Both partners should be encouraged to become involved with the process and be allowed to express their feelings and ask questions. To most couples who desire to initiate TDI, although the issue remains highly personal and confidential, nothing is more helpful than hearing from those who have already experienced TDI and it is highly recommended when such a possibility exists. Secrecy and privacy issues have made it difficult for the couples to gain first-hand exposure to the experience of those who have already experienced TDI. Reports related to the emotional aspects of TDI are often published in scientific journals and may not always be accessible to the couples. It is recommended that both the positive and the negative reports (if any) be provided to and discussed with the couples. Knowledge brings understanding and the expertise to cope with the stress.

Prediction of success after TDI is often difficult; therefore, the couples should have a set plan for their efforts to conceive. Based on the available medical information, method(s) of insemination and treatment, and their emotional and financial tolerance, a plan for the couple could be constructed. The plan should give the couple adequate information about the number of treatment cycles, the cost and a guarded opinion as to the time involved in achieving success. The plan should also include future courses of action in the event the initial plan fails and conception does not occur. Without such a plan, the couple's emotional and financial drain could be enormous.

Genealogical confusion and legality

The issue of biological bewilderment and mental health development have long been the core of discussion in adoption and, more recently, about the children born through TDI. In one study[7], the concept of genealogical bewilderment in children born through TDI was investigated. It was concluded that, where family relationships and attention to the child are adequate, there is no reason why ancestral knowledge should be a prerequisite of mental health. In a controlled quantitative assessment, Kovacs *et al.*[8] compared the psychosocial development of children of the same age and sex.

They found no differences in those children conceived through the TDI method and those conceived naturally. In another study of 54 couples[9] who gave birth to one or more children through TDI it was found that they overwhelmingly preferred TDI, although 72% of them had previously considered adoption. 'The desire to be pregnant and give birth, to have biological and genetic links to the child, and to provide for bonding from the outset were important considerations for many couples in the study'[9]. Czyba and Chevret[10] have written an excellent report on the subject.

Almost all states in the United States have implemented laws that recognize the recipient and her consenting husband as the legal parents. Legislation in these states has established the legitimacy of the offspring by giving any child born through TDI full legal equality with the children conceived naturally. The laws state that a male who donates his semen for the insemination of a female other than his legal wife has no parental rights over the child born as a result of such a procedure.

Evaluation of suitability of applicants

Finally, there is a debate on whether couples considering TDI should also be evaluated for their readiness and fitness, as are adoptive applicants. Many child welfare advocates indicate that they should be evaluated. With the current atmosphere of personal freedom, and the fact that 45 of 100 children born in the mid-1970s in the United States are living in one-parent families of all socioeconomic groups prior to age 18[11], consideration and implementation of such evaluations often prove to be very difficult. Undoubtedly, there should be some degree of observation and evaluation protecting couples from what they may not comprehend under such stressful conditions, as well as, ultimately, the child to be born.

In 1954, Kleegman[1] reported that 19 of 154 patients requesting TDI were rejected because they did not meet the eligibility requirements. Seventeen couples were not accepted because required standards of emotional adjustment were not met. Two couples were not accepted because the husbands were 27 and 29 years older than their wives. Kleegman[1] describes the standards required of the couples as:

(1) each must be mature, well adjusted, and feel they are well married. It must never be considered to 'save our marriage.' That is too much of a burden to place on any child. A shaky marriage is a definite contradiction to donor insemination. (2) The couple must have a true love of children, and should prefer this procedure to adoption. (3) They must be en rapport in regard to their mutual problem(s), and must both prefer this method of solving it.

In some instances, a couple may request to mix the donor and the husband samples for insemination. Although there are reports (see later) that this may not be advisable, the very nature of the request should alert us that the couple may not be fully ready for the procedure. A delay in TDI, combined with additional counseling, may be appropriate.

DONOR SELECTION AND SCREENING

Page 495–6 in the Appendix outlines the criteria for screening sperm donors at our center. There are variations in selection and screening of sperm donors from center to center. The American Fertility Society (AFS) 1993 guidelines[12] for gamete donation describes thoroughly the selection and screening process for sperm donors. The American Association of Tissue Banks (AATB) has adopted similar guidelines, with the exception that testing of the semen be carried out on a weekly basis[13].

It has been our experience, and that of many others, that the frequency of donor testing should be changed to every 2–3 months, without a change in the 60 month quarantine period. Seroconversion for infectious diseases such as HIV, and exposure to *Chlamydia* and herpes, may occur within the 6-month waiting period of the quarantine. Testing every 2–3 months may escalate the costs associated with sperm banking; however, the sooner the seroconversion is detected, the fewer the patients exposed to the samples. Moreover, this would limit the financial loss to the laboratory should it become necessary to discard 6 months of quarantined samples.

Sexually transmitted diseases

Donors must be tested for a variety of sexually transmitted diseases (see page 495 in the Appendix).

Urethral swabs for identification for *Neisseria gonorrhea*, *Chlamydia* species, ureaplasma and genital herpes should be made. If newer polymerase chain reaction (PCR) methods are not available, new techniques such as DNA probes which are much more sensitive than the classical methods should be used, although it must be emphasized that DNA probe tests do not differentiate between the current active infection and inactive stages. Although not very sensitive (68%), culture methods are capable of detecting the active stages. Since rejection of donors with any positive results is recommended, the issue of cultures becomes irrelevant. Weekly tests of semen for gonorrhea should also be conducted (this practice is recommended by the AATB). Each semen sample should be evaluated for the presence of *Trichomonas* and excessive number of round cells (e.g. white blood cells). Samples with *Trichomonas* should be discarded and the donor investigated for the infection. Samples with the round cells >1 million should be evaluated carefully. The issue must be discussed with the donor and attempts made to identify the possible reasons for the high number of round cells. If the number of round cells is not excessive and it is an occasional occurrence, samples should be processed with Percoll to separate the cells and be cryopreserved as 'IUI ready' (see page 503 in the Appendix). Since *Trichomonas* remains inactive at room temperature, semen must be evaluated at or near 37°C.

Urethral swabs are often uncomfortable to donors. However, approval by the Food and Drug Administration (FDA) of a newly developed and very sensitive (95%) urine test for *Chlamydia* DNA using polymerase chain reaction (PCR) has made these easier to conduct more frequently[14]. There are reports that the PCR method can also be used to detect the presence of *Chlamydia* in semen samples of donors shown to be negative using DNA probe methods[15,16]. The detection of *Chlamydia* may prove to be very important in the light of new findings that it may be associated with the development of antisperm antibodies, both in males and females[15]. Additionally, serological testing of the female for *Chlamydia* has been reported to be of more prognostic value for the detection of tubal abnormalities than hysterosalpingography[17]. Since cross-infection is a certainty, identification of *Chlamydia* in donors and donor samples is of great value.

Human immunodeficiency viruses

It is essential to screen all potential semen donors for the presence of antibodies against human immunodeficiency viruses types 1 and 2 (HIV_1 and HIV_2) and for human T-cell lymphotropic virus-1 (HTLV-1). Human T-cell lymphotropic virus is a human type C retrovirus associated etiologically with adult T-cell leukemia and with a demyelinating neurological disorder termed 'tropical spastic paraparesis', or HTLV-1 associated myelopathy. It is endemic in the Caribbean, southeastern Japan and some areas of Africa and the United States. In addition to those patients with the conditions mentioned above, it may also be found in intravenous drug abusers and some healthy individuals. Although serological testing of donors (Appendix 1) is conducted for HIV_1 and HIV_2, the recent trend is toward HIV antigen detection by the PCR method. Detection of HIV antigen combined with frequent serological testing and the 180-day quarantine has made TDI much safer to carry out. Advances in molecular biology and PCR technology have given us the capability of detecting viral and bacterial DNA. In the near future, it may be possible to use fresh semen for TDI again.

It is recommended that tests for most infectious diseases, especially HIV_1 and HIV_2, be repeated every 1–3 months once donors are accepted into the program. It is also recommended that donors be excluded who have positive antibody for HIV_1 and HIV_2, and confirmed to be negative with the Western blot analysis. Many couples considering TDI question whether the 180-day quarantine period is sufficient to eliminate the possibility of HIV transmission. Imagawa *et al.*[18] initially reported that seroconversion after the exposure to HIV may take as long as 42 months. The report created immense interest; however, to date no investigator has been able to confirm this initial finding. The original assumption of delayed seroconversion has been modified and the window period for HIV seroconversion now is believed to be around 45 days[19]. Advocating the use of fresh donor semen, Nachtigall[20] has written an excellent review on the perceived risks of HIV infection though semen and has concluded that, with certain precautions taken into consideration, use of fresh donor semen can be considered relatively safe. He compares the risk of

HIV infection through semen with that of blood transfusion and states that the risk is negligible. Data from blood banks indicate that only one HIV infection has occurred among 4000 men being transfused when undergoing cardiac surgery. Based on these data, the highest risk estimates appear to be around 1:36 000 per unit of blood transfused. Additional data from 17 million blood donations registered at the American Red Cross are indicative of a residual risk for HIV infection of 1:153 000 for both sexes and 1:108 000 for male individuals. This difference is due to the fact that more men than women are infected with HIV. The risk is even lower if donors are from the geographically low risk areas. More recent data put the risk estimate from blood transfusion at 1:225 000 per unit of blood for both genders. Until 1991, a total of 130 000 000 blood products tested for HIV and shown to be negative were used in the United States. Only 20 individuals became positive for HIV from the use of these blood products[20]. Reporting these data, Nachtigall expresses his opinion on the comparison between the risk of HIV infection from blood transfusion and receiving semen from a carefully selected and tested semen donor. He states that the risk of HIV infection through thoroughly tested fresh semen is even less than that of blood transfusion. The risk is lower because, compared to receiving blood, (1) deposition of semen in the vagina or processing it for IUI is less invasive and infectious; (2) compared to blood, semen contains fewer viral particles and white blood cells even in infected individuals; and (3) regular testing of semen donors for many other sexually transmitted diseases leads to the exclusion of high risk donors. The estimated risk for using a single semen sample from a low risk person is about 1:500 000 000; the risk for a single contact between an HIV positive and a seronegative female is <0.3%[20]. In a study of 34 seropositive men, p24 viral antigen was found in peripheral blood of all subjects (100%), whereas the antigen was found in 88% of their sera and only in 32% of their semen. In a similar study of 25 seropositive men, p24 was found in 75% of their blood but in only 16% of their semen. Nachtigall has presented data that the residual risk after HIV antibody testing of a male from the general population is about 1:100 and this risk will reduce to 1:1 000 000 if a face-to-face interview is conducted to explore the risk factors associated with the individual. The risk decreases even further to 1:10 000 000 if the individual is screened for major sexually transmitted diseases and the individual is tested for HIV antigen. The risk is further decreased to 1:1 000 000 000 if an intravaginal insemination is performed. Considering the higher success rate associated with the use of fresh semen and the associated emotional and economical advantages, Nachtigall concludes that we should utilize the extensive experience of blood banks with respect to HIV transmission and revisit the issue of exclusive use of cryopreserved semen for TDI. Fugger *et al.*[21] evaluated 207 seronegative donors for HIV antigen using the PCR method. No individual was found to be positive for the antigen. There has been no report on the predictability of HIV antigen testing with regard to the subsequent HIV seroconversions. However, acknowledging the time lapse required for seroconversion, testing of donors for HIV antigen may be advantageous. As far as answers to the couples' questions are concerned, it must be stated that although such a guarantee cannot be given, a combination of the 180-day quarantine, repeat HIV antibody evaluations at 1–3-month intervals, exclusion of risk group individuals, and perhaps HIV antigen testing, make such transmission less likely. Reports of transmission of HIV to recipients through cryopreserved semen after HIV testing and the 180-day quarantine are lacking. However, in Australia transmission from the cryopreserved semen of a single asymptomatic bisexual donor quarantined for 1–4 months to four of eight patients receiving these samples has been confirmed[22]. However, the other four patients who received cryopreserved samples of the same donor quarantined for 16–17 months remained uninfected[22]. It must be noted that the timing of semen cryopreservation and inseminations was approximately 3 years prior to the time when HIV antibody testing became available. Whether or not longer storage time may be protective against HIV remains to be investigated. Another report[23] is indicative of the seroconversion of one recipient among 176 patients undergoing 710 TDI cycles using fresh donor semen between 1978 and 1985 prior to the time of routine HIV testing. Of samples obtained from six donors, one was found to be HIV positive later upon testing.

Donors' sera should be tested for the presence of

hepatitis B surface antigen, total core antibody and the antibody against hepatitis C. Since elevation of alanine transferase (ALT) could be a prelude to hepatitis C virus (HCV) infection, it should be part of every donor evaluation. However, one note of caution is that the activity of this enzyme decreases upon freezing–thawing of serum[24]. Therefore, ALT tests must be conducted on serum kept at room temperature for only 1 day or refrigerated for a maximum of 3 days.

Cytomegalovirus

Cytomegalovirus (CMV), a member of the herpes virus group, is a major cause of congenital anomalies, surpassing even rubella virus. It is involved in microcephaly and brain damage, deafness, visual defects and occasionally fetal death. Most of the symptomatic cases have been associated with a primary infection acquired by the mother during pregnancy[25]. It has been identified in 2.4–3.2% of semen samples[26–28].

With regard to CMV testing, the recommendation and opinions vary. The American Fertility Society guidelines recommend serological testing of the donor for the presence of anti-CMV antibody (IgG). If the antibody test is positive samples of these donors should be given to seropositive patients only. It is recommended that the donors should also be evaluated for the presence of IgM against CMV and be excluded if positive. For those shown to be positive for the presence of IgG, both urine and semen cultures are also recommended. If either urine or semen cultures are positive, the donor should be rejected. Culture of urine and semen should be performed because it has been reported that the urine cultures could appear falsely to be negative. Some recommend rejection of CMV positive donors[5]. It is reported that there are several heterologous strains of CMV and one test may not represent identification of seropositivity to all strains. A seropositive recipient may be susceptible to these strains. Since more than 60% of the general population is seropositive for CMV[29], whether or not this practice is practical is a matter of debate. Seronegative recipients for CMV should definitely receive seronegative donors' samples. Pregnancy alters cell-mediated immunity as do many viral pathogens; therefore, pregnant women may be more susceptible to the infections by the viral agents and may develop more symptomatic reactions. As a result, CMV seronegative women should be warned to avoid contracting the infection, especially during the first 24 weeks of pregnancy. Young children often contract CMV from other children and pass it on to their parents. Special care must be taken not to have contact with the saliva or urine of young children. All diapers, tissues, glasses, utensils and other potentially contaminated items should be handled carefully. Hands must be washed thoroughly after any contact with these potential sources of contamination.

Karyotyping

With respect to karyotyping, analysis of major mutations for cystic fibrosis (CF) and the human papilloma virus (HPV), opinions vary widely. The American Fertility Society guidelines do not make such evaluations a requirement. Frequency of chromosomal balanced translocations, inversions or low level aneuploidy is about one per 500–1000[6,30]. Frequency of heterozygosity for CF in Caucasians is about one in every 25[31]. Human papilloma virus is a sexually transmitted viral pathogen involving the male urethra[25] and the recent evidence indicates the involvement of Types 16 and 18 HPV as etiologic agents for neoplasia of the female genital tract, such as cervical dysplasia and carcinoma-*in situ* of the vulva[32]. The presence of HPV deoxyribonucleic acid (DNA) in seminal fluid[33] and the detection of HPV gene sequence in sperm (though not proof for the presence of HPV) have been reported[34]. Decision-making with respect to screening of donors for these conditions is very difficult. Matthews *et al.*[35] karyotyped 172 potential donors and found one with a possible chromosomal abnormality. Perez *et al.*[36] reported that the study of 100 potential donors gave no justification for screening donors for chromosomal abnormalities. Selva *et al.*[37] reported that genetic screening of 676 prospective semen donors resulted in exclusion of 3% of candidates, acceptance of 47% with cumulative risk factors (see below) and the acceptance of 50% without restriction. In the absence of very comprehensive genetic screening for many heterozygosities, care must be taken to exclude donors with obvious genetic risks and screen donors with suspicious histories of chromosomal abnormalities, CF or HPV infection. For example, donors with wife, mother or sibling who have had a history of fetal wastage, such as stillborns, anomalous live-borns and repetitive spontaneous abortions should be screened. Although the significance of screening donors for these conditions has been questioned, considering the potential for grave consequences, testing of donors should be available at the request of the recipient.

The value of screening for conditions frequently observed in donors of specific race and ethnic origin cannot be disputed. Individuals of Mediterranean origin and Eastern European ancestry should be tested for β-thalassemia and other hemoglobin abnormalities via hemoglobin electrophoresis at both alkaline and acidic pHs. Individuals of Jewish ethnic origin, especially those of Eastern European descent, should be tested for the deficiency of hexosaminidase A and total (Tay-Sachs), preferably via testing of enzyme deficiency in serum. It is our experience that some French-Canadians may also show a higher incidence for enzyme deficiency. The predominantly Roman Catholic community of Iota, Louisiana, has been shown to have an unusually high incidence of Tay-Sachs. Asians should be screened for α-thalassemia, and blacks for sickle cell and β-thalassemia, both by hemoglobulin electrophoresis.

Additional optional tests, such as blood chemistry profile 12 or 19, urinalysis and culture, and perhaps unannounced urine drug screening (with the initial knowledge of the donor) may also be indicated. Dipstick testing of the urine collected after semen collection may show a trace amount of protein. Therefore, urine samples should be collected using the clean catch method prior to semen collection.

Although sterile collection of semen cannot be done, it should also be screened for excessive bacterial (e.g. group B streptococci) and yeasts/fungal growth (e.g. *Candida albicans*) at regular intervals. Asymptomatic vaginal colonization with group B hemolytic streptococci occurs in 4.6–40.6% of pregnant women[25]. It is a sexually transmitted infection and the transmission by the semen can cause pelvic inflammatory disease. Infection and colonization can lead to conditions such as chorioamnionitis, postpartum endometritis, premature rupture of the membrane and neonatal sepsis, premature labor and delivery[25]. Weekly or biweekly cultures of semen on blood agar and a suitable medium for the fungal growth is recommended. If positive, samples cryopreserved should be discarded. Infection must be investigated and, if there is no reason to become alarmed, the donor may be treated. He can start to donate only after the treatment is complete and the culture results indicate no infection. It is our experience that, with the current methods of cryopreservation and the media used, most of these bacteria will not survive the cryopreservation processes, but this does not make the practice of identifying potential sources of infection insignificant.

Donors should also be asked for their reasoning to become donors. Although the truth may not always be revealed, altruistic reasons or a combination of altruistic and compensatory reasons would be more preferable to compensatory reasons only. Those with unusual and suspicious traits and with extremely low mental capacity should be rejected. The age limit for sperm donors indicated by the AFS guidelines is 40 years, although the upper age limit of 55 years has been suggested[30]. Since advanced paternal age could also contribute to trisomies and some dominant mutations, older donors should be rejected. Proof of the donor's age must be observed.

ASSIGNING DONOR IDENTIFICATION CODES

Traditionally, donors are assigned identifying codes to protect their privacy after they are accepted into the programs. Some donors may be medical students or other professionals who may be in contact with the patients or clients in the future. Concern rises if a donor remembers (knows) his code and happens to meet a child, a patient or a client known to be the result of TDI from the same code that he remembers (knows). Additionally, the possibility of revealing the nature of conception and the donor code to the child by the parents may also exist. In search of his/her biological identity, the child may engage in activities such as contacting the laboratory from which the sample was obtained or even advertising nationally to identify the code. Although these thoughts and occurrences may be improbable and not considered to be significant, in response to these possibilities we have implemented a procedure to avoid informing donors of their assigned identification codes while eliminating the possibility of making the task of donor identification by the laboratory personnel difficult and error-prone.

PERSONALITY AND PSYCHOLOGICAL EVALUATION OF DONORS

Historically, more attention has been paid to match donors' physical characteristics with those of the husband than those of the wife. Nowadays, matches based on psychological and personality profiles are often requested by the couples. When extensive psychological evaluation of the donors is not possible, some basic parameters of donors' personality profiles should be investigated and provided. In one study[38], personality characteristics of 75 sperm donors were assessed using the Cattell 16PF test. It was found that this population of individuals was quite distinct in some personality traits from the general population. Features such as intelligence, boldness, willingness to help and take risks, were notable in the donor group. However, it is highly recommended that prospective donors demonstrating a high degree of 'unusualness', reflecting undesirable traits, those with easily recognizable low mental capacity, and those who are recognizably dependent on the sample compensation be excluded.

Matching donors and recipients

Consideration of physical traits, ethnic origin, blood type and Rh factor are desirable, but not complete. One important, often overlooked factor is the recipient's family medical history. The history must be obtained and, based on all available information, match(es) should be made and suggested to the couples. Submission of a donor list consisting of major physical characteristics, blood type, education and hobbies is not recommended. Undoubtedly, during the initial screening process, the presence of known risk elements in the donors' medical and genetic history will result in their exclusion. However, we must be concerned with more numerous elements that, although they do not constitute reasons for excluding the donors, could present much higher risk if the recipients have similar conditions. In other words, these factors do not constitute real risk unless they are present in both the donor and the recipient. These cumulative risk factors must be avoided. Examples are: selection by the couples of donors with cumulative risk factors which may not be exclusionary (e.g. one parent with late onset hypertension or Graves' disease) similar to those of the recipient (e.g. one or more family members with hypertension). With current knowledge and scientific ability, we are unable to change the genetic profile (being) of the recipient. However, the selection process can be made much safer when all physical and medical aspects of the matching are considered and the confounding factors are avoided. Although the final decision of accepting or rejecting donor matches rests exclusively with the couples, they must be counseled and helped in the selection process. They need such support, medically and emotionally.

Many other factors in the medical history of the recipient may be important for the matching consideration. The recipient's history of blood transfusion should be investigated for possible antibody formation against minor blood group antigens. Although there are remedies if pregnancy is achieved after the initial sensitization, if possible donors should be chosen without such antigens (especially if the antibody titre is shown to be high). Recipients with prevalent conditions such as severe myopia, breast cancer, alcoholism, obesity, allergic reactions, arthritis and autoimmune diseases in the family should be specifically matched with donors devoid of similar conditions. Recent advances in molecular biology have enabled us to gain more knowledge about the factors associated with the polygenic and multifactorial disorders and their risks of inheritance. One of the most striking associations is the increased prevalence of human leukocyte antigens (HLA) DR1/DR2, DQ1, A2, and B27 haplotypes in certain rheumatic diseases. Recipients with a strong history of ankylosing spondylitis exhibit HLA B27 haplotype. Donors with similar HLA have a 90-fold increased risk of developing the condition some time in their lives[30,39]. Hydatidiform mole has been found to be more frequent in women having HLA A1 and is more common in couples with partial compatibility of the B locus[40]. Similarly, the association of other HLA antigens such as DR3 with Graves' disease[39],

DR8 with autoimmune hypothyroidism[41], HLA A10 with the tendency of rheumatic fever to lead to cardiac involvement[42], DR7/DQ2 with seasonal allergic pollenosis[43] and DR3/DR4 with Type I insulin-dependent diabetes[44,45] are some other examples. Whether or not these apparently insignificant factors should seriously be considered is a matter of debate. A recipient with a strong history of such conditions should be informed of possible complications and testing of the donor be performed, if requested.

Since donors are not routinely screened for chromosome abnormalities, Verp[39] questions whether or not it should be considered for all recipients. In a study of 1942 women karyotyped, 21 anomalies were found[39]. Verp[39] also reported on a study that found five of 156 women participating in TDI had chromosomal abnormalities. Combining the two studies, Verp[39] found a 2.1% incidence of chromosomal abnormalities which appears to be high. The high incidence, if real, may be a contributing factor in the couples' infertility.

If possible, all recipients should receive CMV seronegative donor samples. Otherwise, CMV negative donors should be matched with CMV negative recipients. It is also appropriate to test recipients for major infectious (especially sexually transmitted) diseases and immunity against rubella. Association of chlamydial infection with tubal infertility[15] and *Ureaplasma urealyticum* with higher degree of spontaneous abortion[46] are some examples exemplifying the need for screening the recipients for infectious diseases.

Finally, recipients with known major dominant conditions, with recessive X-linked conditions for which there is no prenatal diagnosis, or those presenting with major mental disorders, should be advised not to consider TDI. Recipients may be advised to consider donated eggs or embryos, although it may be very difficult. Some should be advised to remain childless.

Consanguinity and the number of pregnancies from a donor

The issue of consanguinity is one of the major concerns in the minds of couples considering TDI, as well as for healthcare professionals. Not only is it socially undesirable, but offspring resulting from such matings would be at higher risk for genetic disorders and perinatal mortality[6,39]. According to the guidelines of AFS, a limit of 10 pregnancies or less from a donor should be set. In a study of children born through TDI in England[39] it was calculated that, based on 10 pregnancies per donor, only one possible mating could occur every 50–100 years. Others[39] have also reached similar conclusions. In a 1979 survey[39] an annual pregnancy of 6000 to 10 000 was reported. Seventy-seven per cent of the respondents in the survey had never used donors for more than six pregnancies. Approximately 5.7% had used donors for 15 or more pregnancies per donor. In a national survey in 1987[3], the annual pregnancy through TDI was estimated as between 30 000 and 60 000. The risk of unplanned consanguinity depends on a number of factors. With the size of the population involved, the geographic distribution of pregnancies, the mobility of the population and the high frequency of mating across ethnic groups, the risk of involuntary consanguinity should remain negligible. However, a limit of 10–15 pregnancies per donor is highly recommended.

Insemination with donor and husband samples mixed

To become more acceptable to some couples, they may request mixing donor's and husband's samples for insemination. It may be an indication that they have not resolved the issue of using TDI as a solution to their infertility. It is very important to explore any emotional uncertainty about TDI before the procedure is initiated. It is our experience that, if the request is initiated by the wife, the emotional readiness of the couple will be of less concern than when such a request is made by the husband. Most requests of this type initiated by the wife are to demonstrate her concern and often loyalty to the husband.

Additionally, there are reports[6,47] that mixing the samples may facilitate the interaction of agglutinating or immobilizing antibodies present in the husband's semen against the donor sperm, thus rendering them less effective. Quinlivan *et al.*[48] reported a difference between the pregnancy rates in women undergoing TDI based on their sexual intercourse practices around the time of insemination. Those with a sexual abstinence of at least 2 days prior to the scheduled TDI had an 88% pregnancy rate, whereas those without such practice had a rate of 46%. In a study[49] of all pregnancies resulting from TDI (using both fresh and cryopreserved semen) in the past 15 years, it was found that the abortion rate in the couples whose partners 'produced some sperm' was significantly higher (21.8%) than those with azoospermic partners (15.4%). When couples with oligozoospermia were separated based on the degree of oligozoospermia, it was found that those with sperm counts >2 million/mL semen had a significantly higher abortion rate (26.2%) than those with a count of <1 million sperm (11.7%). Using fresh donor semen, Albrecht *et al.*[50] found a fecundity rate of 0.20 in wives whose husbands were azoospermic compared to 0.10 in those whose husbands were oligozoospermic. Kovacs *et al.*[51] also found similar differences. Need *et al.*[52] reported a 9.3% overall rate of preeclampsia in TDI patients, but the rate was much higher in patients whose husbands were oligozoospermic (13.6%). Friedman *et al.*[53], however, found no difference in pregnancy rates when the husband's and donor's samples were mixed, compared with donor semen only. In a series of 227 patients, 34 requested the use of mixed samples and 13 (38%) conceived. Of the 193 remaining patients requesting exclusive use of donor semen, 80 (41%) became pregnant. Although more information from the authors is needed, the data presented by Friedman *et al.*[53] must be interpreted cautiously. Overall low pregnancy rates in both methods, lack of true randomness in the study, presentation of data as pregnancies per patient rather than per cycle, and the fact that two of their seven patients achieved pregnancies when they were switched to donor semen, only make interpretation of the results difficult. Whether or not the presence of antisperm antibodies or other elements in the semen samples of the husband and the donor may have had deleterious effects on each other and on the pregnancy outcome, remain to be elucidated.

Genetic anomalies, spontaneous abortions and ectopic pregnancies in TDI

Nowadays, cryopreserved semen is almost exclusively used for TDI. The question arises as to whether or not cryopreservation and storage of sperm, insemination with cryopreserved sperm and even various methods of ovulation stimulation could result in an increased frequency of anomalous pregnancy or offspring. Verp[39] has reviewed the subject thoroughly and the bulk of our discussion benefits from the review. Conclusions with respect to the anomalies presented in TDI are equivocal and contradictory. There are several reasons for the inconsistency of the reports. In most investigations, no control group matched with the paternal age, genetic history of the parents and the environmental factors exists. In most reports, complete investigation and follow-up of all pregnancies, including stillborns, abortuses, tissue products of early miscarriages and live-borns are not being carried out. In most instances miscarriages, spontaneous abortions, ectopic pregnancies and molar pregnancies falling within the expected normal range are not investigated. Anomalies which may become evident later in life (e.g. sex chromosome anomalies, learning disabilities) are not included. Additionally, often only clinically significant and obvious malformations are investigated and reported. Many of the findings may also be related to the degree of investigators' knowledge, competence and opinion of genetic anomalies (e.g. jaundice as a genetic anomaly without being investigated)[39].

With respect to the genetic damage to spermatozoa as a result of cryopreservation, it is known that cryopreservation reduces motility and damages acrosome, coarse fibers, fibrous sheath, mitochondria and axoneme of spermatozoa[39,54,55]. Whether or not cryopreservation damages spermatozoal DNA leading to new mutations or chromosomal anomalies remains to be fully elucidated. Generally, it is believed that only the 'hardiest sperm' survive cryopreservation. However, sublethal mutations affecting both the pregnancy and the future generation may occur without direct indication[39].

Experimental evidence on the effect of cryopreservation on bovine, human spermatozoa and bacterial DNA do not indicate major genetic damage, at least at the level of gross DNA amount or breaks in DNA strands[39,56–58]. What actually may happen at the nucleotide level remains to be elucidated. Verp *et al.*[59] investigated the outcome of 122 TDI pregnancies and compared it with a control group consisting of infertility patients who conceived with therapies other than TDI. The rate of major and minor anomalies and the incidence of spontaneous abortions or ectopic pregnancies were not different between the two groups. In a summary of 27 studies compiled by Verp[39], similar anomalies were observed in TDI and non-TDI groups. In another study of 502 live-born children conceived through TDI with follow-ups[60], it was concluded that TDI children were at similar risk for congenital anomalies as those in the general, non-therapeutic population. Investigations revealed one chromosomal anomaly, 22 major and 38 minor congenital anomalies, four with syndromic conditions, 5.8% with learning disabilities and 10.5% as gifted children. Spontaneous abortion rate was reported to be about 16.5% and comparison between TDIs using fresh and cryopreserved semen showed no difference with this regard. Higher spontaneous abortion rates in TDI have been reported by some authors[61,62], but evidence indicates that the increase may be related to the maternal age, the cycle number at which conception occurred, the fertility status of the husband and the presence of chlamydial and *Ureaplasma urealyticum* infections[15,46,49]. Higher abortion rates were observed in pregnancies conceived after the twelfth cycle of TDI[60].

Some authors[63], however, reported an increased rate of aneuploidy in offspring born through TDI. In their review of 400 pregnancies, they found three infants with trisomies, while the normal rate should have been 0.6. In another study[64], 2502 TDI pregnancies in Europe were investigated. The number of trisomies found at amniocentesis and at birth was nine compared to the expected normal number of 10.14. However, the authors pointed out that when they excluded three trisomies that had occurred in mothers older than 35, they found a significant increase in the rate of trisomies in pregnancies resulted from TDI. With respect to this finding, Verp[39] argues that setting the age limit at 35 for the association/exclusion of trisomies may not be correct. Had authors excluded trisomies observed in women 34 years or older, then no significant increase in the number of trisomies could be observed.

The rate of non-chromosomal anomalies in pregnancies resulted from TDI has also been investigated. Forse *et al.*[63] reported a higher rate (3.8%) compared to the rate observed in the general population (1.7%). However, another study[64] reported no significant increase in TDI pregnancies. Verp[39] indicates that the review of many reports is indicative of no elevation in the rate of non-chromosomal abnormalities in offspring born through TDI compared to the general population.

CRYOPRESERVATION OF SEMEN: HISTORY

Preservation of biological systems via salting and storage at low temperature has been known to humans since early days of civilization. The scientific and written aspects of preservation began with the work of Boyle[65] in 1663, in his treatise entitled 'New Experiments and Observations Touching Cold'. In 1776, Lazzaro Spallanzani[66,67] reported that semen samples frozen in snow retained spermatozoal motility upon thawing. Later, in the 1820s, John Hunter[65], one of the pioneers of modern cryobiology, expanded Boyle's original work and experimented to cryopreserve complex biological systems. In his failed attempt to cryopreserve, Carps[65] wrote:

> After having exhausted the whole power of life in the production of heat, they froze; but that life was gone could not be known until we thawed them, which was done gradually. But their flexibility they did not recover action, so that they were really dead . . . Till this time I had imagined that it might be possible to prolong life to any period by freezing a person in the frigid zone . . . Like other schemers, I thought I should make my fortune by it, but this experiment undeceived me.

Some of Hunter's original ideas, however, have remained valid today.

In 1866, Paolo Montegazza found that, after thawing of semen stored for a long time at approximately −15°C, a small portion regained motility and suggested establishment of a semen bank for veterinary use and, in addition, for human use to produce legitimate progenies after a husband's death on the battlefield[55,66–69].

In 1937, Jahnel[67] accidentally discovered that a proportion of human spermatozoa survived storage at −79°C (dry ice in acetone slush), −196°C (liquid nitrogen) and −296°C. However, 2 years later, Shettle froze human spermatozoa at the same temperatures, but noted a poor survival rate[67].

Rostand's discovery in the mid-1940s was very important for the science of cryopreservation. He discovered the cryoprotective effects of glycerol (1,2,3 propanetriol, an alcohol) on frog spermatozoa[67]. The method was improved with the discovery by Polge in 1949[68] on the cryoprotective effect of glycerol, propanediol and ethanedial on bovine spermatozoa. The method was applied successfully to the cryopreservation of human spermatozoa and the first three pregnancies as a result of husbands' semen cryopreserved with glycerol in dry ice at approximately –70°C were reported in 1953[69]. Samples cryopreserved for these four cases were all 'normal' and had a survival rate of 53–59%. At the time, it was noted that samples with 'good fertility potential' could survive cryopreservation, whereas those of poor quality could not. This method, it was suggested, could be used as a new criterion for evaluating the fertility potential of a given male[67]. Between 1954 and 1958, there were reports of 27 births through TDI from Japan and the United States[3,70].

In 1962–63, liquid nitrogen vapor was used to cryopreserve semen samples[55]. In 1964, egg yolk citrate buffer as an extender and aid to cryopreservation was introduced and, along with the use of liquid nitrogen vapor, it improved the recovery rate of cryopreserved samples drastically[55].

Since early attempts to cryopreserve semen samples and the use of TDI to achieve pregnancies, many reports have been published on this subject. General reports on cryopreservation[70–72], cryopreservation media[73–76], methods[70–74,77], recovery rates after cryopreservation[74,75,77], possible damage inflicted upon sperm after cryopreservation[74,78–81], success rates for cryopreserved semen samples[82–87] and the male/female ratio upon using cryopreserved semen samples[88–90] are some examples.

Extensive use of donor cryopreserved semen did not come about until the mid-1980s when concern was raised about the transmission of sexually transmitted diseases, such as Acquired Immune Deficiency Syndrome (AIDS) through the use of fresh donor semen. Despite some disadvantages, nowadays, cryopreserved semen samples are used exclusively in TDI in most countries.

Cryopreservation has allowed for the exclusion of the infected samples and has made it easier to schedule TDIs. It has allowed us to perform more inseminations without regard to the donor's schedule or the number of days of abstinence. Additionally, cryopreservation has given couples the choice of having offspring with similar genetic backgrounds if they desire.

PRINCIPLES OF SPERM CRYOPRESERVATION

Long-term storage and preservation of biological systems, such as spermatozoa, can be accomplished. However, such techniques require the arrest of all cellular activities while maintaining the integrity of the structures necessary to restore normal cell function upon their return to physiological conditions. To arrest all cellular activities, cells are exposed to freezing temperatures; however, intracellular water content must be reduced prior to such exposure. Partial removal of intracellular water is carried out to avoid formation of extensive intracellular ice crystals which damage cells and reduce their survival. Partial removal of the water may also help in a more complete arrest of all thermally driven metabolic and enzymatic activities of the cells. Partial removal of the water is accomplished by the addition of a cryoprotectant such as glycerol to the cell mixture (semen), usually in combination with a buffer based medium containing egg yolk (extender, freezing medium) along with the freezing process. When cells are cryopreserved under these controlled conditions, they can be maintained preserved (cryopreserved) at ultra-low temperatures (e.g. –196°C) without much damage. The only reactions that can occur at this temperature are the formation of free radicals and the damage to macromolecules. Possible sources for these reactions and damage at this temperature are the cosmic rays and, more importantly, the terrestrial background ionizing radiation which has not been shown to be significant (0.1 rad/year)[91]. It has been reported that it takes about 3.2×10^4 years for cells cryopreserved in a cryoprotectant such as dimethylsulfoxide (DMSO) to accumulate lethal chromosomal damage to equal one acute dose of X-ray at 22°C[91]. Current storage equipment also further minimizes such possible damage.

Spermatozoa in general are ideal cells to cryopreserve since they are small, usually in high numbers, easily obtained and have very little cytoplasm, containing less total water than many other cells (e.g. oocytes, embryos). To remove or reduce water content of spermatozoa, which also helps to minimize intracellular ice formation during freezing, a variety of organics (cryoprotectants) are used. Some cryoprotectants are permeable (penetrating) and some are non-permeable. Examples of permeable cryoprotectants are glycerol, DMSO, propanediol and some non-permeable ones are sucrose and trehalose. These cryoprotectants, when mixed with cells to be cryopreserved, attract water molecules, leading to an osmotically driven reduction of intracellular water and cell shrinkage (first change in cell volume). If the cryoprotectant used is of the penetrating type, then it can penetrate the cell and the cell can return nearly to its original volume. To cryopreserve cells, addition of cryoprotectant is accompanied by a reduction in temperature (cooling) and eventual freezing to further reduce intracellular water and stop metabolic processes within the cell. As cooling proceeds and the temperature reaches –5° to –15°C, ice nucleation first begins to occur extracellularly. Propagation of ice crystals induces the development of an extracellular solid phase, but the intracellular environment of the cells remains unfrozen but supercooled. Supercooled intracellular water has a higher chemical potential and diffuses out as extracellular water continues to crystallize. Extracellular ice formation does not easily propagate intracellularly because of the barrier represented by the cell 'intact' membrane. Extracellular water molecules usually freeze with the exclusion of solutes and the cells (except in rare cases where deuterium, fluoride, and ammonium can be included)[92]. This results in an increase in concentration of extracellular solutes in the remaining unfrozen solution (extracellular hypertonicity) and further loss of water from cells. This is the second cell volume change resulting from increase in extracellular solute concentration as a result of extracellular ice formation. Additionally, as water exits the cell and freezes, concentration of solutes within the cell also increases; however, this cell dehydration should be kept limited to avoid extensive cell volume loss. This is usually accomplished by a more rapid freezing rate, but this rate must also be set in a fashion that is not too rapid. Too rapid cooling/freezing rate may prevent adequate water (volume) loss by the cell and cause supercooling and excessive intracellular ice formation. Enough time should be given to the cells to become dehydrated while, most importantly, excessive cell shrinkage is avoided (too slow a freezing rate). Accommodating all these changes within a timetable dictated by the freezing protocol is a tremendous task for the cell. Cells must undergo various stages of adjustment to the changes in solute, solvents and temperature around them. Each of these can have effects on the others, as well as on the cells[80]. In summary, during cryopreservation, cells initially shrink when they are exposed to hypertonic cryoprotectants, return back to near normal volume as cryoprotectant penetrates, shrink again as water leaves the cell as extracellular water freezes (during a slow freezing rate) and they may undergo intracellular freezing, if the freezing rate is too rapid. Additionally, cells must go through the same processes when they are thawed[80]. What has been discussed so far are the osmotic events that cells must undergo. A host of other events affect cells during cryopreservation. How these changes and events affect cells and their functional integrity is an extremely important subject to explore. Considering these factors, one wonders how, with our empirical and 'torturous' methods of cryopreservation, these cells survive[80].

Cryoprotectants

Addition of cryoprotective agents, such as glycerol, has been shown to modify, beneficially to some degree, these deleterious effects. Glycerol modifies the physical properties of the solution by lowering its freezing point. In fact, cryopreservation is a process whereby an equilibrium between the ice and the remaining part of a system is established. Addition of glycerol makes it possible to have less ice formed at a specific temperature in order for this equilibrium to be reached. For example, normal saline with an osmolality of 280–290 mOsmol/kg has a freezing point of –0.56°C. At –10°C, approximately 90% of its water must be frozen out in order for an equilibrium between the ice and the remainder of the saline (e.g. salt) is reached. At this temperature, the ice in the system is in equilibrium with a 10 times concentrated solution (the remaining unfrozen part of the saline) with an osmolality of 5300–5400 mOsmol/kg. Addition of a 10% v/v glycerol with an osmolality of approximately 1500 mOsmol/kg to the same saline solution prior to freezing would require freezing of only 68% of the saline water (rather than 90%) in order for the same equilibrium to be reached at −10°C. In this instance, the ice will be in equilibrium with only 3.4 times concentrated solution rather than 10 times concentrated. Additionally, when glycerol replaces intracellular water, it reduces the adverse consequences of excessive cell shrinkage and the phase change during crystallization and cell (membranes) fusion because of the cold temperature. Glycerol may also be a scavenger of free radicals generated during cooling/freezing[65]. Action of cryoprotectants, in general, depends on their ability to permeate cell membranes and replace water. It also depends on the degree of toxicity of the cryoprotectant and the consequence of interaction of cryoprotectants with the cells (see below). To prevent adverse effects of sudden water replacement, it is recommended that glycerol be added slowly to the cell mixture (e.g. semen) to be cryopreserved[93]. To slow down and reduce glycerol toxicity to subcellular metabolism and integrity of the cell, glycerol is allowed to penetrate cells (equilibrate) at a lower temperature than the room temperature (e.g. refrigeration)[93]. In general, the success of cryopreservation is dependent upon factors such as the cell type, cell water permeability and its permeability coefficient, cell surface to volume ratio, type of cryoprotectant (permeating versus non-permeating), concentration of cryoprotectant used, permeability coefficient of the cryoprotectant (1,2 propanediol used to cryopreserve embryos permeates much faster than glycerol), nature of cryoprotectant (DMSO, toxic to sperm), the cooling rate, the freezing rate, storage temperature (ice recrystallization occurs at temperatures above −130°C, so dry ice is not a good medium to keep or ship samples)[94–96], thawing rate, type of vessel used (vials versus straws), amount of sample per vial, and last but not least, the quality of the sample to be cryopreserved (see page 497). The most important conclusion is that 'there is no general recipe for cryopreservation of cells'[97]. Any published protocol must be used exactly for the system for which it was intended. Its application to a different system or under different conditions must be carefully evaluated and redesigned before it is utilized or any conclusion about it is made[97].

Technically, a cryopreservation procedure can be divided into five parts, namely: the addition of cryopreservation medium; equilibration and cooling stage; freezing stage; storage; thawing; and evaluation of the recovery (success) using appropriate methods. Each step has its special relationship to the cell function and metabolism and requires specific handling techniques related to the system to be cryopreserved. For spermatozoa, the cryopreservation medium of choice is glycerol at a concentration of 5% to 10% (usually around 6%). Glycerol is usually added to a buffered medium (freezing medium) containing TES, TRIS and citrate buffers mixed with 20% (v/v) egg yolk and antibiotics[93,98]. The concentration of glycerol in the medium is kept at 12% because the medium usually is mixed with an equal volume of semen, resulting in a 1:1 ratio dilution of the semen and a final glycerol concentration of 6% (v/v). Cryopreservation medium is added slowly to the semen at a rate taking approximately 10–15 min. This allows more gradual loss of water by the cell and replacement of water by the penetrating cryoprotectant. The mixture is refrigerated (4°C) for 30–60 min to allow equilibration and further penetration of the cryoprotectant, and perhaps reducing the possible toxicity of the glycerol to the cell at higher temperatures. The mixture is then aliquoted into properly labeled and refrigerated cryovials (plastic tubes) to a volume of 0.5–0.8 ml per vial. Vials are transferred into a freezing tray for manual freezing or directly into a programmable freezer prior to the refrigeration step. Although several variations of the manual freezing have been published[93,98,99], the simplest one is positioning the vials at 3–4 cm above liquid nitrogen (nitrogen vapor, −190°C) for 20–30 minutes (see page 496). Vials can then be transferred into liquid nitrogen (−196°C) for storage. Several methods for cryopreservation of sperm in programmable freezers have been proposed[70,72,77] (see page 496). Unlike cryopreservation of embryos or oocytes, an automated system for cryopreservation of sperm may not be necessary. Cryosurvival of spermatozoa using an automated system versus the manual method has given inconsistent results[70,93]. More in-depth methods of assessing the success of a cryopreservation technique may lead to development of more successful and refined methods. Using an automated system, a cooling rate of −0.5°C/min from room temperature to −5°C, and a freezing rate of −10°C/min from −5°C to −80° or −90°C, followed by plunging into liquid nitrogen is appropriate. The slower cooling rate of −0.5°C/min allows cells to equilibrate and lose enough intracellular water. Notice that the freezing phase of the protocol mentioned above has a much higher rate of temperature decline than the cooling phase. This is to prevent further water loss from spermatozoa and perhaps minimize excessive stress on the cell membrane. This method has not been shown to be appropriate for cryopreservation of oocytes or embryos because of their higher water content. For these types of cells, as freezing is induced at −6° to −7°C, a slower rate of decline in temperature must be implemented to allow further water loss.

The thawing process

Thawing is another important phase of a cryopreservation procedure. It depends significantly upon the cooling and freezing rates. One of the consequences of a rapid rate of cooling/freezing is the rapid rate of heat removal from the system. As a result, the latent heat released by the initial nucleating sites (ice crystals) as they grow throughout the system becomes insufficient to equal that being removed by cooling. The consequence of this is the formation of small ice nuclei. If a slow method of thawing is applied for this rate of cooling/freezing, in the transition temperature small ice nuclei will grow to larger ones which may damage cells before they are completely thawed. As a rule of thumb, a sample cryopreserved via the quick method must be thawed quickly[89,91,93,100]. Quick thawing can be achieved by placing vials at 37°C for 5–10 min or at 37–42°C for 3 min.

The two most common methods of semen cryopreservation, one automated and the other manual[72], are outlined on page 496, respectively. Our methods of cryopreserving sperm as 'IUI Ready' and preparing cryopreserved samples for IUI are outlined on pages 497–504.

SUCCESS RATES IN TDI

Nowadays, quarantined cryopreserved semen is exclusively used in TDI. It appears that the use of cryopreserved semen is the only constant factor in published reports on the success rates of TDI. Therapeutic donor insemination has primarily been considered as a solution to male infertility or subfertility. As a result many other factors, especially those related to the recipient which could significantly influence the outcome, have been overlooked. Most data from centers performing TDI have been presented as if those receiving therapy formed a homogeneous group. Presence of a variety of factors influencing the results make the comparisons of the success rates almost impossible to evaluate. This has also made it difficult to counsel patients and provide them with a realistic prognosis in terms of duration and outcome of TDI. Some of the factors influencing the pregnancy outcome of TDI are outlined in Table 2. A discussion on the reported success rates using fresh donor semen, comparisons of fresh and cryopreserved donor semen and the rates obtained with cryopreserved only donor semen will follow. Other variables outlined in Table 2 and some recent published reports on their effects on the outcome of TDI will also be discussed.

Success rates with fresh semen

It is generally believed that cryopreserved semen results in lower success rates compared to fresh semen; however, comparative studies have not been uniformly indicative of such difference. Review of the literature on TDI using fresh semen is indicative of the cumulative pregnancy rates comparable to the current controlled studies using cryopreserved semen[1,82,84–87,101–104,111,113,116]. In these studies, TDI success rates using fresh semen in the form of cumulative pregnancies have been reported to be between 70 and 75%, a miscarriage rate of 15–16% and 3.5 as the mean number of cycles to conceive. Using fresh washed donor semen and IUI, Mackenna *et al.*[105] reported a 50% pregnancy rate per patient and 28.6% per cycle for TDI in patients whose partners were azoospermic. They found the results were comparable to the natural conception rate (intercourse) in the control group consisting of fertile couples matched for the age and the timing of insemination. Based on available information from the literature (see later), it appears reasonable to conclude that: (1) cryopreserved semen gives similar results in assisted reproduction techniques such as

Table 2 Factors influencing TDI outcome

- Insemination techniques
  - intravaginal
  - intracervical
  - pericervical (cap)
  - intrauterine
  - intratubal
  - tubal perfusion
  - intrafollicular
  - intraperitoneal
  - *in vitro* procedures
- Sperm preparation methods
  - no preparation (whole semen)
  - sperm washing (with or without swim-up)
  - density gradient (e.g. Percoll)
  - column separations
- Insemination timing
  - BBT, cervical mucus assessment
  - LH surge (serum, urine)
  - ultrasound ± hCG
  - vaginal electrical resistance
  - urinary glycosaminoglycans
- Treatment modality
  - natural cycle
  - clomiphene citrate (CC)
  - FSH/hMG
  - FSH/hMG/GnRHa
  - FSH/hMG/GnRH
- Number of inseminations per cycle
- Number of motile sperm per insemination
- Present and past reproductive history of the female (including duration of infertility)
- Fertility history of the donor
- Fertility status of the husband (oligo? azoospermic?)
- Methods of data analysis

in vitro fertilization (IVF)[85,106–109]; and (2) using TDI, and in the absence of confounding factors (e.g. female factors), the cumulative pregnancy rate using cryopreserved semen is comparable to that of fresh semen, but monthly fecundity may be different. It may not be unreasonable to state that the monthly fecundity may be slightly lower when cryopreserved semen is used for *in vivo* inseminations (e.g. ICI, IUI). This means that it may take more numbers of insemination cycles to achieve pregnancies using cryopreserved semen compared to fresh semen. The number of inseminations required may even be higher if confounding factors such as the female age and her reproductive health care contributory. For *in vitro* inseminations, however, evidence indicates that there is no difference between the fresh and cryopreserved semen samples. In a study[107] of 39 IVF cycles, using fresh donor semen matched with 74 cycles using cryopreserved donor samples, comparable pregnancy rates (39.3% versus 38.5% respectively) were observed.

Success rates with cryopreserved semen

Results obtained from the use of cryopreserved semen in our IVF program are shown in Table 3. Fertilization rates and pregnancy rates are comparable to those of the fresh samples. A retrospective controlled study to assess the use of IVF with cryopreserved donor semen after failed TDI indicated an excellent cumulative pregnancy rate of 83% (n=38, 63 cycles) after four IVF cycles for the group with failed TDI[106]. The control group consisted of patients with only tubal disease undergoing IVF at the same time and matched for age, infertility diagnosis and the number of attempts. The rate for the control group was 59% which was significantly lower than that of the patient group. Gamete intrafallopian transfer (GIFT) was performed on 48 healthy ovulatory females who failed to conceive after nine to 24 cycles of TDI. A pregnancy rate per cycle of 56%, miscarriage rate of 29%, multiple pregnancy of 18% (four twins and one triplet), with no ectopic pregnancies reported[108]. In another study[109], IVF results of 66 patients previously unsuccessful with TDI were reported. A total of 129 IVF trials were performed with either cryopreserved (n=55) or fresh donor semen (n=74). A cumulative ongoing pregnancy rate of 40% after three IVF cycles was reported for both groups. It should be stated that the study was not random and attempts were not made to explore the association of the pregnancy rate with any of the variables in the study.

Fresh versus cryopreserved semen success rates

Review of the success rates reported on the comparison between the fresh and cryopreserved semen is indicative of variability of the results. However, very few random studies have been carried out for this comparison; the success rates appear to be similar in controlled studies. In one study[110], 155 ovulatory patients were randomly grouped to

Table 3 IVF results using cryopreserved donor semen in different age groups

	25–29 years (5 cycles)	*30–34 years (24 cycles)*	*35–39 years (34 cycles)*	*40+ years (17 cycles)*
F/O	97.1%	91.2%	95.1%	98.5%
PR/C	60.0%[a]	45.8%[b]	28.6%[c]	17.6%[d]
PR/T	60.0%[a]	47.8%[b]	29.4%[c]	20.0%[d]
Misc.	0.0[a]	36.4%[b]	30.0%[b]	33.3%[b]
Term	100.0%[a]	30.4%[b]	20.6%[c]	13.3%[d]
Embryo/T	4.0[a]	3.9[a]	3.6[a]	3.4[b]

F/O = fertilization rate per oocyte; PR/C = pregnancy rate per cycle; PR/T = pregnancy rate per transfer; Misc. = miscarriage; Embryo/T = number of embryos per transfer. [a–d] significant from each other, at least at the level of $P<0.05$

receive TDI with either fresh or cryopreserved semen. Pericervical inseminations were performed once on the day of ovulation as assessed by BBT and/or urinary LH surge test. The monthly fecundity rate for the fresh semen was 5.8%, similar to that observed for the cryopreserved semen (5.1%). The average number of cycles per patient was around 4.6, which was not different for the two groups. Cumulative pregnancy rates for the two groups were 52.9% and 65.5%, respectively. Despite the fact that the total number of motile sperm per insemination was significantly higher in TDIs using fresh semen (123 million) compared to cryopreserved semen (24 million), the pregnancy rates were similar between the two groups. Life table analysis of the results of a prospective randomized study reported by Iddenden *et al*[111]. indicated that fresh and cryopreserved semen give a similar cumulative pregnancy rate after six and 12 cycles. Hummel *et al.*[25] reported pregnancy rates per cycle of 12% using fresh and 9.4% using cryopreserved semen.

Authors indicate that the most common causes for failure in patients undergoing TDI is either the female factor or patient dropout. Bordson *et al.*[84] reported similar success rates for fresh and cryopreserved semen used in TDI, comparing a series of 401 TDI cycles (mostly ICIs) monitored using urinary LH surge or ultrasound-timed hCG injection. The monthly fecundity rates were reported as 0.115 for the fresh semen, 0.103 for the cryopreserved semen and 0.113 for the mixed fresh/cryopreserved semen samples (fresh on the first day, cryopreserved for the second day). The most influencing factors in the success rate were the reproductive health and the age of the recipients. 'Healthy' recipients had a fecundity of 0.156 as compared to 0.067 for the recipients with known female factors (e.g. various degrees of endometriosis, pelvic adhesions or ovulatory dysfunction). Those 25 years or younger had the highest fecundity (0.20), those between 26 and 35 years had a rate of 0.10 and for those over 35 years the fecundity rate was 0.087. Authors conclude that a minimum of 40×10^6 motile sperm is needed for TDI using cryopreserved semen. Because of the flaws in the study the results should be interpreted with caution. The trial was not random and patients with known female factors who were grouped together had various degrees of conditions ranging from mild to severe endometriosis, tubal and pelvic adhesions. These patients' responses to TDI may vary greatly depending on the design of the study and the severity and type of the female factor. Moreover, IUIs and ICIs were performed randomly without distinctions being made as to who received what method of insemination.

Using patients as their own controls, Richter *et al.*[82] inseminated patients with fresh and cryopreserved semen in alternate cycles. However, they found that the fresh semen was three times more likely to induce a pregnancy (18.9%) compared with the cryopreserved semen (5%). In a prospective randomized trial[112] of fresh versus cryopreserved sperm, pregnancy results of 198 TDI cycles were compared. Only one insemination per cycle was performed and each patient served as her own control. A maximum of six inseminations per patient were performed, three with fresh and three with cryopreserved semen. Fecundity was 20.6% for the cycles using fresh semen and 9.4% for the cycles using cryopreserved semen. Pericervical inseminations with fresh semen yielded a fecundity rate of 20.3% as compared with 7.8% for the cryopreserved semen. However, IUIs using fresh sperm yielded a similar (21.2%) fecundity, as compared with 15.8% for the cryopreserved sperm. Based on life table analysis for the first three cycles of insemination, fresh sperm yielded a pregnancy rate of 48% ± 10% versus 22% ± 8% for the cryopreserved sperm ($P = 0.05$).

In another study[104], the pregnancy results using fresh and computer controlled cryopreserved donor semen were compared. With a total of 3405 insemination cycles using fresh and 371 cycles using cryopreserved semen, monthly fecundity rates of 11.9% and 5.9%, respectively, were achieved. However, using the life table analysis, a cumulative pregnancy rate of 59.6% for the fresh and 48.6% for the cryopreserved samples were noted (not significantly different). This is one indication that it takes longer to achieve pregnancy using cryopreserved semen and that the dropout rate contributes significantly to the overall success rate achieved with cryopreserved semen.

In a study to determine TDI success rates using cryopreserved semen, Hatasaka *et al.*[86] selected healthy ovulatory single females ($n = 13$) or women whose husbands were azoospermic ($n = 30$). All cryopreserved samples were of similar quality, inseminations were ICI using cervical cap, ovulation was assessed using mid-luteal progesterone and BBT, and the timing was assessed using urinary LH surge in early morning and early evening. Those with early morning surge were inseminated the same day and those with the evening surge were inseminated the next day. With a few exceptions, most patients were inseminated once per cycle and patients were studied for up to eight cycles. Thirty-four (70.1%) of 43 recipients conceived with no insemination complications, ectopic or multiple pregnancies.

Cumulative probability of conception

Based on life table analysis, the overall cumulative probability of conception after eight cycles was found to be 84.0%. Average monthly fecundity from the life table was 19%. All 13 single females conceived within two insemination cycles. Fifty-six percent of pregnancies occurred within the first three cycles of insemination, 23.5% between four and six cycles, and 20.5% between seven and eight cycles. Almost 80% of pregnancies occurred within the first six cycles of insemination. No age or number of insemination cycles were reported. Using cryopreserved semen in 288 cycles of TDI[113], the cumulative probability of conception was reported to be 59% with a monthly fecundity rate of 14.6% (take-home baby rate of 13%). In another study of 751 TDI cycles[114], an average monthly fecundity rate of 16% was reported in patients of all age groups receiving cryopreserved semen. Significantly better pregnancy rates were reported in those aged 34 years or younger. Using cryopreserved donor semen, a combination of LH surge/ultrasound/hCG and IUIs, Silva *et al.*[103] reported a monthly fecundity rate of 24% for total pregnancies and 18% for ongoing pregnancies.

Findings regarding the relationship between TDI success and different methods of insemination have been inconsistent. Some studies find ICI to be as effective as IUI or other methods, while others report the advantages of IUI and other insemination methods over ICI.

Comparative studies of insemination

In comparative studies, many variables influencing the outcome are often ignored. In other studies, the usefulness of a particular method of insemination is evaluated using patients who have failed or not undergone other methods of insemination. Generally, the monthly fecundity for cryopreserved samples used in ICI has been reported to range from 3.9%[83] to 14.6%[115]. The rates for IUI have been reported to be about 9.7% for unstimulated cycles and a range of 15.5%[115] to 24%[103] for stimulated cycles. However many reports indicate that, in patients without the real female factors, ICI may be as effective as IUI[117,118]. Perhaps in the absence of an indication to do otherwise, the practice of two to three cervical inseminations followed by IUI, if ICI is not successful, is not unreasonable. More thorough investigation of the female, a switch to a different donor, and other methods, such as Fallopian tube sperm perfusion[115,123], tubal, intrafollicular, intraperitoneal or *in vitro* assisted production techniques[85,106–109] may be suggested if IUIs fail. In a study (16 of 16) using each patient as her own control[117], TDI conception rates for IUI versus pericervical (ICI/cap) were compared. Twenty-six single unmarried ovulatory women with patent tubes and <40 years of age underwent 81 cycles of inseminations. No more than four cycles of insemination per recipient were performed. Fourteen (54%) of 26 patients conceived, including two (14%) miscarriages within four insemination cycles. Seven (17.5%) patients after IUI and seven (17.1%) after pericervical insemination conceived. It was concluded that the pregnancy rates were similar in both methods, regardless of the order of insemination.

Patton *et al.*[118] compared the relative efficiency of IUIs with washed semen with that of ICIs and found no significant differences despite the fact that the number of motile sperm in ICIs was 10 times higher than IUIs. However, in a randomized prospective study[119], TDI success rates using ICI, IUI and a combination of intratubal and IUI (ITI/IUI) were compared. Cycle fecundity rate was significantly higher for IUI (18.3%) than for ICI (3.9%) or ITI/IUI (7.3%). By life table analysis, the cumulative pregnancy rate of IUI was significantly higher than ICI and ITI/IUI. Pregnancy rates for ICI and ITI/IUI were not different. In another prospective study[83] using each patient as her own control, the results of ICIs and IUIs using cryopreserved donor semen were compared. A total of 154 patients were evaluated who were undergoing 238 IUI and 229 ICI cycles using twice daily quantitative measurements of LH and inseminations on the day of LH peak and the day after. The pregnancy rate per cycle was 9.7% for the IUIs and 3.9% for the ICIs. Abortion and the miscarriage rates for the IUI and ICI were 17.4% and 11.1%, respectively. If all patients continued treatment, the probability of pregnancy for 12 treatment cycles would have been 70.6% for IUIs and 38.2% for ICIs. In a prospective randomized trial[120] it was concluded that, when using cryopreserved semen, IUI outperforms ICI. Monthly fecundity rate for IUI was 23%, whereas the rate for ICI was 5.1%. Authors did not attempt to perform IUIs in those who failed ICIs. In a study of 196 recipients undergoing 1986 TDI cycles (ICIs)[121], 92 conceived giving a pregnancy rate per cycle of 4.6%. Twenty-two (24%) pregnancies occurred within the first three cycles, 29 (31.5%) within cycles four to six, 24 (26%) within seven to 10 cycles and 17 pregnancies (18%) with more than 11 cycles of insemination. In another study[122], about 75% of all pregnancies occurred within the first three cycles and 94% within the first six cycles of insemination.

Fallopian tube sperm perfusion

Fallopian tube sperm perfusion (FSP) is another method of insemination whereby a large volume (usually around 4 mL) of sperm suspension is used for the insemination. Kahn *et al.*[115] reported a pregnancy rate per cycle of 27.9% in 172 TDI treatment cycles. Ovarian stimulation was carried out in all cycles. The pregnancy rate declined significantly from the first attempt (34.1%) to the fourth attempts (14.3%). The rate was significantly higher in women with three to five mature follicles compared to those with two or fewer follicles. Cycles in which hCG was administered on day 11 or later had significantly higher pregnancy rates than those in which hCG was administered on day 10. There was no difference in the pregnancy rate with respect to the number of motile sperm per insemination. In another prospective randomized study[123], FSP results were compared with those of IUIs. The group receiving FSP had a significantly higher pregnancy rate per cycle (26.9%) and the number of motile sperm used in each insemination ($52 \pm 5 \times 10^6$) compared to the group receiving IUIs (9.8% and $28 \pm 3 \times 10^6$, respectively). Authors indicated that FSP is superior to IUI and the number of motile sperm per insemination may be one of the factors responsible for the higher success rate using FSP. In an earlier study[115], however, the same group found no relationship between the number of motile sperm inseminated (8 million versus 30 million) and the pregnancy outcome.

In another study[124], 29 refractory patients with azoospermic husbands and with a history of unsuccessful TDI (ICI, mean of 13.6, median of 9.5 and range of two to 39 cycles), were inseminated intratubally following thorough investigation of tubal patency and normal external tubal anatomy. Pelvic ultrasound examinations were carried out from the time of LH rise to monitor the follicle growth. Rise in LH was established with its determinations in serum and by a rise in serum progesterone greater than twice the previous level. Using at least 50 000 washed/swim-up motile sperm cells in 30 mL medium, inseminations were carried out within 30–46 h after the start of LH rise. Of the 50 cycles, 46 were catheterized successfully and six conceived giving an overall fecundity of 0.12. In 27 of the attempted cycles, the dominant follicle was still present at the time of insemination and this was the case in five of six pregnancies. Authors indicate that, since the number of motile sperm per tube in gamete intrafallopian transfer is around 100 000, increasing the number of sperm in this procedure may further improve the pregnancy rate.

Methods of sperm preparation

Exclusive reports of the influence of sperm preparation methods on cryopreserved donor semen and on TDI outcome are very few[125]. However, several lines of evidence related to fresh semen reviewed in an excellent article written by Mortimer[126] pointing to the fact that the methods of sperm preparation could significantly influence the outcome of artificial insemination may also very well be applicable to the cryopreserved semen. This is not an unreasonable assumption, because cryopreserved spermatozoa may have been functionally impaired and the same care must be taken in processing them as suggested for samples with poor quality.

In evaluating the methods of sperm preparation, attention must be paid to understand the mechanism of each separation technique and the potential influence the technique may have on sperm recovery and function. The ideal sperm preparation technique is fairly rapid, simple, inexpensive, and enables us to recover the highest number of purely motile sperm with normal function and morphology without inflicting excessive damage to spermatozoa. To this date, it is not clear which method of sperm preparation is the most suitable for TDI and other assisted reproduction techniques. With some modifications, the evidence and methodology presented in the literature on fresh samples can also be applied to cryopreserved semen. A sperm rise (swim-up) method was introduced by Drevious in 1971[127]; however, one-, two- and even three-step semen dilution and washing was the first method employed for sperm preparation methods applied to early *in vivo* and *in vitro* techniques[126].

Using fresh semen, a simple (one-step) sperm dilution and washing was used in the first reported case of human oocyte *in vitro* fertilization and a double dilution/wash (two-step) method in the first IVF clinical pregnancy in the world. The methods were subsequently used in many centers for assisted reproduction. The washing method is still being used in many centers for simple techniques such as artificial insemination. Earlier scientific thoughts were that the most motile fraction of spermatozoa is the portion capable of fertilization and, as knowledge was gained, that certain natural and pathological components of semen could interfere with sperm ability to fertilize attention was directed towards separation of this fraction for assisted reproduction. It was logical to think that, since the most functionally normal sperm is the one which is motile, attempts were made to let sperm migrate from the washed sperm pellet and be separated. Besides the earlier work of Drevious[127], there was a report in 1981[126] of the development of a swim-up migration method from the washed sperm pellet to separate the motile fraction of sperm. The method gained more acceptance, gave desirable results with fertilization *in vitro*, and was also widely used for artificial inseminations (e.g. TDI). However, as time passed and more knowledge was gained, the indications for assisted reproduction techniques grew to include categories such as idiopathic and male factor infertilities. Compared with the better samples used in cases of tubal infertility, samples of lower quality were used in an attempt to assist male factor and idiopathic infertility cases. For the first time, the failure of assisted reproduction techniques could easily be associated with the sperm[126].

Since sperm migration (e.g. swim-up) techniques were used in these categories, methods were explored to improve the recovery rate of the motile fraction from the poor quality samples, and to inflict the least damage to sperm and obtain a pure, supposedly highly fertile subpopulation of sperm. Benefiting from earlier works, Aitken *et al.*[128], in 1988, for the first time presented clear evidence that the induction of sperm iatrogenic complications could be related to the laboratory method of sperm preparation and these complications could facilitate sperm dysfunction, damage the 'normal' fraction of sperm, and cause the failure of sperm to fertilize[126]. Authors pointed to the fact that most semen samples from subfertile patients contain excess number of round cells (e.g. neutrophils, macrophages and round spermatids). They also showed that there are some subpopulations of sperm in the semen with inherent problems of producing excess amounts of reactive oxygen species, inability to detoxify these species, or a combination of both. They reported that the centrifugation and pelleting steps applied to whole semen to prepare the swim-up fraction causes these sperm cells with impaired function, as well as all other components of semen, such as round cells and cytoplasmic droplets/debris, to come into close contact with the 'normal' spermatozoa and eventually damage them. Under these suitable conditions, the production of reactive oxygen species such as superoxide and hydroxyl free radicals can cause peroxidation of membrane phospholipids. Cytokines and free radicals produced by some round cells could also further inflict damage to the 'normal' sperm subpopulation trapped in the pellet[126,128,129]. Buch *et al.*[129] reported that, in semen samples that are simply washed to pellet spermatozoa, one-third of membrane lipid peroxidation activity could be attributable to the proinflammatory cytokines interleukin-1 (IL-1 α and β) and to tumor necrosis factor α secreted by white blood cells present in the semen. In search of a selective method to separate and identify these sperm subpopulations, and prevent direct contact among these fractions, Aitken *et al.*[128] applied Percoll gradient centrifugation technique to the semen samples. They discovered that the defective and damaging subpopulation of sperm has a lower density (higher cytoplasmic volume, cytoplasmic droplets and coating envelopes)[130], and is separated in the 40–50% (low density) fraction of the Percoll gradient. Review of the literature indicates that the swim-up method has been used successfully in many assisted reproduction techniques. As Mortimer[126] stated, the question arises as to how the success of these samples can be explained when the technique has its major inherent problem. The answer is that the method may be suitable for a sample with a very high number of 'normal' sperm and very low levels of non-spermatozoal contaminants. Most subfertile and low quality semen samples do not meet such criteria and processing of these samples requires careful attention in selecting a method which minimizes peroxidative and cytokinetic damages and protects both 'normal' and those spermatozoa with 'borderline' quality[126]. The success rate could have also been higher had cryopreserved samples been processed using a less damaging method.

Methods of sperm preparation

There has been a variety of methods of sperm preparation applied in TDI and other assisted reproduction techniques. Direct swim-up from semen into a nutrient medium with or without further washing of the separated sperm[125,126,131], direct swim-up into a hyaluronidase-based medium (Sperm Select), column separations (e.g. Sephadex)[125] and sperm density gradient centrifugation methods such as Percoll, Ficoll and Nycodenz are some examples of the methods currently used to process samples for TDI. However, Percoll gradient centrifugation has been shown to be the most practised and suitable. Originally described by Suarez *et al.*[132], Percoll use for IVF was first reported in 1986 by Hyne *et al.*[133]. Percoll separation technique was used for cases of poor IVF results obtained by using swim-up samples prepared from washed pellets. A significantly higher fertilization rate was obtained and some pregnancies were achieved. In 1989, another group[134] reported a much higher pregnancy rate with the Percoll processed samples compared to those prepared by swim-up, despite the fact that the cleavage rates between the two groups were similar. Additionally, samples processed differently in prior failed IVF attempts were able to fertilize eggs when processed with Percoll[134]. In another report[135], to obtain motile sperm fractions for IUIs using cryopreserved donor semen, separations via Percoll density gradient and the swim-up in Menezo B2 were compared. Recovery of motile sperm using the Percoll method was consistently higher (1.7×10^6) compared to the swim-up method (0.77×10^6). Authors reported that the Percoll method was superior because the number of motile sperm per insemination in the stimulated cycles was significantly contributory to the pregnancy outcome[135]. In another study[130] it was reported that, based on the electronmicroscopy evaluations, spermatozoa separated from the 90% fraction of Percoll were highly motile and lacked coating envelopes (cytoplasmic coating indicative of poorer quality) than was observed on the sperm cells in the lower density fractions (at the interface of 47–90% layers). Authors concluded that the Percoll method is superior in isolating a highly pure fraction of motile sperm with normal function, excellent morphology and fully condensed chromatin. Le

Lannou *et al.*[136] reported that the sperm morphology and nuclear maturity (condensed chromatin) was superior in fractions of motile sperm obtained via Percoll separation compared to the swim-up method. It is not clear whether sperm cells with fully condensed chromatin are functionally more 'normal'; however, Tanphaichitr *et al.*[130] reported that, morphologically, those with fully condensed chromatin have more oval and regular head shape. Percoll separation has also been shown to remove a major part of bacterial contamination from the semen. In a study of 20 grossly contaminated samples processed by Percoll[137], 14 were found to be free of bacteria and the remaining processed samples had very low contamination.

Cryopreserved–thawed samples using Percoll separation

Methods of preparing cryopreserved samples for TDI have varied from a simple thaw with no special preparative technique (ICI) to a simple wash (one-step or two-step) with or without swim-up. Based on the fact that the simple wash and swim-up techniques do not address the issue of iatrogenic damage in an already compromised (cryopreserved) sample, their use for TDI samples is not recommended. Results of Percoll separation using cryopreserved samples have not been consistent[125], mainly because of the errors in handling the samples. In processing the cryopreserved samples for TDI, one very important factor must be remembered. Cryopreserved–thawed samples (mixture of semen and cryopreservation medium) have a high osmolality that can reach as high as 700–900 mOsmol/kg compared to the normal osmolality of around 285. To process a cryopreserved–thawed sample for sperm separation by the Percoll method, the sample must be thawed and a buffer-based medium with normal osmolality added to it. Care must be taken to add the buffer very slowly in order to avoid sudden exposure of sperm cells to a low (normal) osmolality environment. Osmolal shock to an already compromised cell is very real, although the indication of such shock may not be immediately observed; it may exert its effect hours after the insemination has been completed in the form of drastic motility or other functional loss. It is also important to add the diluting medium to the thawed sample prior to the loading on top of the Percoll layers. One alternative is to use a hyperosmolal (350–400 mOsmol/kg) Percoll medium. Using hyperosmolal Percoll, our preliminary results have shown a much higher recovery of the motile sperm fraction from cryopreserved samples. The influence of this method of recovery on the pregnancy outcome remains to be found.

Ovulation detection

In an attempt to improve TDI success rates several methods of detecting ovulation are being used. In a retrospective study of inseminations over a 2-year period[138], administered to women participating in a TDI program showed no significant difference between four different methods of ovulation detection with respect to the pregnancy outcome. Inseminations carried out several hours before or after the ovulation appeared to have no significant influence on the pregnancy outcome. However, in another study[83] it was found that, based on one TDI per cycle, the optimal time for insemination differed when IUI or ICI was utilized. The highest pregnancy rate per cycle following single ICI was when inseminations were carried out 0–10 h after the LH peak (as measured quantitatively twice daily). The optimal time for single IUIs was somewhat later, 10–20 h after the LH peak. In a randomized prospective study[139], it was found that home urinary LH detection was as effective as clinic methods (e.g. ultrasound). The practice did not affect significantly the pregnancy outcome of TDI. Another prospective randomized study[140] found timing based on BBT to be as effective as timing based on urinary LH surge (insemination the day after the surge). In another study[141], it was found that a substantial number of women with LH surge do not demonstrate sonographic evidence of ovulation until the second day after detection of the urinary LH surge. This evidence was associated with the clinical pregnancy rates in the study. A prospective randomized study of 264 TDI cycles monitored with LH surge kit and one ICI, or monitored based on previous cycle length and BBT and two ICIs, found a monthly fecundity rate of 0.123 for the first group and 0.053 for the second group (not significantly different). However, financially, it was more advantageous for the patients to use LH surge kits[142].

Miscarriage rates in TDI

The effects of treatment modalities on the success or miscarriage rates in TDI have also been investigated. In general, females with no history of ovulatory dysfunction or evidence of tubal diseases conceive sooner than those who are treated. However, those receiving stimulations may achieve the same likelihood of pregnancy as females with normal ovulatory function, but at a slower rate. In a study[143] of miscarriage rates between patients receiving TDI with a natural cycle versus those stimulated with menotropin, a significantly higher spontaneous abortion rate (28.5%) was observed in women with treatment cycles compared with those with natural cycles (11.7%). Whether or not the higher abortion rate is purely related to the treatment modality, surveillance bias or the hidden subsets in the patient groups influencing the results remains to be further studied. Gagliardi[144] reported that patients with ovulatory dysfunction (not normal ovulatory females) who did not conceive with hMG/IUI could benefit significantly by the addition of GnRHa to their controlled ovarian hyperstimulation regimens.

Pregnancy rates per TDI cycle

Effects of the number of inseminations per cycle on the TDI pregnancy outcome have also been investigated. In a prospective randomized study[145], pregnancy rates per treatment cycle of controlled ovarian hyperstimulation (COH) patients receiving one IUI per cycle were compared with those of COH patients receiving two IUIs. No significant differences were observed. In another study of normal ovulatory 25–40-year-old patients[146] (mean 34±1) randomized via patients' preference, 113 cycles of TDI using one ICI (on the day after LH surge) were compared with 100 cycles with two ICIs (on the day of and the day after LH surge). The monthly fecundity rate for those with one ICI was 0.06 and the rate for those with two ICIs was 0.21 which was significantly higher. The estimated cumulative probability of conception for six cycles in this study was reported to be 32% for the first group and 78% for the second group, indicating that the group with two consecutive ICIs had a significantly higher conception rate. However, in another prospective randomized study[83], the success rate for one or two inseminations was dependent upon the method of insemination. Patients with IUI had a pregnancy rate per cycle of 11.6% for two inseminations and 7.0% for one insemination ($P<0.05$). With the ICI, a pregnancy rate per cycle of 4.3% for two inseminations and 3.7% for one insemination was obtained (not significantly different).

It is a common belief that the quality of the sample and the number of motile sperm used in TDI can have a significant effect on the success rate. Although an adequate number of motile sperm must be provided, a minimum for the number of motile sperm to achieve success has not consistently been established. Using fresh semen and IUI, Dodson *et al.*[147] reported that no pregnancies occurred when $<1\times10^6$ motile spermatozoa were used for inseminations. However, the pregnancy rates for inseminations with 1–5 million motile sperm and >20 million (17% versus 16%, respectively) were not different. Byrd *et al.*[83] reported that the pregnancy outcome using cryopreserved semen following IUI and ICI was highly dependent upon the number of motile spermatozoa used for inseminations. The minimum number of motile spermatozoa required to obtain optimal pregnancy rates was found to be 6–15 million for IUIs and 50–100 million for ICIs. In the same study, it was found that the post-thaw motility of the sample could also significantly influence the pregnancy rate. Cryopreserved semen samples with the post-thaw motility of ≤30% had the lowest rate (5.5% for IUI) compared to those with the post-thaw motility of 30% to 50% (15.4%, IUI) and those with the post-thaw motility of >50% (27.2% IUI).

Our study of cervical inseminations using cryopreserved donor semen samples indicated that the highest number of pregnancies occurred when patients were inseminated with 40 million motile sperm[148]. In a study with a pregnancy rate per cycle of 24.8%[135], pregnant women were recipients of a significantly higher number of motile sperm (1.64×10^6) compared to non-pregnant counterparts (1.1×10^6). It was concluded that inseminations with 1.5×10^6 motile sperm at a maximum plasma estradiol level of 1100 pg/mL would result in an optimal pregnancy rate without increasing the possibility of multiple gestations. Pregnancy occurred in four of our TDI patients who returned for a second pregnancy and were inseminated (IUI with 2–8 million motile sperm) at their request with suboptimal samples from the same donors for their first children. These samples had not been given to other patients because they had a post-thaw motility of <25% with <10 million motile sperm per vial.

Scott *et al.*[113] evaluated characteristics of 33 cryopreserved ejaculates that resulted in pregnancy and 137 that did not after they were normalized via a square root transformation method. No statistical differences were observed between the two groups with regard to variables, such as percentage motility of the original sample or that of the post-thaws, and the number of motile sperm per insemination (5–28 million for pregnancies and 4.7–21 for non-pregnancies). In a self-controlled random study of 99 TDI cycles[146], patients were inseminated intracervically with a range of 20–60 million motile sperm. No significant difference was observed between the pregnant and non-pregnant groups with respect to the number of motile sperm inseminated. In a 15-year retrospective study[149], correlation between semen variables and the pregnancy outcome for 10 796 treatment cycles of TDI was assessed. The pregnancy rate per cycle for TDI was 8.9%. By logistic regression, sperm count in the fresh semen, normal morphology, post-thaw motility and post-thaw motility index explained 28% of the variance of the pregnancy rates.

Other factors related to donors including sperm motility in the fresh semen, donor age, weight and reproductive hormones were not contributory. It was concluded that sperm concentration, morphology and post-thaw motility are the most important factors for the selection of highly fertile donors, and that the pragmatic approach of discontinuing donors with reasonable number of failures (20–50) should continue. Using Fallopian tube sperm perfusion, Kahn *et al.*[115] found no difference in pregnancy rates between inseminations with 8–10 million motile sperm and those with 30 million or greater.

Female reproductive health and age

The contribution of females to the success or failure of TDI cannot be disputed. Female reproductive health and age have been shown to have a major impact on the success rate in TDI[84,114,150,151]. Even distribution of body fat in the female has been shown to have more significant effect on the pregnancy outcome than the female age or obesity[152]. A 0.1 unit increase in waist/hip ratio has shown to lead to a 30% decrease in the probability of conception per cycle after adjustment for age, obesity, reasons for TDI, cycle length and regularity, smoking and parity. In a study of 154 patients undergoing 467 TDI cycles, Byrd *et al.*[83] reported that females with no known infertility factor had a pregnancy rate of 14.9% for IUI and 7.5% for ICI. Those with ovulatory disorders had a rate of 6.1% for IUI and 2.2% for ICI. A very low pregnancy rate was observed in patients with endometriosis and an even lower rate in those with several infertility problems.

In a study of 751 married woman with azoospermic partners undergoing TDI[153], it was found that age was one of the most important factors influencing success rates. The estimated critical age for 'fall' in fecundity was approximately 31. After 12 cycles of TDI, the probability of pregnancy for women aged 31 or more was 0.54 compared to 0.74 for those <25 years of age. This difference between the two age groups disappeared after 24 cycles of TDI. The probability of having a healthy baby also decreased based on age. Authors concluded that, after the age of 31, the probability of conception decreases, but this decrease may be partially compensated for by continuing inseminations for more cycles. However, the chance of having a healthy baby is reduced by almost 50% in older females (>31) compared to those aged 25 years or younger.

In a prospective study of 26 infertile women who failed to conceive after nine or more cycles of TDI[150], it was found that 42% of recipients had retarded endometrium. Additionally, morphometric analyses revealed significant differences in the glandular component of the endometrium between this group and the control (fertile) group. In a study of 2998 TDI treatment cycles[151], it was found that gravidity did not influence the pregnancy outcome, but females <30 years of age had significantly higher pregnancy rates than those >30. The cumulative pregnancy rates for those aged 30 years or younger after three, six and 12 cycles of treatment were 21%, 40% and 62%, respectively. The rates for those >30 years were 17%, 26% and 44%, respectively, for the same number of cycles. In an attempt to provide the prognostic guidelines for TDI patients, it was found that recipients with treated endometriosis and ovulatory dysfunction had a significantly higher fecundity (0.093 and 0.091, respectively) than those with other infertility factors (0.021), such as fibroids, tubal disease or a combination of several infertility factors[154]. In this study, females with no infertility factor whose husbands were azoospermic had the highest fecundity (0.178).

Relationship of fertility status to basic semen parameters

Attempts have been made to identify and relate the fertility status of semen donors to characteristics such as their reproductive hormones and basic semen parameters. Findings have not been very successful in this respect. No single semen parameter in the fresh or cryopreserved semen has been found to be an excellent indication of a donor's fertility potential. In a study to identify such a parameter, Byrd *et al.*[83] reported that there was no difference between sperm count and percent motility in the fresh and cryopreserved semen of donors who achieved the highest number of pregnancies after 15 IUI cycles and those who did not. Based on computerized semen analysis data, the only significant factors differentiating the two groups of donors were the post-thaw linearity, straight-line velocity and lateral head displacement, which were found to be significantly higher in the group with the highest number of pregnancies. It is our experience that, although the higher post-thaw outcome is desirable with respect to the number of motile sperm survived/recovered, it has no major positive bearing on pregnancy outcome. In other words, not all samples with good cryosurvival may produce pregnancies.

Fertility status of the husband has also been reported to be associated with the pregnancy outcome of TDI[49–51,60,154]. It has been demonstrated that the wives of azoospermic individuals have a higher fecundity rate (0.20) compared to those whose husbands are oligozoospermic (0.10). Abortion rates and the incidence of pre-eclampsia have been reported to be higher in TDI patients with oligozoospermic husbands than those with azoospermic partners[49,52]. In another study[154], evaluation of 207 females participating in TDI revealed that those with no female factor and with azoospermic partners had the highest fecundity (0.178) compared to those with no female factor but with subfertile partners (0.036). Byrd *et al.*[83] indicated that the highest pregnancy rate was observed following IUI in women with no known female infertility and with azoospermic husbands (16.4%, $n=73$ cycles versus 9.7% for the entire group of patients). This may indicate a possible negative influence imposed by the subfertile male partner, a female factor yet to be identified (subsets within an apparently homogeneous group), and elimination from the group because of spontaneous conception in highly fertile females with subfertile partners.

Methods of data analysis and reporting

Methods of data analysis and reporting are other important factors when evaluating the success rate of TDI[6]. Success rates reported in terms of cumulative pregnancy rate, pregnancy rate per cycle and the total pregnancy rate in the form of pregnancy rate per patient or pregnancy rate per case (since some patients may return for a second pregnancy) could present very conflicting data. Often, patients starting in subsequent courses of treatment after the first successful attempt may or may not be included in the reports, without any mention of such inclusion or exclusion. Pregnancy for initial and subsequent courses could differ significantly, with the second conception occurring more rapidly. Reports of total number of pregnancies may appear falsely higher than the pregnancy rate per cycle. For example, five pregnancies resulting from 10 patients undergoing 40 cycles of insemination gives a pregnancy rate per patient of 50%, whereas the rate per cycle would be 12.5%. Life table analysis for the dropouts, discontinuations because of early successes or cessation of treatment is not always carried out. This may influence significantly the reported results. DiMarzo *et al.*[155] reported that the monthly fecundity rate using fresh donor semen for 3405 insemination cycles was found to be 11.9%, which was significantly different from the rate of 5.9% obtained for 371 cycles using cryopreserved semen. However, when life table analysis was performed, the cumulative pregnancy rate for the fresh semen was found to be 59.6% compared to 48.6% for the cryopreserved semen. Although statistics on take-home babies and pregnancy losses are a must in reporting TDI success, this is not often considered by the investigators. In some reports, it is unclear whether or not biochemical pregnancies have been included in the report of overall success rate. This is very important because of the fact that there have been some reports[156] of the slow excretion of exogenous hCG and the resultant false biochemical pregnancies observed in some patients. All of these variables influencing the outcome may result in incorrect reporting. Additionally, different forms of calculating and reporting the outcome make the comparison studies extremely difficult to carry out.

References

1. Kleegman, J. S. (1954). Therapeutic donor insemination. *Fertil. Steril.*, **5**, 7–31
2. Arny, M. and Quagliarello, J. R. (1987). History of artificial insemination. A tribute to Sophia Kleegman, M. D. *Semin. Reprod. Endocrinol.*, **5**, 1–3
3. US Congress, Office of Technology Assessment (1988). *Infertility: Medical and Social Changes, OTA-BA-358.* (Washington, DC: US Government Printing Office)
4. Schorer, L. R., Collins, R. L. and Richards, S. (1992). Psychological aspects of donor insemination evaluation and follow-up of recipient couples. *Fertil. Steril.*, **57**, 583–90
5. Loy, R. A. and Seibel, M. M. (1990). Therapeutic insemination. In Seibel, M. (ed.) *Infertility, A Comprehensive Text*, ch. 14, pp. 199–215. (Norwalk: Appleton and Lange)
6. Batzer, F. R. and Corson, S. L. (1987). Indications, techniques, success rates and pregnancy outcome: new directions with donor insemination. *Semin. Reprod. Endocrinol.*, **5**, 45–57
7. Humphrey, M. and Humphrey, H. (1987). A fresh look at genealogical bewilderment. *Br. J. Med. Psych.*, **59**, 133–40
8. Kovacs, G. T., Mushin, D., Kane, H. and Baker, H. W. G. (1993). A controlled study of the psychosocial development of children conceived following insemination with donor semen. *Hum. Reprod.*, **8**, 788–90
9. Daniels, K. R. (1994). Adoption and donor insemination: factors influencing couples' choices. *Child Welfare*, **78**, 5–13
10. Czyba, C. J. and Chevret, M. (1979). Psychological reactions of couples to artificial insemination with donor sperm. *Int. J. Fertil.*, **24**, 240–5
11. Strong, C. and Schinfeld, S. J. (1985). The single woman and artificial insemination by donor. *J. Reprod. Med.*, **29**, 293–9
12. The American Fertility Society. (1993). Guidelines for gamete donation. *Fertil. Steril.*, **59** (Suppl.), **1**, 1S–9S
13. American Association of Tissue Banks. (1992). *Technical Manual for Tissue Banking: Reproductive Cells and Tissues.* (1350 Beverly Rd., Suite 220A, McLean, VA 22101)
14. Randall, T. (1993). New tools ready for chlamydia diagnosis, treatment, what teams need education most. *J. Am. Med. Assoc.*, **269**, 2716–18
15. Witkins, S., Jeremias, J., Grifo, J. A. and Ledger, W. J. (1993). Detection of chlamydia trachomatis in semen by the polymerase chain reaction in male members of infertile couples. *Am. J. Obstet. Gynecol.*, **168**, 1457–62
16. Van den Brule, A. J. C., Hemrika, D., Walboomers, J., Raaphorst, P., Amstel, N., Bleker, O. P. and Meijer, C. (1993). Detection of chlamydia trachomatis in semen of artificial insemination donors by polymerase chain reaction. *Fertil. Steril.*, **59**, 1098–104
17. Dabekausen, Y., Evers, J., Land, J. and Stals, F. S. (1994). *Chlamydia trachomatis* antibody testing is more accurate than hysterosalpingography in predicting tubal factor infertility. *Fertil. Steril.*, **61**, 833–7
18. Imagawa, D. T., Lee, M. H., Wolinsky, S. M., Sano, K., Morales, F., Kwok, S., Sninsky, J. J., Parunag, G., Nishanian, P.g., Giorgi, J., Fahey, J. L., Dudley, J., Visscher, B. R. and Detels, R. (1989). Human immunodeficiency virus Type 1 infection in homosexual men who remain seronegative for prolonged periods. *N. Engl. J. Med.*, **320**, 1458–62
19. Imigawa, D. T. and Detels, R. (1991). HIV-1 in seronegative homosexual men. *N. Engl. J. Med.*, **325**, 1250–1
20. Nachtigall, R. D. (1994). Donor insemination and human immunodeficiency virus: a risk/benefit analysis. *Am. J. Obstet, Gynecol.*, **170**, 1692–8
21. Fuggers, E. F., Maddalena, A. and Schulman, J. D. (1993). Results of retroactive testing of human semen donors for cystic fibrosis and human immunodeficiency virus by polymerase chain reaction. *Hum. Reprod.*, **9**, 1435–7
22. Greenblatt, O. R. M., Handsfield, H. H., Sayers, M. H. and Holmes, K. K. (1986). Screening therapeutic insemination donors for sexually transmitted diseases: overview and recommendations. *Fertil. Steril.*, **46**, 351–64
23. Chiasson, M. A., Stoneburger, R. L. and Joseph, S. C. (1990). Human immunodeficiency virus transmission through artificial insemination. *J. AIDS*, **3**, 69–72
24. Hohnadel, D. C. (1989). Enzymes. In Kaplan, L. A. and Pesce, A. J. (eds.) *Clinical Chemistry: Theory, Analysis and Correction*, ch. 48, p. 783. (St Louis: C. V. Mosby Co.)
25. Hummel, W. P. and Talbert, L. M. (1989). Current management of a donor insemination program. *Fertil. Steril.*, **51**, 919–30

26. Long, D. J. and Kumner, J. F. (1972). Demonstration of cytomegalovirus infection in semen. *N. Engl. J. Med.*, **287**, 756–8
27. Yow, M. D., Williamson, D. W. and Leeds, L. J. (1988). Epidemiologic characteristics of cytomegalovirus infection in mothers and their infants. *Am. J. Obstet. Gynecol.*, **158**, 1189–95
28. McGowan, M. P., Hoges, K., Kovacs, G. T. and Leydon, J. A. (1983). Prevalence of cytomegalovirus and herpes simplex virus in human semen. *Int. J. Androl.*, **6**, 331
29. Huang, E.-S. and Kowalik, T. F. (1993). Consideration toward elucidating the mechanism of HCMV pathogenesis. In Becker, Y., Darai, G. and Huang, E.-S. (eds.) *Molecular Aspects of Human Cytomegalovirus Diseases*, p. 5 (Berlin: Springer-Verlag)
30. Jalbert, P., Leonard, C., Selva, J. and David, G. (1989). Genetic aspects of artificial insemination with donor semen. The French CECOS Federation Guidelines. *Am. J. Med. Genet.*, **33**, 269–75
31. Anderson, R. R., Brooks, K. A., Lemke, A., Uhlmann, W. and Valverde, K. (1990). *Genetic Testing for Cystic Fibrosis: A Handbook for Professionals*. (Wallingford, PA: National Society of Genetic Counselors)
32. Crum, C. P., Braun, L. A., Shah, K. V., Fu, Y., Levine, R. U., Fenoglio, C. M., Richart, R. M. and Townsend, D. E. (1982). Vulvar epithelial neoplasia: correlation of nuclear DNA content in the presence of human papilloma virus (HPV) structural antigen. *Cancer*, **49**, 468–71
33. Ostrow, R. S., Zachow, K. R., Niimura, M., Okagaki, T., Muller, S., Bender, M. and Faras, A. J. (1986). Detection of papilloma virus DNA in human semen. *Science*, **231**, 731–3
34. Chan, P. J., Su, B. C., Kalugdan, T., Seraj, I. M., Tredway, D. R. and King, A. (1994). Human papilloma virus gene sequence in washed human sperm deoxyribonucleic acid. *Fertil. Steril.*, **61**, 982–5
35. Matthews, C. D., Ford, J. H., Peek, J. C. and McEvoy, M. (1983). Screening of karyotype and semen quality in an artificial insemination program: acceptance and rejection criteria. *Fertil. Steril.*, **40**, 648–54
36. Perez, M. D. M., Marina, S. and Egozcue, J. (1990). Karyotype screening of potential sperm donors for artificial insemination. *Hum. Reprod.*, **5**, 282–5
37. Silva, J., Leonard, C., Albert, M., Auger, J. and David, G. (1986). Genetic screening for artificial insemination by donor (AID): Results of a study of 676 semen donors. *Clin. Genet.*, **19**, 389–96
38. Handelsman, D. J., Dunn, S. M., Conway, A. J., Boylan, L. M. and Jansen, R. P. S. (1985). Psychological and attitudinal profiles in donors for artificial insemination. *Fertil. Steril.*, **43**, 95–101
39. Verp, M. S. (1987). Genetic issues in artificial insemination by donor. *Semin. Reprod. Endocrinol.*, **5**, 59–68
40. Souka, A. R., Khalifa, A., Zaki, S., Rocca, M. and Ghonem, I. (1993). Human leukocyte antigen in hydatidiform mole. *Int. J. Gynaecol. Obstet.*, **41**, 257–60
41. Cho, D. Y., Chung, J. H., Shung, Y. K., Chang, Y. B., Han, H., Lee, J. B., Lee, H. K. and Koh, C. S. (1993). A strong association between thyrotropin receptor-blocking antibody-position atrophic autoimmune thyroiditis and HLA-DR8 and HLA-D9B1*0302 in Koreans. *J. Clin. Endocrinol. Metab.*, **77**, 611–15
42. Olmez, U., Turgay, M., Ozenirler, S., Tutkak, H., Duzgun, N., Duman, M. and Tokgoz, G. (1993). Association of HLA Class I and II antigens with rheumatic fever in a Turkish population. *Scand. J. Rheumatol.*, **22**, 49–52
43. Cardaba, B., Vilches, C., Martin, E., de Andres, B., del-Pozo, V., Hernandez, D., Gallardo, S., Fernandez, J. C., Villalba, M., Rodriguez, R. and Basomba, A. (1993). DR7 and DQ2 are positively associated with immunoglobulin-E response to the main antigen of olive pollen in allergic patients. *Hum. Immunol.*, **38**, 293–9
44. Huang, H. S., Huang, M. J. and Huang, C. C. (1992). Assessment of the association of HLA-DR314 heterozygotes with diabetes mellitus and non-diabetic diseases. *J. Formos. Med. Assoc.*, **91**, 233–6
45. Groop, L. and Bottazzo, G. F. (1994). Genetic susceptibility to non-insulin-dependent diabetes. *Br. Med. J.*, **308**, 534
46. Gray, D. J., Robinson, H. B., Malone, J. and Thorson, R. B. Jr. (1993). Adverse outcome in pregnancy following amniotic fluid isolation of ureaplasma urealyticum. *Obstet. Gynecol. Surv.*, **48**, 451–3
47. Quinlivan, W. L. G. and Sullivan, M. (1977). The immunologic effects of husband's semen on donor spermatozoa during mixed insemination. *Fertil. Steril.*, **18**, 448–50
48. Quinlivan, W. L. G. and Sullivan, M. (1977). Spermatozoa antibodies in human seminal plasma as a cause of failed artificial donor insemination. *Fertil. Steril.*, **28**, 1082–5
49. Amuzu, B. J. and Shapiro, S. S. (1993). Variation in spontaneous abortion rate relates to the indication for therapeutic donor insemination. *Obstet. Gynecol.*, **82**, 128–31
50. Albrecht, B. H., Cramer, D. and Schiff, I. (1991). Factors influencing the success of artificial insemination. *Fertil. Steril.*, **37**, 791–7
51. Kovacs, G. T., Leeton, J. F., Matthews, C. D., Steigrad, S. J., Saunders, D. M., Jones, W. R., Lyneham, R. and McMaster, R. (1982). The outcome of artificial insemination compared to the husband's fertility status. *Clin. Reprod. Fertil.*, **1**, 295–9
52. Need, J. A., Bell, B., Meffin, E. and Jones, W. R. (1983). Pre-eclampsia in pregnancies from donor inseminations. *J. Reprod. Immunol.*, **5**, 329–38
53. Friedman, S. (1980). Artificial insemination with donor semen mixed with semen of the infertile husband. *Fertil. Steril.*, **33**, 125–8
54. Mahadevan, M. M. and Trounson, A. O. (1984). Relationship of fine structure of sperm head to fertility of frozen human semen. *Fertil. Steril.*, **41**, 287–93

55. Brotherton, J. (1990). Cryopreservation of human semen. *Arch. Androl.*, **25**, 181–95
56. Sherman, J. K. (1973). Synopsis of the use of frozen human semen since 1964: state of the art of human semen banking. *Fertil. Steril.*, **24**, 397–412
57. Ackerman, D. R. and Sod-Moriah, U. A. (1968). DNA content of human spermatozoa after storage at low temperatures. *J. Reprod. Fertil.*, **17**, 1–7
58. Ashwood-Smith, M. J., Trevino, J. and Warby, C. (1972). Effect of freezing on the molecular weight of bacterial DNA. *Cryobiology*, **9**, 141–3
59. Verp, M. S., Cohen, M. R. and Simpson, J. L. (1983). Necessity of formal genetic screening in artificial insemination by donor. *Obstet. Gynecol.*, **62**, 474–9
60. Amuzu, B., Ladova, R. and Shapiro, S. S. (1990). Pregnancy outcome, health of children, and family adjustment of the donor insemination. *Obstet. Gynecol.*, **75**, 899–905
61. Varma, T. R. and Patel, R. H. (1987). Outcome of pregnancy following investigation and treatment of infertility. *Int. J. Gynaecol. Obstet.*, **25**, 113–20
62. Virro, M. R. and Shewchu, A. B. (1984). Pregnancy outcome in 242 conceptions after artificial insemination with donor sperm and effects of maternal age on the prognosis for successful pregnancy. *Am. J. Obstet. Gynecol.*, **148**, 518–24
63. Furse, R. A., Ackman, C. F. D. and Fraser, F. C. (1985). Possible teratogenic effects of artificial insemination by donor. *Clin. Genet.*, **28**, 23–6
64. Fédération Française des CECOS, Mattei, J. F. and Le Mare, C. B. (1983). Genetic aspects of artificial insemination by donor (AID). Indications, surveillance, and results. *Clin. Genet.*, **23**, 132–8
65. Fuller, B. J. (1991). The effect of cooling on mammalian cells. In Fuller, B. J. and Grout, B. W. W. (eds.) *Clinical Applications of Endocrinology*, pp. 1–21. (Boca Raton: CRC Press)
66. Triano, V. (1980). Artificial insemination and semen banks in Italy. In Daniel, A. and Price, W. (eds.) *Human Artificial Insemination and Semen Preservation*, p. 51. (New York: Plenum Press)
67. Bunge, R. G., Keettel, W. C. and Sherman, J. K. (1954). Clinical use of frozen semen. Report of four cases. *Fertil. Steril.*, **5**, 520–9
68. Bunge, R. G. and Sherman, J. K. (1954). Frozen human sperm. *Fertil. Steril.*, **5**, 193–4
69. Bunge, R. G. and Sherman, J. K. (1953). Fertilizing capacity of frozen-human spermatozoa. *Nature*, **172**, 767–8
70. Sherman, J. K. (1990). Cryopreservation of human semen. In Keel, B. A. and Webster, B. W. (eds.) *Handbook of the Laboratory Diagnosis and Treatment of Infertility*, ch. 13, pp. 224–59. (Boca Raton: CRC Press)
71. Sherman, J. K. (1978). Bibliography (with review) on artificial insemination and cryopreservation of human semen. *Biogr. Reprod.*, **32**, 401–4, 485–8
72. Serafini, P. and Marrs, R. P. (1986). Computerized staged-freezing technique improves sperm survival and preserves penetration of zona-free hamster ova. *Fertil. Steril.*, **5**, 854–8
73. Weidel, L. and Prins, G. S. (1987). Cryosurvival of human spermatozoa in eight different buffer systems. *J. Androl.*, **8**, 41–7
74. Bell, M., Wang, R., Hellstrom, W. J. G., Sikka, S. C. (1993). Effect of cryoprotective additives and cryopreservation protocol on sperm membrane lipid peroxidation and recovery of motile human sperm. *J. Androl.*, **14**, 472–8
75. Centola, G. M., Raibertas, R. F., Mattos, J. H. (1992). Cryopreservation of human semen: comparison of cryoprotectives, sources of variability, and prediction of post-thaw survival. *J. Androl.*, **13**, 383–8
76. Mahadevan, M., Trounson, A. O. (1983). Effect of cryoprotective media and dilution methods on the preservation of human spermatozoa. *Andrologia*, **15**, 355–66
77. Critser, J. K., Huse-Benda, A. R., Aaker, D. V., Ameson, B. W., Ball, G. D. (1987). Cryopreservation of human spermatozoa. I. Effects of holding procedure and seeding on motility, fertilizability, and acrosome reaction. *Fertil. Steril.*, **47**, 656–63
78. Alvarez, J. G., Storey, B. T. (1992). Evidence of lipid peroxidation damage and loss of superoxide dismutase activity as a mode of sublethal cryodamage to human sperm during cryopreservation. *J. Androl.*, **13**, 232–41
79. Lasso, J. L., Noiles, E. E., Alvarez, J. G., Storey, B. T. (1994). Mechanism of superoxide dismutase loss from human sperm cells during cryopreservation. *J. Androl.*, **15**, 255–65
80. Hammerstedt, R. H., Graham, J. J., Nolan, J. P. (1990). Cryopreservation of mammalian sperm: what we ask them to survive. *J. Androl.*, **11**, 73–87
81. Alvarez, J. G. and Storey, B. T. (1993). Evidence that membrane stress contributes more than lipid peroxidation to sublethal cryodamage in cryopreserved human sperm: glycerol and other polyols as sole cryoprotectant. *J. Androl.*, **14**, 199–208
82. Richter, M. A., Haning, R. V. and Shapiro, S. S. (1984). Artificial donor insemination: fresh versus frozen semen; the patient's versus her own control. *Fertil. Steril.*, **41**, 277–80
83. Byrd, W., Bradshaw, K., Carr, B., Edman, C., Odom, J. and Ackerman, G. (1990). A prospective randomized study of pregnancy rates following intrauterine and intracervical insemination using frozen donor sperm. *Fertil. Steril.*, **53**, 521–7
84. Bordson, B. L., Ricci, E., Dunaway, H., Taylor, S. N. and Carole, D. N. (1986). Comparison of fecundability with fresh and frozen semen in therapeutic donor insemination. *Fertil. Steril.*, **46**, 466–9
85. Morshedi, M., Oehninger, S., Veeck, L. L., Ertunc, H., Bocca, S. and Acosta, A. A. (1990). Cryopreserved/thawed semen for *in vitro* fertilization: results from fertile donors and infertile patients. *Fertil. Steril.*, **54**, 1093–9

86. Hatasaka, H. H., Hect, B. R. and Jeyendran, R. S. (1993). Absolute male factor infertility. A useful method for evaluating the efficacy of cryopreserved semen. *J. Reprod. Med.*, **38**, 692–4
87. Kovacs, G., Baker, G., Burger, H., DeKretser, D., Lording, D. and Lee, J. (1988). Artificial insemination with cryopreserved donor semen: a decade of experience. *Br. J. Obstet. Gynaecol.*, **95**, 354–60
88. Bromwich, P., Kilpatrick, M. and Newton, J. R. (1978). Artificial insemination with frozen stored donor semen. *Br. J. Obstet. Gynaecol.*, **85**, 641–4
89. Corson, S. L. and Batzer, F. R. (1987). Human gender selection. *Semin. Reprod. Endocrinol.*, **5**, 81–9
90. David, G., Czyglik, F., Mayaux, M. J., Martin-Boyce, A. and Schwartz, D. (1980). Artificial insemination with frozen sperm: protocol, method of analysis, and results of 1188 women. *Br. J. Obstet. Gynaecol.*, **87**, 1022–8
91. Mazur, P. (1984). Freezing of living cells: mechanisms and implications. *Am. J. Physiol.*, **247**, C-125–42
92. Grout, B. W. N. (1991). The effects of ice formation during cryopreservation of clinical systems. In Fuller, B. J. and Grout, B. W. W. (eds.) *Clinical Applications of Cryobiology*, pp. 81–93. (Boca Raton: CRC Press)
93. Wolf, D. P. and Patton, P. E. (1989). Sperm cryopreservation: state of the art. *J.* In Vitro *Fertil. Embryo Transf.*, **6**, 315–17
94. Brockbank, K. G. M., Carpenter, J. F. and Dawson, P. E. (1992). Effects of storage temperature on viable bioprosthetic heart valves. *Cryobiology*, **29**, 537–42
95. Karow, A. M. (1981). Biophysical and chemical consideration in cryopreservation. In Karow, A. M. and Pegg, D. E. (eds.) *Organ Preservation for Transplantation*, pp. 113–41. (New York: Dekker)
96. Walker, R. H. (1992). Pilot surveys for proficiency testing of semen analysis. Comparison of dry ice versus liquid nitrogen shipments. *Arch. Pathol. Lab. Med.*, **116**, 423–4
97. Bernard, A. G. (1991). Freeze preservation of mammalian reproduction cells. In Fuller, B. J. and Grout, B. W. W. (eds.) *Clinical Application of Cryobiology*, pp. 149–68. (Boca Raton: CRC Press)
98. Mahony, M. C., Morshedi, M., Scott, R. T., DeVilliers, A. and Erasmus, E. (1989). Role of spermatozoa cryopreservative in assisted reproduction. In Acosta, A. A. and Kruger T. F. (eds.) *Human Spermatozoa in Assisted Reproduction*, pp. 310–8. (Baltimore: Williams and Wilkins)
99. Jouannet, P., Frydman, R., Van Steirteghem, A., Wolf, J. P., Czyglik, F. and Van Den Abeel, E. (1990). Cryopreservation and infertility. In Seibel, M. M. (ed.) *Infertility, a Comprehensive Text*, ch. 37, pp. 525–38. (Norwalk: Appleton and Lange)
100. Schneider, U. (1986). Cryobiological principles of embryo freezing. *J.* In Vitro *Fertil. Embryo Transf.*, **3**, 3–9
101. Smith, K. D., Rodriguez-Rigau, L. J. and Steinberger, E. (1981). The influence of ovulatory dysfunction and timing of insemination on the success of artificial insemination donor with fresh or cryopreserved semen. *Fertil. Steril.*, **36**, 497–502
102. Brown, C. A., Boone, W. R. and Shapiro, S. S. (1988). Improved cryopreserved semen fecundability in an alternating fresh-frozen artificial insemination program. *Fertil. Steril.*, **50**, 825–7
103. Silva, P. D., Meisch, J. and Schauberger, C. W. (1989). Intrauterine insemination of cryopreserved donor semen. *Fertil. Steril.*, **52**, 243–5
104. DiMarzo, S. J., Huang, J., Kennedy, J. F., Villanueva, B., Hebert, S. A. and Young, P. E. (1990). Pregnancy rates with fresh versus computer-controlled cryopreserved semen for artificial insemination by donor in a private practice setting. *Am. J. Obstet. Gynecol.*, **102**, 1483–90
105. MacKenna, A. I., Zegers-Hochschild, F., Fernandez, E. O., Fabres, C. V., Huidobro, C. A. and Guadairama, A. R. (1992). Intrauterine insemination: critical analysis of a therapeutic procedure. *Hum. Reprod.*, **7**, 351–4
106. Robinson, J. N., Lockwood, G. M., Dokras, A., Egan, D. M., Ross, C. and Barlow, D. H. (1993). A controlled study to assess the use of *in vitro* fertilization with donor semen after failed therapeutic donor insemination. *Fertil. Steril.*, **59**, 353–8
107. Yavetz, H., Hessing, J. B., Niv, Y., Amil, A., Brok, Y., Yovel, I., David, M. P., Peyser, M. R., Yogev, L., Homonnai, Z. and Paz, G. (1991). The efficacy of cryopreserved semen versus fresh semen for *in vitro* fertilization/embryo transfer. *J.* In Vitro *Fertil. Embryo Transf.*, **8**, 145–8
108. Cefalu, E., Cittadini, E., Balmaceda, J. P., Guastella, C., Ord, T., Rojas, F. J. and Asch, R. H. (1988). Successful gamete intrafallopian transfer following failed artificial insemination donor: Evidence for a defect in gamete transport. *Fertil. Steril.*, **50**, 279–82
109. Englert, Y., Delvigne, A., Vekemans, M., Lejeune, B., Henlisz, A., DeMaertelaer, G. and Leroy, F. (1989). Is fresh or frozen semen to be used in *in vitro* fertilization with donor sperm? *Fertil. Steril.*, **51**, 661–4
110. Keel, B. A. and Webster, B. W. (1989). Semen analysis data from fresh and cryopreserved donor ejaculates: comparison of cryoprotectants and pregnancy rates. *Fertil. Steril.*, **52**, 100–5
111. Iffenden, D. A., Sallam, J. C. and Collins, W. P. (1985). A prospective randomized study comparing fresh semen and cryopreserved semen for artificial insemination by donor. *Int. J. Fertil.*, **30**, 54–6
112. Subak, L. L., Adamson, C. D. and Boltz, N. L. (1992). Therapeutic donor insemination: a prospective randomized trial of fresh versus frozen sperm. *Am. J. Obstet. Gynecol.*, **166**, 1597–64
113. Scott, S. G., Mortimer, D., Taylor, P. J., Leader, A. and Pattinson, H. A. (1990). Therapeutic donor

insemination with frozen sperm. *Can. Med. Assoc. J.*, **143**, 273–8
114. Stovall, D. W., Toma, S. K., Hammond, M. G. and Talbert, L. M. (1991). The effect of age on female fecundity. *Obstet. Gynecol.*, **77**, 33–6
115. Kahn, J. A., Von During, V., Sunde, A. and Molne, K. (1992). Fallopian tube sperm perfusion used in donor insemination program. *Hum. Reprod.*, **7**, 806–12
116. Melzer, H. (1991). Artificial human donor insemination as a treatment possibility for sterile couples at the gynecologic clinic of the Chemnitz 'Friedrich Wolf' District Hospital. *Zentralb. Gynakol.*, **113**, 7–12
117. Peters, A. J., Hecht, B., Wentz, A. C. and Jeyendran, R. S. (1993). Comparison of the methods of artificial insemination on the incidence of conception in single unmarried women. *Fertil. Steril.*, **59**, 121–4
118. Patton, P. E., Burry, K. A., Novy, M. J. and Wolf, D. P. (1990). A comparative evaluation of intracervical and intrauterine routes in donor therapeutic insemination. *Hum. Reprod.*, **5**, 263–5
119. Hurd, W. W., Randolph, J. F., Ansbacher, R., Menge, A. C., Ohl, D. A. and Brown, A. N. (1993). Comparison of intracervical, intrauterine, and intratubal techniques for donor insemination. *Fertil. Steril.*, **59**, 339–42
120. Patton, P. E., Burry, K. A., Thurmond, A., Novy, M. J. and Wolf, D. P. (1992). Intrauterine insemination outperforms intracervical insemination in a randomized controlled study with frozen donor semen. *Fertil. Steril.*, **57**, 559–64
121. Tyler, E. T. (1993). The clinical use of frozen semen banks. *Fertil. Steril.*, **24**, 413–16
122. Friberg, J. and Gemzell, C. (1977). Sperm freezing and donor insemination. *Int. J. Fertil.*, **22**, 148–54
123. Khan, J. A., Sunde, A., Koskemies, A., Von During, V., Sordal, T., Christensen, F. and Molne, K. (1993). Fallopian tube sperm perfusion (FSP) versus intrauterine insemination (IV) in the treatment of unexplained infertility: a prospective randomized study. *Hum. Reprod.*, **8**, 890–4
124. Jansen, R. P., Anderson, J. C., Radonic, I., Smit, J. and Sutherland, P. D. (1988). Pregnancies after ultrasound-guided fallopian insemination with cryostored donor semen. *Fertil. Steril.*, **49**, 920–2
125. Drobnis, E. Z., Zhony, C. O. and Overstreet, J. W. (1991). Separation of cryopreserved human semen using Sephadex columns, washing, or Percoll gradients. *J. Androl.*, **12**, 201–8
126. Mortimer, D. (1991). Sperm preparation techniques and iatrogenic failures of *in vitro* fertilization. *Hum. Reprod.*, **6**, 173–6
127. Drevius, L. O. (1971). The 'sperm rise' test. *J. Reprod. Fertil.*, **24**, 427–32
128. Aitken, R. J. and Clarkson, J. S. (1988). Significance of reaction oxygen species and antioxidants in defining the efficacy of sperm preparation techniques. *J. Androl.*, **9**, 367–76
129. Buch, J. P., Kolon, T. F., Maulik, N., Kreutzer, D. L. and Das, D. K. (1994). Cytokines stimulate lipid membrane peroxidation of human sperm. *Fertil. Steril.*, **62**, 186–8
130. Tanphaichitr, N., Millette, C. F., Agulnick, A. and Fitzgerald, L. M. (1988). Egg penetration ability and structural properties of human sperm prepared by Percoll-gradient centrifugation. *Gamete Res.*, **20**, 67–81
131. Mortimer, D., Mortimer, S. T. (1992). Methods of sperm preparation for assisted reproduction. *Ann. Acad. Med. Singapore*, **21**, 517–24
132. Suarez, S. S., Wolf, D. P. and Meizel, S. (1986). Induction of the acrosome reaction in human spermatozoa by a fraction of human follicular fluid. *Gamete Res.*, **14**, 107–21
133. Hyne, R. V., Stojanoff, A., Clarke, G. N., Lopata, A. and Johnston, W. I. H. (1986). Pregnancy from *in vitro* fertilization of human eggs after separation of motile spermatozoa by density gradient centrifugation. *Fertil. Steril.*, **45**, 93–6
134. Guerin, J. F., Mathieu, C., Lornage, J., Pinatel, M. C. and Boulieu, D. (1989). Improvement of survival and fertilizing capacity of human spermatozoa in an IVF programme by selection of discontinuous Percoll gradients. *Hum. Reprod.*, **4**, 798–804
135. Wainer, R., Merlet, F., Bailly, M., Aegeter, P., Triblats, S., Roussel, C. and Bisson, J. P. (1993). Retrospective evaluation of an intrauterine insemination program with donor. *Contracept. Fertil. Sex.*, **21**, 839–43
136. LeLannou, D. and Blanchard, Y. (1988). Nuclear maturity and morphology of human spermatozoa selected by Percoll density gradient centrifugation or swim-up procedure. *J. Reprod. Fertil.*, **84**, 551–6
137. Bolton, V. N., Warner, R. E. and Braude, P. (1986). Removal of bacterial contaminants from semen for *in vitro* fertilization or artificial insemination by the use of buoyant density centrifugation. *Fertil. Steril.*, **46**, 1128–32
138. Brook, P. F., Barratt, C. L. and Cook, I. D. (1994). The more accurate timing of insemination with regard to ovulation does not create a significant improvement in pregnancy rates in a donor insemination program. *Fertil. Steril.*, **61**, 308–13
139. Robinson, J. N., Lockwood, G. M., Dalton, J. D., Franklin, P. A., Farr, M. M. and Barlow, D. H. (1992). A randomized prospective study to assess the effect of the use of home urinary luteinizing hormone detection on the efficiency of donor insemination. *Hum. Reprod.*, **7**, 63–5
140. Odem, R. R., Durso, N. M., Long, C. A., Pidenda, J. A., Strickler, R. C. and Gast, M. J. (1991). Therapeutic donor insemination: a prospective randomized study of scheduling methods. *Fertil. Steril.*, **55**, 976–82
141. Pearlstone, A. C. and Surrey, E. S. (1994). The temporal relation between the urine LH surge and sono-

graphic evidence of ovulation: determinants and clinical significance. *Obstet. Gynecol.*, **83**, 184–8

142. Federman, C. A., Dumesic, D. A., Boone, W. R. and Shapiro, S. S. (1990). Relative efficiency of therapeutic donor insemination using a luteinizing hormone monitor. *Fertil. Steril.*, **54**, 489–92
143. Ransom, M. X., Bohrer, M., Blotner, M. B. and Kemmann, E. (1993). The difference in miscarriage rates between menotropin-induced and natural cycle pregnancies is not surveillance related. *Fertil. Steril.*, **59**, 567–70
144. Gagliardi, C. L. (1993) Utility of gonadotropin-releasing hormone agonists in programs of ovarian hyperstimulation with intrauterine insemination. *Clin. Obstet. Gynecol.*, **36**, 711–18
145. Ransom, M. D., Blotner, M. D., Bohrer, M., Corson, G. and Kemmann, E. (1994). Does increasing frequency of intrauterine insemination improve pregnancy rates significantly during super ovulation cycles? *Fertil. Steril.*, **61**, 303–7
146. Centola, G. M., Mattox, J. H. and Raubertas, R. F. (1990). Pregnancy rates after double versus single insemination with frozen donor sperm. *Fertil. Steril.*, **54**, 1089–92
147. Dodson, W. C. and Haney, A. F. (1991). Controlled ovarian hyperstimulation and intrauterine insemination for treatment of infertility. *Fertil. Steril.*, **55**, 457–67
148. Irianni, F. M., Morshedi, M., Oehninger, S. and Acosta, A. A. (1992). Therapeutic donor insemination (TDI): The Norfolk experience. *Assist. Reprod. Technol./Andrology*, (S), 35–47
149. Johnston, R. C., Kovacs, G. T., Lordin, D. H. and Baker, H. W. (1994). Correlation of seven variables and pregnancy rates for donor insemination. A 15-year retrospective study. *Fertil. Steril.*, **61**, 355–9
150. Li, T. C., Klentzeris, L., Burratt, C., Warren, M. A., Cooke, S. and Cook, I. D. (1993). A study of endometrial morphology in women who failed to conceive in a donor insemination programme. *Br. J. Obstet. Gynacol.*, **100**, 935–8
151. Shenfield, F., Doyle, P., Valentine, A., Steele, S. J. and Tan, S. L. (1993). Effects of age, gravidity and male infertility status on cumulative conception rates following artificial insemination with cryopreserved donor semen: analysis of 2,998 cycles of treatment in one centre over 10 years. *Hum. Reprod.*, **8**, 60–4
152. Zaadstra, B. M., Seidell, J. C., Van Noord, P. A., te-Velde, E. R., Habbena, J. D., Vrieswijk, B. and Karbaat, J. (1993). Fat and female fecundity: prospective study of effect of body fat distribution on conception rates. *Br. Med. J.*, **306**, 484–7
153. Van Noord, P. A., Zaadstra, B. M., Looman, C. W., Alsbach, H., Habbema, J. D., te Velde, E. R. and Karbaat, J. (1991). Delaying childbearing effect of age on fecundity and outcome of pregnancy. *Br. Med. J.*, **301**, 1361–5
154. Chauhan, M., Barrah, C. L. R., Cooke, S. M. S. and Cooke, I. D. (1989). Difference in the fertility of donor insemination recipients – a study to provide prognostic guidelines as to its success and outcome. *Fertil. Steril.*, **51**, 815–9
155. DiMarzo, S. J., Huang, J., Kennedy, J. F., Villanueva, B., Hebert, S. A. and Young, P. E. (1990). Pregnancy rates with fresh versus computer-controlled cryopreserved semen for artificial insemination by donor in a private practice setting. *Am. J. Obstet. Gynecol.*, **162**, 1483–90
156. Maier, D. B. and Metzger, D. A. (1992). Slow excretion of exogenous human chorionic gonadotropin stimulating repeated pregnancies and pregnancy losses. *Fertil. Steril.*, **59**, 1363–6
157. Ord, T. (1993). Techniques of sperm processing. Handbook for the postgraduate course (IV): *Technological Advances in the Diagnosis and Management of Male Infertility*, Twenty-sixth Annual Postgraduate Course, American Fertility Society, 9–14 October, pp. 19–33

Artificial insemination 2: using the husband's sperm

30

W. Ombelet, A. Cox, M. Janssen, H. Vandeput and E. Bosmans

INTRODUCTION

Artificial insemination with husband's semen (AIH) has been used in clinical medicine for more than 200 years in the treatment of infertile couples. The first documented application of AIH was done in London in the 1770s by John Hunter[1]. A patient with severe hypospadias was advised to collect, in a warmed syringe, the semen (which escaped during coitus) and inject the sample into the vagina. J. M. Sims[2] reported his findings of post-coital tests and 55 inseminations in the mid-1800s, but artificial insemination (AID) only became very popular after the introduction of sperm donation. For many years, homologous artificial inseminations were only indicated in cases of physiological and psychological dysfunction, such as retrograde ejaculation, vaginismus, hypospadias and impotence. With the routine use of post-coital tests other indications were added, such as hostile cervical mucus and immunological causes with the presence of anti-spermatozoal antibodies in the cervical mucus. Previous studies by Settlage *et al.*[3] were very disappointing regarding the capacity of motile spermatozoa to reach the oviduct. According to this report, only 0.1% of spermatozoa placed in the upper vagina were also present in the cervical canal 1 h after insemination. Even more striking was the finding that only one in every 14 million motile sperm deposited in the vagina reached the site of fertilization in the oviduct. A very important reduction in sperm number (5–6×) along the length of the female reproductive tract was previously described by Mortimer *et al.*[4]. The term AIH covers a wide range of different techniques. Washed or unwashed semen can be used and inseminated at various levels in the female reproductive tract. The insemination can be done intravaginally, intracervically, pericervically using a cap, intrauterine, intratubal or directly intraperitoneal. Most studies refer to intrauterine insemination (IUI) which seems to be an easy and better way of treatment. The rationale for the therapy of artificial insemination is the increase of gamete density at the site of fertilization[5]. The theroretical advantage of IUI over intravaginal techniques may be due to the increasing number of sperm arriving at the fertilization site, even when sperm or cervical mucus abnormalities are present. The increasing use of AIH in idiopathic and male infertility is mainly the result of the refinement of techniques for the preparation of washed motile spermatozoa as they were used in *in vitro* fertilization (IVF) procedures. Washing procedures seem to be necessary to remove prostaglandins, infectious agents and antigenic proteins. These techniques should also result in the removal of non-motile spermatozoa and round cells, either immature germ cells or leukocytes. This may be important, since the latter release lymphokines and/or cytokines that may reduce sperm fertilizing ability. Sperm preparation techniques also decrease the role of free oxygen radicals, another important factor for human sperm function *in vitro* and *in vivo*[6].

Several reports emphasize the value of semen preparation techniques (swim-up procedure, Percoll and miniPercoll gradient techniques) in selecting a sperm population with a better motility and morphology index[5,7–9].

These facts may indicate that intrauterine insemination of washed sperm can have a beneficial effect on the number of motile and morphologically normal spermatozoa at the ovulation site. However, the use of AIH remains controversial and the literature is still very confusing[10–18]. The population treated by AIH is very heterogeneous and ovulation induction regimens, semen preparation techniques and insemination procedures vary widely.

Table 1 Genk AIH Program: general data

Number of couples	412	
Number of cycles	1163	
cancelled	63	(5.4%)
completed	1100	(94.5%)
Mean number of inseminations per cycle	1.97	(range 1–2)
Duration of infertility (months)	33	(range 12–190)
Age of patients (years)		
male	31.4	(range 22–57)
female	29.2	(range 18–43)
Number of cycles		
primary infertility	812	(73.8%)
secondary infertility	288	(26.2%)

Especially in cases of idiopathic and male subfertility, the debate continues. The present study summarizes the data of 1100 artificial intrauterine inseminations at the Genk Institute for Fertility Technology in Genk, Belgium.

MATERIALS AND METHODS

During a period of 64 months, from September 1988 until December 1993, homologous artificial insemination was used in 412 subfertile couples during 1100 treatment cycles. Eleven hundred and sixty-three cycles were started, of which 63 were canceled (28 because of inadequate and 35 because of excessive ovarian response with a high risk of ovarian hyperstimulation and/or multiple pregnancies). A total of 2167 inseminations were performed with a mean of 1.9 (range 1–2) AIHs per cycle. We never performed three consecutive AIH cycles in order to give the couple some psychological rest. The average subfertility period for our couples was 33 months (range 12–190) with a mean age of 31.4 years for men (range 22–57) and 29.2 years for their partners (range 18–43) (Table 1). All patients had undergone an infertility work-up including ultrasound monitoring of folliculogenesis, luteal phase concentrations of progesterone, hysterosalpingogram indicating a normal uterine cavity and at least one patent tube and a midcycle post-coital test. Antisperm antibody measurements (ELISA, IBL, RE 52029, Eurogenetics, Tessenderlo, Belgium) of both partners were examined and male subfertility was diagnosed when sperm abnormalities were found on at least two recent sperm examinations. Semen specimens were collected by masturbation in a specimen container after an abstinence period of 2–4 days for the first sample and 24 h for the second sample. It was delivered to the laboratory within 1 h of collection and after complete liquefaction the semen was analyzed according to the WHO guidelines[19], except for the sperm morphology. For this important parameter we used the strict criteria as described by Kruger *et al.*[20].

A laparoscopy and hysteroscopy were performed when endometriosis was suspected, with a history of previous abdominal surgery or when the hysterosalpingogram revealed no clear diagnosis of bilateral tubal patency.

PATIENT SELECTION: INDICATION FOR AIH

The couples were grouped into four major categories: unexplained infertility; female factor including cervical factor, endometriosis and ovulatory dysfunction; male factor only; and the combination of male and female factors.

1. Unexplained infertility was considered if no abnormalities could be found during the infertility work-up.

2. Female factor:
   a. *Cervical factor:* this diagnosis was only made when a well-timed post-coital test was negative (<3 motile sperm/high power field) and no signs of infection or cervical antisperm antibodies were present. Often an anatomic defect, mostly after a previous conization, could be detected.
   b. *Endometriosis:* in almost 50% of our patients a laparoscopy was performed, mostly because endometriosis was suspected after history of patient's complaints. We classified our patients according to the revised AFS guidelines[21].
   c. *Ovulatory dysfunction:* patients with a history of oligomenorrhea or amenorrhea, an abnormal basal body temperature (BBT) chart and abnormal findings midcycle (ultrasonography, hormonal) were categorized as having ovulatory disorders.

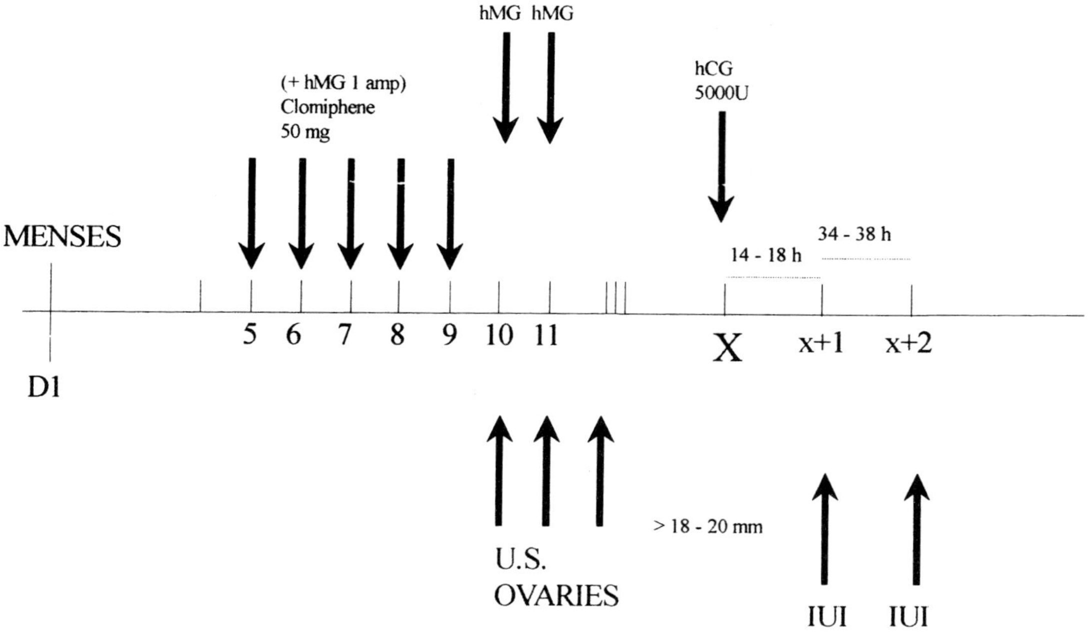

Figure 1 Genk AIH Program: practical scheme of a treatment cycle (U.S. denotes ultrasonographic measurement of follicles, IUI intrauterine insemination)

3. Male factor:
   A male factor was diagnosed if sperm concentration was <20 mill/mL, total motility (grade a+b)<50%, and sperm morphology <9% normal forms according to the strict criteria.

   Moderate and severe OTA (oligo-, terato-, asthenozoospermia) was diagnosed if three of the following results were present:

   (a) Moderate OTA: <20 mill/mL
   <25% grade a motility
   <50% grade a+b motility
   <9% normal forms

   (b) Severe OTA: <10 mill/mL
   <10% grade a motility
   <20% grade a+b motility
   <5% normal forms

   Regarding immunological factors, only the patients with a positive mixed antiglobulin reaction (MAR test >40%) were taken into account.

4. Combined female and male factor.

OVARIAN STIMULATION

All our patients received follicular stimulation medication. The first choice treatment was the clomiphene citrate–human chorionic gonadotropin (CC-hCG) regimen. A daily dose of 50 mg was given for 5 days starting on days 3–5 of the cycle. In those patients with a history of clomiphene resistance, or in cases where no pregnancy occurred after two or more AIH treatment cycles, we always used the combination of CC 50 mg and 75 units of human menopausal gonadotropin (hMG) every day from day 5 to day 9 (CC-hMG-hCG regimen). At the 10th day of the cycle, all patients attended our clinic for follicular ultrasonography and serum estradiol determination. Additional hMG (75 or 150 units) was given during the following days if the ovarian response was insignificant. In both regimens, hCG 5000 units were given when the average diameter of the dominant follicle was more or equal to 19 mm (Figure 1). In 39 cycles, we used a combination of GnRH analogues and hMG. In all these patients, an *in vitro* fertilization procedure was planned but canceled because of insufficient ovarian response (<three follicles with an average of 15 mm or more).

INSEMINATION PROCEDURE

In 1072 cycles, two high intrauterine inseminations were done on two consecutive days in the periovulatory period. The inseminations were timed 14–18 h and 36–40 h post-hCG (Figure 1). The washed motile fraction was inserted up to the uterine fundus and the sperm were gently expelled into the uterine cavity. Subsequently the catheter was withdrawn and the patient remained in supine position for 30 min after the insemination. We always used a Frydman catheter. In 37 cases the procedure was very difficult and the insemination could only be performed after cervical dilatation. Moderate bleeding was noted in 22 treatment cycles.

SEMEN EXAMINATION AND PREPARATION

As already mentioned every semen sample was analyzed after complete liquefaction according to the WHO guidelines, except for sperm morphology. Sperm morphology was assessed according to the strict criteria[20,22,23]. At least 200 spermatozoa situated in more than five different fields were evaluated and the percentage of sperm cells with complete normal forms were defined as the morphology index. A hypo-osmotic swelling test according to Jeyendran *et al.*[24] was always done. A mixed antiglobulin reaction (MAR) test for immunoglobulin IgG was performed on all semen samples to detect the presence of antisperm antibodies. This test was considered positive if >40% of spermatozoa demonstrated immunoglobulin attachment. Sperm were prepared by the conventional swim-up technique. After liquefaction all fresh semen samples were diluted with 5 mL Earle's balanced salt solution (EBSS) supplemented with penicillin, streptomycin and pyruvate (1 mL sample to 2 mL EBSS) and centrifuged at 200***g*** for 10 min. The pelleted spermatozoa were centrifuged once more after resuspension in supplemented EBSS. Supernatants were discarded again. For normal semen specimens (count >20 million/mL and total motility >40%) the pellets were gently layered over with 2 mL EBSS supplemented with penicillin, pyruvate and 0.3% human serum albumin and incubated at 37°C. The most motile fraction was selected by gentle aspiration of 1–1.5 mL of the supernatant. Sperm concentration and motility were counted once again. Finally, this fraction was concentrated to 0.3 mL by centrifugation. For subnormal sperm samples (count <20 million/mL and an initial total motility <40%) we performed only one wash procedure, followed by centrifugation of the pellets on a miniPercoll gradient (1 mL 95%–1 mL 50% Percoll) at 200***g*** for 20 min. The 95% fraction was recovered and washed twice with EBSS + penicillin and pyruvate. The pellet was resuspended in 1 mL EBSS + 0.3% human serum albumin. Motility and concentration were determined and the samples were also concentrated to 0.3 mL.

DEFINITION OF PREGNANCIES

Chemical and clinical pregnancies were taken into account. Clinical pregnancies were defined by a normal gestational sac at 6 weeks of pregnancy on vaginal ultrasonography. The pregnancy was considered to be 'ongoing' if clinical and ultrasound parameters looked normal beyond 20 weeks of gestation.

Statistics

Receiver operating characteristic (ROC) curve analysis was used to determine the predictive power of different sperm parameters. Group mean differences were ascertained by means of paired *t*-test, analysis of variance (ANOVA), multivariate ANOVA (MANOVA) and linear discriminant analysis (LDA). The differences between non-conceptional and conceptional cycles were tested by a paired *t*-test for unpaired samples and by chi-square tests after classification of patients in function of semen analysis results in contingency tables.

RESULTS

AIH yielded a total of 149 pregnancies in 1100 treatment cycles. A conception rate of 13.5% per cycle was observed, although in 900 cycles (81.8%) a male factor could be demonstrated. The cycle fecundity per couple was 36.2% after a mean of 1.8 cycles (range 1–6). A baby take-home rate of 10.2% per treatment cycle and a chemical and clinical abortion rate of 23.8% were noted.

The pregnancy rate (PR) per cycle (cycle fecun-

Table 2 Life table analysis for all patients undergoing AIH (1100 cycles)

Cycle number	*Number of patients*	*Conceptions*	*Withdrawals (%)*	*Conception rate per cycle (%)*	*Cumulative probability of conception*
1	454	81	92 (24.6)	17.8	0.17
2	281	32	55 (22.1)	11.4	0.26
3	194	26	65 (38.6)	13.4	0.35
4	103	7	56 (58.3)	6.8	0.40
5	40	2	20 (50.0)	5.0	0.43
6	18	1	7 (38.8)	5.5	0.46
>6	10	0			

Table 3 Cycle fecundity by female's age and duration of infertility

Age (years)	*Conception rate per cycle*	*Fecundity*	*Duration of infertility (months)*	*Conception rate per cycle*	*Fecundity*
<25	9/65	0.13	<24	60/291	0.20*
25–29	69/475	0.14	25–47	57/507	0.11
30–34	55/436	0.12	48–71	21/182	0.11
35–39	16/115	0.13	72–95	7/54	0.12
>39	09	0.00	>95	4/66	0.06*

*Chi-square statistics, *P*<0.05

Table 4 Type of ovulation induction (chi-square statistics, *P*<0.05)

Type of stimulation	*Number of cycles (%)*	*Total (%)*	*Number of pregnancies*		
			Single	*Twins*	*Triplets*
CC-hCG*	548	55 (10.0)†	55	—	—
CC-hMG-hCG*	508	90 (17.7)†	75	13	2
GnRH-hMG-hCG*	39	4 (10.2)	2	2	—
Pure FSH-hCG*	5	0	—	—	—
	1100	149	132 (88.6)	15 (10.0)	2 (1.4)

*CC=clomiphene citrate, hCG=human chorionic gonadotropin, hMG=human menopausal gonadotropin, GnRH=gonadotropin releasing hormone analogue, FSH=follicle stimulating hormone. †Chi-square statistics, *P*<0.05

dity) is shown in Table 2. The PR was significantly higher in the first treatment cycle (17.9% for cycle one versus 10.5% for cycles two to six *P*<0.001).

Regarding the duration of infertility, the patients with an infertility period of 12–24 months scored significantly better than those with an infertility problem for more than 2 years (PR 20.6% versus 10.6%, *P*<0.0001) (Table 3). We were unable to demonstrate the influence of female age on the conception rate in this study. A cycle fecundity of 13.9% (16/115) in patients of 35–39 years old was not different from patients less than 30 years old (78/540 or 14.4%) (Table 3).

Table 4 shows the cycle fecundity among the different ovarian stimulation protocols. For gonadotropin stimulation cycles a higher PR was found compared to clomiphene (only) stimulated cycles (17.7% versus 10.0%, *P*<0.0001). All twin (15 or 10%) and triplet pregnancies (two or 1.4%) occurred after using hMG for ovulation induction.

Cycle fecundity of AIH performed in canceled IVF cycles did not differ from the planned AIH cycles (Table 5). Although an easy insemination seems to yield a better prognosis per cycle compared to difficult inseminations, the difference was not statistically significant (Table 6).

The indication for AIH was not helpful in predicting pregnancy rates in this study. The con-

Table 5 Influence of a difficult or easy insemination procedure on cycle fecundity

	Cycles	*Pregnancies*	*Conception rate per cycle (%)*
Easy	1041	142	15.8*
Difficult	59	7	11.9

*Not significant

Table 6 Cycle fecundity for 'canceled IVF' versus 'planned AIH' treatment cycles

	Cycles	*Pregnancies*	*Conception rate per cycle (%)*
Canceled IVF	101	11	10.9*
Planned AIH	999	138	13.8

*Not significant

ception rates per cycle were 11.1% for idiopathic infertility, 13.3% for female factor only, 11.8% for male factor only and 16.5% for combined male and female factor, respectively (Table 7).

A history of secondary infertility yielded no better prognosis than the primary infertility group (PR per cycle 13.5% and 13.4%, respectively).

Individual sperm parameters were of no value in predicting conception using the ROC curve. The use of ROC curve analysis is a very good method to compare the different diagnostic tests that are used for the same purpose, in this case the prediction of pregnancy during an AIH cycle. The ROC curve for an ideal diagnostic test result reaches the upper left-hand corner, whereas a parameter with no diagnostic value appears as a 45-degree line through the origin.

Figure 2 clearly shows that none of our investigated sperm parameters showed any predictive or diagnostic value. Multivariate analysis of variance (MANOVA) and linear discriminant analysis (LDA) were performed on different sperm factors (semen volume, morphology index, total count, sperm concentration, motility (total grade a+b or grade a motility only), total motile sperm after washing, hyperactive and grade a motility after washing) as discriminating variables. By means of MANOVA no significant separation was detected between conceptional and non-conceptional cycles ($F=0.9$, Wilk's $X=0.95$, d.f. = 13/280, $P=0.5$). LDA showed no significant separation of both groups. After dividing the patients into different groups (normal, moderate and severely abnormal) for all investigated sperm factors only a morphology score of <5% normal forms, a hypo-osmotic swelling test score (HOS) of <40%, a total motile count of 300 000 or less spermatozoa after washing and a percentage of <10% hyperactive + grade a motility after washing indicate a bad prognosis regarding cycle fecundity (Figure 3). A total motility score of <40% yielded a PR of 8.6%, less than the 14.5% of the control group (motility >40%) ($P<0.05$). We also compared the conceptional cycles (CC-group, 149

Table 7 Different indications and results of 1100 AIH cycles in 412 couples

Indication	*Number of cycles (%)*	*Pregnancies*	*% Pregnancies/cycle*
• Idiopathic	72 (6.5)	8	11.1
• Female factor	128 (11.6)	17	13.3
cervical	29 (2.6)	2	6.9
endometriosis	57 (5.2)	7	12.2
ovulatory	42 (3.8%)	8	19.0
• Male Factor	526 (47.8)	62	11.8
oligo	7 (0.6)	1	14.3
astheno	36 (3.3)	1	2.7
terato 1 (5–8% normal)	136 (12.4)	17	12.5
terato 2 (0–4% normal)	147 (13.4)	14	9.5
moderate OTA*	71 (6.4)	12	16.9
severe OTA*	129 (11.7)	17	13.1
• Combined (female & male)	374 (34.0)	62	16.5
Total	1100 (100%)	149	13.5

*OTA = oligo, astheno, teratozoospermia

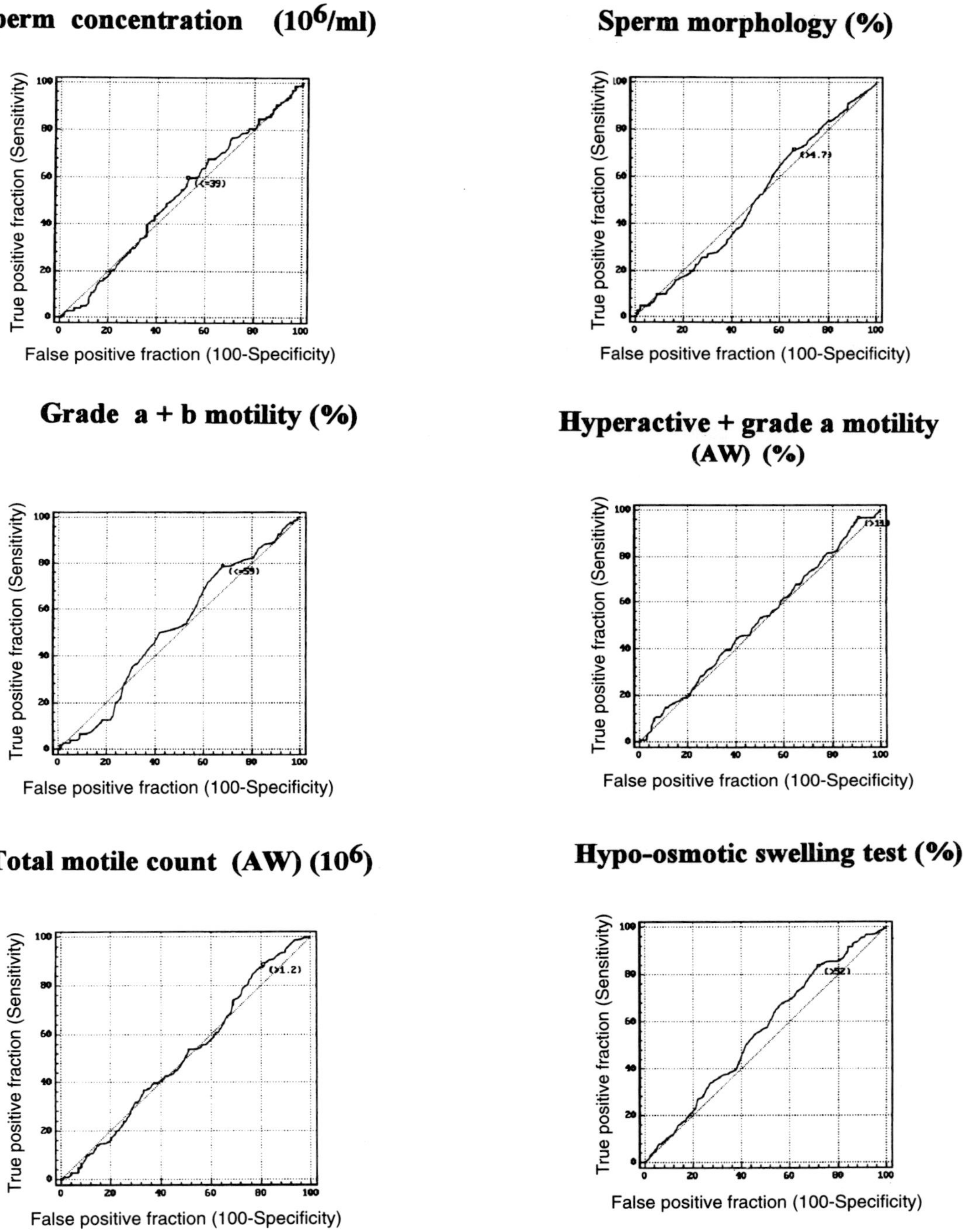

Figure 2 Receiver operating characteristic (ROC) analysis of six different semen parameters measured on sample of day 1. AW denotes for 'after washing'; ° = criterion value corresponding with the highest accuracy (minimal false negative and false positive results)

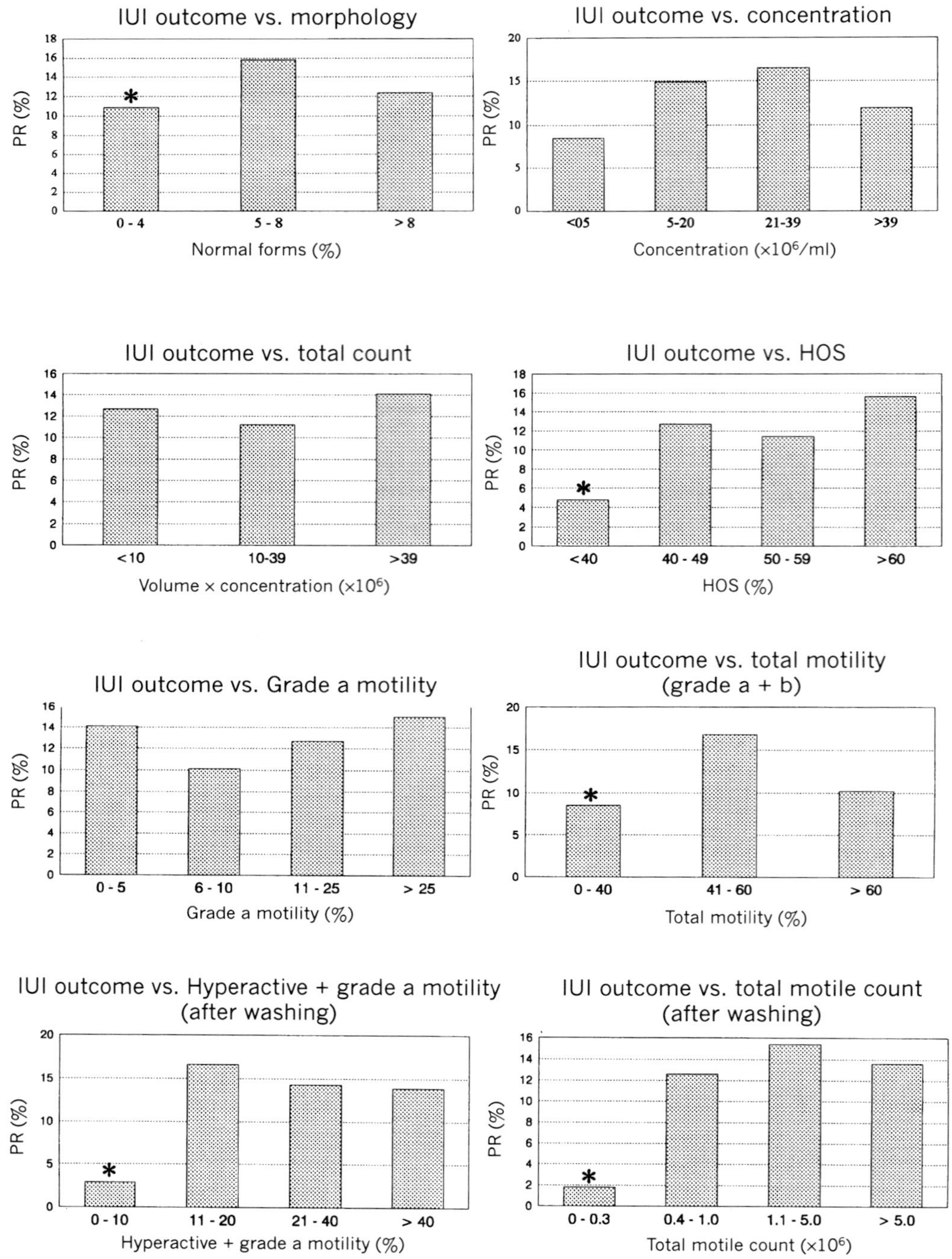

Figure 3 Analysis of eight different semen parameters (PR denotes pregnancy rate per cycle, HOS denotes hypo-osmotic swelling test). *Differences statistically significant by Chi-square and Fisher exact probability test $P<0.05$

Table 8 Comparison of the characteristics of the pregnant and the non-pregnant AIH-cycles

	NCC‡-group (154) (mean ± SD)	*CC†-group (149) (mean ± SD)*	*Statistics**
Age (years) (F)	29.6 ± 3.6	29.5 ± 3.6	NS
Age (years) (M)	31.9 ± 5.2	31.5 ± 4.7	NS
Duration of infertility (months)	39.0 ± 28.5	32.5 ± 27.0	NS
Semen factors			
Volume (mL)	3.2 ± 1.5	3.4 ± 1.7	NS
Concentration (mill/mL)	56.2 ± 51.5	47.0 ± 45.5	NS
Morphology	7.1 ± 3.9	7.3 ± 4.4	NS
Grade a motility (%)	23.3 ± 15.4	20.9 ± 14.5	NS
Total motility (Grade a + b) (%)	51.8 ± 16.5	51.0 ± 13.4	NS
FIT-test (%)	59.3 ± 19.6	61.8 ± 18.1	NS
Hyper + good (after washing) (%)	47.7 ± 22.7	49.0 ± 22.1	NS
Total motile count (mill)	8.9 ± 10.3	8.1 ± 9.7	NS

*Differences between CC and NCC cycles were tested by paired *t*-test for unpaired samples; $P<0.05$, NS = not significant; †CC = conceptional cycle; ‡NCC = non-conceptional cycle of couples completing at least 3 AIH cycles

cycles) with all non-conceptional cycles (NCC-group: 154 cycles) of couples completing at least three consecutive AIH cycles. The following parameters were examined: female and male age, duration of infertility and different semen parameters. As shown in Table 8 there was no significant difference (X ± SD) between the studied conceptional and non-conceptional cycles.

Figure 4 summarizes the follow-up of our 412 couples. We found a surprisingly low number of natural conceptions during this 64-month period (35 or 8.5%). The high number of male infertility probably attributes to this low figure. Unsuccessful AIH cycles were followed by IVF or GIFT procedures in 35.4% of our patients. Of this group of patients, 56.2% became pregnant within three treatment cycles. A large number of patients withdrew after the fourth AIH cycle (20% after cycle five, 55.5% after cycle six). Some of these patients refused to continue with other techniques of assisted reproduction.

PREGNANCY OUTCOME

In our series of patients, we achieved 149 pregnancies. They were complicated by two ectopic pregnancies (1.3%), 14 chemical (9.4%) and 21 clinical abortions (14.0%). Ninety-five patients delivered and seventeen preganancies are still ongoing (beyond 20 weeks' gestation). The increase in the observed rate of early miscarriages in AIH patients may be related to factors responsible for the subfertility (luteal phase defects, genetic defects), or may be due to the very early detection of pregnancies in this study population. We noticed a surprisingly high amount of intrauterine growth retardation for singleton pregnancies (15/95 or 15.8%). This incidence is much higher than the normal rate of this complication, even for patients with the same age and parity in our institute, as described earlier[25]. Our multiple pregnancy number was 17 (11.4%) including 15 twin and two triplet pregnancies.

COMPLICATIONS

None of our patients required hospitalization because of severe ovarian hyperstimulation (OHSS) despite the presence of ovulatory disorders in 11% of them, which is believed to be the most important predisposing factor for OHSS. This was probably due to the careful monitoring of serum estradiol (E_2) concentrations and ultrasound monitoring of the number and size of ovarian follicles. Human chorionic gonadotropin was withdrawn when E_2 reached a level of 1200 pg/mL or more and, under these circumstances, we advised the couple to refrain from intercourse during the following days.

Pelvic inflammatory disease, another complication of intrauterine catheterization, was found in one patient. We did not use prophylactic antibiotics in our institute and we agree with others that it will be difficult to prove the effectiveness of prophylactic antibiotics for AIH due to this low incidence of salpingitis[5,15,26]. Another disadvantage of AIH may be

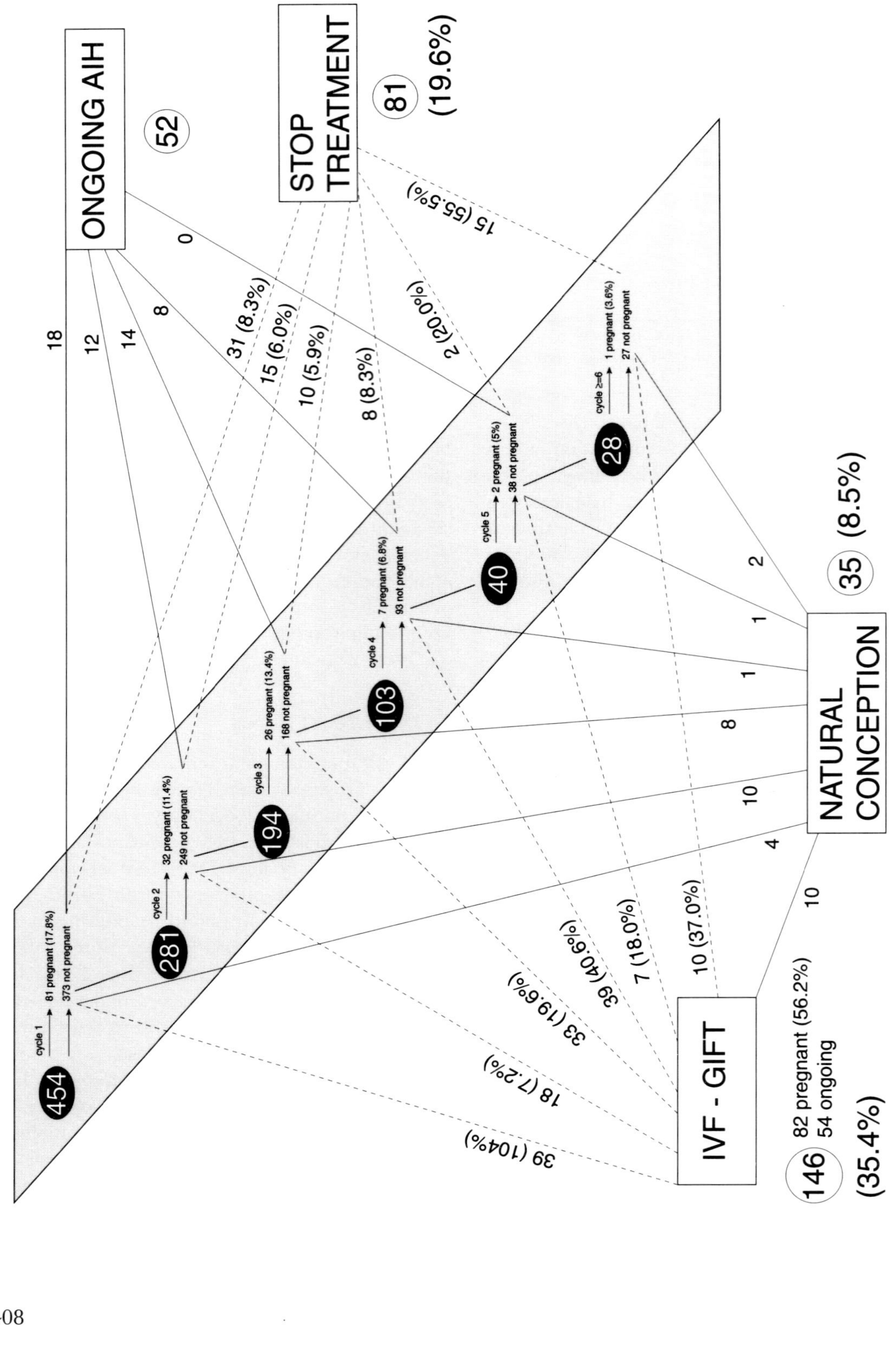

Figure 4 Genk AIH Program: follow-up study of 412 couples

the possible increase in titers of antisperm antibodies in the women post-insemination. With normal intercourse only tens of hundreds of spermatozoa reach the peritoneal cavity. Using AIH techniques, the introduction of large numbers of sperm may lead to an increased risk of sensitization, although the literature remains controversial regarding this issue[27,28]. In this series, we did not evaluate the serum antibody titer before and after AIH.

DISCUSSION

At present, conflicting claims are often made regarding the efficacy and merits, use and abuse of different methods of assisted procreation. The clinical value of artificial insemination with husband's sperm remains controversial, at the least. Nevertheless, all clinicians working in the field of human reproduction have to admit that there is still a need for a simple, less expensive and acceptable treatment that offers a reasonable success rate. The treatment with AIH should be of great value for patients rejecting the more expensive and aggressive assisted reproduction techniques (GIFT, IVF, ZIFT), at least if similar results can be obtained with the same selection of patients. Especially in small infertility clinics or in a general gynecological practice, this simple technique of AIH may be available to all physicians working in unsophisticated circumstances.

In this series, we almost always used ovulation induction medication (CC-hCG, CC-hMG, hCG or GnRH analogs-hMG-hCG) during AIH treatment cycles. The difference in cycle fecundity between the different regimens, in favor of the gonadotropins, has been described previously[29–35]. The enhanced conception rate with the use of gonadotropins (compared to the CC-hCG regimen) can be attributed to the increased number of fertilizable oocytes. Nevertheless, we had no multiple pregnancies after CC-hCG, indicating the value of this stimulation regimen for a large number of subfertile couples starting AIH procedures (stepwise treatment to avoid a high number of unwanted multiple pregnancies). We almost always performed two intrauterine inseminations on two consecutive days post-hCG. According to the literature, no definite statement can be made whether or not two inseminations per cycle are necessary[29,36–38]. We preferred intrauterine insemination because this technique seems to be more successful than intravaginal or intracervical (cap) inseminations[39] and is less aggressive than intraperitoneal inseminations. The risk of infection after intrauterine catheterization is negligible, since the development of new methods of semen preparation. Female age was of no value in predicting conception in our study, as described before in a male infertility group[40]. The first AIH cycle was the most successful in this study. The observation of a significant decline in cycle fecundity after the third well-timed AIH cycle does not agree with other studies, although some authors report the same phenomenon after the fourth treatment cycle[26,41–43]. Regarding the predictive value of different sperm factors on cycle fecundity, the literature is confusing[44,45]. Our results did not support the value of individual semen parameters in predicting conception in AIH cycles. In our hands a total motile sperm count of >300 000 spermatozoa after sperm preparation seems to be necessary to justify AIH treatment. An ongoing pregnancy rate of almost 10% was reached even when only 400 000–500 000 motile spermatozoa were recovered after washing procedure. With a total count of <10 million sperm cells in the initial sample, our PR per cycle was 12.7%. These data are in contrast with other studies reporting the poor prognosis with AIH for oligozoospermic males[11,46,47].

A score of at least 10% hyperactive + grade a motility after washing procedure seems to be of value in predicting conception after AIH. The hypo-osmotic swelling test and sperm morphology according to the strict criteria were also helpful in predicting success. According to the literature the use of strict criteria appears to increase the correlation between sperm morphology and success or failure in IVF[48–51]. The need for *in vivo* studies concerning this semen parameter is crucial. In this series we found a significant difference in cycle fecundity comparing the 'poor-prognosis' (<5% normal forms) with the 'good-prognosis' group (5–8% normal forms). Our cutoff point at 9% was calculated statistically by reviewing 162 IVF cycles in our center[52]. However, using the ROC curve analysis individual semen parameters showed to be of limited or no value in predicting conception rates. This finding might be explained by the large amount of variables influencing the pregnancy rates in individuals. According to our results derived from a large prospective study, at least three AIH cycles might be beneficial for most patients with patent tubes, taking into account that this technique is simple, relatively non-invasive and probably more cost-effective than IVF or GIFT procedures. Although some reports question the value of AIH for male subfertility and rather prefer GIFT as a first choice treatment[53,54], our results do support the belief that AIH is a useful method in the treatment of male infertility, a confirmation of many other studies[55–58]. The general applicability of AIH as a 'front line' treatment for non-tubal infertility should be considered and validated in further prospective controlled studies.

CONCLUSIONS

(1) AIH is a simple and non-invasive technique with a very low complication rate. AIH can be performed without expensive infrastructure.

(2) No difference in success after AIH was observed between the primary and secondary infertility group.

(3) The negative predictive value of the duration of infertility as an exclusion criterion for selecting couples for AIH treatment was only valid for an infertility period of more than 8 years.

(4) In AIH highest success rates are observed for the first attempt and PR only drops significantly after the third treatment cycle.

(5) Below the age of 40 years, female age was not predictive concerning conception rate per cycle after AIH treatment.

(6) Ovulation stimulation with gonadotropins yields better results after AIH treatment compared to the clomiphene treated cycles, taking into account the higher incidence of moderate ovarian hyperstimulation and multiple pregnancies.

(7) The withdrawal rate of patients only became important after the sixth AIH cycle.

(8) Failure in four consecutive AIH cycles is no negative predictor for further IVF or GIFT attempts.

(9) Applying AIH after canceling an IVF procedure resulted in a PR of almost 11%, which justifies this approach after IVF cancellation in women with at least one patent tube.

(10) No individual semen parameter can predict success in AIH using the statistical approach of the ROC analysis.

(11) If >300 000 motile spermatozoa with a motility of at least 10% (grade a + hyperactive) can be obtained in the washed insemination sample, AIH can be considered as a valuable first choice treatment in all cases of moderate and severe male subfertility before starting more invasive techniques of assisted reproduction.

References

1. Siegler, S. L. (1944). *Fertility in Women*, p. 403. (Philadelphia: J. B. Lippincott)
2. Sims, J. M. (1873). *Uterine Surgery*, p. 365. (New York: William Wood and Co.)
3. Settlage, D. S. F., Motoshima, M. and Tredway, D. R. (1972). Sperm transport from the external cervical os to the fallopian tubes in women: a time and quantitation study. *Fertil. Steril.*, **24**, 655–61
4. Mortimer, D. and Templeton, A. A. (1982). Sperm transport in the human female reproductive tract in relation to semen analysis characteristics and time of ovulation. *J. Reprod. Fert.*, **64**, 401–8
5. Allen, N. C., Herbert, C. M., Maxcon, W. S., Rogers, B. J., Diamond, M. P. and Wentz, A. C. (1985). Intrauterine insemination: a critical review. *Fertil. Steril.*, **44**, 568–80
6. Aitken, R. J. and Clarkson, J. S. (1987). Cellular basis of defective sperm function and its association with the genesis of reactive oxygen species by human spermatozoa. *J. Reprod. Fertil.*, **81**, 459–69
7. Bornman, M. S., Sevenster, C. B. v. O., de Milander, C., Otto, B. S. and Olivier, I. (1988). The effect of semen processing on sperm morphology. *Andrologia*, **21**, 117–19
8. Hoing, L. M., Devroey, P. and Van Steirteghem, A. C. (1986). Treatment of infertility because of oligo–astheno–teratozoospermia by transcervical

intrauterine insemination of motile spermatozoa. *Fertil. Steril.*, **45**, 388–91

9. Kerin, J. F. P., Peek, J., Warnes, G. M., Kirby, C., Jeffrey, R., Matthews, C. D. and Cox, L. W. (1984). Improved conception rate after intrauterine insemination of washed spermatozoa from men with poor quality semen. *Lancet*, **1**, 533–4
10. Adamson, D. G., Subak, L. L., Boltz, N. L. and McNulty, M. (1991). Failure of intrauterine insemination in a refractory infertility population. *Fertil. Steril.*, **56**, 361–3
11. Confino, E., Friberg, J. F., Dudkiewicz, A. B. and Gleicher, N. (1986). Intrauterine inseminations with washed human spermatozoa. *Fertil. Steril.*, **46**, 55–60
12. Hewitt, J., Cohen, J., Krishnaswamy, V., Fehilly, C. B., Steptoe, P. C. and Walters, D. E. (1985). Treatment of idiopathic infertility, cervical mucus hostility, and male infertility: artificial insemination with husband's semen or *in vitro* fertilization? *Fertil. Steril.*, **44**, 350–5
13. Ho, P.-C., Poon, I. M. L., Chan,. S. Y. W. and Wang, C. (1989). Intrauterine insemination is not useful in oligo-asthenospermia. *Fertil. Steril.*, **51**, 682–4
14. Ho, P.-C., So, W.-K., Chan, Y.-F. and Yeung, W. S.-B. (1992). Intrauterine insemination after ovarian stimulation as a treatment for subfertility because of subnormal semen: a prospective randomized controlled trial. *Fertil. Steril.*, **58**, 995–9
15. Horvath, P. M., Bohrer, M., Shelden, R. M. and Kemmann, E. (1989). The relationship of sperm parameters to cycle fecundity in superovulated women undergoing intrauterine insemination. *Fertil. Steril.*, **52**, 288–94
16. Johnson, L., Hemmings, R. and Tulandi, T. (1992). Comparison of intrauterine insemination, intracervical insemination, and timed intercourse in women treated with human menopausal gonadotropins. *Int. J. Fertil.*, **37**, 218–21
17. Mills, M. S., Eddowes, H. A., Cahill, D. J., Fahy, U. M., Abuzeid, M. I. M., McDermott, A. and Hull, M. G. R. (1992). A prospective controlled study of *in-vitro* fertilization, gamete intra-Fallopian transfer and intrauterine insemination combined with superovulation. *Hum. Reprod.*, **7**, 490–4
18. Yovich, J. L. and Matson, P. L. (1988). The treatment of infertility by the high intrauterine insemination of husband's washed spermatozoa. *Hum. Reprod.*, **3**, 939–43
19. World Health Organization. (1980). *Laboratory Manual for the Examination of Human Semen and Sperm–Cervical Mucus Interaction.* (Singapore: Press Concern)
20. Kruger, T. F., Menkveld, R., Stander, F. S. H., Lombard, C. J., Van der Merwe, J. P., Van Zyl, J. A. and Smith, K. (1986). Sperm morphologic features as a prognostic factor in *in vitro* fertilization. *Fertil. Steril.*, **46**, 1118–23
21. American Fertility Society. (1985). Revised American Fertility Society Classification of endometriosis. *Fertil. Steril.*, **43**, 351–2
22. Kruger, T. F., Acosta, A. A., Simmons, K. F., Swanson, R. J., Matta, J. F. and Oehninger, S. (1988). Predictive value of abnormal sperm morphology in IVF. *Fertil. Steril.*, **49**, 112–17
23. Menkveld, R., Stander, F. S. H., Kotze, T. J. vW., Kruger, T. F. and Van Zyl, J. (1990). The evaluation of morphological characteristics of human spermatozoa according to stricter criteria. *Hum. Reprod.*, **5**, 586–92
24. Jeyendran, R. S., Van der Ven, H. H., Perez-Palaez, M., Grabo, B. G. and Zaneveld, J. D. (1984). Development of an assay to assess the functional integrity of the human sperm membrane and its relationship to other semen characteristics. *J. Reprod. Fertil.*, **70**, 219–28
25. Ombelet, W., Fourie, F. le R., Vandeput, H., Gielen, J., Van Waes, A., Vlasselaer, J. and Bosmans, E. (1992). Conception following assisted procreation techniques: A high risk pregnancy is born. *Hum. Reprod.*, **7** (Suppl. 2), 181
26. Dodson, W. C. and Haney, A. F. (1991). Controlled ovarian hyperstimulation and intrauterine insemination for treatment of infertility. *Fertil. Steril.*, **55**, 457–67
27. Bronson, R. A., Cooper, G. W. and Rosenfeld, D. (1984). Sperm antibodies: their role in infertility. *Fertil. Steril.*, **42**, 171–83
28. Moretti-Rojas, I., Rojas, F. J., Leisure, M., Stone, S. C. and Asch, R. H. (1990). Intrauterine inseminations with washed human spermatozoa does not induce formation of antisperm antibodies. *Fertil. Steril.*, **53**, 180–2
29. Aboulghar, M. A., Mansour, R. T., Serour, G. I., Amin, Y., Abbas, M. A. and Salah, I. M. (1993). Ovarian superstimulation and intrauterine insemination for the treatment of unexplained infertility. *Fertil. Steril.*, **60**, 303–6
30. Crosignani, P. G., Walters, D. E. and Soliani, A. (1991). The ESHRE multicentre trial on the treatment of unexplained infertility: a preliminary report. *Hum. Reprod.*, **6**, 953–8
31. DiMarzo, S. J., Kennedy, J. F., Young, P. E., Hebert, S. A., Rosenberg, D. C. and Villanueva, B. (1992). Effect of controlled ovarian hyperstimulation on pregnancy rates after intrauterine insemination. *Am. J. Obstet. Gynecol.*, **166**, 1607–13
32. Hurst, B. S., Tjaden, B. L., Kimball, A., Schlaff, W. D., Damewood, M. D. and Rock, J. A. (1992). Superovulation with or without intrauterine insemination for the treatment of infertility. *J. Reprod. Med.*, **37**, 237–41
33. Irianni, F. M., Ramey, J., Vaintraub, M. T., Oehninger, S. and Acosta, A. A. (1993). Therapeutic intrauterine insemination improves with gonadotropin ovarian stimulation. *Arch. Androl.*, **31**, 55–62
34. Karlstrom, P.-O., Bergh, T. and Lundkvist, O. (1993).

A prospective randomized trial of artificial insemination versus intercourse in cycles stimulated with human menopausal gonadotropin or clomiphene citrate. *Fertil. Steril.*, **59**, 554–9
35. Serhal, P. F., Katz, M., Little, V. and Woronowski, H. (1988). Unexplained infertility – the value of Pergonal superovulation combined with intrauterine insemination. *Fertil. Steril.*, **49**, 602–6
36. Centola, G. M., Mattox, J. H. and Raubertas, R. F. (1990). Pregnancy rates after double versus single insemination with frozen donor semen. *Fertil. Steril.*, **54**, 1089–92
37. Ransom, M. X., Blotner, M. B., Bohrer, M., Corsan, G. and Kemmann, E. (1994). Does increasing frequency of intrauterine insemination improve pregnancy rates significantly during superovulation cycles? *Fertil. Steril.*, **61**, 303–7
38. Silverberg, K. M., Johnson, J. V., Olive, D. L., Burns, W. N. and Schenken, R. S. (1992). A prospective, randomized trial comparing two different intrauterine insemination regimens in controlled ovarian hyperstimulation cycles. *Fertil. Steril.*, **57**, 357–61
39. Hurd, W. W., Randolph, J. F., Ansbacher, R., Menge, A. C., Ohl, D. A. and Brown, A. N. (1993). Comparison of intracervical, intrauterine, and intratubal techniques for donor insemination. *Fertil. Steril.*, **59**, 339–42
40. Horbay, G. L. A., Cowell, C. A. and Casper, R. F. (1991). Multiple follicular recruitment outcomes compared by age and diagnosis. *Hum. Reprod.*, **6**, 947–52
41. Friedman, A. J., Juneau-Norcross, M., Sedensky, B., Andrews, N., Dorfman, J. and Cramer, D. W. (1992). Life table analysis of intrauterine insemination pregnancy rates for couples with cervical factor, male factor, and idiopathic infertility. *Fertil. Steril.*, **55**, 1005–7
42. Kerin, J. and Quinn, P. (1987). Washed intrauterine insemination in the treatment of oligospermic infertility. *Semin. Reprod. Endocrinol.*, **5**, 23–33
43. Kirby, C. A., Flaherty, S. P., Godfrey, B. M., Warnes, G. M. and Matthews, C. D. (1991). A prospective trial of intrauterine insemination of motile spermatozoa versus timed intercourse. *Fertil. Steril.*, **56**, 102–7
44. Bolton, V. N., Braude, P. R., Ockenden, K., Marsh, K., Robertson, G. and Ross, L. D. (1989). An evaluation of semen analysis and *in-vitro* tests of sperm function in the prediction of the outcome of intrauterine AIH. *Hum. Reprod.*, **4**, 674–9
45. Francavilla, F., Romano, R., Santucci, R. and Poccia, G. (1990). Effect of sperm morphology and motile sperm count on outcome of intrauterine insemination in oligozoospermia and/or asthenozoospermia. *Fertil. Steril.*, **53**, 892–7
46. Hull, M. E., Magyar, D. M., Vasquez, J. M., Hayes, M. F. and Moghissi, K. S. (1986). Experience with intrauterine insemination for cervical factor and oligospermia. *Am. J. Obstet. Gynecol.*, **154**, 1333–8
47. Nachtigall, R. D., Faure, N. and Glass, R. H. (1979). Artificial insemination of husband's sperm. *Fertil. Steril.*, **32**, 141–7
48. Acosta, A. A., Oehninger, S., Morshedi, M., Swanson, R. J., Scott, R. and Irianni, F. (1988). Assisted reproduction in the diagnosis and treatment of the male factor. *Obstet. Gynecol. Surv.*, **44**, 1–18
49. Enginsu, M. E., Dumoulin, J. C. M., Pieters, M. H. E. C., Bras, M., Evers, J. L. H. and Geraedts, J. P. M. (1991). Evaluation of human sperm morphology using strict criteria after Diff-Quik staining: correlation of morphology with fertilization *in vitro*. *Hum. Reprod.*, **6**, 854–8
50. Oehninger, S., Acosta, A. A., Kruger, T. F., Veeck, L. L., Flood, J. and Jones, H. W. (1988). Failure of fertilization in *in vitro* fertilization: The 'occult' male factor. *J.* In Vitro *Fertil. Embryo Transf.*, **5**, 181–7
51. Ombelet, W., Fourie, F. le R., Vandeput, H., Bosmans, E., Cox, A., Janssen, M. and Kruger, T. F. (1994). Teratozoospermia and *in vitro* fertilization: A randomized prospective study. *Hum. Reprod.*, **9**, 1479–84
52. Ombelet, W., Cox, A., Janssen, M. and Bosmans, E. (1991). *In vitro* fertilization and embryo transfer: predictive value of five different sperm factors. *Hum. Reprod.*, **6** (Suppl. 1), 314
53. Murdoch, A. P., Harris, M., Mahroo, M., Williams, M. and Dunlop, W. (1991). Gamete intrafallopian transfer (GIFT) compared with intrauterine insemination in the treatment of unexplained infertility. *Br. J. Obstet. Gynaecol.*, **98**, 1107–11
54. Robinson, D., Syrop, C. H. and Hammitt, D. G. (1992). After superovulation–intrauterine insemination fails: the prognosis for treatment by gamete intrafallopian transfer/pronuclear stage transfer. *Fertil. Steril.*, **57**, 606–12
55. Sunde, A., Kahn, J. and Mohne, K. (1988). Intrauterine insemination. *Hum. Reprod.*, **3**, 97–9
56. Sunde, A., Kahn, J. A. and Mohne, K. (1988). Intrauterine insemination: a European collaborative report. *Hum. Reprod.*, **3** (Suppl. 2), 69–73
57. Tarlatzis, B. C., Bontis, J., Kolibianakis, E. M., Sanopoulou, T., Papadimas, J., Lagos, S. and Mantalenakis, S. (1991). Evaluation of intrauterine insemination with washed spermatozoa from the husband in the treatment of infertility. *Hum. Reprod.*, **6**, 1241–6
58. Tucker, M. J., Chan, Y. M., Wong, C. J. Y., Leong, M. K. H. and Leung, C. K. M. (1991). Routine intrauterine insemination, and the effect of spermatozoal washing as assessed by computer-assisted semen analyzer. *Int. J. Fertil.*, **36**, 113–20

Assisted fertilization

31

A. Van Steirteghem, H. Joris, P. Nagy, J. Liu, A. Wisanto, E. Van Assche, I. Liebaers and P. Devroey

INTRODUCTION

For more than a decade, *in vitro* fertilization (IVF) has been successful in the treatment of couples with long-standing infertility due to tubal disease, unexplained and male-factor infertility and endometriosis. It has been well documented that the results of IVF in male infertility are not as good as those in patients with normal spermatozoa. This is obvious in the 1991 results from the American Society for Assisted Reproductive Technology[1]. It is common in IVF for tubal infertility that 60–70% of the inseminated cumulus–oocyte complexes should be normally fertilized, while in andrological infertility, this fertilization rate is only 20–30%. Failure of fertilization may occur in 30% of the cycles. The lower the number of normally fertilized oocytes, the less chance of available embryos, so that patients may have no embryos for transfer[2]. Modifications of standard IVF techniques, such as insemination with larger numbers of sperm, *in vitro* culture in tubes, and pooling oocytes together in one or more culture tubes have been reported successful in the treatment of severe male-factor infertility[3,4]. Nevertheless, it has been the experience of all centers for reproductive medicine, including our own, that a certain number of couples with male-factor infertility cannot be helped by standard IVF treatment. After insemination, even with high numbers of motile spermatozoa, the number of 2-pronucleiv (PN) oocytes is either zero or <5%. Furthermore, a sizeable number of couples cannot be accepted for IVF if the number of progressively motile spermatozoa in the ejaculate is below a certain threshold number, such as 500 000.

In the past five years, assisted fertilization procedures have been developed in order to circumvent the barriers to sperm access to the ooplasm, namely the zona pellucida and the ooplasmic membrane. Pregnancies and births have been reported after partial zona dissection (PZD) and subzonal insemination (SUZI). The clinical use of PZD has decreased recently because the efficacy of this procedure, especially in terms of normal fertilization, is limited[5]. Several groups have abandoned PZD because it is considered too inconsistent[6,7]. The microinjection of about 5–20 spermatozoa into the perivitelline space has been applied in many clinics for patients with fertilization failure in one or more standard IVF cycles and for patients with extremely impaired semen characteristics. It has been the experience of most groups that the monospermic fertilization rate in SUZI is about 20% of the microinjected metaphase-II oocytes[5,8–12]. Several factors have been reported to influence the results of SUZI, such as a stable and supportive environment for the oocyte, which is minimally distorted during SUZI[13], the percentage of acrosome defects in the semen[14] and the percentage of acrosome-free spermatozoa in the sperm suspension used for microinjection[15]. SUZI has also been carried out successfully with cryopreserved sperm obtained from a patient with seminoma and severe oligoasthenospermia[16]. When fertilization fails following SUZI it is possible to repeat the procedure in order to achieve fertilization, embryonic development and pregnancy[17]. A pregnancy has also been reported after oocytes were replaced after SUZI into the Fallopian tube[18].

The success rates of PZD and SUZI have remained moderate: the normal fertilization rate (2-PN oocytes) has never exceeded 20–25% of the micromanipulated oocytes; only two-thirds of the patients usually have a transfer of a low number of embryos, resulting in a reduced pregnancy and take-home baby rate[10,19–23]. More recently, our group has reported pregnancies and births obtained after replacement of embryos generated by a novel procedure of assisted fertilization, i.e. intracytoplasmic sperm injection (ICSI)[11,12,24–26]. In rabbits and cattle, embryos obtained by ICSI had already been transferred to recipient mothers and live offspring had resulted[27]. The centers in Norfolk, Virginia and Singapore have reported that 2-PN oocytes were observed in 30 oocytes after ICSI was carried out in 143 oocytes; the replacement of four zygotes in two women and of 11 embryos in seven women failed to result in pregnancy[23,28]. The results of the first 600 cycles of assisted fertilization by SUZI and ICSI at the Brussels Free University Centre, as well as a controlled comparison on 144 oocytes in 11 cycles, indicated that the normal fertilization rate after ICSI was substantially higher than after SUZI, while further *in vitro* cleavage to transferable or freezable embryos was quite similar for the two procedures. The higher fertilization rate resulted in more embryos for replacement after ICSI and high implantation rates have been obtained. These results led us to adopt ICSI as routine treatment for assisted fertilization from August 1992 onward.

This report describes the outcome of 1189 cycles of ICSI with ejaculated sperm performed at the Brussels Free University Centre for Reproductive Medicine from October 1991 to December 1993. Several aspects of the ICSI procedure will be described in detail, such as (1) patient selection and management; (2) ovarian stimulation and oocyte handling; (3) semen evaluation and preparation; (4) the ICSI procedure itself; (5) oocyte damage after ICSI; (6) the pronuclear status after ICSI; (7) embryo development and transfer and freezing of supernumerary embryos; (8) the establishment of pregnancy; and (9) the current results of prenatal diagnosis and prospective follow-up of the children born after ICSI. The initial results of ICSI in patients with obstructive azoospermia will also be reviewed.

PATIENT SELECTION AND MANAGEMENT

Couples selected for ICSI suffered from long-standing infertility. Two categories of couples were treated in these 1189 treatment cycles:

(1) Couples who had undergone at least one, but more frequently two, three or more cycles of standard IVF attempts in our center or in a referring center; after juxtaposition of the cumulus–oocyte complexes with 5000 progressively motile spermatozoa per droplet of 25 μL (i.e. 200 000 spermatozoa/mL), fertilization had not occurred or had occurred in fewer than 5% of the oocytes; and

(2) Couples with semen parameters that were too impaired to be accepted for standard IVF because fewer than 500 000 progressively motile spermatozoa were present in the total ejaculate. ICSI can also be used for couples with obstructive azoospermia due to congenital absence of the vas deferens or failed vasovasostomy and vasoepididymostomy; this application of ICSI will be summarized at the end of this chapter.

The couples were fully informed about the novelty of the ICSI procedure and about its many unknown aspects. After extensive counseling, the couples agreed and signed a consent form to have prenatal diagnosis and to participate in a prospective follow-up of the children born after ICSI.

The ICSI procedure was reviewed and approved by the institutional ethical committee of the University Hospital and Medical School.

Ovarian stimulation and oocyte handling

Ovarian stimulation was carried out by a desensitizing protocol of the intranasally administered gonadotropin-releasing hormone agonist (GnRHa) buserelin (Suprefact; Hoechst, Frankfurt, Germany) in association with human menopausal gonadotropins (hMG; Humegon from Organon, Oss, The Netherlands, or Pergonal from Serono, Geneva, Switzerland). Human chorionic gonadotropins (hCG; Pregnyl from Organon or Profasi from Serono) were administered if at least two or three follicles measured >17 mm in diameter and serum estradiol concentrations were >1000 ng/L[29]. The supplementation of the luteal phase was started on the day after hCG administration and consisted of natural micronized progesterone 600 mg per day intravaginally in three divided doses (Utrogestan; Piette, Brussels, Belgium)[30,31].

Oocyte retrieval was carried out by vaginal ultrasound-guided follicular puncture 36 h after administration of the ovulation-inducing dose (10 000 IU) of hCG. In all, 14 795 cumulus–oocyte complexes were retrieved in these 1189 cycles, i.e. a mean of

12.4 complexes per cycle. The inspection of these complexes under the inverted microscope at 40× or 100× magnification revealed that in almost all cases the cumulus and corona cells were well dispersed. These complexes were transferred into 5 mL Falcon tubes with 1 mL of pre-equilibrated Earle's medium and transported in a thermobox at 37°C to the microinjection laboratory, which is located at a distance of about 500 m.

The cells of the cumulus and corona radiata were removed by incubation for less than one minute in HEPES-buffered Earle's medium with about 60 IU hyaluronidase/mL. The removal of the cumulus cells was enhanced by aspiration of the cumulus–corona–oocyte complexes in and out of hand-drawn glass pipettes with two different diameters: first, with an opening of 250 to 300 μm, and then with an opening of 200 μm. Afterwards, the oocytes were rinsed several times in droplets of HEPES-buffered Earle's and B_2 medium and then carefully observed under the inverted microscope at 200× magnification. This included an assessment of the zona pellucida and the oocyte, as well as noting the presence or absence of a germinal vesicle or the first polar body. Besides the assessment of nuclear maturity, the cytoplasm of the oocyte was examined for the presence of vacuoles or other abnormalities in the texture of the ooplasm. Of the 14 795 complexes, 14 143 (95.6%) contained an intact oocyte with an intact zona pellucida and clear cytoplasm. Analysis of the nuclear status of the intact oocytes revealed 85% metaphase-II oocytes which had extruded the first polar body, 11% germinal-vesicle-stage oocytes and 4% metaphase-I oocytes which had undergone breakdown of the germinal vesicle but had not yet extruded the first polar body. The oocytes were then incubated in 25 μL microdrops of B_2 medium covered by lightweight paraffin oil at 37°C in an atmosphere of 5% O_2, 5% CO_2 and 90% N_2. Nuclear maturity was assessed again just prior to the microinjection procedure. ICSI was carried out on all metaphase-II oocytes. ICSI was not carried out in two treatment cycles where no metaphase-II oocytes were observed.

Semen evaluation and preparation

Before the start of the treatment cycle, semen analysis and a semen selection procedure were carried out to verify whether enough spermatozoa were present to carry out the ICSI procedure. Semen analysis included the assessment of conventional semen characteristics by well-established procedures. The time of ejaculation as well as the duration of liquefaction at 37°C were recorded; the outcome of liquefaction was recorded on a semi-quantitative scale: normal liquefaction (0), slightly viscous (1) or very viscous (2). In case of very viscous semen the ejaculate was passed through a 21G needle. The semen volume was measured after transfer into a graduated test tube. Sperm density in 10^6 per mL was determined in a Makler or Neubauer counting chamber. The percentages of four different categories of motility were assessed in the same counting chamber by evaluating, if possible, at least 100 spermatozoa. The morphology was assessed by strict Kruger criteria after Diff-Quik staining. At least 100 spermatozoa were evaluated. Using an automatic device we recorded: (1) normal spermatozoa, (2) abnormal heads, (3) abnormal midpieces or (4) abnormal tails. The presence of other cells was also recorded and in the remarks it was also possible to make a note of possible abnormalities in acrosome size. Semen values were considered normal if (1) sperm concentration was at least 20×10^6 mL, (2) progressive sperm motility was at least 40% and (3) normal sperm morphology was at least 14%. The distribution of the semen characteristics of the 1189 freshly ejaculated sperm samples is summarized in Table 1. Oligo-astheno-teratozoospermia was present in 50% of the cycles, two abnormal sperm parameters were noticed in 29% of the cycles and a single sperm defect was noticed in 15% of the cycles. Conventional semen parameters were normal in 6% of the cycles per-

Table 1 Sperm characteristics of 1189 ICSI cycles with ejaculated sperm

Normal sperm (%)	77 cycles	(6)
Single sperm defect (%)	177 cycles	(15)
oligozoospermia	49 cycles	
asthenozoospermia	64 cycles	
teratozoospermia	64 cycles	
Double sperm defects (%)	345 cycles	(29)
oligo-teratozoospermia	145 cycles	
astheno-teratozoospermia	92 cycles	
oligo-asthenozoospermia	108 cycles	
Triple sperm defects (%)		
oligo-astheno-teratozoospermia	590 cycles	(50)

taining to patients who had unsuccessfully undergone at least two previous IVF cycles with a sufficient number of oocytes.

The preparation of the ejaculated sperm for ICSI involved the following steps. The seminal fluid was removed from the semen by washing in a 10 mL Falcon tube with Earle's medium containing 3% BSA fraction V (Sigma, St Louis, MO, USA), centrifuging at 1800***g*** for 5 min and removing the supernatant. The further selection procedure of the spermatozoa depended upon the number of motile spermatozoa present in the semen. The sperm selection was done through three or two layers of Percoll. Three layers of Percoll (90%–70%–50%) were used if at least 5 million/mL spermatozoa with a motility of 40% were present; two Percoll layers (95%–47.5%) were used for the other semen samples. The volume of the different Percoll gradients was 0.6 mL in a 5 mL Falcon tube. The sperm suspension was put on top of the lowest density gradient. After centrifugation at 300***g*** for 20 min, the bottom layer was aspirated with a long plastic tip mounted on a Gilson pipette into a 5 mL Falcon tube. This tube was filled with Earle's medium and centrifuged at 1800***g*** for 5 min. The supernatant was removed and 200 μL of Earle's medium was added to the pellet. The sperm suspension was then kept in the 37°C incubator (5% CO_2, 5% O_2, 90% N_2) until the intracytoplasmic injection of the oocytes[32].

ICSI procedure

The holding and injection pipettes were made of glass capillary tubes (Drummond Scientific Company, Broomall, PA, USA) of 78 mm length and an inner and outer diameter of 0.69 mm and 0.97 mm. These glass capillaries were cleaned by (1) sonication for 30 min in pure water (Milli-RO and Milli-Q, Millipore, Bedford, MA, USA) with 2% (vol/vol) detergent (7X-PF O-MATIC, Flow Laboratories, Irvine, Scotland) and (2) rinsing in running Milli-Q water for 30 min. Both cleaning steps were repeated before drying and sterilizing the pipettes in a hot-air oven (100°C for 6 h; Memmert type ULE 500). The second sonication was done in water without detergent. The glass pipettes were obtained by drawing thin-walled glass capillary tubes (Drummond Scientific Company) using a horizontal microelectrode puller (Flaming/Brown micropipette puller model P-97; Sutter Instrument Company, Navato, CA, USA). The holding pipette was cut and fire-polished on a microforge (MF-9 Microforge; Narishige, Tokyo, Japan) to obtain an outer diameter of 60 μm and an inner diameter of 20 μm. To prepare the injection pipette, the pulled capillary was opened on a microgrinder (EG-4 Micro-Grinder, Narishige) to an outer diameter of 7 μm and an inner diameter of 5 μm; the bevel angle was 50°. This grinding step required about 3 min and the whetstone of the grinder was humidified by slow water drip during the procedure. The microforge was used to make a sharp spike on the injection pipette and to bend the edge of the holding and injection pipettes to an angle of about 45° in order to facilitate the injection procedure in the Petri dish.

Just prior to the injection procedure, the sperm fraction was concentrated by washing in a 1.5 mL Eppendorf tube containing Earle's medium. This tube was centrifuged at 1800***g*** for 5 min. The supernatant was removed and the pellet was resuspended in 20–50 μL of medium. One μL of this sperm fraction was added to 2–4 μL of a 1 g/10 mL polyvinylpyrrolidone (PVP, Sigma) solution in HEPES-buffered Earle's medium containing 0.5% (w/v) BSA (Fraction V, Sigma). The PVP solution was filtered through an 0.8 μm filter (Millipore) and stored at 4°C for a maximum of 3 weeks.

The 3–5 μL sperm-PVP droplet was placed in the center of a Petri dish (Falcon type 1006) and was surrounded by eight 5 μL droplets of HEPES-buffered Earle's medium with 0.5% crystalline BSA. These droplets were covered by about 3.5 mL of lightweight paraffin oil.

The ICSI procedure was carried out on the heated stage (37°C; THN-60/16 and MS100 Controller from Linkam Scientific Instruments, Surrey, UK) of an inverted microscope (Diaphot; Nikon Corporation, Tokyo, Japan) at 400× magnification using a Hoffman Modulation Contrast System (Modulation Optics Inc., Greenvale, NY, USA). The microscope was equipped with a Nikon F-601M camera for still pictures and a video camera (DXC-755 P; Sony Corporation, Tokyo, Japan) that allows the procedure to be followed on a Trinitron color video monitor (PVM-1443MD, Sony).

The microscope was equipped with two coarse positioning manipulators (3D Motor Driven Coarse

Control Manipulator MM-188, Narishige) and with two three-dimensional hydraulic remote-control micromanipulators (Joystick Hydraulic Micromanipulator MO-188, Narishige). The holding and injection pipettes were fitted to a tool holder and were connected by Teflon tubing (CT-1, Narishige) to a micrometer-type microinjector (IM-6, Narishige). Solution delivery was controlled via a 1 μL resolution vernier micrometer. A single immobilised spermatozoon was selected from the central droplet and was aspirated tail first into the tip of the injection pipette. The Petri dish was then moved in order to visualize an oocyte in one of the droplets surrounding the sperm suspension. The oocyte was immobilized by slight negative pressure exerted on the holding pipette. The polar body was held at 12 or 6 o'clock and the micropipette was pushed through the zona pellucida and the oolemma into the ooplasm at 3 o'clock. A single spermatozoon was injected into the ooplasm with around 1 pL of medium. The injection pipette was withdrawn gently and the injected oocyte was released from the holding pipette. The aspiration of a single spermatozoon and injection into the ooplasm were repeated until all metaphase-II oocytes were injected. The injected oocytes were then washed in B_2 medium and transferred into 25 μL droplets of B_2 medium covered by lightweight paraffin oil. The Petri dishes with the oocytes were incubated in an incubator (B5060 EK/02; Heraeus, Hanau, Germany) at 37°C with 5% O_2, 5% CO_2 and 90% N_2.

Oocyte damage and pronuclear status after ICSI

The further handling of the injected oocytes was similar to our standard IVF procedure. About 16–18 h after microinjection, the oocytes were observed under the inverted microscope at 200 or 400× magnification for any sign of damage which may have been due to the ICSI procedure and for the presence of one, two or three pronuclei. In these 1189 cycles, ICSI was carried out on 11 971 metaphase-II oocytes, i.e. a mean of 10.1 oocytes per cycle. The number of intact oocytes after ICSI was 10 601 (88.6% of the injected oocytes). The mean number of successfully injected oocytes was 8.9 per treatment cycle.

Fertilization was considered normal when two clearly distinct pronuclei containing nucleoli were present. The presence of one pronucleus or three pronuclei was noted together with the presence of one, two or fragmented polar bodies. If a single pronucleus was observed, a second evaluation was carried out about 4 h later in order to see whether the pronuclear status had changed. The number of normally fertilized oocytes was 7203, i.e. 67.9% of the successfully injected oocytes, 60.2% of the injected metaphase-II oocytes and 48.7% of the retrieved cumulus–oocyte complexes.

The number of abnormally fertilized oocytes was 438 1-PN oocytes (4.1% of the intact oocytes) and 492 3-PN oocytes (4.6% of the intact oocytes). In our microinjected 1-PN oocytes, pronuclear status was reassessed a few hours after the initial observation. In contrast to our standard IVF program, no change in pronuclear status was observed at the time of the second microscopic observation[33]. If these oocytes cleave they are not transferred. This relative activation may be due to mechanical or chemical factors. As a matter of practical policy the concentration of hyaluronidase that is used to remove the cumulus and corona cells around the oocyte is low, and we are limiting the exposure to hyaluronidase to <1 min. It may be a surprise to observe 3-PN oocytes after the injection of only one spermatozoon into the ooplasm. We carefully observed the polar bodies at the time of fertilization and it is obvious that the three pronuclei were mostly due to non-extrusion of the second polar body at the time of fertilization.

As indicated in Table 2, the damage and normal fertilization rates after ICSI were not different for the four categories of semen used to carry out ICSI. The percentage of intact oocytes varied from 87.9% to 89.4% of the total oocytes and the normal fertilization rate from 74.1% to 65.4% of the intact oocytes. The exceptional circumstances in which none of the injected oocytes were normally fertilized occurred when (1) only one metaphse-II oocyte was available for ICSI, (2) only totally immotile spermatozoa were available for the injection, (3) gross abnormalities were present in the oocytes, (4) round-headed spermatozoa were injected, and (5) when all oocytes were damaged by the injection procedure. Some of these patients achieved fertilization in a subsequent cycle.

Table 2 Number of intact oocytes, fertilization and cleavage after ICSI

Semen	*No. of cycles*	*No. eggs injected*	*Intact (%)*	*2-PN (%)*	*Embryos*	
					Transferrable (%)	*Transferred or frozen (%)*
Normal	77	769	89.1	71.4	71.2	64.0
Single defect	177	1729	87.9	74.1	75.3	66.2
Double defect	345	3534	89.4	68.5	77.0	69.6
Triple defect	590	5939	88.2	65.4	74.4	66.3
Totals	1189	11971	88.6	67.9	75.1	67.1

These high fertilization rates have been constant in a busy clinical program of five or seven ICSI cycles per day, as well as three to four standard IVF procedures. It is, in fact, not unusual for the ICSI results to equal or even exceed the standard IVF results when such data are reviewed at the authors' weekly clinical laboratory review meeting. These results have been achieved where the ICSI procedure has been carried out by a team of two physician-scientists, one senior technician and five medical technologists. It is the authors' conviction that such results can be consistently obtained if great care is taken with optimal conditions for the many factors involved in the assisted reproduction procedures involving ICSI.

Embryo development, embryo transfer and cryopreservation

The embryo cleavage of the two-pronuclear oocytes was evaluated after a further 24 h of *in vitro* culture. The cleaving embryos were scored according to the equality of size of the blastomeres and the number of anucleate fragments. These embryos were classified into three categories according to the percentage of anucleate fragments: (1) excellent type-A embryos (without anucleate fragments); (2) good-quality type-B embryos (between 1% and 20% of the volume filled with anucleate fragments); and (3) fair-quality type-C embryos (between 21% and 50% anucleate fragments). Cleaved embryos with less than half of their volume filled with anucleate fragments were eligible for transfer. Up to two, three or, exceptionally, four embryos were loaded with a few microliters of Earle's medium into a Frydman catheter and transferred into the uterine cavity. Embryo replacement was usually performed about 48 h after the microinjection procedure. If supernumerary embryos with <20% anucleate fragments were available, they were cryopreserved on day 2 or day 3 after oocyte retrieval using the slow-freezing protocol with dimethylsulfoxide[34,35].

The total number of embryos of sufficient quality to be transferred (<50% anucleate fragments) was 5409, i.e. 75.1% of the 2-PN oocytes, 51.0% of the successfully injected oocytes, 45.2% of the injected metaphase-II oocytes and 36.6% of the retrieved cumulus–oocyte complexes. As indicated in Table 2, there was no difference in the percentage of transferable embryos in the four semen categories.

The total number of embryos which were actually transferred or frozen (<20% anucleate fragments) was 4833, i.e. 67.1% of the 2-PN oocytes, 45.6% of the successfully injected oocytes, 40.4% of the injected metaphase-II oocytes and 32.7% of the retrieved cumulus–oocyte complexes.

As indicated in Table 3, there was no difference in the distribution of embryos of types A, B or C when ICSI was carried out with sperm with normal semen parameters, with one, two or three semen anomalies. In the four groups of semen parameters, the percentage of excellent type-A embryos varied from 8.3% to 10.0%, the percentage of good quality type-B embryos from 48.7% to 55.9% and the percentage of fair quality type-C embryos from 10.4% to 12.7%.

Embryo quality after ICSI and after standard IVF was compared in 801 ICSI cycles and 1031 standard IVF cycles carried out concomitantly in 1993 (Table 4). There was no significant difference in the distribution of embryo quality when 2-PN oocytes were cultured for 24 h *in vitro*.

Table 3 ICSI and embryo development in relation to the sperm parameters from ejaculated sperm

Sperm parameters	*Cycles*	*2-PN*	*Type-A embryos*	*Type-B embryos*	*Type-C embryos*
Normal	77	489	42 (8.6%)	238 (48.7%)	62 (12.7%)
1 Anomaly	177	1126	93 (8.3%)	599 (53.2%)	142 (12.6%)
2 Anomalies	345	2164	216 (10.0%)	1210 (55.9%)	224 (10.4%)
3 Anomalies	590	3424	305 (8.9%)	1828 (53.4%)	391 (11.4%)

Table 4 Embryo quality after ICSI and standard IVF

	ICSI	*IVF*
Cycles	801	1031
2-PN oocytes	4546	5125
Type-A embryos (0% fragmentation)	460 (10.1%)	852 (16.6%)
Type-B embryos (1%–20% fragmentation)	2462 (54.2%)	2652 (51.7%)
Type-C embryos (21%–50% fragmentation)	490 (10.8%)	455 (8.9%)
Type-D embryos (>50% or complete fragmentation)	1134 (24.9%)	1166 (22.8%)

The freezing of at least one supernumerary embryo was possible in 517 of the 1189 cycles (43.5%). The percentages of cycles with freezing were: 42.9% in cycles with normal semen; 45.8% in cycles with a single sperm defect; 47.5% in cycles with two sperm defects; and 40.5% in cycles with triple sperm defects.

An embryo replacement was possible in 1085 of the 1189 treatment cycles (91.3%). This is a high transfer rate for couples with previous fertilization failure in standard IVF or with sperm characteristics too poor to be included in IVF. As indicated in Table 5, the percentage of transfers was similar in the four groups of semen parameters; the transfer rate varied from 93.3% to 89.7% of the cycles. The distribution of transfers with one, two, three or more embryos was also similar in the four groups of semen parameters. Except for some patients older than 40 years of age, the number of embryos replaced was limited to a maximum of three.

The number of patients with positive serum hCG was 428, i.e. 39.5% pregnancy rate per transfer and 36.0% per started cycle. As indicated in Table 6, the pregnancy rate was especially high when an elective transfer of two embryos was carried out and when three embryos were transferred. A comparison was made in the pregnancy rates per transfer in IVF and ICSI in patients in whom two or three embryos were replaced (Table 7). For both procedures the pregnancy rate was substantially higher when an elective transfer of two embryos was carried out than when only two embryos were available for replacement. Very high pregnancy rates were observed in IVF and ICSI when an elective transfer of two embryos or a transfer of three embryos was carried out.

The ICSI results were analyzed separately in

Table 5 ICSI and number of embryos transferred in relation to the sperm parameters from ejaculated sperm

Sperm parameters	*Cycles*	*Transfers n (%)*	*1 n (%)*	*2 n (%)*	*3 n (%)*	*>3 n (%)*
Normal	77	70 (90.9)	5 (7.1)	21 (30.0)	41 (58.6)	3 (4.3)
1 Anomaly	177	164 (92.7)	13 (7.9)	53 (32.3)	93 (56.7)	5 (3.0)
2 Anomalies	345	322 (93.3)	26 (8.1)	127 (39.4)	166 (51.6)	3 (0.9)
3 Anomalies	590	529 (89.7)	51 (9.6)	187 (35.3)	277 (52.4)	14 (2.7)

Table 6 Embryo transfer after ICSI with ejaculated sperm

Cycles	1189	
Transfers (%)	1085	(91%)
Pregnancies/transfers (%)		
1 embryo	11/95	(12%)
2 embryos	41/153	(27%)
2 embryos (elective)	97/234	(42%)
3 embryos	136/304	(45%)
3 embryos (elective)	134/274	(49%)
>3 embryos	9/25	(36%)
	428/1085	(39.5%)
% Clinical pregnancies or deliveries/transfer	330	(30.4%)

patients with extremely impaired semen parameters: cryptozoospermia (57 cycles), 100% asthenozoospermia (66 cycles) and 100% teratozoospermia (48 cycles). As indicated in Table 8, normal fertilization, cleavage and clinical pregnancy rates were lower in patients with total asthenozoospermia, but these differences reached statistical significance only for the 2-PN fertilization rate. It is clear from these data that ICSI can also be successful in couples considered sterile because of cryptozoospermia, total asthenozoospermia or total teratozoospermia.

One hundred and twenty couples who had frozen embryos after ICSI were scheduled for the replacement of cryopreserved embryos. After thawing 413 embryos, 218 (52.8%) were replaced in 101 embryo transfers (84.2%) of the scheduled procedures. Twenty-two pregnancies were established in 101 transfers, corresponding to a total pregnancy rate of 21.8% per transfer. The clinical pregnancy rate was 12.9% per transfer and the delivery rate was 5.9% per transfer. The high incidence of preclinical abortions (40.9%) after transfer of human embryos cryopreserved after ICSI requires extension of the series[35].

ICSI in patients with obstructive azoospermia

ICSI was also carried out in couples with obstructive azoospermia due to congenital bilateral absence of the vas deferens or failed vasovasostomy and vasoepididymostomy. Epididymal fluid was collected by microsurgical procedure on the same day as the oocyte retrieval procedure[36]. The epididymal fluid was diluted in 1 mL HEPES-buffered Earle's medium and examined for the presence of some motile spermatozoa. The MESA procedure was continued until enough motile spermatozoa were harvested. The tubes containing motile spermatozoa were centrifuged at 1800***g*** for 5 min. The combined pellets were put on a two-layer Percoll gradient and then further processed in the same way as the ejaculated sperm samples. If more sperm samples were available than required for the ICSI

Table 7 Elective transfer of two or three good-quality embryos in IVF and ICSI

Embryos replaced	*IVF*		*ICSI*	
	Transfers	*Pregnancies (%)*	*Transfers*	*Pregnancies (%)*
2	105	23[a] (22)	112	26[c] (23)
2 (elective)	208	101[a,b] (49)	230	94[c] (41)
3	233	86[b] (37)	276	121 (44)
3 (elective)	221	98 (44)	201	97 (48)

[a]$P<0.0001$; [b]$P<0.01$; [c]$P<0.001$

Table 8 ICSI and extremely impaired semen

	Cryptozoospermia	*100% astheno*	*100% terato*
Cycles	57	66	48
Oocytes	601	678	488
Intact after ICSI (%)	516 (86)	611 (90)	436 (89)
2-PN oocytes (%)	320[a] (62)	316[a] (52)	259[a] (68)
Transferred or frozen (%)	236 (74)	197 (62)	198 (67)
Clinical pregnancies	15 (26)	8 (12)	13 (27)

[a]$P<0.05$

procedure, they were frozen by standard sperm freezing procedures[37]. ICSI was sometimes carried out with frozen–thawed epididymal sperm. Immediately after thawing, the sperm suspension was put on top of a two-layer Percoll gradient and then processed as described above for ejaculated sperm. A testicular biopsy was performed when no spermatozoa were found in several MESA attempts or where the epididymis was absent after previous surgery. The testicular biopsy specimens were shredded in HEPES-buffered Earle's medium and then centrifuged at 300***g*** for 5 min. For ICSI, motile spermatozoa were aspirated from a droplet containing the sperm suspension. The median number of spermatozoa recovered was 46×10^6 for freshly collected epididymal sperm, 150 000 for frozen–thawed epididymal sperm and 540 000 for testicular sperm. Total and progressive motility rates were 12% and 2% for freshly collected epididymal sperm, while very few motile spermatozoa were recovered in frozen–thawed epididymal sperm and testicular sperm.

ICSI was carried out with freshly collected epididymal sperm in 49 cycles, frozen–thawed epididymal sperm in 10 cycles and testicular sperm in 17 cycles. The number of metaphase-II oocytes injected with epididymal sperm was 759 and the number of oocytes injected with testicular sperm was 242. After ICSI the percentages of intact oocytes was 90.0% for epididymal sperm and 89.7% for testicular sperm. The number of intact oocytes which were normally fertilized was 48.5% for epididymal sperm and 49.8% for testicular sperm. The percentages of 2-PN oocytes which developed to transferable embryos were 60.7% for epididymal sperm and 61.1% for testicular sperm. The percentage of treatment cycles resulting in an embryo transfer was 89.8% for epididymal sperm and 76.5% for testicular sperm. The percentage of clinical pregnancies or deliveries per transfer was 34.0% for epididymal sperm and 38.5% for testicular sperm.

Prenatal diagnosis and pediatric follow-up

Because of the novelty of ICSI, the couples were asked after extensive counseling to adhere to the follow-up conditions which include genetic counseling, agreement to prenatal testing and participation in a prospective clinical follow-up study of the children[38].

Table 9 Outcome of ICSI (evaluation date 14 June 1994)

• Number of pregnancies including replacement of frozen-thawed embryos	743
• Prenatal karyotypes	
total	353
fresh embryos replaced	345
cryopreserved embryos	8
normal 46,XX or 46,XY	345
in vitro or tissue limited aberrations	2
benign familial structural aberrations	5
Klinefelter karyotype after cryopreservation	1
• Number of children born (total)	339
Fresh embryos	333
ICSI with ejaculated sperm	326
ICSI with fresh epididymal sperm	6
ICSI with frozen–thawed epididymal sperm	1
• Cryopreserved embryos	6

At the time of writing (June 1994) the number of pregnancies (positive serum hCG) after ICSI-embryos were replaced was 743, including 44 pregnancies after replacement of frozen–thawed embryos (Table 9). After chorionic villus sampling or amniocentesis, 353 fetal karyotypes were obtained. The sex ratio was close to the expected 50/50 distribution. There was one abnormal karyotype: a 47,XXY Klinefelter karyotype after the replacement of a frozen–thawed embryo; the parents elected to interrupt the pregnancy. So far, 339 children have been born: (1) 326 after the replacement of embryos after ICSI with fresh ejaculated sperm; (2) six after ICSI with fresh epididymal sperm; (3) one after ICSI with frozen–thawed epididymal sperm; and (4) six after replacement of frozen-thawed supernumerary embryos. The number of major congenital malformations is listed in Table 10. Ten major congenital malformations were observed in these 339 children, i.e. 2.9% of the children; this percentage is not different from the percentage of abnormalities observed after natural conception or after standard IVF procedure. Six of these 10 major congenital malformations occurred in multiple pregnancies, five in twin pregnancies and one in a triplet pregnancy.

Although there is no indication of an increase in major congenital malformations after replacement

Table 10 Major congenital malformations after ICSI (evaluation date 14 June 1994)

- Ten major congenital malformations (i.e. 2.9% of 339 children born)
- Malformations in singleton pregnancies
  - cheilognathopalatoschisis and duplication of the kidney
  - malformation of the left hip and left leg
  - hypospadias
  - tetralogy of Fallot
- Malformations in twin pregnancies
  - two children with palatoschisis (dizygotic twins)
  - femur–fibula–ulna syndrome
  - hernia diaphragmatica
  - Down's syndrome
- Malformations in triplet pregnancy
  - holoprosencephaly in one child, two other children normal

of embryos obtained after ICSI, it is important to continue this careful prospective follow-up study of the children in different centers practicing ICSI. This is one of the goals of the 'Task Force on ICSI' established by the European Society of Human Reproduction and Embryology (ESHRE).

CONCLUSION

Intracytoplasmic sperm injection can now be considered a successful new treatment for couples with long-standing severe male-factor infertility, including obstructive azoospermia due to congenital bilateral absence of the vas deferens, failed reversal of vasectomy or absent epididymis.

ACKNOWLEDGMENTS

The authors are indebted to their many colleagues of the Centre for Reproductive Medicine and the Centre for Medical Genetics. Special thanks to Geertrui Bocken, Bart Desmet, An Vankelecom, Petra Van Lerberghe and Heidi Van Ranst of the microinjection team, to research nurses Andrea Buysse and Marleen Magnus for collecting the data on pregnancy and pediatric follow-up, to Frank Winter of the Language Education Centre for editing the manuscript, and to Viviane De Wolf for typesetting the manuscript. This work is supported by grants from the Belgian Fund for Medical Research and from Organon International.

References

1. Society for Assisted Reproductive Technologies. (1993). Assisted Reproductive Technology in The United States and Canada: 1991 Results from the Society for Assisted Reproductive Technology Generated from the American Fertility Society Registry. *Fertil. Steril.*, **59**, 956–62
2. Tournaye, H., Devroey, P., Camus, M., Staessen, C., Bollen, N., Smitz, J. and Van Steirteghem, A. C. (1992). Comparison of *in-vitro* fertilization in male and tubal infertility: a 3 year survey. *Hum. Reprod.*, **7**, 218–22
3. Ordt, T., Patricio, P., Balmaceda, J. P. and Asch, R. H. (1993). Can severe male factor infertility be treated without micromanipulation. *Fertil. Steril.*, **60**, 110–15
4. Hammitt, D. G. (1993). Treatment of male-factor infertility by *in vitro* insemination with high concentrations of motile sperm. *Semin. Reprod. Endocrinol.*, **11**, 72–82
5. Cohen, J., Adler, A., Alikano, M., Ferrara, T. A., Kissin, E., Reing, A. M., Suzman, M., Talansky, B. E. and Rosenwaks, Z. (1993). Assisted fertilization and abnormal sperm function. *Semin. Reprod. Endocrinol.*, **11**, 83–94
6. Tucker, M., Wiker, S. and Massey, J. (1993). Rational approach to assisted fertilization. *Hum. Reprod.*, **8**, 1778
7. Fishel, S., Dowell, K., Timson, J., Green, S., Hall, J. and Klentzeris, L. (1993). Micro-assisted fertilization with human gametes. *Hum. Reprod.*, **8**, 1780–4
8. Imoedemhe, D. A. G. and Sigue, A. B. (1993). Subzonal multiple sperm injection in the treatment of previous failed human *in vitro* fertilization. *Fertil. Steril.*, **59**, 172–6
9. Lippi, J., Mortimer, D. and Jansen, R. P. S. (1993). Sub-zonal insemination for extreme male factor infertility. *Hum. Reprod.*, **8**, 939–44
10. Palermo, G., Joris, H., Devroey, P. and Van Steirteghem, A. C. (1992). Induction of acrosome reaction in human spermatozoa used for subzonal insemination. *Hum. Reprod.*, **7**, 248–54
11. Palermo, G., Joris, H., Derde, M. P., Camus, M., Devroey, P. and Van Steirteghem, A. C. (1993). Sperm characteristics and outcome of human assisted fertilization by subzonal insemination and intracytoplasmic sperm injection. *Fertil. Steril.*, **59**, 826–35

12. Van Steirteghem, A. C., Liu, J., Nagy, Z., Joris, H., Tournaye, H., Liebaers, I. and Devroey, P. (1993). Use of assisted fertilization. *Hum. Reprod.*, **8**, 1784–5
13. Garrisi, G. J., Chin, A. J., Dolan, P. M., Nagler, H. M., Vasquez-Levin, M., Navot, D. and Gordon, J. W. (1993). Analysis of factors contributing to success in a program of micromanipulation-assisted fertilization. *Fertil. Steril.*, **59**, 366–74
14. Wolf, J. P., Dugot, B., Kunstmann, J. M., Frydman, R. and Jouannet, P. (1992). Influence of sperm parameters on outcome of subzonal insemination in the case of previous IVF failure. *Hum. Reprod.*, **7**, 1407–13
15. Obasaju, M. F., Venier, W. C., Carson, R. S. and Ying, Y. (1993). The effect of sperm preparation methods on the fertilization rate of oocytes microinseminated by subzonal sperm injection. *Hum. Reprod.*, **8**, 1886–91
16. Levron, J., Lightman, A., Stein, D. W., Brandes, J. M. and Itskovitz-Eldor, J. (1992). Pregnancy after subzonal insertion of cryopreserved spermatozoa from a patient with testicular seminoma. *Fertil. Steril.*, **58**, 839–40
17. Wiker, S. R., Tucker, M. J., Wright, G., Malter, H. E., Kort, H. I. and Massey, J. B. (1993). Repeated sperm injection under the zona following initial fertilization failure. *Hum. Reprod.*, **8**, 467–9
18. Imoedemhe, D. A. G., Sigue, A. B. and Luciano, E. C. (1993). Successful twin pregnancy and delivery after microinseminated oocyte fallopian transfer for male factor infertility. *Fertil. Steril.*, **59**, 662–3
19. Cohen, J., Malter, H., Wright, H., Kort, H., Massey, J. and Mitchell, D. (1989). Partial zona dissection of human oocytes when failure of zona pellucida penetration is anticipated. *Hum. Reprod.*, **4**, 435–42
20. Cohen, J., Talansky, B. E., Malter, H., Alikani, M., Adler, A., Reing, A., Berkeley, A., Graf, M., Davis, O., Liu, H., Bedford, J. M. and Rosenwaks, Z. (1991). Microsurgical fertilization and teratozoospermia. *Hum. Reprod.*, **6**, 118–23
21. Cohen, J., Alikani, M., Adler, A., Berkerly, A., Davis, O., Ferrara, T. A., Graf, M., Grifo, J., Liu, H. C., Malter, H. E., Reing, A. M., Suzman, M., Talansky, B. E., Trowbridge, J. and Rosenwaks, Z. (1992). Microsurgical fertilization procedures: The absence of stringent criteria for patient selection. *J. Assist. Reprod. Genet.*, **9**, 197–206
22. Fishel, S., Timson, J., Lisi, F. and Rinaldi, L. (1992). Evaluation of 225 patients undergoing subzonal insemination for the procurement of fertilization *in vitro*. *Fertil. Steril.*, **57**, 840–9
23. Ng, S. C., Bongso, A. and Ratnam, S. S. (1991). Microinjection of human oocytes: a technique for severe oligo-astheno-teratozoospermia. *Fertil. Steril.*, **56**, 1117–23
24. Palermo, G., Joris, H., Devroey, P. and Van Steirteghem, A. C. (1992). Pregnancies after intracytoplasmic injection of single spermatozoon into an oocyte. *Lancet*, **340**, 17–18
25. Van Steirteghem, A. C., Liu, J., Joris, H., Nagy, Z., Janssenswillen, C., Tournaye, H., Derde, M. P., Van Assche, E. and Devroey, P. (1993). Higher success rate by intracytoplasmic sperm injection than by subzonal insemination. Report of a second series of 300 consecutive treatment cycles. *Hum. Reprod.*, **8**, 1055–60
26. Van Steirteghem, A. C., Nagy, P., Joris, H., Liu, J., Staessen, C., Smitz, J., Wisanto, A. and Devroey, P. (1993). High fertilization and implantation rates after intracytoplasmic sperm injection. *Hum. Reprod.*, **8**, 1061–6
27. Iritani, A. (1991). Micromanipulation of gametes for *in vitro* assisted fertilization. *Mol. Reprod. Dev.*, **28**, 199–207
28. Veeck, L. L., Oehninger, S., Acosta, A. A. and Muasher, S. J. (1990). Sperm microinjection in a clinical *in vitro* fertilization program. *Proceedings of the 45th Annual Meeting of the American Fertility Society*, 13–16 November, 1989; San Francisco; Birmingham, Alabama; American Fertility Society
29. Smitz, J., Devroey, P., Camus, M., Deschacht, J., Khan, I., Staessen, C., Van Waesberghe, L., Wisanto, A. and Van Steirteghem, A. C. (1988). The luteal phase and early pregnancy after combined GnRH-agonist/hMG treatment for superovulation in IVF or GIFT. *Hum. Reprod.*, **3**, 585–90
30. Smitz, J., Devroey, P., Faguer, B., Bourgain, C., Camus, M. and Van Steirteghem, A. C. (1992). A prospective randomized comparison of intramuscular or intravaginal progesterone as a luteal phase and early pregnancy supplement. *Hum. Reprod.*, **7**, 168–75
31. Smitz, J., Bourgain, C., Van Waesberghe, L., Camus, M., Devroey, P. and Van Steirteghem, A. C. (1993). A prospective randomized study on oestradiol valerate supplementation in addition to intravaginal micronized progesterone in buserelin and hMG-induced superovulation. *Hum. Reprod.*, **8**, 40–45
32. Liu, J., Nagy, Z., Joris, H., Tournaye, H., Devroey, P. and Van Steirteghem, A. C. (1994). Intracytoplasmic sperm injection does not require special treatment of the spermatozoa. *Hum. Reprod.*, **9**, 1127–30
33. Staessen, C., Janssenswillen, C., Devroey, P. and Van Steirteghem, A. C. (1993). Cytogenetic and morphological observations of single pronucleated human oocytes after *in-vitro* fertilization. *Hum. Reprod.*, **8**, 221–3
34. Camus, M., Van den Abbeel, E., Van Waesberghe, L., Wisanto, A., Devroey, P. and Van Steirteghem, A. C. (1989). Human embryo viability after freezing with dimethylsulfoxide as a cryoprotectant. *Fertil. Steril.*, **51**, 460–5
35. Van Steirteghem, A. C., Van der Elst, J., Van den Abbeel, E., Joris, H., Camus, M. and Devroey, P. (1994). Cryopreservation of supernumerary multicellular human embryos obtained after intracytoplasmic sperm injection. *Fertil. Steril.*, **62**, 775–80

36. Silber, S., Nagy, Z. P., Liu, J., Godoy, H., Devroey, P. and Van Steirteghem, A. C. (1994). Conventional IVF versus ICSI (intracytoplasmic sperm injection) for patients requiring MESA (microsurgical sperm aspiration). *Hum. Reprod.*, **9**, 1705–9
37. Verheyen, G., Pletincx, I. and Van Steirteghem, A. C. (1993). Effect of freezing method, thawing temperature and post-thaw dilution/washing on motility (CASA) and morphology characteristics of high-quality human sperm. *Hum. Reprod.*, **8**, 1678–84
38. Bonduelle, M., Desmyttere, S., Buysse, A., Van Assche, E., Schiettecatte, J., Devroey, P., Van Steirteghem, A. C. and Liebaers, I. (1994). Prospective follow-up study of 55 children born after subzonal insemination and intracytoplasmic sperm injection. *Hum. Reprod.*, **9**, 1765–9

Epididymal microaspiration and *in vitro* fertilization

P. Patrizio, R. H. Asch and T. Ord

INTRODUCTION AND HISTORICAL BACKGROUND

Historically in 1985, there was the first documentation of a human pregnancy, obtained by *in vitro* fertilization (IVF) using epididymal sperm retrieved from a man with a failed vasectomy reversal[1]. In 1987, the concept of retrieving epididymal sperm for IVF was successfully applied to men with congenital absence of the vas deferens[2], and in 1988 the first two births from embryos generated with epididymal sperm were reported[3].

Since then, the use of epididymal sperm in assisted reproduction has steadily increased and currently many centers worldwide are using epididymal sperm aspiration as the treatment of choice for obstructive azoospermia not amenable to surgical correction, and have reported pregnancies and live births[4–9].

Table 1 lists the most common indications for epididymal microaspiration. Congenital absence of the vas deferens (CAVD) and multiple failed vasectomy reversal attempts have so far been the most frequent indications for microepididymal sperm aspiration (MESA) and IVF. It is estimated that CAVD has an incidence of 1–2% of all the cases of male factor infertility and 10–25% of all the obstructive azoospermias[10,11]. Epidemiological data indicate that 25–30% of male infertility is due to azoospermia and of these 40% recognize an obstructive process. Translated in numbers and calculating a population of 1 million infertile couples with male factor infertility, of the about 300 000 men with azoospermia, 120 000 have some kind of obstruction that is identified as CAVD in about 25 000 cases. By adding to these numbers the cases of obstructive azoospermia due to iatrogenic conditions (mainly failed vasectomy reversal attempts) there is a final population of patients candidate for MESA and IVF in the range of 250 000 patients[12].

Table 1 Indications for MESA and IVF

- Congenital absence of the vas deferens (CAVD)
- Inoperable ejaculatory ducts or distal vasal obstruction
- Post-inflammatory obstructions (TBC, gonorrhea, etc.)
- Failed vasectomy reversal
- Radical cysto-prostatectomy
- Spinal cord injuries – ejaculatory dysfunction

The approach to this type of infertility is multidisciplinary including: controlled ovarian hyperstimulation, transvaginal oocyte aspiration, microsurgical epididymal sperm aspiration, *in vitro* fertilization, lately with intracytoplasmic sperm injection (ICIS) and, finally, tubal or uterine embryo transfer. Since the first two steps of the entire treatment are common for any of the assisted reproductive technologies (ARTs), we will describe the diagnostic and therapeutic strategies involved in MESA and IVF. In this chapter, however, we will first summarize some of the preliminary basic science studies on epididymal sperm physiology in obstructive conditions and then will detail the surgical technique and the clinical results achieved with epididymal sperm microaspiration.

SUMMARY OF BASIC SCIENCE STUDIES RELATED TO HUMAN EPIDIDYMAL SPERM

The development of the MESA procedure and its clinical evolution has contributed to expand our knowledge on some of the physiological mechanisms operating in the human epididymis and on epididymal sperm in cases of obstructive azoospermia. In this section, the following subjects will be summarized:

(1) Spermatogenesis, epididymal sperm ultrastructure, disposal mechanisms and epididymal anatomy

(2) Immunological mechanisms

(3) Etiology of CAVD

Spermatogenesis, epididymal sperm ultrastructure, sperm disposal mechanisms and epididymal anatomy

Spermatogenesis

In men with CAVD spermatogenesis is normal and so is the endocrine testicular activity. The testicular biopsies which proved the existence of normal spermatogenesis were evaluated by quantitative analysis[13]. This method allows the determination of sperm production and an accurate extrapolation of the actual number of sperm that would have been present in the ejaculate if no obstruction existed[14]. In the original study it was found that in each of the 22 cases examined, the spermatogenesis was adequate although the frequency distribution of sperm production was lower than one would expect in a normal population of patients. Furthermore, no cases of maturational arrest were observed. Another interesting finding was the lack of relationship between testicular sperm production, quality of epididymal sperm retrieved microsurgically and their *in vitro* fertilization capacity. There was, in fact, no significant improvement in the percentage of active forward motile sperm in men with high testicular sperm count and, similarly, there was no better fertilization rate over cases showing less sperm count.

Morphological ultrastructure

The morphological ultrastructure of sperm retrieved from the vasa efferentia or the most proximal segments of the caput epididymis was consistently better than of those retrieved from the more distal segments of the epididymis, where the majority of sperm were necrotic and degenerated[15]. The vasa efferentia or proximal caput sperm displayed nuclei, acrosomes and flagella similar to ejaculated sperm, although some of them still showed the presence of a small cytoplasmic droplet in the posterior aspect of the head. Epididymal sperm retrieved from sites closer to the obstruction always revealed degenerative changes with karyorrhexis and karyolysis, swelling of the flagellar mitochondria and fragmentation of their plasma membranes.

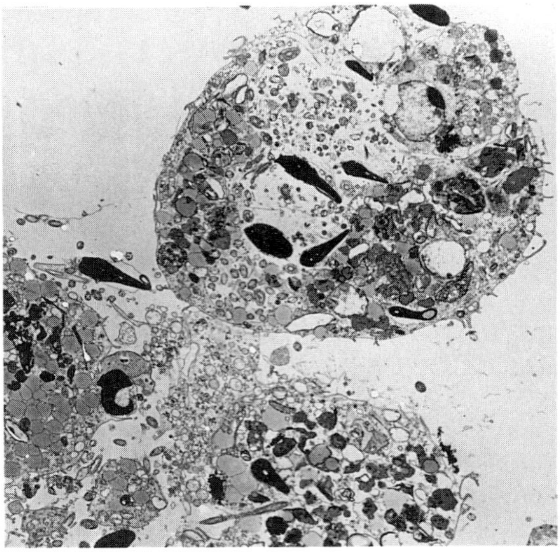

Figure 1 Electronmicroscopy photograph of macrophages after phagocytosis of epididymal sperm from the proximal caput

Sperm disposal mechanisms

Concerning sperm disposal mechanisms, it was clear that in areas near to the obstruction, where the number of degenerated and necrotic sperm was at the peak, the number of macrophages was also high[16]. Characteristically these macrophages (see Figure 1) were exceedingly large and laden with sperm remnants barely recognizable within their cytoplasm. Upon completion of their sperm phagocytosis they underwent degeneration and release of the numerous lipid droplets packed in their cytoplasm. On the other hand, in the most proximal segments of the excurrent pathways, the number of macrophages was minimal and also their size was less impressive than of those observed in the distal portions.

Such information has led to direct sperm aspiration procedures in the most proximal portions of the caput epididymis or vasa efferentia in order to retrieve the most motile and already reproductively competent sperm.

Epididymal anatomy in men with CAVD

Concerning the epididymal anatomy in men with CAVD, it has been observed that the epididymis has different degrees of development and the muscle layer is generally hypertophic due to the chronic obstruction[16,17]. In the majority of the cases the epididymis is formed either by the proximal portion of the caput alone or with a small proximal portion of the corpus, perhaps reflecting early developmental arrest or reabsorption of the mesonephric or Wolffian duct. Few patients have development of the caput, the entire corpus and a small representation of the cauda of the epididymis. Clinically, we correlated the epididymal length with the *in vitro* fertilization results[18]. Interestingly, men with an epididymis longer than 4 cm (caput and portions of the corpus) had a significantly better IVF rate compared to men with shorter, <2 cm, epididymis (24% versus 7%, respectively). Although this observation could seem to support the theory of epididymal transit, it must be mentioned that regardless of the epididymal length, sperm microaspiration was always performed in the proximal caput. Therefore, the better fertilization rate could be explained by assuming that a longer epididymis allows the arrival of 'fresher' waves of sperm while in a short epididymis the system is congested and occupied by old, senescent sperm.

Immunological mechanisms

It is well known that men with obstructive azoospermia due to vasectomy have high incidence of serum antisperm antibodies (ASA). Very few studies investigated the immunological response of obstructive azoospermia due to congenital blockages. A total of four studies was carried out in patients undergoing epididymal sperm microaspiration because of CAVD. The first study showed that men with CAVD have a lower incidence of serum antisperm antibodies when compared to men with vasectomy (29% versus 80%) and the same low incidence was also found by testing epididymal sperm directly[7,17].

One of the possible explanations for this low level of sperm autoimmunity was thought to be due to a different sperm antigenicity of men with CAVD since their sperm usually cannot complete the epididymal transit. The second immunological study proved[19], however, that human epididymal sperm retrieved from the vasa efferentia have the same surface antigenic epitopes, detectable by immunobinding, as ejaculated sperm and that this antigenic immunocompetence is acquired within the testes before their epididymal transit. Therefore, the low incidence of ASAs in men with CAVD does not reflect a different sperm antigenicity. It is possible that sperm exposure to the immune system is minimal or, alternatively, it is likely that active lymphocyte immunosuppression may exist within the testes, thus preventing autoimmunity.

The third immunological study addressed the question of whether the presence of ASAs on epididymal sperm used for IVF might have a detrimental effect upon their *in vitro* fertilization capacity[20]. At the time of oocyte insemination, sperm retrieved from the proximal caput epididymis and vasa efferentia of 45 patients were tested by direct immunoblot testing. Sixteen patients (35%) were found positive and of these 11 (69%) fertilized at least one oocyte that successively cleaved with an overall fertilization rate of 16% and five (31%) pregnancies were documented. In the negative group, 15 of 29 patients (52%) achieved fertilization, the overall fertilization rate was 21% and five pregnancies (18%) ensued.

In conclusion, no relationship between the presence of ASAs, class of immunoglobulin, site of antibody location on epididymal sperm, titer of binding and subsequent fertilization and pregnancy rates was found, therefore, autoimmunity to epididymal sperm should not be considered as a reason for failed fertilization.

The fourth and final immunological study evaluated the concept of whether repetitive attempts of sperm aspiration could have an impact in evoking new sperm autoimmunity in men with obstructive azoospermia[21].

During sperm retrieval blood–sperm exposure is unavoidable; therefore, it might be possible to speculate about formation of ASAs after each procedure or especially after repetitive attempts. This study showed that after performing two, three or four MESA attempts, patients who were originally negative for ASAs remained negative despite sperm antigenic exposure, leading to the assumption that there is a population of men, perhaps genetically predisposed, who are non-immunological responders to their sperm antigens and, therefore, MESA

Table 2 Overall genetic screening results for CF mutations in three generations

CF mutations	*Patients*	*Wives*	*Fathers*	*Mothers*	*Offspring*
DF508	22	1	3	4	3
W1282X	10	—	—	1	—
N1303K	1	—	—	1	—
G542X	1	—	—	—	—
1717G.A	1	—	1	—	—
R553X	1	—	—	—	—
R117H	—	1	2	2	—
R553X/R117H	1	—	—	—	—
R117H/R117H	1	—	—	—	—
DF508/R117H	4	—	—	—	—
Total	42/66	2/49	6/15	8/19	3/13
Incidence	(64%)	(4%)	(41%)		(23%)

can be safely repeated without the risk of creating new sperm autoimmunity.

Etiology of congenital absence of the vas deferens

For a long time the etiology of CAVD has been unknown. Recently, a common link between this peculiar form of male infertility and cystic fibrosis (CF) has been found[22,23]. Genetic screening for CF was offered to 66 men with CAVD, their wives, some of their parents and to 13 offspring generated with MESA+IVF. The results are listed in Table 2. The genetic study revealed that 42 (64%) patients were positive for CF mutations and thus identified as having a mild form of CF disease. In these patients, the CF gene expression exclusively affected the development of portions of the mesonephric duct, since no other symptoms or signs typical of CF were present. Recently, extensive analysis of the entire gene sequence revealed new mutations in the CF gene[24] and a particular variant, called 5T, specific for patients with CAVD[25]. With this additional testing, the incidence of CF mutations, (compound heterozygotes and homozygotes) rose to 75%, although 25% of patients with CAVD still show no mutations. It is now clear that congenital absence of the vas deferens is due to an autosomal recessive condition inherited by sons of the parents who are carriers for different CF mutations.

This discovery prompted the offering of genetic counseling to each couple interested in MESA+ IVF when CAVD is a factor in their infertility. The risk of having a child with CF is extremely small (0.3%) if the wives are CF negative, while the risk is more difficult to assess when wives are found CF positive[23].

DIAGNOSTIC ITER IN OBSTRUCTIVE AZOOSPERMIA

(1) Complete medical history

(2) Physical examination

(3) Semen analysis

(4) Hormonal and immunological tests

(5) Genetic screening for cystic fibrosis

(6) Testicular biopsy

(7) Vasogram

In general, to facilitate the differential diagnosis of the azoospermia, and to select the proper treatment, the schematic approach shown in Table 3 is used.

EPIDIDYMAL MICROASPIRATION

Surgical technique

The surgical aspect of the MESA procedure is relatively simple. After exposure of the scrotal content, at a magnification varying between 6 and 40× using an operating microscope, a loop of epididymal tubule is chosen for the aspiration and carefully denuded of the periadventitial tunica. Bearing in mind the results of the ultrastructural study[14], it is safe to recommend the most proximal portion of the caput epididymis as the 'best bet' for less senescent and better quality sperm. After a very careful

Table 3 Schematic approach to differential diagnosis of azoospermia and treatment selection

	CAVD	*Acquired obstruction*	*Testicular failure*	*Ejaculatory dysfunction*
Semen volume	low	NL–low	NL	low
PH	acid	NL	NL	NL
Fructose	absent	present–low	present	present
Sperm in postcoital Urine	absent	absent	absent	present
FSH	NL	NL	high	NL
Testicular biopsy	NL	NL	abnormal	NL
Treatment	MESA+IVF	MESA+IVF+ vasoepididymostomy	donor sperm insemination spermatid injection	IUI or IVF or MESA+IVF

hemostasis, the epididymal tubule is longitudinally incised and the outflowing fluid is collected in a 22 Medicut needle attached to a tuberculin syringe containing small aliquots of human tubal fluid (HTF) to avoid the risk of drying out the sample (see Figure 2). Each specimen is then promptly handed to the biologist and assessed for presence, quality and quantity of sperm. The information from the laboratory serves as guidance for the surgeons regarding whether to continue the aspiration in the same place or move to a different (usually more proximal) location. At times, it is necessary to perform sperm microaspiration from the vasa efferentia since the specimens from the proximal caput epididymis exhibit extremely poor sperm quality.

The retrieval is completed when the biologist estimates that there are enough sperm for IVF or, alternatively, when no more fluid is obtainable from any place of the epididymis of both sides. At this point, in order to preserve intact the chances for a future sperm aspiration attempt, the epididymal tubules are closed with 10-0 nylon and the periadventitial tissue with 9-0 nylon. Indeed, in a few cases MESA procedure has been repeated up to four or even five times and no technical difficulties in retrieving sperm were encountered, and the identification of previous stitches helped in recognizing the best site for aspiration. It must be said that it is possible to encounter cases where no sperm are found, despite dissection and aspiration at the level of the vasa efferentia. In these instances, a rete testis blockage must be presumed since the spermatogenesis process as seen in testicular biopsies is normal.

Recently, these unexpected failures of sperm retrieval have been managed by performing testicular biopsies and extracting sperm to be used in conjunction with subzonal or oocyte intracytoplasmic injection[26–28].

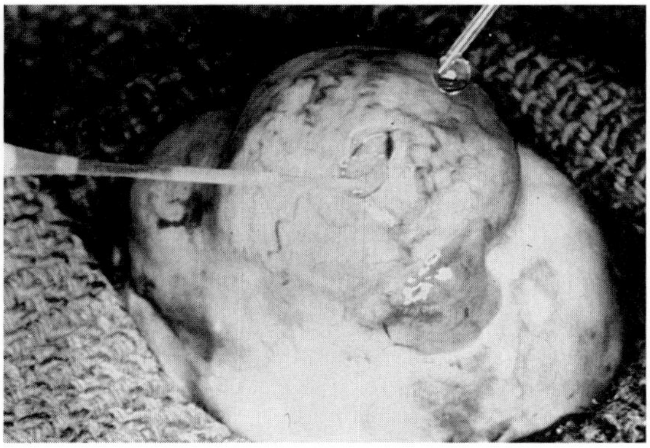

Figure 2 Photograph showing a proximal caput epididymal tubule longitudinally incised and aspiration of blood-free epididymal fluid

The role of the IVF laboratory

The second and certainly the most important step for the establishment of the fertilizing ability of epididymal sperm is the role played by the IVF laboratory (see Appendix for complete details)[29]. There is no doubt that epididymal sperm has worse motility, progression and morphology than ejaculated sperm. Further, although a great deal of attention is paid in trying to avoid blood contamination during the surgery, the epididymal aspirates are frequently contaminated with red blood cells, debris and macrophages. In order to obtain clean sample suitable to be used for IVF, new methodologies of sperm processing and handling had to be created.

Table 4 Overall IVF results with MESA procedure

	Group 1 CAVD	*Group 2 Acquired azoospermia*
No. patients	132	25
No. cycles	164	28
No. with motile sperm	160	23
No. with fertilization	82	14
No. oocytes	2916	324
No. embryos (fert. rate %)	369 (13)*	99 (31)*
No. pregnancies**	22	4
No. pregnancy wastage	7	0
No. with frozen embryos	20	6

*$P<10^{-6}$; **Pregnancy rate per cycle 14% in both groups, pregnancy rate per transfer 28% in CAVD, 33% in acquired azoospermia

The idea of the MiniPercoll by Ord[29] for the treatment of these samples has improved the fertilization rate over classic methods of swim-up or wash and resuspension, since the minigradient of Percoll allows not only the recovery of blood-free sperm, but also a good number of normal and motile sperm. In addition, during the last 2 years, pentoxifylline and 2-deoxyadenosine, both acting by allowing more availability of ATP, have also been used in conjunction with MiniPercoll in order to improve the epididymal sperm fertilization rate[30].

The IVF process *per se* does not differ from standard IVF cases except that with epididymal sperm, the cumulus-denuded oocytes are inseminated with a higher number of sperm, varying upon availability between 300 000 and 1.5 million. The resulting embryos are transferred preferentially to the Fallopian tubes via laparoscopy, 40–48 h after insemination. If excess embryos are available, they can be safely frozen and utilized subsequently for replacement cycles.

CLINICAL RESULTS

Table 4 summarizes the clinical results with fertilization and pregnancy rate for 192 cycles of MESA and IVF procedures. The patients are divided into two groups according to the etiology of their obstruction. Group 1 ($n=164$) comprised men with CAVD, group 2 ($n=28$) were men with acquired obstruction such as vasectomy reversal failure, epididymal blockages, post-surgical ejaculatory failure and vas deferens scarring. The overall fertilization rate was 15%, but in keeping the groups separated, there was a much higher fertilization rate in patients with acquired obstruction (31% versus 13%, $P<10^{-6}$), although the sperm aspiration site was always the proximal head of the epididymis.

There was still a statistical difference in fertilization rate when the IVF data were analyzed taking into account only patients who achieved fertilization. In patients with CAVD the fertilization rate was 25% and in patients with acquired azoospermia, the fertilization rate was 42% ($P<10^{-6}$). In men with CAVD, by comparing sperm parameters values between patients who did and did not fertilize, except for a lower motility, there was no apparent explanation. In men with acquired azoospermia, on the other hand, a clear discriminant factor for successful fertilization was the number of sperm and the total motile count. In fact, men who fertilized had a sperm count of 53.8 ± 4.4 million while the values of those who failed to fertilize were 12.3 ± 4.9 million and 1.6 ± 0.4 million, respectively, with P values of <0.04 and <0.01, respectively.

In group 1 there was a total of 22 pregnancies of which five were twin gestation. Twenty patients had excess embryos available for cryopreservation and up to the present seven replacement cycles have been performed yielding two pregnancies with singleton live births[31].

In group 2 there were four pregnancies of which one was multiple (triplets). Six patients had excess embryos for cryopreservation. In both groups excess sperm was cryopreserved.

CONCLUSION

Epididymal sperm are now used routinely in IVF for particularly selected cases of male factor infertility. Since in several mammalian species sperm must pass through the epididymis prior to acquiring fertilizing capacity, it was assumed that the same concept should be applied to humans. The clinical results published during the last 7 years have, in contrast, indicated that human epididymal sperm can fertilize *in vitro* and the resulting embryos can generate live births. There are, however, some limiting factors to overcome: first, epididymal sperm of men with CAVD have an overall low (<20%) IVF rate. Further, it is impossible to predict fertilization based upon the common parameters of count, motility, progression and morphology. Curiously, with repeated attempts of epididymal microaspiration, the fertilization results can be predicted according to the very first procedure.

Epididymal sperm of men with acquired obstructive azoospermia have a significantly better IVF rate (31% in acquired azoospermia versus 13% in CAVD). Further, in this group of patients, the chances of successful fertilization are directly related to the total number of motile sperm retrieved.

A recent study[32], aimed at evaluation of the existence of a possible correlation between IVF results and the presence and type of CF mutations in men with CAVD, found that patients with the most severe mutation, Delta F-508, have the worst IVF results. Briefly, it was demonstrated that the fertilization rate was 7% if men had genotype Delta F-508, versus 21% for patients with other mutations, 23% for patients with CAVD but no detectable CF mutations, and 31% in patients without CAVD. These results led to the conclusion that CF gene activity may play an important role during spermatogenesis, and men with CAVD and genotype Delta F-508 might have biochemically defective epididymal sperm (alteration of CI-channel) and an impairment in their fertilization function.

The advent of intracytoplasmic sperm injection (ICSI)[33,34] has undoubtedly renewed the hope of improving the fertilization rate of epididymal sperm. In our own experience, however, the preliminary results have shown an improvement in the fertilization rate (35%), but not yet improvement in the pregnancy rate (30%). Of great interest is the use of ICSI in conjunction with testicular sperm. Two recent MESA cases were treated by injection of testicular sperm retrieved from testicular biopsies because of rete testis blockage in one, and absent epididymis in the other. In the first case, two of six oocytes (33%) were fertilized and cleaved; in the second case, 12 of 24 (50%) oocytes were fertilized and cleaved; however, no pregnancies ensued. Another advantage in the use of ICSI is the possibility of offering sperm cryopreservation in every case of MESA, thus limiting the number and the need of repetitive surgical procedures. When the number of sperm is extremely small, they can be frozen 24 h after insemination. In our experience, upon thawing 24-h-old frozen sperm, a few survived and were used for microinjection which gave origin to two embryos, but no pregnancy resulted.

The use of sperm from testicular biopsy is extremely exciting. The first pregnancy has been recently reported[28] and thus it is theoretically possible to offer treatment also to the most difficult cases of obstruction (rete testis). Additionally, if the successful use of testicular sperm is confirmed by other centers, it is possible to predict that the rapid and less invasive testicular biopsies might replace the entire MESA procedure.

References

1. Temple Smith, P. D., Southwick, G. J., Yates, C. A., Trounson, A. O. and De Krester, D. M. (1985). Human pregnancy by *in vitro* fertilization (IVF) using sperm aspirated from the epididymis. *J.* In Vitro *Fertil. Embryo Transf.*, **2**, 119–22
2. Silber, S. J., Ord, T., Borrero, C., Balmaceda, J. P. and Asch, R. H. (1985). New treatment for infertility due to congenital absence of vas. *Lancet*, **2**, 850
3. Patrizio, P., Ord, T., Silber, S. J., Balmaceda, J. P. and Asch, R. H. (1988). Two births after microsurgical epididymal sperm aspiration in congenital absence of the vas deferens (letter). *Lancet*, **2**, 1364
4. Silber, S., Ord, T., Balmaceda, J. P., Patrizio, P. and Asch, R. H. (1990). Congenital absence of the vas deferens: Studies on the fertilizing capacity of the human epididymal sperm. *N. Engl. J. Med.*, **323**, 1788–92
5. Olar, T. T., La Nasa, J., Dickey, R. P., Taylor, S. N. and Curole, D. N. (1990). Fertilization of human oocytes by microinjection of human sperm aspirated from the caput epididymides of an individual with obstructive azoospermia. *J.* In Vitro *Fertil. Embryo Transf.*, **7**, 160–4
6. Schoysman, R., Bertin, G., VanDerZwalmen, P. and Segal, L. (1990). Utilization du sperme epididymaire dans un programme de fecondation *in vitro*. *Prog. Androl.*, **3**, 137–45
7. Patrizio, P. and Asch, R. H. (1992). Epididymal sperm in assisted reproduction. *Ann. N.Y. Acad. Med.*, **21**, 533–7
8. Marmar, J. L., Corson, S. L., Batzer, F. R., Gocial, B. and Go, K. (1993). Microsurgical aspiration of sperm from the epididymis: A mobile program. *J. Urol.*, **149**, 1368–73
9. Rosen, E. G. and Nagler, H. M. (1993). Treatment options for patients with congenital vasal agenesis: Spermatocele to microsurgical epididymal sperm aspiration. *Asst. Reprod. Rev.*, **3**, 255–60
10. Patrizio, P. and Asch, R. H. (1993). Intratubal gamete and embryo transfer in male infertility. In Rajfer, J.

(ed.) *Common Problems in Infertility and Impotence*, pp. 137–48. (Year Book Medical Publisher)

11. Jequier, A. M., Amel, I. D. and Bullimore, N. J. (1985). Congenital absence of the vasa deferentia presenting with infertility. *J. Androl.*, **6**, 15–19
12. Asch, R. H. and Silber, S. J. (1991). Microsurgical epididymal sperm aspiration and assisted reproductive techniques. *Ann. N.Y. Acad. Sci.*, **626**, 101–10
13. Silber, S. J., Patrizio, P. and Asch, R. H. (1990). Quantitative evaluation of spermatogenesis by testicular histology in men with congenital absence of the vas deferens undergoing epididymal sperm aspiration. *Hum. Reprod.*, **5**, 89–93
14. Silber, S. J. and Rodriguez-Rigau, L. J. (1981). Quantitative analysis of testicle biopsy: Determination of partial obstruction and prediction of sperm count after surgery for obstruction. *Fertil. Steril.*, **36**, 480–95
15. Asch, R. H., Patrizio, P. and Silber, S. J. (1992). Ultrastructure of human sperm in men with congenital absence of the vas deferens: Clinical implications. *Fertil. Steril.*, **58**, 190–3
16. Patrizio, P. (1989). Spermatogenesis, sperm disposal mechanisms and immunology in congenital absence of vas deferens. In Capitanio, G. L., Asch, R. H., Croce, S. and De Cecco, L. (eds.) *GIFT: From Basics to Clinics*, Vol. 63, pp. 25–36. (New York: Raven Press, Serono Symposia Publications)
17. Patrizio, P., Moretti-Rojas, I., Ord, T., Balmaceda, J. P., Silber, S. and Asch, R. H. (1989). Low incidence of antisperm antibodies in men with congenital absence of the vas deferens. *Fertil. Steril.*, **52**, 1018–21
18. Patrizio, P., Ord, T., Silber, S. J. and Asch, R. H. (1994). Correlation between epididymal length and fertilization rate in men with congenital absence of the vas deferens. *Fertil. Steril.*, **61**, 265–8
19. Patrizio, P., Bronson, R., Silber, S. J., Ord, T. and Asch, R. H. (1992). Testicular origin of immunobead reacting antigens in human sperm. *Fertil. Steril.*, **57**, 183–6
20. Patrizio, P., Silber, S. J., Ord, T., Moretti-Rojas, I. and Asch, R. H. (1992). Relationship of epididymal sperm antibodies to their *in vitro* fertilization capacity in men with congenital absence of the vas deferens. *Fertil. Steril.*, **58**, 1006–10
21. Patrizio, P., Ord, T., Silber, S. J., La, A. T., Rojas, F. J. and Asch, R. H. (1992). Repetitive attempts of sperm aspiration and *in vitro* fertilization in men with congentical absence of the vas deferens on development of antisperm antibodies. *Presented at the 48th Annual Meeting American Fertility Society*, New Orleans, LA, October–November 1992, S22, pp. 0–048
22. Anguiano, A., Oates, R. H., Amos, J. A., Dean, M., Gerrard, B., Stewart, C., Maher, T. A., White, M. B. and Milunsky, A. (1992). Congenital bilateral absence of the vas deferens: A primarily general form of cystic fibrosis. *J. Am. Med. Assoc.*, **67**, 1794–7
23. Patrizio, P., Asch, R. H., Handelin, B. and Silber, S. J. (1993). Aetiology of congenital absence of the vas deferens: Genetic study of three generations. *Hum. Reprod.*, **8**, 215–20
24. Zielenski, J., Patrizio, P., Markiewicz, D., Asch, R. H. and Tsui, L. C. (1995). Identification of two mutations (S50Y, 4173delC) in the CFTR gene from patients with CAVD. *Hum. Mutation*, in press
25. Zielenski, J., Patrizio, P., Corey, M., Hardelin, B., Markiewicz, D., Asch, R. H. and Tsui, L-C. (1995). CFTR gene variants for patients with congenital absence of vas deferens. *Am. J. Hum. Genet.*, in press
26. Schoysman, R., VanDerZwalmen, P., Nijs, M., Segal-Bertine, G. and VanDe Casseye, M. (1993). Successful fertilization by testicular spermatozoa in an *in vitro* fertilization programme (letter). *Hum. Reprod.*, **8**, 1339–40
27. Craft, I., Bennett, V. and Nicholson, N. (1993). Fertilizing ability of testicular spermatozoa (letter). *Lancet*, **342**, 864
28. Schoysman, R., VanDerZwalmen, P., Nijs, M., Segal, L., Segal-Bertin, G., Geerts, L., VanRoosendaal, E. and Schoysman, D. (1993). Pregnancy after fertilization with human testicular spermatozoa (letter). *Lancet*, **342**, 1237
29. Ord, T., Patrizio, P., Marello, E., Balmaceda, J. P. and Asch, R. H. (1990). MiniPercoll: A new method of semen preparation for IVF in severe male factor infertility. *Hum. Reprod.*, **5**, 987–9
30. Ord, T., Marello, E., Patrizio, P., Balmaceda, J. P., Silber, S. J. and Asch, R. H. (1992). The role of the laboratory in the handling of the epididymal sperm for assisted reproductive technologies. *Fertil. Steril.*, **57**, 1103–6
31. Patrizio, P., Silber, S. J., Ord, T., Marello, E., Balmaceda, J. P. and Asch, R. H. (1992). Replacement of frozen embryos generated from epididymal sperm: The first two pregnancies. *Hum. Reprod.*, **7**, 652–3
32. Patrizio, P., Ord, T., Silber, S. J. and Asch, R. H. (1993). Cystic fibrosis mutations impair the fertilization rate of epididymal sperm from men with congenital absence of the vas deferens. *Hum. Reprod.*, **8**, 1259–63
33. Palermo, G., Joris, H., Derde, M. P., Camus, M., Devroey, P. and Van Steirteghem, A. C. (1993). Sperm characteristics and outcome of human assisted fertilization by subzonal insemination and intracytoplasmic sperm injection. *Fertil. Steril.*, **59**, 826–35
34. Van Steirteghem, A. C., Liv, J., Joris, H., Nagy, Z., Janssenswillen, C., Tournaye, H., Derde, M. P., Van Assche, E. and Devroey, P. (1993). Higher success rate by intracytoplasmic sperm injection than subzonal insemination. Report of a second series of 300 consecutive cycles. *Hum. Reprod.*, **8**, 1055–60

Systemic treatment of sperm defects 33

A. A. Acosta

INTRODUCTION

Systemic medical treatment to improve testicular and sperm functions has been extensively, and for the most part, empirically tried. Evaluation of the sperm function(s) has changed dramatically since the introduction of Assisted Reproduction Technologies (ART) in the field of Andrology; the focus was changed from measuring sperm parameters in the semen analysis, and using pregnancy induction and rates in the female as endpoints, to a more direct evaluation of tests of sperm function (Table 1), of egg and sperm interaction under the laboratory conditions of ART and of implantation, pregnancy and abortion rates using these methodologies.

The success of systemic medical treatment of testicular dysfunctions is high when cases of secondary testicular deficiency (hypogonadotropic hypogonadism, hyperprolactinemia, thyroid disorders and different variants of congenital adrenal hyperplasia) are diagnosed[1]. In those cases, the use of appropriate etiologic therapy renders excellent results. Unfortunately, those cases represent a small number of patients within the total population of testicular dysfunctions.

A completely different situation arises when 'idiopathic oligozoospermia' due to primary testicular deficiency is diagnosed. In this category, extensive gaps in the knowledge of the pathophysiological characteristics of the hypothalamic–pituitary–testicular axis and of the intratesticular regulators and modulators of spermatogenesis, lack of reliable tests to evaluate the different portions of the axis and, mainly, the intratesticular pathophysiology makes systemic medical treatment empirical in most cases, and clinical results extremely difficult to assess. We will review briefly in this presentation:

(1) The pathophysiology of the hypothalamic–pituitary–testicular axis in patients with idiopathic oligo-astheno-teratozoospermia;

(2) The tests to evaluate the hypothalmic–pituitary–testicular axis and their clinical significance;

(3) The systemic medical treatments and their results in natural reproduction; and

(4) The systemic medical treatments and their results in assisted reproduction.

Table 1 Tests of sperm function

Acrosin content
ATP
Reactive oxygen species (ROS)
Cervical mucus penetration
Evaluation of acrosome status
Triple staining
Ligands
Immunological
Hypo-osmotic swelling test
Hamster zona-free oocyte, human spermatozoa penetration assay (SPA)
Hemizona assay

PATHOPHYSIOLOGY OF THE HYPOTHALAMIC–PITUITARY TESTICULAR AXIS IN PATIENTS WITH IDIOPATHIC OLIGO-ASTHENO-TERATOZOOSPERMIA

The classical description of a hypothalamic luteinizing hormone-releasing hormone (LHRH) pulse generator modulated by suprahypothalamic (adrenergic, cholinergic, dopaminergic and opioidergic) influences and stimulating, through the GnRH mediator, gonadotropin synthesis, storage and release is certainly well known. The action of those gonadotropins (follicle-stimulating hormone [FSH] and luteinizing hormone [LH]) on the gonads, as well as the intracellular, ultra-short, short and long feedback mechanisms of FSH and LH regulations have been already described and are not within the scope of this review. In spite of all the research done in these areas, major gaps exist in the human in regard to many potential functional steps of this stimulatory–modulatory system, mainly in reference to the intratesticular control mechanisms. Some of the intratesticular peptides found and described in different compartments of the testes have physiological significance and function; others, although known to be present in testicular cells, have not yet been found to have physiological relevance[2].

Research attempts to establish the pathophysiological basis for idiopathic oligo-astheno-teratozoospermia are scanty and the information produced of doubtful clinical use.

Pulse generator characteristics

The characteristics of the pulse generator in normal, young, fertile males are well established[3,4]. Matsumoto *et al.*[5] investigated the status of the LHRH pulse generator in males with hypogonadotrophic eunuchoidism and in patients with idiopathic oligo-azoospermia and elevated FSH levels. These males, of whom approximately 20% have elevated serum FSH and normal serum LH and testosterone levels[6], showed a reduced LH pulse frequency[5] with no significant differences from controls in LH pulse amplitude and total and free testosterone and estradiol levels[7,8]. Pulsatile administration of LHRH at normal frequencies restores FSH levels to the normal range, without significant changes in serum LH, testosterone and estradiol levels[9,10]. When physiological pulses of LHRH were administered for a prolonged period of time (12 months or more) using 5 μg every 90 min, LH levels were significantly increased, FSH levels decreased and testosterone and estradiol levels were elevated; all changes reversed to previous patterns when treatment was stopped. Azoospermia and severe oligozoospermia (<1 million sperm/mL) did not improve. One subject with less severe oligozoospermia did not show a sustained improvement, but his wife became pregnant after 3 months of LH–RH therapy. In two others, sperm production did not improve[5]. Similar results were published by Bals-Pratsch *et al.*[11]. Wagner *et al.*[12] reported an increase in motile sperm density after LHRH therapy in males with severe idiopathic oligozoospermia (sperm counts <10 million/mL). Aulitzky *et al.*[13] also found significant increase in sperm density with three pregnancies in males with a less severe degree of spermatogenic damage, increased spontaneous LH pulse frequency, and elevated serum FSH levels. According to these uncontrolled studies there may be a subpopulation of idiopathic oligo-asthenozoospermic males showing an abnormal pulse generator function that could be improved by prolonged pulsatile LHRH administration, although the identification criteria for these males by diagnostic testing are not clear.

The decrease in LHRH pulse frequency in these patients has not been found by other investigators. Wu *et al.*[14] studied the physiology of gonadotropin secretion in a group of infertile males with idiopathic azoospermia or oligo-asthenozoospermia and found no significant differences with a control group. Pulse interval was increased in patients with normal FSH and LH. Total testosterone, but not free testosterone index was decreased in the infertile population. Bennet *et al.*[15] studied 51 patients with idiopathic oligospermia and 10 control subjects, and found the immunoactive LH pulse frequency higher and the mean bioactive to immunoactive LH ratio lower in the infertile male group. Even in patients with elevated FSH, these authors found an increased mean LH pulse frequency, in agreement with Booth *et al.*[16], but in disagreement with the previously mentioned researchers. The authors believe that the defect is primarily in the testes and not at higher levels of the hypothalamic–pituitary–testicular axis. Similar conclusions were reached by Avril-Ducarne[17] that ascribed the mechanism of oligospermia with isolated high FSH level to an abnormal feedback of testicular gonadopeptides and steroids. In a group of 23 patients with oligospermia, high FSH levels and normal LH and testosterone values, they found decreased mean testosterone, decreased mean LH (baseline and LHRH-stimulated), increased area under the LH pulsatility curve, normal frequency and increased amplitude in half of the patients, while the other half showed reduced frequency and increased amplitude. Pulsatile administration of LHRH did not restore a normal FSH–LH ratio; therefore, the authors conclude that it is not a suitable treatment.

Interference with FSH action by anti-gonadotropin antibodies, specifically anti-FSH antibodies, were investigated in 29 infertile males with azoospermia or oligo-astheno-teratozoospermia, and in eight normal controls. In this small group of patients, no evidence of FSH blocking antibodies was found[18].

Few studies have tried to elucidate the possible abnormalities in the intratesticular environment. Fredricsson *et al.*[19] have reported prepubertal phosphorous metabolism in infertile males with a defect in the 17-hydroxylation step and subsequent derangement in androgen synthesis; concomitant changes at the level of the lamina propria were found.

Growth hormone-releasing hormone

A growth hormone-releasing hormone (GHRH)-like mRNA is present in the testes of rats and humans[20,21]. Srivastava *et al.*[22] demonstrated that immunoreactive GHRH-like mRNA is synthesized in early spermatogenic cells, but not in mature sperm. Its role in spermatogenesis is unknown, but its existence may open a window of opportunity for its therapeutic utilization.

Bergmann *et al.*[23] described abnormal tight junctions between Sertoli cells and spermatogonia in ectopic positions within the seminiferous epithelium associated with elevated FSH levels.

Namiki *et al.*[24] have found abnormalities at the testicular FSH receptor level in infertile males, and Buch *et al.*[25] characterized the defect at the binding step activity.

Endocrine investigation

Endocrine investigation of the seminal plasma compartment of infertile males has disclosed an increase in estradiol values[26]; the significance of this finding is not fully understood. Estradiol seems to impair spermatogenesis[27,28], but clinical trials that try to decrease estradiol production in patients with idiopathic oligo-astheno-teratozoospermia have rendered conflicting results and it is unknown whether the estradiol (E_2) elevation is the consequence or the cause of the spermatogenic disturbance.

Inhibin concentration

Inhibin concentration in peripheral plasma or in seminal fluid has been proposed as an indicator of testicular dysfunction, using established radioimmunoassays or *in vitro* bioassay methods. Scott and Burger[29] reported negative correlation between immunoreactive inhibin in seminal plasma and peripheral FSH levels in azoospermic patients; peripheral serum immunoreactive inhibin showed no correlation with normal FSH levels in men with idiopathic oligozoospermia or azoospermia[30]. No decrease of inhibin was found in Kleinfelter's patients[30] or in idiopathic hypogonadotropic hypogonadism[31].

Transferrin concentration

Transferrin concentration in seminal plasma has also been used as an indicator of Sertoli cell function, and low levels of transferrin have been correlated with low sperm density and poor sperm function in terms of fertilizing ability of human oocytes in the *in vitro* system[32]. Irisawa *et al.*[33] investigated the concentration of transferrin in seminal plasma in 94 male patients attending an infertility clinic, including patients with Kleinfelter's syndrome, varicocele, azoospermia, oligozoospermia and normozoospermia. Patients with obstructive azoospermia were excluded. The transferrin levels by radioimmunoassay were higher in the normozoospermia group and correlated with the concentration of spermatozoa; it did not correlate with the motility of the sample. Those levels were inversely correlated with serum levels of LH, FSH and prolactin, similar to the results obtained by Tagaki *et al.*[34]. Fuse *et al.*[35] concluded that transferrin levels may be indicative of the physiopathology of the germ cells, but it is not a distinctive marker of the fertility of an individual. Cek *et al.*[36] found significantly lower levels of seminal plasma transferrin in the infertile male group than in the fertile counterpart.

Papadimas *et al.*[37] found a decrease of seminal plasma transferrin levels only in cases of azoospermia and not in other sperm quality disorders; levels correlated with sperm count, seminal fluid volume and LH levels.

LDH isoenzymes

Lactate dehydrogenase (LDH) isoenzymes have also been tried as markers of sperm quality. LDH-X has been demonstrated to be specific of human spermatozoa, and it has been reported to be absent in patients with azoospermia. Keltimlidis[38] investigated LDH-X and found that it was absent in males with testicular chromosomal aberrations, history of mumps orchitis, obstructive azoospermia and idiopathic seminiferous tubular failure and in oligozoospermic males with sperm concentrations $<15\times10^6$ sperm/mL. The concentration of LDH-X in oligo-asthenozoospermia is reduced when compared with values of males with normal sperm counts. LDH-X is present in primary spermatocytes, and is found exclusively in spermatozoa at the level of the inner membrane of the mitochondrial cristae[39]. Noguera Velasco *et al.*[40] found a good correlation between levels of LDH-C_4 activity and fertility potential, and also with sperm density.

Cytogenic studies of peripheral blood karyotypes or of germ cell line karyotypes, although potentially valuable, cannot be used yet in the clinical decision-making process.

TESTS OF EVALUATION OF THE HYPOTHALAMIC–PITUITARY–TESTICULAR AXIS: CLINICAL SIGNIFICANCE

The endocrine evaluation of pituitary gonadotropins (FSH, LH) and prolactin (PRL), of testicular steroids (testosterone [T] and estradiol) and of one of the main peptides, inhibin, has been the most commonly used hormone panel intended to determine whether testicular failure resides at the central or testicular level. When gonadotropins are elevated, the diagnosis of primary testicular failure is confirmed. Nevertheless, in a substantial number of cases, failure is at the testicular level and gonadotropins are within normal limits, or slightly elevated; therefore, the test is clinically useful only when it is abnormal.

On the other hand, evaluation of semen using the classical parameters is no longer accurate, since function of the sperm in terms of fertilizing ability is not taken into account, except in an indirect fashion.

A detailed discussion of each one of these tests is not within the scope of this review, but an attempt will be made to put some of them into proper perspective.

The addition of bioactive FSH determination to the most commonly used radioimmunoassay test has been evaluated by different groups. Jockenhövel *et al.*[41] showed a good correlation between the two, both in infertile males and males with proven fertility, using the Sertoli cell aromatase bioassay to measure bioactive FSH, and a two-site fluoroimmunoassay to evaluate immunoreactive FSH. They were clearly elevated in patients with Kleinfelter syndrome, non-obstructive azoospermia, maldescended testes and patients with severe oligozoospermia, but were minimally elevated in infertile males with moderate oligozoospermia and with normal sperm counts. The bioactive to immunoreactive FSH ratios were reduced in all groups except the patients with normal sperm counts when compared with the fertile population. The authors concluded that the immunoreactive FSH determination is enough for clinical purposes, that there is a reduction of the bioactive/immunoreactive FSH ratio in the infertile population, and that some men may secrete immunoreactive FSH with reduced bioactivity. The determination of bioactive FSH is not available in the majority of the clinical laboratories; it is a very elaborate test and needs strict quality control to be significant. Therefore, the identification of the group of males that secrete an FSH with reduced bioactivity is still elusive to the clinician. Wang *et al.*[42] reached a similar conclusion in regard to the bio/immuno FSH ratio in infertile males. Jockenhövel *et al.*[41] also found decreased serum testosterone levels and increased levels of LH resulting in significantly reduced testosterone/LH ratios, when compared with normal fertile males. Individual patients in the different groups showed a discrepancy between bio-FSH and immuno-FSH levels.

Similar investigation done by Fauser *et al.*[43], using a different bio-FSH assay, achieved similar results, except that these authors were unable to find decreased bioactivity of FSH in oligospermia and azoospermia.

When qualitative and quantitative analyses of seminiferous epithelium are performed in testicular biopsies[44], significant reduction in the mean number of spermatids is present in patients with high gonadotropin levels; meanwhile, the mean numbers of B-spermatogonia and preleptotene spermatocytes were significantly elevated in comparison with normogonadotropic males. The authors propose that high levels of FSH produce hyperactivation of spermatogonia designed to compensate the quantitative decrease in gamete production.

Endocrine determinations

The question of the usefulness of endocrine determinations in patients with testicular dysfunction is still unanswered, and the need for stimulation (hormone load) and suppression tests in the investigation of the infertile male patient is questionable, to say the least. Tests proposed have been GnRH, thyroid-releasing hormone (TRH), adrenocorticotropic hormone (ACTH) and human chorionic gonadotropin (hCG) stimulation assays. Gerhard *et al.*[45] performed a wide variety of tests – GnRH, TRH and ACTH – in a sizeable population of 225 male members of infertile couples, and investigated E_2, thyroid-stimulating hormone (TSH), prolactin, testosterone, dehydrotestosterone, androstenedione, 17-hydroxypregnenolone, 17-hydroxyprogesterone, dehydroepiandrosterone, dehydroepiandrosterone sulfate, cortisone and 21-desoxycortisone. Basal and stimulated LH values were found to have a highly significant correlation with all routine semen parameters (concentration, motility, and morphology) with better correlation of stimulated LH values than the basal ones. Basal FSH showed an even better correlation with semen parameters. The authors suggest that basal FSH and estradiol concentration, as well as stimulated LH, testosterone and prolactin determinations should be included in the evaluation of male infertility. Similar conclusions were reached by the same group in 1992[46].

Human chorionic gonadotropin–Leydig cell stimulation test

The use of the hCG–Leydig cell stimulation test is also subject to controversy. Itoh *et al.*[47] utilized this test and the response of the testes in terms of testosterone and estradiol levels and E_2/T ratio, in human subjects with different degrees of testicular dysfunction (male infertility, aged males, Kleinfelter's syndrome, and hypogonadotrophic hypogonadism). An increase in the serum E_2/T ratio was found in subfertile males, oligozoospermia and azoospermia in comparison with normal adult males; the results were significantly lower in males with Kleinfelter's syndrome and hypogonadotropic hypogonadism. The authors conclude that, in cases of oligozoospermia characterized by an LH level of 13.7 mIU/mL or less, a sperm concentration of 5×10^6/mL or more, and an increasing rate in the serum E_2/T of 4.01 or less, the therapeutic efficacy is superior. Interestingly, Burger *et al.*[48] studied the effect of hCG treatment for 3–6 months, and then hCG combined with FSH for 1–5 months in males with hypogonadotropic hypogonadism. They noticed that hCG, with or without FSH, caused a rise in inhibin and testosterone, supporting previous observations that LH, as well as FSH, plays a role in the regulation of inhibin or inhibin-related peptides in men.

The use of these tests must be put in the context of the patient's history, physical examination and seminal findings. In the case of the azoospermic patient, the differential diagnosis includes testicular failure and ductal obstruction; testicular biopsy is the final tool for a definitive diagnosis. Proper use of physical findings (testicular size and palpatory evidence of presence or absence of epididymis and vas deferens), and the use of gonadotropins (mainly FSH) may help to avoid testicular biopsy. Patients with normal or slightly elevated FSH and at least one normal-sized testicle and vas deferens should have testicular biopsy for final diagnosis; those with clear elevation of FSH or non-palpable epididymis and/or vas have testicular failure and ductal agenesis, respectively, and testicular biopsy is not warranted[49]. In the oligo-astheno-teratozoospermic individual, the diagnostic algorithm is not that simple, and the application of similar diagnostic tools (history and physical examination, semen analysis interpretation and endocrine evaluation by basal endocrine levels, and stimulation and suppression tests) do not offer the same degree of sensitivity and specificity. A systematic elimination of sexual and/or ejaculatory dysfunctions, immunological problems, seminal plasma abnormalities, iatrogenic causes, systemic and/or environmental factors, genital anomalies, acquired testicular factors, varicocele and infection lead to the final diagnosis of idiopathic oligo-astheno-teratozoospermia[50].

The question now is, 'do we have any medical treatment for this condition?'

SYSTEMIC MEDICAL TREATMENTS AND RESULTS IN NATURAL REPRODUCTION

We will restrict the discussion to medical treatment of male infertility due to idiopathic oligo-asthenoteratozoospermia. As stated before, the lack of knowledge of the pathophysiological mechanisms involved and the fact that few endpoints are available in natural reproduction, namely sperm analysis and pregnancy, makes the evaluation of results extremely difficult.

Gonadotropin-releasing hormone (GnRH) therapy

Pulsatile administration of GnRH in the treatment of idiopathic oligo-astheno-teratozoospermia has not been widely tried. Schwarstein *et al.*, in 1978 and 1982[51,52], had already determined that that therapy showed no efficacy. Although it is successful in the treatment of hypothalamic hypogonadism, limitations due to the need for using micropumps and injections through the subcutaneous or intravenous route for several months makes compliance difficult for patients. Furthermore, the very few series published do not seem to indicate real benefit in this kind of treatment, even when an abnormal pulsatile pattern is identified. Even when elevated FSH levels were restored to normal by normal frequency of LHRH pulsatile administration, no as well as the lack of stimulation of the Sertoli-germ cell compartment, which is the main sector compromised in this population, has many clinicians favoring a combined gonadotropin protocol. Lunenfeld *et al.*[55] used a combination of hMG–hCG (75 IU i.m. daily for 90 days, and 5000 IU every 5 days for 90 days, respectively) in patients showing normal basal FSH levels, low response to acute GnRH stimulation test trying to exclude cases of primary testicular failure, low normal LH levels, and low normal T values. Response was obtained in an excellent percentage of cases (62.5–83.3%) according to the different parameters considered. Schellen and Bruinse[53] presented similar results with a slightly different therapeutic schedule (225 IU of hMG and 2000 IU of hCG twice weekly for 13 weeks). Isidori[56], using similar criteria for selection and therapeutic regimens, obtained 85% improvement in spermatogenesis and 30% pregnancies in the partners. Schill *et al.*[57] found that the endocrine parameters, including GnRH stimulation tests, were no different in responders and non-responders except for testosterone levels which, when low, indicated a favorable response. A significant improvement in count and motility was found and 50% pregnancy rate was obtained in the responder group versus 19% in the non-responder group. The authors concluded that the treatment is efficient in a small proportion of cases. Isidori *et al.*[58] and Conte *et al.*[59,60] have tried to individualize and define better criteria to select cases for this type of medical treatment. Among the central causes of male hypogonadism, they recognized an 'inadequate gonadotropin secretion', either of a quantitative or qualitative nature; within the qualitative abnormalities, pulsatile anomalies and gonadotropins of abnormal biological activity are mentioned. Causes for inefficient gonadotropin secretion are abnormalities in the neurotransmission or neuromodulation of the hypothalamic pulse generator improvement was noticed in individuals with azoospermia or severe oligozoospermia (<1 million sperm/mL) although, in isolated cases, pregnancies were obtained[5,11]. Other authors reported an increase in motile sperm density with isolated pregnancies occurring[12,13]. Furthermore, when used in combination with hCG[53], the results were unsatisfactory.

Some of the results obtained have already been described in the section on the pathophysiology of the hypothalamic–pituitary–testicular axis.

No clearcut criteria to identify the patient population prone to respond to this therapy have been established.

Mastrogiacomo *et al.*[54], working with patients having hypogonadotropic hypogonadism, hypothesized that, by using LHRH, the recovery phase goes through several stages: (1) functional recovery of Leydig cells, followed by improved function of seminal vesicles and prostate; (2) recovery of epididymal function, perhaps subsequent to tubular function improvement; (3) recovery of Sertoli cell function, which, even in this population, is more difficult.

Gonadotropin treatment

The gonadotropin treatment of the idiopathic oligo-astheno-teratozoospermia has been attempted on empirical basis with discouraging results and isolated successes. Human chorionic gonadotropin has been the commonly used agent for many years. The fact that its action is only directed toward stimulation of the Leydig cell and increase in T production, which in the majority of these cases is normal or slightly decreased; the potential for down-regulation of the hypothalamic–pituitary axis, and the failure to demonstrate a clear effect in this type of patient, from suprahypothalamic levels due to stress, toxic and pharmacological agents. Within the peripheral causes at the interstitial or tubular compartment level the authors mention receptor, Sertoli cell gap junctions, enzymatic and protein synthesis defects. Based on these hypothetical pathophysiological mechanisms, the authors recommend application of gonadotropic therapy to patients with (1) normal or low gonadotropin levels by radioimmunoassay; (2) reduced response to the GnRH test; (3) normal prolactin levels; (4) low bioactivity of LH and FSH with a low bio/immuno ratio; (5) abnormal pulsatility studies using naloxone or clomiphene tests. At the same time, peripheral abnormalities should be evaluated by biochemical, structural and immunological studies of the seminal fluid, response to the hCG test and testicular histology looking for spermatogenic arrest after the spermatocyte stage, absence of thickening of the basal membrane of the tubule, absence of vascular or inflammatory damage and absence of antitesticular or antisperm antibodies. Using these selection criteria, 26% of idiopathic oligozoospermics can be treated with gonadotropins, according to the authors' experience. The therapeutic protocol proposed is a combination of hCG (4000 IU/weekly) and hMG or pure FSH (225 IU/weekly) for 3 months. After a 2-month interval, the course can be repeated. In cases selected by this criterion, 85% showed an improvement of spermatogenesis, including the theoretical fertility potential (membrane lipooxygenase, acrosine content, lipid peroxidation, chromatin heterogeneity, swelling test, seminal LDH-X, triple staining, ATP, computerized velocimetry and sperm penetration in cervical mucus) and 37.7% spontaneous pregnancy rate was achieved.

Growth hormone

Several studies in experimental animals have shown an augmentation effect of growth hormone (GH) on the gonadotropins' action at the testicular level[61–63], as well as potentiating the effect of gonadotropins in the regulation of testicular insulin growth factor-I[64]. Receptors for GH have been identified by Sertoli and Leydig cells[63]. LH is the main gonadotropin triggering synthesis of IGF-I by the Leydig cells[65], and of their IGF-I receptors[66]. There is no definite evidence that GH plays a role in the stimulation of spermatogenesis[67]. IGF-I, on the other hand, may be an important regulator of steroidogenesis and spermatogenesis[67]. Based on these physiological findings, and on some encouraging reports on the improvement of ovarian response during gonadotropin stimulation when GH was added, the combined protocol was tried in stimulation of spermatogenesis[68,69]. The treatment was applied to males with hypogonadotropic hypogonadism who failed to respond to either LHRH or hMG plus hCG. When hGH was added (4 IU three times per week for 24 weeks), three patients increased T secretion, two produced adequate sperm and one impregnated his wife. This treatment modality needs to be applied to patients with oligo-astheno-teratozoospermia to see if improved results are obtained.

The number of series reported in the literature of idiopathic oligo-astheno-teratozoospermia treated by gonadotropins are few; they are uncontrolled series, and therefore the real value of the treatment methodology is questionable.

Anti-estrogen treatment

Clomiphene citrate therapy

The two agents most commonly used are clomiphene citrate and tamoxifen. The mechanism of action seems to be at the hypothalamic level, where they bind competitively to estrogen receptors and inhibit the negative feedback of estrogens; the final result is an increase in GnRH and secondarily of FSH and LH, which in turn improve testicular stimulation in both compartments: interstitial and tubular. Wieland *et al.*[70], in 1972, treated randomly, in an uncontrolled study, men with idiopathic oligozoospermia ($<20\times10^6$ sperm/mL) showing 'elevated levels of FSH and LH' but normal levels of testosterone using cisclomiphene; they found an increase in LH and T over control values, but an unpredictable response in semen parameters. Masala *et al.*[71] investigated the effect of the administration of 100 mg daily dose of clomiphene citrate in patients with idiopathic oligospermia and normal volunteers; a significant increase in plasma immunoreactive LHRH, gonadotropins and testosterone values were noted in both groups without significant differences in their response.

Several uncontrolled studies have found a beneficial effect of clomiphene administration to idiopathic oligo-astheno-teratozoospermic males in terms of sperm production and motility[72,73]. A review by Sorbie and Perez-Marrero[74] also indicated a possible beneficial effect; similar selection criteria to those outlined for gonadotropin treatment should be used.

Check *et al.*[75] decided to use clomiphene therapy in an empirical fashion in the male partner of couples with unexplained infertility in spite of normal semen parameters, in a randomized study using ascorbic acid treatment as control. No significant changes were found after clomiphene therapy in terms of semen parameters, but a better pregnancy rate was reported in the treated group (58% versus 16%). A similar study using a prospective randomized protocol was carried out by the Scottish Infertility Group[76] and no significant differences were found. Micic and Dotlic[77] ran a randomized study treating oligospermic males with normal or low FSH levels and infertility lasting for more than 2 years, with 50 mg clomiphene citrate for 6–9 months, and compared the results with an untreated group. Sperm density was improved in almost 30% of the treated patients and seven pregnancies were established, a significantly better result than in the untreated arm of the study in which only 7% showed improvement of semen parameters and no pregnancies occurred. Another randomized study was done by Sokol *et al.*[78], who found no significant differences in terms of semen parameters, results of sperm penetration assay and pregnancy rates between treated and placebo group.

The World Health Organization (WHO)[79] conducted a double-blind trial for the treatment of idiopathic male infertility with clomiphene citrate. This multicentric randomized double-blind study involved 190 couples with a pure male factor represented by idiopathic impairment of semen quality. Patients received 25 mg clomiphene citrate daily, or placebo for 6 months. No significant differences in treatment results between the two groups were found during the time of treatment. No useful criteria were found to help identify those patients who will respond favorably to the medication. This study concurs with the results of several other randomized series which failed to demonstrate an improvement in the pregnancy rate following this therapy.

Tamoxifen therapy

Tamoxifen has become a more common treatment for this condition, and there are many reports in the literature on its effect with results that are either inconclusive or even contradictory[80–86]. Although the main action of anti-estrogens is undoubtedly at the level of the hypothalamus, there is some evidence in the literature[87] indicating the presence of specific nuclear estradiol receptors at the testicular level, which may suggest a possible action of anti-estrogens also on the gonad. Smals *et al.*[88] have indicated that tamoxifen may suppress the gonadotropin-induced 17α-hydroxyprogesterone accumulation in normal males, leading to an improvement in the production of testosterone; other reports[89,90] indicate no testicular action of these medications.

Damber *et al.*[91] studied the effect of tamoxifen adminstered to 17 male patients (20 mg/day for 6 to 9 months) and investigated the response of LH, FSH, progesterone, 17α-hydroxyprogesterone, testosterone, estradiol-17β, prolactin and serum hormone binding globulin (SHBG); furthermore, an hCG stimulation test was performed before treatment and after one month of therapy. During treatment, serum concentrations of LH, FSH, progesterone, 17α-hydroxyprogesterone, testosterone and estradiol-17β increased. No changes were found in the response to hCG stimulation test, and the sperm density, motility and morphology improved. Sterzik *et al.*[84] evaluated 29 men with idiopathic oligozoospermia including the results of hamster ova penetration assay, and the hypo-osmotic swelling test as tests of sperm function. The same dose of tamoxifen was used for 3 months, and the endocrine evaluation included LH, FSH, testosterone, estradiol and prolactin. Significant increases of LH, FSH, testosterone and estradiol were noticed. Prolactin was not modified. No significant improvement in conventional semen parameters, hamster oocyte penetration assay, or hypo-osmotic swelling test was found. Krause *et al.*[82] published a placebo-controlled randomized study of 76 men with sperm counts of $2–20 \times 10^6$ sperm/mL, sperm motility between 20% and 50% and sperm morphology between 50% and 80% abnormal forms. Patients with varicocele, testicular maldescent or genital infections were excluded. Thirty-nine patients were in the tamoxifen arm, and 37 patients in the placebo arm of the study. Only testosterone levels increased significantly. FSH showed a slight increase without statistical significance, and LH showed no differences between groups. The increase in sperm count was not significant. There was no modification of motile and abnormal sperm forms; in five patients in the tamoxifen-treated group and in three of the placebo group, a conception in the female partner was recorded within 9 months of treatment. It is difficult to understand in this study why the authors persisted in the administration of tamoxifen at the same dose, when almost no modifications were found in FSH and LH. In a follow-up study on the fertility of these couples[89], they confirmed the previous results.

Breznik and Borko[92] followed 69 oligozoospermic males for a 4-year period (27 had no treatment, 22 took tamoxifen and 20 had clomiphene treatment). The pregnancy rate was no different in the treated and untreated groups.

Ain Melk *et al.*[93] did a prospective, randomized, double-blind study with crossover using tamoxifen (20 mg a day) and placebo for 6 months in 16 infertile men with idiopathic oligozoospermia. A significant increase in plasma FSH, LH, E_2 and T with no modifications of PRL and TSH levels, LHRH stimulation test and SPA, as well as semen analysis, showed no differences.

O'Donovan *et al.*[94], in a very recent meta-analysis of published randomized controlled trials, found a suggestion that anti-estrogen treatment works. Few side-effects in the male using the doses described previously have been reported[95].

The controversy over tamoxifen treatment continues, and unless clearcut guidelines, criteria for patient selection and well-designed protocols are put in place, we will be unable to establish the real efficiency of this treatment.

Kallikrein treatment

The kallikrein–kinin system involves a precursor, kininogen, and a final effector, kinin, with two enzymic systems triggering conversions: kininogenases (kallikreins) and kininases. Kallikrein stimulates the release of the kinins, which will be degraded by kininases in a short time. The doses of kallikrein administered vary, but they are around 600 kU daily for 3 months. Berzin *et al.*[96] investigated the effect of kallikrein on endogenous sperm ATP content, calcium and magnesium levels, and on routine semen parameters. Twenty-five males with a history of infertility, lasting 1–14 years (mean 5.2 years) were included in the study after ruling out varicoceles and genitourinary infections. The authors defined improvement as a two-fold increase in sperm count and/or >8% increase in normal morphology and/or >15% increase in motility, and >20% improvement in viability. Thirteen patients improved under treatment (four in terms of morphology, two in motility results and five in viability figures). ATP levels dropped significantly in the whole group and in the group of responders, but did not change in the group of non-responders. Calcium and magnesium levels did not change. The authors ascribe the drop in ATP levels to greater ATP utilization, and suggest that initial high levels of ATP in spermatozoa may be useful as a predictor of response to kallikrein.

Hofmann *et al.*[97], using the same dose of kallikrein in 70 subfertile males, observed an increase in the count.

Izzo *et al.*[98] performed a placebo-controlled double-blind trial on kallikrein effect in patients with oligo-asthenozoospermia using the same dose of kaillikrein as previously mentioned. Semen volume and mean sperm motility increased significantly. The sperm concentration also increased but was not statistically significant, and a true increase in the percentage of morphologically normal spermatozoa was found in the treated group. No changes were observed in the placebo-controlled group. An endocrine panel (FSH, LH, testosterone, prolactin, T3 and T4) showed no changes in either group.

Three conceptions occurred in the treated group (two during treatment and one thereafter), with no pregnancies in the control group. Micic[99] used a randomized protocol in 120 men with oligoasthenozoospermia and genital infections who were treated with antibiotics for 8–12 weeks, and 64 of them received kallikrein for 3 months. A significant improvement in count, motility and morphology was observed in both groups, but the improvement in motility and morphology was significantly higher in the kallikrein-treated group; the pregnancy rate was also higher in this group. In a second study, Micic *et al.*[100] presented a randomized control series that showed significant improvement in motility and morphology after treatment. O'Donovan *et al.*[94], using a meta-analysis, found a possible significant beneficial effect of the treatment.

Haidl and Schill[101] studied the structure of the sperm midpieces and tails before and after kallikrein treatment in 60 andrologic patients with significant improvement in sperm motility after therapy. A decrease in tail abnormalities characteristic of epididymal dysfunctions was observed.

Keck *et al.*[102] published a double-blind randomized, placebo-controlled trial and were unable to demonstrate any beneficial effect of kallikrein in conventional semen parameters, computerized analysis and pregnancy rates.

A combination of tamoxifen and kallikrein treatment was reported by Maier and Hienert[103]. In an earlier study, the authors[104] confirmed previous results that the main action of tamoxifen on sperm parameters was on concentration with very little, if any, improvement in motility and morphology. Therefore, they decided to study a group of 67 patients with a combination of tamoxifen (main action on sperm density) and kallikrein (main action on motility) to determine whether the combination of agents improved these two sperm parameters. Patients were selected because of a count <20 million and a 2-h motility test of <50%, independent of the morphology studies and the sperm swelling test. Patients with other genital pathology were excluded and the endocrine profile (FSH, LH, prolactin, testosterone and estradiol) had to be normal. Patients had an average duration of infertility of 2.4 years. One group of patients was treated with 30 mg/day of tamoxifen alone (33 cases) and a second group had a similar treatment with the addition of 600 KU/daily (34 patients). Both groups showed a significant increase in sperm density after 3 months. The group treated with a combination protocol also showed significant improvement of sperm motility. Sperm morphology and sperm swelling tests were not affected substantially. Four pregnancies occurred in each group during the period of observation (12 weeks). The effect is expressed mainly in patients with an initial density of >10 million/mL.

Gerhard *et al.*[105] studied the effect of kallikrein added to semen in an AIH program. No improvement in pregnancy rates were observed and the kallikrein added specimens showed an improved initial motility in half of the patients, but after 2 h a capillary tube test showed earlier deterioration of motility in those samples. The authors concluded that addition of kallikrein to semen seems to be unnecessary for AIH.

Androgen treatment

Androgen therapy has used testosterone (suppositories, transdermal administration and/or nasal route, subcutaneous implants of pellets or capsules and injectables, using esters: propionate, enanthate, cypionate) and oral compounds: methyltestosterone, mesterolone, fluoxymesterone. In theory, it could also be given by intratesticular injections or implants. It is extremely difficult to reach high intratesticular concentrations of testosterone by any one of these routes and therefore, if the Leydig cell compartment is valid, therapy with hCG is much more efficient. Hepatotoxicity has been demonstrated in some derivatives, such as methyltestosterone or fluoxymesterone. An exception is a DHT derivative, mesterolone, which is able to reach high concentrations within the seminiferous tubules and therefore has been proposed for the treatment of oligo-astheno-teratozoospermia. Another orally active derivative is testosterone undecanoate.

Androgen therapy can be used in high doses to suppress tubular testicular function and obtain temporary oligozoospermia, or even azoospermia, allowing function to *rebound* after treatment is stopped. Real efficacy of this therapy has not been proven, and in some cases rebound does not occur and the patient continues with severe oligozoospermia after treatment is stopped. High-dose androgen therapy is also accompanied by side-effects. Low-dose androgen treatment has not demonstrated significant benefits and therefore is not used for cases of idiopathic oligo-astheno-teratozoospermia.

Testosterone undecanoate effects have been studied by Gregoriou *et al.*[106] within a placebo-controlled design. A significant increase in DHT levels, a marginal improvement in sperm morphology, a significant decrease in FSH values and a non-significant reduction in LH values were demonstrated. Four pregnancies were obtained in the treatment arm and none in the placebo group. The authors concluded that there was a demonstrable positive effect. Pusch[107] studied 30 patients with normogonadotropic oligospermia and 30 with sperm densities between 40 and 210×10^6 sperm/mL using 120 mg T undecanoate per os for 100 days in a double-blind placebo-controlled trial. Significant improvements were found in the treated group as far as sperm morphology was concerned (head and tail malformations) as well as sperm density; motility was unchanged. No differences in pregnancies were noted. Comhaire[108], in a double-blind study, used high dose (240 mg/day) T undecanoate and found increased concentrations of dihydrotestosterone and the DHT/T ratio in peripheral blood, suppression of LH levels and a tendency to decreased FSH concentrations. Unfortunately, he concluded that the medication was not effective in the treatment of males with idiopathic testicular failure.

Dehydrotestosterone, another possible therapeutic agent, can be administered transdermally, orally, or parenterally in cases of male infertility. Gerris *et al.*[109] investigated the effect of mesterolone in 52 patients with this problem during a 12-month period (150 mg/day) in a placebo-controlled protocol. Mesterolone is a terminal DHT derivative that is not converted to estrogens, does not have hepatotoxicity and does not affect FSH and LH levels. Mesterolone seemed to be a good candidate for androgen treatment. In this study, no effect on fertility of men with idiopathic testicular failure was demonstrated. The Scottish Infertility Group[110] published a prospective randomized trial of 9 months' treatment with mesterolone or vitamin C in 368 males of an infertile marriage. No differences in the pregnancy rates were found between groups, even when only males with low–normal T and low sperm density were considered. The World Health Organization (WHO)[111] did another prospective randomized double-blind study in males with primary idiopathic testicular failure or idiopathic low sperm motility. The study was considered unsatisfactory because of low statistical power; a doubtful improvement in pregnancy rate was seen and a new study was initiated to try to clarify the issue. O'Donovan *et al.*[94] used meta-analysis to evaluate the available trials and found no differences between treatment and control groups.

Aromatase inhibitors

This medication has been used on the assumption that inhibiting testicular estradiol production, which can be detrimental to the germinal epithelium[27,28,112] is beneficial, and that excess estrogens can decrease testosterone biosynthesis by inhibiting steroidogenic enzymes[113]. Since the original publication of Vigersky and Glass[114], several other uncontrolled studies have been published indicating a possible benefit of this medication.

Clark and Sherins[115], in a well designed double-blinded, randomized, placebo-controlled trial with cross-over, showed no changes in E_2 and T concentrations and a 15–20% increase in LH and FSH on drug therapy. SHBG was decreased by 30% and free testosterone was significantly increased by 36%. Mean concentration of 17-hydroxyprogesterone was elevated by about 90% and prolactin concentrations were unchanged. Total sperm counts, sperm density, motility, morphology and testicular size showed no consistent changes. None of the wives became pregnant during the study. Therefore, the theoretical advantages of this treatment have not been demonstrated in the clinical work.

Folinic acid

This treatment has been recently proposed by an Italian group as a possible therapeutic approach to the 'round cell idiopathic syndrome'[116]. In a dose of 15 mg a day for 3 months, it has been implicated in improving pregnancy rates, sperm density, motility and number of round cells that are reduced with an increase in spermatozoa/round cell ratio. This isolated report has not used an adequate protocol to prove its point.

SYSTEMIC MEDICAL TREATMENTS AND RESULTS IN ASSISTED REPRODUCTION

With this dismal background of hormone therapy in idiopathic oligo-astheno-teratozoospermia, we need to approach treatment for the male factor using assisted reproduction technologies. The results reported with the use of this treatment in the male factor face a major problem, namely, the lack of a uniform definition of what constitutes a male factor when assisted reproduction technologies are utilized.

Definition and characterization of male factor in assisted reproduction

The World Health Organization (WHO), in its third edition[117], has re-stated criteria for normality that were described in the previous edition (Table 2), with a reduction in the percentage of normal forms in specimens that could be considered normal. The reason for the reduction is explained in the footnote but, nevertheless, the figure does not conform with the results obtained in the publications quoted[89]. It should be pointed out that the information tries only to establish criteria for normal semen and according to WHO interpretation, those normal values do not intend to express minimum requirements for fertilization. Therefore, the WHO criteria allow us to establish solely that the male is normal or subnormal, but do not permit us to try to predict his fertility potential. Minimal semen parameters for fertility prediction have been proposed by other groups[118]. The WHO criteria therefore allow us to divide the male population into two categories: normal and subnormal based on sperm quality. The subnormal category is the one in which the female partner should be exhaustively investigated before assigning the couple's infertility to the male factor. However, once investigation has been performed, treatment has failed and assisted reproduction is used, part of this population will behave as normal males in the *in vitro* fertilization system. These patients should not be included in the reports as male factors in assisted reproduction, because using these advanced technologies they behave as normal males.

Table 2 Normal values for basic semen analysis and optimal tests. Reproduced with permission of World Health Organization[117]

Standard tests	
volume	2.0 mL or more
pH	7.2–8.0
sperm concentration	20×10^6 spermatozoa/mL or more
total sperm count	40×10^6 spermatozoa per ejaculate or more
motility	50% or more with forward progression (categories 'a' and 'b') or 25% or more with rapid progression (category 'a') within 60 min of ejaculation
morphology	30% or more with normal forms[a]
vitality	75% or more live, i.e. excluding dye
white blood cells	Fewer than 1×10^6/mL
immunobead test	Fewer than 10% spermatozoa with adherent particles
mixed antiglobulin reaction (MAR)	Fewer than 10% spermatozoa with adherent particles
Optional tests	
α-Glucosidase (neutral)	20 mU or more per ejaculate
zinc (total)	2.4 μmol or more per ejaculate
citric acid (total)	52 μmol or more per ejaculate
acid phosphatase (total)	200 U or more per ejaculate
fructose (total)	13 μmol or more per ejaculate

[a]Although no clinical studies have been completed, experience in a number of centers suggests that the percentage of normal forms should be adjusted downwards when more strict criteria are applied. An empirical reference value is suggested to be 30% or more with normal forms

In our group, we investigated the mean total and normal fertilization rates (excluding delayed fertilization and polyspermia) and subtracted two standard deviations from it to determine what can be considered the minimum total fertilization rate, and the minimum normal fertilization rate in our normal male and female gamete populations. The figures obtained in the Norfolk program closely match the figures obtained at the Tygerberg program in South Africa (50% and 35%, respectively).

Therefore, our definition of male factor in assisted reproduction allows us to include in this category only those patients that show fertilization rates below 50% and 35%, when the preovulatory oocytes obtained from the female partner (metaphase IIs and late metaphase Is) appear normal[119].

A second threshold needs to be developed in this abnormal population to differentiate what we call a 'severe male factor in assisted reproduction': those patients that will not fertilize in the Embryology Laboratory. Norfolk criteria for this threshold include sperm density of <5 million sperm/mL, <10% motility, <4% normal forms, swim-up recovery rate below 1.5 million sperm and a hemizona assay index below 36%[120]. Most probably, these patients will not fertilize or will fertilize very poorly in the *in vitro* system and, therefore, need to be placed in a different program. Assisted fertilization using insemination by microdroplet or cytoplasmic sperm microinjection (ICSI) or empiric systemic medical treatment trying to improve sperm quality as much as possible can be attempted.

Possibilities of gonadotropin treatment for severe male factor in assisted reproduction

When a diagnosis of severe male factor in assisted reproduction is made, as previously defined, or when a previous *in vitro* fertilization attempt has demonstrated that, in spite of the presence of morphologically normal preovulatory oocytes, fertilization did not occur, the need for a solution to this serious problem arises. Assisted fertilization by using microdroplets or micromanipulation, mainly in the form of intracytoplasmic sperm injection (ICSI), seem to be ways to solve it.

On the other hand, very few efforts have been made in assisted reproduction to determine whether the use of systemic treatment can improve either the classical semen parameters quantitatively or qualitatively, or the sperm fertilizing ability in the *in vitro* system.

It is interesting to note that most patients in this category show a normal hypothalamic–pituitary–Leydig cell axis as judged by basal serum levels of LH, T and T/LH ratio, or at the very most, a subtle subclinical deficiency of the Leydig cell compartment which seems to be compensated with mild increase in the LH output, with a subsequent modification of the T/LH ratio. It has been demonstrated in the non-human primate that testosterone and FSH are necessary for quantitatively and qualitatively normal spermatogenesis.

The introduction of pure FSH (classical, ultrapure, or recombinant) allows a more direct approach to stimulation of the testicular tubular component without major disturbance of the interstitial (Leydig cell) compartment, when the latter is clearly normal by presently available tests. In Djungarian hamsters rendered hypogonadotropic by exposure to short-day photoperiods, FSH alone stimulated spermatogenesis up to the level of spermatids[121]. In a second study using the same experimental model[122], administration of FSH produced qualitatively normal spermatogenesis with sperm present in the epididymides in spite of low intratesticular T, suggesting that FSH is also able to restore spermiogenesis and spermiation. Pescosolido *et al.*[123] have proposed treatment with pure FSH in patients with idiopathic moderate oligo-asthenozoospermia, using 75 IU of FSH daily for 3 months. Patients with moderate oligo-asthenozoospermia (mean sperm concentration $20–29\times10^6$ sperm/mL before therapy) responded more favorably than those with severe ($10–19\times10^6$ sperm/mL), or even more severe sperm defects ($<9\times10^6$ sperm/mL) that did not respond. Similarly, patients with extreme asthenozoospermia (<10%) did not respond to treatment.

In theory, the use of pure FSH will certainly provide adequate endocrine stimulation to the Sertoli cell and it may enhance FSH-dependent functions, including spermatogenesis in cases in which there is deficient FSH stimulation due to abnormal gonadotropin secretion in pattern or quality, or when there is mild or partial Sertoli cell deficiency. Other FSH-dependent functions that can be improved are: production of adenosine 3′,5′-cyclic monophosphate (cAMP), most important androgen binding proteins, inhibin, ceruloplasmin, transferrin and plasminogen activator. Santiemma *et al.*[124] investigated the response of the human Sertoli cell *in vitro* to the addition of human FSH and found a three-fold increase in cAMP and also an increase in ABP. Avoiding using LH in these circumstances will prevent tampering with the hypothalamic–pituitary–Leydig cell axis and testosterone levels, and will also prevent the possibility of increasing estrogen levels which may not be favorable in early spermatogenesis[14,27,112].

With this in mind, we performed an experimental clinical trial in Norfolk[120,125] to determine the effects of pure FSH treatment on endocrine and semen parameters in patients with severe male factor in assisted reproduction, to assess the potential of this therapy to either improve the classical parameters of the semen analysis in this population, or to enhance sperm fertilizing ability in the *in vitro* system. Two groups of severe male factor patients were evaluated: (1) patients with previous failed fertilization in IVF attempts; and (2) cases fulfilling the criteria for poor or no fertilization, as previously indicated. The results obtained in this preliminary experimental clinical trial have been confirmed in studies from other centers and at the present time a cooperative, prospective, randomized analysis is being done in Europe by four groups of investigators to try to validate those results[126].

It is important to emphasize that these results are only applicable to assisted reproduction and until further validation is obtained, they should still be considered in an experimental phase.

The patients participating in this experimental clinical trial are divided into two groups: (1) patients that did not fertilize in previous attempts in the IVF system (secondary group); and (2) patients that fulfill the criteria of severe male factor in assisted reproduction previously mentioned, and therefore, were considered as having very poor chances for fertilization (primary group). An extensive evaluation in terms of comparing basal endocrine values (LH-RIA and bioassay, prolactin [PRL], E_2, T, T/LH, and E_2/T ratios) and basal semen analysis, including concentration, motility and morphology was performed in order to compare the two populations, and no significant differences were found.

The dose of pure FSH selected and used in this study was 150 IU delivered by i.m. injections three times a week for at least 3 months. Some other groups have used 225 IU and the results do not seem to be different.

The patients had a careful review of all medical records and surgical treatments, and a complete physical examination.

A battery of endocrine tests (FSH-RIA, LH-RIA, FSH bioassay and LH bioassay, PRL-RIA, T-RIA and E_2-RIA) was obtained before treatment and during the second, fourth and eighth weeks of therapy. Semen samples were obtained simultaneously with the blood samples in most patients, and in all of them before treatment was started and after its completion. Sperm analysis including sperm density, motility, mean velocity, mean linearity, motility index and total motile sperm fraction by computerized method and volume, pH and morphology estimated manually was performed. The IVF attempts followed the regular Norfolk procedure, and only preovulatory oocytes (metaphase IIs or late metaphase Is) were considered in the evaluation. Sperm concentration at insemination was routinely increased in the male factor population before and after FSH treatment from $5–10\times10^4$ sperm/mL/oocyte in 3 mL of insemination medium used when normal males were considered, to $5\times10^5–1\times10^6$ sperm/mL/oocyte. As demonstrated by our group, the increase of sperm concentration at insemination during IVF is the most efficient way to improve fertilization rate in patients with normal morphology <14% by strict criteria. When the number of sperm available was not enough to follow the protocol, the retrieved oocytes were put together in the well of a microtiter dish (0.3–1.0 mL) and inseminated with the entire number of sperm recovered after swim-up separation. Examination of the oocytes was performed 16 hours thereafter, and if two pronuclei were not visualized a new sperm sample was requested and reinsemination performed. Investigation of pronuclear formation continued and either delayed fertilization or lack of fertilization was diagnosed. If normal fertilization occurred, pre-embryos were transferred to the uterine cavity at 42–44 h after insemination, usually between the two- and four-cell stages. The research protocol and the consent forms were approved by the Institutional Review Board of the Eastern Virginia Medical School, and an Investigative New Drug (IND) application was filed with the Food and Drug Administration (FDA) for this particular use of pure FSH.

The patients were divided according to the basal FSH levels in different categories. Patients showing normal basal FSH values (5–15 mIU/mL; within three standard deviations of the mean for a control group of normal fertile donors), and patients with elevated FSH (16 mIU/mL or over). Prolactin levels did not show any significant changes. Basal E_2 levels were also similar. Basal T/LH ratios decreased as basal FSH-RIA levels increased, as an expression of

Table 3 Fertilization rates of preovulatory oocytes before and after follicle stimulating hormone (FSH) treatment

FSH status	*Group*	*No. of oocytes inseminated*	*No. of oocytes fertilized*	*Normal fertilization rate (%)*
Normal (5–15 mIU/mL)	Primary			
	after FSH Secondary	197	103	52.2
	before FSH	190	16 (9 abnormal)	3.6[a]
	after FSH	218	109	50[a]
Elevated (≥16 mIU/mL)	Primary			
	after FSH	105	52	49.5
	Secondary			
	before FSH	7	0	0
	after FSH	13	6	46
Total		533[b]	270[b]	50.6

[a]$P<0.001$; [b]secondary post-FSH and primary

Table 4 Total and term pregnancy outcome with follicle stimulating hormone (FSH) therapy (primary and secondary groups)

Basal FSH levels	*Group*	*No. of patients*	*No. of cycles*	*No. of embryo transf.*	*Total no. of preg.*	*No. of term preg.*	*Term preg. rates*
Normal (5–15 mIU/mL)	Primary	22	35	23	8	7	30% cycle 31% transf.
	Secondary	27	39	30	10	8**	20.5% cycle 27% transf.
Elevated (>15 mIU/mL)	Primary	6	14	10*	4	3**	21.4% cycle 30% transf.
	Secondary	3	4	2	—	—	(0%)
Total		58	87	63	22	18	20.6% cycle 28.5% transf.

*Donated oocytes; **1 twin pregnancy

greater LH than T increase in these patients. Nevertheless, these trends were not significantly different. Neither RIA nor bio-LH changed significantly, nor was the ratio modified. The RIA/FSH levels were significantly higher in the post-treatment group, and bioactive FSH levels increased after treatment, but the difference did not reach statistical significance. Bio-immune FSH ratios were lower than those of control. Sperm concentration, motility and morphology did not change significantly in any of the groups and subgroups previously established. Substantial change was found in the secondary treatment group in terms of fertilization rates per oocyte (Table 3), and as a direct consequence, the pregnancy rate improved dramatically in this treatment group (Table 4). The primary group had very similar fertilization and pregnancy rates (Tables 3, 4).

No significant differences in any parameter were found in the patients who became pregnant versus those who did not.

In general, one-third of the patients seemed to respond to this treatment and corrected the fertilization problem. Isolated cases that had been treated for longer periods of time have shown increasingly better results when IVF was repeated. A critical threshold seems to exist when the sperm morphology using strict criteria is below 1%. Very few patients fertilized after treatment when the proportion of normal forms was below that threshold. The minimum number of available sperm after separation that resulted in pregnancy was 700 000, so there is a minimal critical mass of sperm that needs to be present for the treatment to be effective.

The abortion rate was similar to the abortion rate of our program in patients with normal sperm. Similar results were found by Bartoov *et al.*[127] in

Israel, in 31 infertile males in whom electronmicroscopy analysis of the sperm before and after FSH treatment (percent of normally formed sperm cells, intact acrosome, karyoplasm, head shape, axoneme and tail shape) showed significant improvement of the head subcellular organelles after therapy. Nine patients (29%) exhibited positive fertility index values post-treatment, and seven of them improved the fertilization rate dramatically. Two female partners conceived spontaneously[127].

On the other hand, Pinkas *et al.*[128], using the same treatment in patients who were selected for micromanipulation, and in whom the critical mass of sperm available is certainly minimal, showed no effect of the FSH treatment, validating our conclusion that unless there is an adequate threshold of valid sperm available (critical mass), the treatment will not improve the results.

CONCLUSIONS

Evaluation of the sperm has experienced fundamental changes since the advent of assisted reproductive technologies; we understand now, for instance, that sperm function and performance can be improved without major changes in the old classical parameters.

Idiopathic oligo-astheno-teratozoospermia, that represents the majority of the cases seen in clinical practice, continues to be a puzzling problem to basic scientists and clinicians.

The attempts to study the pathophysiology of the hypothalamic–pituitary–testicular axis in these patients have not been very successful. In terms of hypothalamic–pituitary function some patients seem to have a reduced LH pulse frequency, but in other patients a normal or even an increased pulse frequency has been described. Restoration of normal pulses corrects the problem in very few patients, and the majority of the investigators believe that these alterations are secondary to testicular dysfunction and abnormal feedback mechanisms rather than being primary etiological motivators.

The possibility of abnormal gonadotropin production, mainly different isotypes with aberrations of α- or β-subunits and/or glycosylation determining subsequent deficient testicular action has been postulated.

At the testicular level, abnormalities of enzymic systems within the steroidogenic process, abnormalities of the FSH receptor and/or the androgen receptor or of post-receptor steps (mild forms of androgen insensitivity syndrome), as well as the possibility of aberrations in the intratesticular non-steroidal peptides, either those present with a known function, or those present with an unknown function, have been mentioned and considered.

Investigation of the seminal plasma components does not allow to further the understanding of the clinical picture.

Early extensive studies of peripheral blood karyotypes in the most severe degrees of this problem have shown abnormal chromosome complements in a low percentage of these patients, without clear evidence of a cause and effect relationship.

The endocrine evaluation of these patients has not made any substantial progress. The main indicator of primary testicular deficiencies, namely FSH, is elevated in only a small portion of this population. It is possible that the addition of bioactive FSH determinations may detect another small fraction, as well as identify abnormal gonadotropins; but these techniques cannot be utilized in the majority of the clinical laboratories. The stimulation and suppression tests, although theoretically useful in defining another small group of patients that may have subclinical conditions, have not been demonstrated to be of help in the majority of cases; they are costly and cumbersome and, for the most part, are unable to predict the response to treatment.

The policy to minimize the number of testicular biopsies in cases of oligo-astheno-teratozoospermia, which is still valid and used by the majority of the clinicians, should perhaps change in the future. The possibility of obtaining useful biopsies by fine-needle aspiration with minimal trauma to the testes may allow researchers to look carefully at the testicular microenvironment, mainly at the Sertoli cell/germ cell complex, to investigate the morphology and function of their components. Even if this part of the problem is clarified, the chances that we can modify the intratesticular conditions in the foreseeable future do not seem to be encouraging.

The gaps in knowledge in the two previously mentioned areas, namely the understanding of the pathophysiology and the lack of accurate tests, have put the clinicians in a very difficult position in regard to treatment. The majority of treatments proposed – pulsatile administration of GnRH, gonadotropin stimulation and anti-estrogens – are aimed at improving the quantity and quality of testicular stimulation. The majority of the trials have not been done using sound experimental designs and the number of patients treated was relatively small; therefore, the statistical power and significance are very weak; even when series are pooled and meta-analysis is used, the conclusions are still unreliable. Although gonadotropins specifically directed to stimulate the intratubular compartment have been developed, results have not changed. In the majority of these patients, the hypothalamic–pituitary–Leydig cell axis does not seem to be severely compromised, but the intratesticular testosterone concentrations have not been determined; therefore, the question remains unanswered. Furthermore, very few groups have been actively involved in the use of gonadotropins. A small group within the patients with oligo-astheno-teratozoospermia have been found to be candidates for gonadotropin treatment with only 80% of them showing improvement in some of the tests and 30% achieving spontaneous pregnancies. The attempt to add growth hormone to the gonadotropin protocols is encouraging, but has not been successful or applied to enough numbers of patients with this problem. The cost of these regimens is also of concern.

The use of anti-estrogens is perhaps the most common treatment utilized. Due to lower cost of the medication and the easy administration, it has gained popularity among clinicians, but only a small group of this entire population seems to respond to treatment. Perhaps this therapy should be used as a screening treatment to determine the group that may respond when no contraindications are found. In any event, the true nature of the therapy and the results should always be made available and clear to the patient.

The kallikrein treatment has been directed to improve the situation of patients with predominant asthenozoospermia. Here again, very few groups have worked with this medication, and it is not available in the United States. The idea of using a combination of anti-estrogens and kallikrein is theoretically attractive, but certainly needs to be applied under proper experimental design conditions to be able to answer the question of its usefulness.

Androgen therapy and aromatase inhibitors have not demonstrated efficacy.

The advent of assisted reproduction and assisted fertilization has simplified, and perhaps oversimplified, the treatment of the male factor by reducing the number and quality of sperm necessary for fertilization and pregnancy to figures that are negligible. Nevertheless, although this represents a tremendous breakthrough in solving the infertility problem, it has some negative aspects. This oversimplification may lead to an overuse of the procedure, assuming that other centers can achieve the same results obtained by the leading groups. We want to avoid this possibility. A tremendous challenge to the clinicians and scientists, therefore, is to establish clearcut thresholds to indicate the need for assisted fertilization. In borderline cases, it is still the responsibility of the clinician to give the embryologists the best quality sperm for oocyte insemination and in those cases it is justified, in my view, to try some of the simpler medical treatments to see if that goal is achievable.

The other negative consequence of the use of assisted fertilization is perhaps to diminish even further the interests of the basic scientists and the clinicians to search for the etiologic basis of oligo-astheno-teratozoospermia.

We need to be reminded that the number of centers that will achieve excellence in assisted fertilization capabilities is and will be relatively small, and therefore, 'Why?' ought to be a key question in the minds of patients, clinicians and scientists when dealing with the problem of oligo-astheno-teratozoospermia in the foreseeable future.

The need for a common language in assisted reproduction to define a male factor is another crucial issue.

If the results obtained in this field with the use of FSH are confirmed, we still have another therapy available before jumping into the less available and technologically very difficult methods of assisted fertilization. Having found a solution to the problem does not preclude the need for understanding it. If we forget this basic principle, clinicians and scientists would have lost the battle to technology.

References

1. Steinberger, E. (1986). Critical assessment of treatment results in male infertility. In Santen, R. J. and Swerdloff, R. S. (eds.) *Male Reproductive Dysfunction*, pp. 373–86. (New York: Marcel Dekker)
2. Spiteri-Grech, J. and Nieschlag, E. (1993). Paracrine factors relevant to the regulation of spermatogenesis – a review. *J. Reprod. Fertil.*, **98**, 1–14
3. Talbot, J. A., Rodger, R. S., Shalet, S. M., Littley, M. D. and Robertson, W. R. (1990). The pulsatile secretion of bioactive luteinizing hormone in normal adult men. *Acta Endocrinol. Copenh.*, **22**, 643–50
4. Veldhuis, J. D., Evans, W. S., Urban, R. J., Rogol, A. D. and Johnson, M. L. (1988). Physiologic attributes of the luteinizing hormone pulse signal in the human. Cross-validation studies in men. *J. Androl.*, **9**, 69–77
5. Matsumoto, A. M., Gross, K. M., Sheckter, C. B. and Bremmer, W. J. (1990). The luteinizing hormone-releasing hormone pulse generator in men: abnormalities and clinical management. *Am. J. Obstet. Gynecol.*, **163**, 1743–52
6. de Kretser, D. M., Berger, H. G., Fortune, D., Hudson, B., Long, A. R., Paulsen, C. A. and Taft, H. P. (1972). Hormonal, histological and chromosomal studies in adult males with testicular disorders. *J. Clin. Endocrinol. Metab.*, **35**, 392–401
7. Gross, K. M., Matsumoto, A. M., Southworth, M. B. and Bremmer, W. J. (1985). Evidence for decreased luteinizing hormone-releasing hormone pulse frequency in men with selective elevations of follicle-stimulating hormone. *J. Clin. Endocrinol. Metab.*, **60**, 197–202
8. Wagner, T. O. F., Brabant, G., Warsch, F. and von Zur Mühlen, A. (1984). Slow pulsing oligospermia. *Acta Endocrinol. Copenh.*, **264** (Suppl.), 152 (abstr.)
9. Gross, K. M., Matsumoto, A. M., Berger, R. E. and Bremmer, W. J. (1986). Increased frequency of pulsatile luteinizing hormone-releasing hormone administration selectively decreases follicle-stimulating hormone levels in men with idiopathic azoospermia. *Fertil. Steril.*, **45**, 392–6
10. Hönigl, W., Knuth, U. A. and Nieschlag, E. (1986). Selective reduction of elevated FSH levels in infertile men by pulsatile LR-RH treatment. *Clin. Endocrinol.* (Oxf.) **24**, 177–82
11. Bals-Pratsch, M., Knuth, U. A., Hönigl, W., Klein, H. M., Bergman, M. and Nieschlag, E. (1989). Pulsatile GnRH-therapy in oligozoospermic men does not improve seminal parameters despite decreased FSH levels. *Clin. Endocrinol. (Oxf.)* **30**, 549–60
12. Wagner, T. O. F. and von Zur Mühlen, A. (1987). Slow pulsing oligospermia: treatment by long time pulsatile LH-RH therapy. In Wagner, T. O. F. and Filicori, M. (eds.) *Episodic Hormone Secretion: From Basic Science to Clinical Application*, p. 197. (Hemelin, West Germany: T. M. Verlag)
13. Aulitzky, W., Frick, J. and Hadziselimovic, F. (1989). Pulsatile LH-RH therapy in patients with oligozoospermic and disturbed LH pulsatility. *Int. J. Androl.*, **12**, 265–72
14. Wu, F. C. W., Taylor, P. L. and Sellar, R. E. (1989). LH-RH pulse frequency in normal and infertile men. *J. Endocrinol.*, **123**, 149–58
15. Bennet, A., Bujan, L., Plantavid, M., Barbe, P., Caron, P. and Louvet, J. P. (1991). Luteinizing hormone pulse frequency and *in vitro* bioactivity in male idiopathic infertility. *Fertil. Steril.*, **55**, 612–18
16. Booth, J. D., Merriam, G. R., Clark, R. V., Loriaux, D. L. and Sherins, R. J. (1987). Evidence for Leydig cell dysfunction in infertile men with a selective increase in plasma follicle-stimulating hormone. *J. Clin. Endocrinol. Metab.*, **64**, 1194–204
17. Avril-Ducarne, C., Kuhn, J. M., Bastit, P., Bisson, P., Aubert, H. and Wolf, L. M. (1990). Dynamique de la sécrétion gonadotrope dans les oligospermies á FSH isolément élevée. *Presse Med.*, **19**, 1791–4
18. Simoni, M., Paschlke, R. and Nieschlag, E. (1993). A search for circulating immunoglobulins blocking follicle-stimulating hormone action in male idiopathic infertility. *Int. J. Androl.*, **16**, 129–35
19. Fredricsson, B., Carlstrom, K. and Pleon, L. (1989). Steroid metabolism and morphologic features of the human testis. *J. Androl.*, **19**, 43–9
20. Berry, S. A. and Pescovitz, O. H. (1988). Identification of a GHRH-like substance and its messenger RNA in rat testis. *Endrocrinology*, **123**, 661–3
21. Berry, S. A., Srivastava, C. H., Rubin, L. R., Phipps, W. and Pescovitz, O. H. (1992). Growth hormone releasing present in human testis and placenta. *J. Clin. Endocrinol. Metab.*, **75**, 281–4
22. Srivastava, C. H., Collard, M. W., Rothrock, J. K., Peredo, M. J., Berry, S. A., Pescovitz, O. H. (1993). Germ cell localization of a testicular growth hormone-releasing hormone-like factor. *Endocrinology*, **133**, 83–9
23. Bergmann, M., Nashan, D. and Nieschlag, E. (1989). Pattern of compartmentation in human seminiferous tubules showing dislocation of spermatogonia. *Cell Tissue Res.*, **256**, 183–90
24. Namiki, M., Koide, T., Okuyama, A., Sonoda, T., Itatani, H., Miyake, A., Aono, T., Terada, N. and Matsumoto, K. (1984). Abnormality of testicular FSH receptors in infertile men. *Acta Endocrinol.*, **106**, 548–55
25. Buch, J. P., Lipschultz, L. I. and Smith, R. G. (1991). Evidence for altered receptor-binding activity of serum follicle stimulating hormone in male infertility. *Fertil. Steril.*, **55**, 358–62
26. Bujan, L., Mieusset, R., Audran, F., Lumbroso, S.

and Sultan, C. (1993). Increased oestradiol level in seminal plasma in infertile men. *Hum. Reprod.*, **8**, 74–7

27. Franchimont, P., Millet, D., Vendrely, E., Letawe, J., Legros, J. J. and Netter, A. (1972). Relationships between spermatogenesis and serum gonadotropin level in azoospermia and oligospermia. *J. Endocrinol.*, **34**, 1003–8
28. Wu, F. C. W., Swanston, I. A. and Baird, D. T. (1982). Raised plasma oestrogens in infertile men with elevated levels of FSH. *Clin. Endrocrinol.*, **16**, 39–47
29. Scott, R. S. and Burger, H. (1981). An inverse relationship exists between seminal plasma inhibin and serum follicle-stimulating hormone in man. *J. Clin. Endocrinol. Metab.*, **52**, 796–803
30. de Kretser, D. M., McLachlan, R. I., Robertson, D. M. and Burger, H. G. (1989). Serum inhibin levels in normal men and women with testicular disorders. *J. Endocrinol.*, **120**, 517–23
31. Sheckter, C. B., McLachlan, R. I., Tenover, J. S., Matsumoto, A. M., Burger, H. G., de Kretser, D. M. and Bremmer, W. J. (1988). Stimulation of serum inhibin concentrations by gonadotropin-releasing hormone in men with idiopathic hypo-gonadotropic hypogonadism. *J. Clin. Endocrinol. Metab.*, **67**, 1221–4
32. Sueldo, C., Marrs, R. P., Berger, T., Kletsky, O. A. and O'Brien, T. J. (1984). Correlation of semen tranferrin concentration and sperm fertilizing capacity. *Am. J. Obstet. Gynecol.*, **150**, 528–30
33. Irisawa, C., Nakada, T., Kubota, Y., Sasagawa, I., Adachi, Y. and Yaguchi, H. (1993). Transferrin concentration in seminal plasma with special reference to serum hormone levels in infertile men. *Arch. Androl.*, **30**, 13–21
34. Tagaki, Y., Kumamoto, Y. and Watanabe, Y. G. (1989). Study of Sertoli cell function in male infertility: relationship between seminal plasma transferrin and seminal plasma inhibin activity. *Japan J. Fertil. Steril.*, **34**, 214–24
35. Fuse, H., Satomi, S., Okumura, M. and Katayama, T. (1992). Seminal plasma transferrin concentration: relationship with seminal parameters and plasma hormone levels. *Urol. Int.*, **49**, 158–62
36. Cek, M., Curgul, S., Ertas, M., Sozer, T. and Alpacar, Z. (1992). Seminal transferrin levels in seminal plasma of fertile and infertile men. *Urol. Int.*, **49**, 218–21
37. Papadimas, I., Papadopoulou, F., Ioannidis, S., Katsaveli, R., Tarlatzis, B., Bontis, I. and Mantalenakis, S. (1992). Seminal plasma transferrin in infertile men. *Arch. Androl.*, **28**, 125–33
38. Keltimlidis, K., Papadimas, J., Bontis, J. and Mantalenakis, S. (1989). LDH isoenzymes in semen of infertile men. *Arch. Androl.*, **22**, 77–84
39. Markert, C. L. (1963). Lactate dehydrogenase isoenzymes: Dissociation and recombination of subunits. *Science*, **140**, 1329–31
40. Noguera Velasco, J. A., Tovar Zapata, I., Martinez Hernandez, P., Perez Albacete, M., Tortosa Oltra, J. and Parrilla Patricio, J. J. (1993). Lactic dehydrogenase-C_4 activity in seminal plasma and male infertility. *Fertil. Steril.*, **60**, 331–5
41. Jockenhövel, F., Khan, S. A. and Nieschlag, E. (1989). Diagnostic value of bioactive FSH in male infertility. *Acta Endocrinol. Copenh.*, **121**, 802–10
42. Wang, C., Dahl, K. D., Leung, A., Chan, S. Y. W., Hsueh, A. J. W. (1987). Serum bioactive follicle-stimulating hormone in men with idiopathic azoospermia and oligospermia. *J. Clin. Endocrinol. Metab.*, **65**, 629–33
43. Fauser, B. C. J. M., Bogers, J. W., Hop, W. C. J. and de Jong, F. S. H. (1990). Bioactive and immunoreactive FSH in serum of normal and oligospermic men. *Clin. Endocrinol.*, **32**, 433–42
44. Kula, K. (1991). Hyperactivation of early steps of spermatogenesis compromises meiotic insufficiency in men with hypergonadotrophism. A possible quantitative assay for high FSH/low testosterone availabilities. *Andrologia*, **23**, 127–33
45. Gerhard, I., Lenhard, H. K., Eggert-Kruse, W. and Runnebaum, B. (1991). Hormone load tests in infertile male patients. *Arch. Androl.*, **27**, 129–47
46. Gerhard, I., Lenhard, H. K., Eggert-Kruse, W. and Runnebaum, B. (1992). Routine hormone load tests are unnecessary in infertile men. *Andrologia*, **24**, 219–26
47. Itoh, N., Kumamoto, Y. and Maruta, H. (1992). Studies on the production rate of estradiol in the testis in male infertility studies of the predictive values on therapeutic efficacy in patients with oligozoospermia. *Nippon Naibunpi Gakkai Zasshi*, **68**, 1276–93
48. Burger, H. G., Tiu, S. C., Bangah, M. L. and de Kretser, D. M. (1990). Human chorionic gonadotrophin raises serum immunoreactive inhibin levels in men with hypogonadotrophic hypogonadism. *Reprod. Fertil. Dev.*, **2**, 137–44
49. Jarow, J. P., Espeland, M. A. and Lipshultz, L. I. (1989). Evaluation of the azoospermic patient. *J. Urol.*, **142**, 62–5
50. Comhaire, F. H. (1992). An approach to the management of male infertility. *Baillière's Clin. Endocrinol. Metab.*, **6**, 435–50
51. Schwarzstein, L., Aparicio, N. J. and Schally, A. V. (1982). D-tryptophan-6-luteinizing hormone-releasing hormone in the treatment of normogonadotropic oligoastheno-zoospermia. *Int. J. Androl.*, **5**, 171–8
52. Schwarzstein, L., Aparicio, N. J., Turner, D., De Turner, E. A., Premoli, F. and Schally, A. V. (1978). D-Leucine-6-luteinizing hormone-releasing hormone ethylamide in the treatment of normogonadotropic oligoasthenospermia. *Fertil. Steril.*, **29**, 332–5
53. Schellen, T. M. C. M. and Bruinse, H. W. (1980). Evaluation of the treatment with gonadotropic hormones in cases of severe and moderate oligozoospermia. *Andrologia*, **12**, 174–8
54. Mastrogiacomo, I., Motta, R. G., Botteon, S., Bonanni, G. and Schiesaro, M. (1991). Achievement

of spermatogenesis and genital tract maturation in hypogonadotropic hypogonadic subjects during long-term treatment with gonadotropins or LHRH. *Andrologia*, **23**, 285–9

55. Lunenfeld, B., Olchovsky, D., Tadir, Y. and Glezerman, M. (1979). Treatment of male infertility with human gonadotrophins: selection of cases, management and results. *Andrologia*, **11**, 331–6
56. Isidori, A. (1990). Gonadotropin therapy in the male. In Matson, J. and Lieberman, B. A. (eds.) *Clinical IVF Forum*, pp. 140–50. (Manchester: Manchester University Press)
57. Schill, W.-B., Jüngst, D., Unterburger, P. and Braun, S. (1982). Combined hMG/hCG treatment in subfertile men with idiopathic normogonadotrophic oligozoospermia. *Int. J. Androl.*, **5**, 467–77
58. Isidori, A. (1981). A modern approach to the gonadotropin treatment in oligozoospermia. *Andrologia*, **13**, 187–97
59. Conte, D., Nordio, M., Romanelli, F. and Isidori, A. (1991). Hormonal treatment of the infertile male. *Clin. Adv. Androl.*, **1**, 1–11
60. Conte, D., Romanelli, F. and Isidori, A. (1990). Terapia con gonadotropine della sterilità maschile idiopatica. *Minerva Endocrinol.*, **15**, 91–4
61. Chandrashekar, V., Bartke, A. and Wagner, T. E. (1988). Endogenous human growth hormone (GH) modulates the effect of gonadotropin-releasing hormone on pituitary function and the gonadotropin response to the negative feedback effect of testosterone in adult male transgenic mice bearing the human GH gene. *Endocrinology*, **123**, 2717–22
62. Closset, J., Dombrowica, D., Vandenbroeck, M. and Henne, G. (1991). Effect of bovine, human and rat growth hormones on immature hypophysectomized rat testis. *Growth Regul.*, **1**, 29–37
63. Lobie, P. E., Breipohl, W., Garcia Aragon, J. and Waters, M. J. (1990). Cellular localization of the growth hormone receptor/binding protein in the male and female reproductive systems. *Endocrinology*, **126**, 2214–21
64. Spiteri-Grech, J., Bartlett, J. M. and Nieschlag, E. (1991). Regulation of testicular insulin-like growth factor I in pubertal growth hormone-deficient male rats. *J. Endocrinol.*, **131**, 279–85
65. Naville, D., Chatelain, P. G., Avallet, O. and Saez, J. M. (1990). Control of production of insulin-like growth factor-I by pig Leydig and Sertoli cells cultured alone or together. Cell–cell interactions. *Mol. Cell Endocrinol.*, **70**, 217–24
66. Nagpal, M. L., Wang, D., Calkins, J. H., Chang, W. and Lin, T. (1991). Human chorionic gonadotropin up-regulates insulin-like growth factor-I receptor gene expression of Leydig cells. *Endocrinology*, **129**, 2820–6
67. Spiteri-Grech, J. and Nieschlag, E. (1992). The role of growth hormone and insulin-like growth Factor I in the regulation of male reproductive function. *Hormone Res.*, **38** (suppl. 1), 22–7
68. Jacobs, H. S., Bouchard, P., Conway, G. S., Homburg, R., Lahlou, N., Mason, B., Ostergaard, H., Owen, E. J. and Shoham, Z. (1991). Role of growth hormone in infertility. *Hormone Res.*, **36** (suppl.), 61–5
69. Shoham, Z., Conway, G. S., Ostergaard, H., Lahlou, N., Bouchard, P. and Jacobs, H. S. (1992). Cotreatment with growth hormone for induction of spermatogenesis in patients with hypo-gonadotropic hypogonadism. *Fertil. Steril.*, **57**, 1044–51
70. Wieland, R. G., Ansari, A. H., Klein, D. E., Doshi, N. S., Hallberg, M. C. and Chen, J. C. (1972). Idiopathic oligospermia: control observations and response to cisclomiphene. *Fertil. Steril.*, **23**, 471–4
71. Masala, A., Delitala, G., Alagna, S., Devilla, L. and Lotti, G. (1978). Effect of clomiphene citrate on plasma levels of immunoreactive luteinizing hormone-releasing hormone, gonadotropin, and testosterone in normal subjects and in patients with idiopathic oligospermia. *Fertil. Steril.*, **29**, 424–7
72. Jones, T. M., Fang, V. S., Rosenfeld, R. L. and Schoenberg, H. W. (1980). Parameters of response to clomiphene citrate in oligospermic men. *J. Urol.*, **124**, 53–5
73. Rönnberg, L. (1980). The effect of clomiphene citrate on different sperm parameters in men with idiopathic oligozoospermia. *Andrologia*, **12**, 261–5
74. Sorbie, P. J. and Perez-Marrero, R. The use of clomiphene citrate in male infertility. *J. Urol.*, **131**, 425–9
75. Check, J. H., Chase, J. S., Nowroozi, K., Wu, C. H. and Adelson, H. G. (1989). Empirical therapy of the male with clomiphene in couples with unexplained infertility. *Int. J. Fertil.*, **34**, 120–2
76. Scottish Infertility Group: Abel, B. J., Carswell, G., Elton, R., Hargreave, T. B., Kyle, K., Orr, S., Rogers, A., Baxby, K. and Yates, A. (1982). Randomized trial of clomiphene citrate treatment and vitamin C for male infertility. *Br. J. Urol.*, **54**, 780–4
77. Micic, S. and Dotlic, R. (1985). Evaluation of sperm parameters in clinical trial with clomiphene citrate of oligospermic men. *J. Urol.*, **133**, 221–2
78. Sokol, R., Steiner, B., Bustillo, M., Petersen, G. and Swerdloff, R. (1988). A controlled comparison of the efficacy of clomiphene citrate in male infertility. *Fertil. Steril.*, **49**, 865–70
79. World Health Organization. (1992). A double-blind trial of clomiphene citrate for the treatment of idiopathic male infertility. *Int. J. Androl.*, **15**, 299–307
80. Comhaire, F. (1976). Treatment of oligospermia with tamoxifen. *Int. J. Fertil.*, **21**, 232–8
81. Fauser, B. C. J. M., Dony, J. M. J., Doesburg, W. H. Thomas, C. M. G. and Rolland, R. (1984). Short- and long-term hormonal effects of a single dose of 50 mg tamoxifen administered to normal males. *Andrologia*, **16**, 465–70
82. Krause, W., Holland-Moritz, H. and Schramm, P.

(1992). Treatment of idiopathic oligozoospermia with tamoxifen – a randomized controlled study. *Int. J. Androl.*, **15**, 14–18
83. Schill, W. B. and Landthaler, M. (1980). Tamoxifen treatment of oligozoospermia. *Andrologia*, **12**, 546–8
84. Sterzik, K., Rosenbusch, B., Grab, D., Heyden, M., Lichtenberger, K. and Wolf, A. (1991). Die behandlung der oligozoospermie mit tamoxifen führt zu keiner verbessenrung der spermienqualität. *Zentbl. Gynäkol.*, **113**, 683–8
85. van Bergeijk, L., Gooren, L.J. G., van der Veen, E. A. and de Vries, C. P. (1985). Effects of short- and long-term administration of tamoxifen on hCG-induced testicular steroidogenesis in man: no evidence for an oestradiol-induced steroidogenic lesion. *Int. J. Androl.*, **8**, 28–36
86. Willis, K. J., London, D. R., Bevis, M. A., Butt, W. R., Lynch, S. S. and Holder, G. (1977). Hormonal effects of tamoxifen in oligospermic men. *J. Endocrinol.*, **73**, 171–8
87. Murphy, J. B., Emmot, R. C., Hicks, L. L. and Walsh, P. C. (1980). Estrogen receptors in the human prostate, seminal vesicle, epididymis, testis and genital skin: a marker for estrogen-responsive tissues? *J. Clin. Endocrinol. Metab.*, **50**, 938–48
88. Smals, A. G. H., Pieters, G. F. F. M., Drayer, J. I. M., Boers, G. H. J., Benraad, T. J. and Kloppenborg, P. W. C. (1980). Tamoxifen suppresses gonadotropin-induced 17-alpha-hydroxyprogesterone accumulation in normal men. *J. Clin. Endocrinol. Metab.*, **51**, 1026–9
89. Krause, W., Hübner, H. M. and Wichmann, U. (1985). Treatment of oligozoospermia by tamoxifen: no evidence for direct testicular action. *Andrologia*, **17**, 285–90
90. Sterzik, K., Rosenbusch, B., Mogck, J., Heyden, M. and Lichenberger, K. (1993). Tamoxifen treatment of oligozoospermia: a re-evaluation of its effects including additional sperm function tests. *Arch. Gynecol. Obstet.*, **252**, 143–7
91. Damber, J.-E., Abramsson, L. and Duchek, M. (1989). Tamoxifen treatment of idiopathic oligozoospermia: effect of hCG-induced steroidogenesis and semen variables. *Scand. J. Urol. Nephrol.*, **23**, 241–6
92. Breznik, R. and Borko, E. (1993). Effectiveness of anti-estrogens in infertile men. *Arch. Androl.*, **31**, 43–8
93. Ain Melk, Y., Belisle, S., Carmel, M. and Tetreault, J.-P. (1987). Tamoxifen citrate therapy in male infertility. *Fertil. Steril.*, **48**, 113–17
94. O'Donovan, P. A., Vandekerckhove, P., Lilford, R. J. and Hughes, E. (1993). Treatment of male infertility: is it effective? Review and meta-analysis of published randomized controlled trials. *Hum. Reprod.*, **8**, 1209–22
95. Gerner, E. W. (1989). Ocular toxicity of tamoxifen. *Ann. Ophthalmol.* **21**, 420–3
96. Berzin, M., Bilgeri, Y. R., Zanzinger, A., Wing, J., Kalk, W. J. and Mendelsohn, D. (1987). The effect of kallikrein on spermatozoal ATP and other semen parameters. *Andrologia*, **19**, 273–7
97. Hofmann, N., Schöenberger, A. and Gall, H. (1975). Untersuchungen zur kallikrein-behandlung männlicher fertilität-sstörungen. *Ze Hautkr.*, **50**, 1003–12
98. Izzo, P. L., Canale, D., Bianchi, B., Meschini, P., Esposito, G., Menchini Fabris, G. F., Fasani, R. and Ohnmeiss, H. (1984). The treatment of male subfertility with kallikrein. *Andrologia*, **16**, 156–61
99. Micic, S. (1988). Kallikrein and antibiotics in the treatment of infertile men with genital tract infections. *Andrologia*, **20**, 55–9
100. Micic, S., Tolić, C. and Dotlić, R. (1990). Kallikrein therapy of infertile men with varicocele and impaired sperm motility. *Andrologia*, **22**, 179–83
101. Haidl, G. and Schill, W. B. (1993). Changes of sperm tail morphology after kallikrein treatment. *Arch. Androl.*, **31**, 1–8
102. Keck, C., Behreh, M., Jockenhövel, F. and Nieschlag, E. (1994). Ineffectiveness of kallikrein in treatment of idiopathic male infertility: a double-blind, randomized, placebo-controlled trial. *Hum. Reprod.*, **9**, 325–9
103. Maier, U. and Hienert, G. (1990). Tamoxifen and kallikrein in therapy of oligoastheno zoospermia: results of a randomized study. *Eur. Urol.*, **17**, 223–5
104. Maier, U., Kratzik, C. and Spona, J. (1985). Tamoxifen in der behandlung der oligozoospermie. Ergebnisse bei 200 sufertilen männern. *Annual Meeting of the Austrian Society for Sterility and Fertility*, Vienna
105. Gerhard, I., Roth, B., Eggert-Kruse, W. and Runnenbaum, B. (1990). Effects of kallikrein on sperm motility, capillary tube test and pregnancy rate on an AIH program. *Arch. Androl.*, **24**, 129–45
106. Gregoriou, O., Papadias, C., Gargaropoulos, A., Konidaris, S., Kontogeorgi, Z. and Kalampokas, E. (1993). Treatment of idiopathic infertility with testosterone undecanoate. A double blind study. *Clin. Exp. Obstet. Gynecol.*, **20**, 9–12
107. Pusch, H. H. (1989). Oral treatment of oligozoospermia with testosterone–undecanoate: Results of a double-blind placebo-controlled trial. *Andrologia*, **21**, 76–82
108. Comhaire, F. (1990). Treatment of idiopathic testicular failure with high-dose testosterone undecanoate: a double-blind pilot study. *Fertil. Steril.* **54**, 689–93
109. Gerris, J., Comhaire, F., Hellemans, P., Peeters, K. and Schoonjans, F. (1991). Placebo-controlled trial of high-dose mesterolone treatment of idiopathic male infertility. *Fertil. Steril.*, **55**, 603–7
110. Scottish Infertility Group: Hargreave, T. B., Kyle, K. F., Baxby, K., Rogers, A. C. N., Scott, R., Tolley, D. A., Abel, B. J., Orr, P. S. and Elton, R. A. (1984). Randomized trial of mesterolone versus vitamin C for male infertility. *Br. J. Urol.*, 740–4
111. World Health Organization Task Force on the

Diagnosis and Treatment of Infertility. (1989). Mesterolone and idiopathic male infertility: a double-blind study. *Int. J. Androl.*, **12**, 254–64

112. Ciaccio, L. A., Joseph, A. A. and Kinel, F. A. (1978). Direct inhibition of testicular function in rats by estriol and progesterone. *J. Steroid Biochem.*, **9**, 1257–9
113. Onoda, M. and Hall, P. F. (1981). Inhibition of testicular microsomal cytochrome P-450 (17α-hydroxylase/C-17, 20-lyase) by estrogens. *Endocrinology*, **109**, 763–7
114. Vigersky, R. A. and Glass, A. R. (1981). Effects of testolactone on the pituitary–testicular axis in oligozoospermic men. *J. Clin. Endocrinol. Metab.*, **52**, 897–902
115. Clark, R. V., Sherins, R. J. (1989). Treatment of men with idiopathic oligozoospermic infertility using the aromatase inhibitor, testolactone results of a double-blinded, randomized, placebo-controlled trial with crossover. *J. Androl.*, **10**, 240–7
116. Bentivoglio, G., Melica, F. and Critoforoni, P. (1993). Folinic acid in the treatment of human male infertility. *Fertil. Steril.*, **60**, 698–701
117. World Health Organization. (1992). *WHO Laboratory Manual for the Examination of Human Semen and Sperm–Cervical Mucus Interaction*, 3rd edn., pp. 43–4. (Cambridge: Cambridge University Press)
118. Van Zyl, J. A., Menkveld, R., Kotze, T. J. W. and Van Nickerk, J. A. (1976). *Proceedings of the 17th International Urology Congress, Johannesburg*, 25–30 July. Diffusion Doin, Paris, **2**, 263–71
119. Acosta, A. A. (1992). Male factor in assisted reproduction. *Infertil. Reprod. Med. Clin. North Am.*, **3**, 487–503
120. Acosta, A. A., Oehninger, S., Ertunc, H. and Philput, C. (1991). Possible role of pure human follicle-stimulating hormone in the treatment of severe male-factor infertility by assisted reproduction: preliminary report. *Fertil. Steril.*, **55**, 1150–6
121. Niklowitz, P., Khan, S., Bergmann, M., Hoffman, K. and Nieschlag, E. (1989). Differential effects of follicle-stimulating hormone and luteinizing hormone on Leydig cell function and restoration of spermatogenesis in hypophysectomized and photoinhibited Djungarian hamsters (*Phodopus sungorus*). *Biol. Reprod.*, **41**, 871–80
122. Lerchl, A., Sotiriadou, S., Behre, H. M., Pierce, J., Weinbauer, G. F., Kliesh, S. and Nieschlag, E. (1993). Restoration of spermatogenesis by follicle-stimulating hormone despite intratesticular testosterone in photoinhibited hypogonadotropic Djungarian Hamsters (*Phodopus sungorus*). *Biol. Reprod.*, **49**, 1108–16
123. Pescosolido, D., Curatola, A., Gentili, S., Magiera, M. G. and Decio, R. (1985). A new gonadotropin treatment for idiopathic moderate oligoasthenospermia. *Acta Eur. Fertil.*, **16**, 129–32
124. Santiemma, V., Rosati, P., Guerzoni, C., Mariani, S., Beligotti, F., Magnanti, M., Garufa, G., Galoni, T. and Fabbrini, A. (1992). Human Sertoli cells *in vitro*: morphological features and androgen-binding protein secretion. *J. Steroid Biochem. Mol. Biol.*, **43**, 523–9
125. Acosta, A. A., Khalifa, E. and Oehninger, S. (1992). Pure human follicle-stimulating hormone has a role in the treatment of severe male infertility by assisted reproduction. Norfolk's total experience. *Hum. Reprod.*, **7**, 1067–72
126. Baker, G., Brinsden, P., Jouannet, P., Loumaye, E., Van Steirteghem, A. and Winston, R. (1993). Treatment of severe male infertility with pure follicle-stimulating hormone (FSH): the need for a properly controlled multi-center trial. *Hum. Reprod.*, **8**, 500–1
127. Bartoov, B., Lunenfeld, B., Eltes, F., Lederman, H. and Lunenfeld, E. (1993). Sperm quality of subfertile male before and after Metrodin treatment. (Abstr.) *Annual Meeting of the Israeli Fertility Association*, 21–22 April
128. Pinkas, H., Amit, S., Rufas, O., Stein, A., Ovadia, J. and Fisch, B. (1993). FSH treatment of infertile men: its effect on fertilization rate in micromanipulation. (Abstr.). *Annual Meeting of the Israeli Fertility Association*, 21–22 April

Sperm collection for assisted reproduction in ejaculatory dysfunction

34

D. A. Ohl and J. Sønksen

INTRODUCTION

Assisted reproduction in cases of ejaculatory dysfunction has been receiving a great deal of attention in the last several years. This is not because ejaculatory dysfunction is a prevalent etiology of male infertility. Indeed, only 2% of men presenting for male infertility in one large series suffered ejaculatory dysfunction as a cause of their subfertility[1]. Rather, the recent excitement is because of development, study and improvement of techniques which allow induction of ejaculation and initiation of pregnancies by men who previously had no other treatment options.

In this chapter we will review the normal physiology of ejaculation and discuss pathophysiological conditions in which ejaculatory dysfunction represents the major cause of inability to conceive. We will then discuss historical and current methods to retrieve sperm from men with anejaculation and review recent results from these procedures.

OVERVIEW OF NORMAL EJACULATORY FUNCTION

The ejaculatory reflex is a complex set of events culminating in projectile expulsion of semen from the urethra. There are several neurophysiologic components of this reflex[2].

There are two major afferent stimuli for the ejaculatory reflex. One is from tactile stimulation of the genitals. Manipulation of the penis during sexual intercourse or masturbation results in neural transmission into the sacral spinal cord via the dorsal nerves of the penis. The tranmissions travel cephalad to the ejaculatory center in the thoracolumbar cord. Conditions which impair sensory afferents in this area may cause delayed or absent ejaculation. Under certain circumstances (e.g. penile vibratory stimulation), genital afferent stimulation alone is sufficient to initiate an ejaculatory reflex without input from higher neural centers.

The second, and more poorly understood, input into the ejaculatory reflex is that arising from the cerebral cortex. Visual, psychogenic and possibly sleep-related erotic stimuli are processed here and sent through descending pathways to the thoracolumbar spinal cord where they are co-ordinated with input from the genital afferents in initiating the reflex response. In certain instances (e.g. nocturnal emission), the higher centers are capable of initiating the ejaculatory reflex without input from the genitals.

The ejaculatory reflex is co-ordinated at the thoracolumbar cord. Sympathetic efferents arise from spinal levels T11–L2. The fibers course into the sympathetic chain ganglia and then merge into the inferior mesenteric/hypogastric plexus. Input from both sympathetic chains contributes to the plexus. The hypogastric nerves carry the neural impulses into the pelvis toward the ejaculatory organs where they synapse to short adrenergic neurons near or in the wall of these structures. In the pelvis, the sympathetic and parasympathetic fibers travel in close anatomic proximity. However, they remain functionally different, as demonstrated by the fact that penile erectile function (parasympathetic) and ejaculatory function (sympathetic) may suffer different degrees of functional impairment.

The ejaculatory organs are the epididymis, vas deferens, seminal vesicles, prostate and the bladder neck/internal urinary sphincter. In response to sexual stimulation, sperm is transported from its storage site in the cauda epididymis distally into the vas deferens[3]. During the ejaculatory reflex, the vas deferens further propels sperm very rapidly through the ejaculatory ducts into the posterior urethra. At the ejaculatory ducts the sperm are joined by fluid from the seminal vesicles and prostate and sympathetic stimulation of these organs causes contraction and emptying of their contents. The expulsion of seminal fluid into the urethra is termed *seminal emission*. The bladder neck's function during ejaculation is to close tightly to assure that sperm is propelled toward the ejaculatory ducts. Failure of adequate bladder neck closure results in retrograde ejaculation into the bladder.

At the time of seminal emission there are also ill-defined sensations of genital and psychic pleasure, collectively termed *orgasm*. The psychic component of orgasm is poorly understood. It has been thought by some that distention of the posterior urethra by seminal emission causes the genital sensation of orgasm, but experience with men who experience orgasm without seminal emission, who usually report a normal sensation of orgasm, suggests that genital pleasure is a component of the central reflex.

Immediately after seminal emission into the posterior urethra, rhythmic contractions of the bulbocavernosus and ischiocavernosus muscle and rhythmic relaxation of the external sphincter create *projectile ejaculation* from the urethral meatus. As mentioned above, tight contraction of the bladder neck prevents retrograde ejaculation into the bladder and creates the 'back wall' for the force of the projectile phase of the reflex. These muscles are under the control of somatic fibers arising from the pudendal nerve. Nevertheless, the rhythmic contractions are not under voluntary control during the ejaculatory reflex. It has been suggested that these rhythmic contractions may be a reflex response to distention of the posterior urethra by seminal fluid, but experience in men with orgasm but no seminal emission would again suggest otherwise. Typically, such men have rhythmic contractions and the sensation of projectile ejaculation despite total absence of seminal emission.

In summary, the ejaculatory reflex has afferent input from genital tactile sensation from the dorsal nerves of the penis and also from erotic stimuli from higher centers. Efferent outflow for the reflex is from sympathetic fibers arising from the thoracolumbar spinal cord. The sympathetic nervous system is responsible for seminal emission and bladder neck closure. Projectile ejaculation is controlled by somatic nerve fibers.

EJACULATORY DYSFUNCTION – CLINICAL SETTINGS

Premature ejaculation

Premature ejaculation is a condition where a man is unable to delay the ejaculatory reflex until the desired time. Men with this condition may ejaculate very shortly after vaginal penetration, and in such situations premature ejaculation creates sexual difficulties. It should be remembered also that although many have attempted to create a definition that would be applicable to all men[4], premature ejaculation is only a *problem* when defined as such by the couple. If the couple is sexually satisfied, then it need not be treated. Sex therapy (see below) is the treatment in men/couples desiring treatment.

In severe cases, the premature ejaculation may occur *prior to* vaginal penetration. It is in these couples that an obvious fertility problem arises. The initial treatment is also sex therapy and equivalent good results are seen. Failing improvement with therapy, the sperm can be retrieved and utilized for artificial insemination. If no other factors leading to infertility complicate the situation, couples may be counseled on collection of the ejaculate, aspiration into a syringe, and timed vaginal insemination at home. In a couple unwilling and/or incapable of doing this, then semen can be collected and used for artificial insemination in a fertility clinic setting.

Treatment of premature ejaculation is generally very successful with response rates of 90%. Exercises involving stopping masturbation or sexual activity just prior to the threshold of ejaculation and restarting after the sensation abates (stop–start technique) results in progressively longer periods of delaying ejaculation[5]. Application of a noxious stimulus, typically a firm squeeze of the glans penis, just prior to reaching the ejaculatory threshold (the 'squeeze technique') may aid in preventing the orgasm from occurring during this training period.

Men with premature ejaculation can nearly always be managed by the above-mentioned techniques and should not be considered for ejaculation induction procedures.

Idiopathic anejaculation

Idiopathic anejaculation is a condition in which a neurologically normal man is unable to achieve orgasm and ejaculation during sexual activity[6]. Usually patients present with a history of never having been able to ejaculate during sexual activity; hence, the synonym of primary anejaculation. Most men with idiopathic anejaculation have intermittent nocturnal emissions with a frequency of several days to several weeks between episodes.

Because such men are neurologically normal, and because nocturnal emissions are characteristically present, this condition has also been termed *psychogenic anejaculation.* One must remember, however, that there may be some subtle neurological abnormalities leading to the condition. Indeed, we have treated a patient with a lipoma of his distal spinal cord and tethered cord syndrome who was initially diagnosed with psychogenic anejaculation. He successfully fathered a child through electroejaculation.

Nevertheless, most men with idiopathic anejaculation probably have a psychogenic etiology. Further evidence to support a psychogenic source is correlation to anxiety disorders, sexually repressive upbringing and other psychological problems[6]. Therefore, the initial treatment is sex therapy or psychotherapy. Treatment is aimed at increasing erotic stimulation and decreasing anxiety during sexual activity. Occasionally tricyclic antidepressants and alcohol are used in mild to moderate amounts. Masturbation exercises and erotic imagery may be suggested. Unfortunately, results with sex therapy and psychotherapy in idiopathic anejaculation are not very good. Couples who suffer infertility from idiopathic anejaculation, and who have failed psychotherapy or sex therapy, may be considered candidates for electroejaculation[6].

Retrograde ejaculation

Retrograde ejaculation is caused by inability of the bladder neck to close tightly enough during the ejaculatory reflex to prevent retrograde flow of emitted semen into the bladder. Common etiologies are listed in Table 1.

Anatomic conditions are usually the result of a surgical procedure which disrupts the internal sphincter mechanism/prostate area. Prostatic and bladder neck surgeries to relieve urinary obstruction (e.g. transurethral prostatectomy) are the typical operations seen.

Table 1 Etiologies of retrograde ejaculation

Anatomic etiologies
TURP
Y–V plasty of bladder
injury to bladder neck
urethral stricture distal to ejaculatory ducts
Pharmacological etiologies
antihypertensives (e.g. prazosin)
BPH drugs (terazosin)
antipsychotics (trazodone)
Neurogenic etiologies
incomplete spinal cord injury
myelodysplasia
multiple sclerosis
retroperitoneal surgery (RPLND or aortic surgery)
diabetic neuropathy
sympathectomy

Drugs which create retrograde ejaculation possess α-adrenergic blocking activity. Although bladder neck contraction may be adequate without the medication, α-blockade of the sympathetic nerves responsible for bladder neck activity may result in ineffectual closing during the ejaculatory process.

Neurogenic etiologies impair sympathetic outflow enough to prevent effective bladder neck closure but not enough to prevent seminal emission. Neurogenic sources of retrograde ejaculation are usually slowly progressive conditions leading to peripheral or central autonomic neuropathy, such as in diabetic neuropathy or multiple sclerosis. These patients have an initial period of retrograde ejaculation when sympathetic nerve dysfunction is moderate, and eventually develop total absence of ejaculation when the autonomic dysfunction is more severe. Men with acute neurological lesions such as spinal cord injury or retroperitoneal lymph node dissection (RPLND) will usually experience total absence of seminal emission rather than simply retrograde ejaculation.

Men with retrograde ejaculation are initially treated with sympathomimetic agents (Table 2) to stimulate more effective contraction of the bladder neck during ejaculation[7–9]. If this therapy results in antegrade expulsion of adequate numbers of motile sperm, then timed intercourse is suggested. If pharmacological treatment is unsuccessful, couples may be treated with sperm retrieval from the bladder, processing and artificial insemination or other assisted reproductive technologies. Techniques for

Table 2 Sympathomimetic therapy regimens

Phenylpropanolamine	75 mg b.i.d.
Imipramine	75–100 mg q.h.s. (initiate and withdraw slowly)
Ephedrine	25 mg q.i.d.

the removal of retrograde ejaculate from the bladder are discussed later in this chapter and in the Appendix.

While some reports have suggested surgical repair of anatomic defects of the bladder neck[10,11], this seems unjustified with current methods of achieving pregnancy by lesser means.

Absence of seminal emission/anejaculation

When seminal emission is totally absent due to pathophysiological conditions, infertility results and is more difficult to treat than the above-mentioned conditions. The reasons for anejaculation are varied and present in different ways. Common etiologies of anejaculation will be discussed below.

Spinal cord injury

For several decades it has been a widespread belief that individuals with a spinal cord injury (SCI) are permanently and completely impotent and infertile. Fortunately, many investigations have shown that this is not true[12,13]. Previously published studies on baseline sexual function in SCI men are difficult to interpret and compare due to several methodological inconsistencies. However, we can draw some general conclusions from that literature.

Erectile and ejaculatory function

Erectile function may be impaired in the spinal cord-injured man and this may contribute to infertility by impairing normal sexual intercourse and semen delivery. The reported frequency of reflexogenic, psychogenic or mixed erection in SCI men ranges from 54% to 95% whereas the frequency of erection sufficient for coitus ranges from 5% to 75%[12]. In general, it has been noted that erection is more common among men with incomplete spinal lesions, upper motor neuron lesions and lesions located higher in the cord[14]. Even though the knowledge of these parameters makes possible a general prognosis, it does not necessarily provide an accurate prognosis of future sexual function in the individual case[15]. Also, even though erectile function may be present to some degree, the inconsistent timing of erections and short duration seen commonly in SCI men limit the man's ability to engage in sexual intercourse.

In attempting to determine the frequency of normal *ejaculatory function* among SCI men methodological differences are again encountered in the literature. Most studies rely only on history from the patient, without an examination of the purported semen specimen. In some studies, dribbling 'emission' has been included, but not in other studies[16] and the rare investigation has searched for retrograde ejaculation. Despite these limitations, the literature would suggest that the frequency of ejaculation in SCI men ranges from 0 to 55%[13]. The frequency of ejaculation is higher among SCI men with incomplete cord lesions, with lower motor neuron lesions, and with lesions lower in the spinal cord[14].

Fertility potential

The best information on fertility potential of the untreated SCI man is obtained from reports of spontaneous procreation. Unfortunately, there are also problems here. Paternity has not been verified, pregnancy rates are difficult to ascertain and prognostic indicators (such as characteristics of the spinal injury) are impossible to extract. Furthermore, information on the sperm quality from spontaneous ejaculation in SCI men is virtually non-existent[13].

In three other studies involving 592 SCI men 12 pregnancies were reported, but no information about number of live births was given[17–19]. In six more recent papers, 274 liveborn children were reported to have been fathered by 1102 SCI men without medical assistance[20–25]. However, 205 of these pregnancies (fathered by 108 SCI men) were from Guttmann's series, in which only those who successfully initiated a pregnancy were reported[23].

Autonomic dysreflexia

The problem of autonomic dysreflexia during sexual activity and ejaculation induction in SCI men deserves mention here because of clinical implications. This condition may be experienced by patients whose lesions are at or above T6 spinal cord level. A normal ejaculatory reflex or a noxious stimulus such as vibratory stimulation or electroejaculation[26–30] may induce excessive activation of the sympathetic nervous system. Symptoms include flushing, sweating and sudden pounding headache due to rapid increase in the blood pressure, sometimes to very dangerous levels[31].

When an episode of autonomic dysreflexia begins it is essential to eliminate the initiating stimulus, such as stopping the ejaculation induction procedure. A quick response may prevent the need for further treatment. If the blood pressure remains at a dangerous level then emergent antihypertensive therapy is necessary, such as sublingual nifedipine, or intravenous nitroprusside or alpha blockers. In SCI men with a history of autonomic dysreflexia and/or cord lesions at or above T6, it is recommended to administer prophylactically the calcium channel blocker, nifedipine, by sublingual route, 10–15 min prior to initiating an ejaculation induction procedure[29,30].

Testicular cancer/retroperitoneal lymph node dissection

Fertility in men with testicular cancer may be due to three types of etiologies: pretreatment subfertility (an ill-defined phenomenon), treatment-related subfertility (e.g. chemotherapy, radiation therapy) and ejaculatory dysfunction due to retroperitoneal lymph node dissection (RPLND)[32]. It is this third category which will be discussed in this section.

Classic bilateral RPLND for testicular cancer results in ejaculatory dysfunction in the majority of cases[33,34]. During the surgery portions of the sympathetic chains and the inferior mesenteric/hypogastric plexus are removed, effectively removing the efferent limb of the ejaculatory reflex. Newer nerve-sparing procedures have been developed to avoid one sympathetic chain and the crucial portions of the inferior mesenteric plexus below the inferior mesenteric artery. When a successful nerve-sparing procedure is done for minimal disease, preservation of ejaculation now approaches 100% in men with low stage disease[35]. In men with extensive disease in which a more radical lymph node removal must be done, and in some men undergoing an attempted nerve-sparing procedure, ejaculatory dysfunction still results.

Most men with ejaculatory dysfunction from RPLND have total absence of seminal emission[36] rather than retrograde ejaculation. These men report normal erections and normal sensation of orgasm, including rhythmic contractions of the periurethral muscles, mimicking projectile antegrade ejaculation. This may lead the evaluating physician to assume incorrectly the presence of retrograde ejaculation. There are no other neurological deficits from RPLND other than loss of seminal emission.

These men are tried on sympathomimetic agents to induce antegrade or retrograde ejaculation. If successful, they are treated accordingly. Failing sympathomimetic therapy, ejaculation induction can be considered. Since the efferent phase of the ejaculatory reflex is absent, a procedure which does not require an intact reflex arc is necessary. Therefore, vibrator stimulation does not work in these men, and the only successful treatment to retrieve sperm without surgery is electroejaculation.

Diabetic neuropathy

Diabetic neuropathy may cause autonomic dysfunction in multiple areas of the body[37]. Erectile dysfunction is the most common sexual problem related to diabetic neuropathy[38], but ejaculatory dysfunction may also occur[39,40]. Since diabetic neuropathy is a progressive condition such men usually see, first, a decrease in ejaculate volume, followed by development of retrograde ejaculation and finally absence of seminal emission. Men with early onset anejaculation from diabetic neuropathy will commonly respond to sympathomimetic agents for several months until further worsening of the neuropathy leads to a relapse.

If the diabetic neuropath has persistent absence of seminal emission despite therapy, electroejaculation can be considered. Vibratory stimulation has a very low likelihood of success, because the efferent limb of the reflex is usually affected by the neuropathy.

Multiple sclerosis

In multiple sclerosis (MS) sexual dysfunction is common[41], but the presentation and course are quite variable. Remissions and relapses, which are common in MS, may lead to resolution and recurrence of ejaculatory dysfunction. Therefore, no sweeping conclusions may be reached concerning the appropriate therapy for ejaculatory dysfunction in these patients. If there is relatively good preservation of neural function sympathomimetics may be tried, proceeding to electroejaculation if this fails[42]. If the patient is effectively a paraplegic or quadriplegic, vibrator ejaculation or electroejaculation may be appropriate, depending on the specific characteristics of the spinal cord dysfunction.

Other neurological conditions

Any pathophysiological condition which impairs components of the normal ejaculatory reflex may cause ejaculatory dysfunction. We have treated men with anejaculation due to myelodysplasia, syringomyelia, rectal surgery, staging laparotomy for Hodgkin's disease with sampling of retroperitoneal nodes, placement of an aortic graft and 'senile' anejaculation (poor penile sensation and inability to ejaculate) and loss of penile sensation from penile surgery. To characterize their dysfunction adequately, a complete history, physical examination and laboratory testing is necessary and the treatment plan tailored to meet specific needs.

TECHNIQUES TO RETRIEVE SPERM IN EJACULATORY DYSFUNCTION

Retrieval of sperm in premature and idiopathic anejaculation

In men with premature ejaculation, there is usually no difficulty in the man producing a semen specimen himself. This can be by masturbation or with sexual activity at home. Ejaculation is directed into a specimen container and processed as it would be for any artificial insemination procedure.

The situation is not as simple in men with idiopathic anejaculation. As mentioned above, many of these men will have frequent nocturnal emissions. In couples wishing to avoid electroejaculation, a non-spermicidal condom may be placed upon going to sleep at night during the wife's fertile period. If the man experiences frequent nocturnal emissions he may be lucky enough to experience an ejaculate at the appropriate time, and the sperm can be used for artificial insemination. In most cases, however, this will not occur and electroejaculation will be necessary[6].

Sperm retrieval in men with retrograde ejaculation

In men with retrograde ejaculation who are neurologically normal, the post-orgasm urine can be collected and utilized for artificial insemination. The specimen may be obtained by voiding or by catheterization of the bladder. We prefer urethral catheterization for several reasons. First, the bladder is catheterized prior to orgasm to assure absolutely complete emptying of all the urine to minimize urinary contact of the sperm. Second, a buffered sperm-friendly medium can be instilled into the bladder to optimize sperm viability in the hostile environment[40,43]. Third, the post-orgasm catheterization allows complete emptying of the bladder and irrigation with the media to allow suspension and complete removal of intravesical sperm. The catheterization and irrigation procedures should be performed with caution to avoid trauma and subsequent contamination of the specimens with red blood cells.

Men are prepared with 1.5 g of sodium bicarbonate taken orally 12 h and 2 h prior to the procedure to alkalinize any urine produced between the two catheterizations. Fluids are restricted for 6 h prior to the procedure to reduce the urine production during the procedure.

We concede that the above maneuvers are controversial. Shangold *et al.*[44] had patients drink several glasses of water several hours prior to the sperm retrieval in an attempt to optimize osmolality. They and others[45] suggest that spontaneous voiding is as effective as catheterization. Nevertheless, our bias is that decreasing the amount of actual urine contact is more effective than attempting to change the chemical contents of the urine produced. Many patients cannot void after emptying their bladder only a few minutes previously. The catheter circumvents this problem. With our methodology the post-orgasm 'urine' specimen consists of nearly pure semen and media, with very little urine contamination in most cases.

Specimens obtained from the bladder are transported without delay to the laboratory where washing is performed immediately to separate the urine from the sperm. Subsequent standard separation techniques (e.g. Percoll, etc.) prepare the sperm for insemination or other assisted reproduction technology (ART) procedures.

There are several case reports of pregnancies occurring from insemination of processed retrograde ejaculates, but very few series of patients. Urry *et al.*[45] reported that of 12 men with retrograde ejaculation, seven had occasions where sperm of adequate motility were present. These seven men underwent sperm retrieval and intrauterine insemination (IUI) with their spouses and six couples conceived. Therefore, approximately half of the men seeking treatment were able to effect a pregnancy, and 86% of those attempting IUI were successful. In working with eight couples, van der Linden *et al.*[46] were able to achieve 12 pregnancies by artificial insemination with a cycle of fecundity of 44%. Interestingly, in this group there were four spontaneous abortions in the 12 pregnancies (33%).

Nearly all case reports and series in the literature have utilized IUI or more invasive/expensive procedures to effect pregnancy. Pregnancies have been reported with direct intraperitoneal insemination (DIPI)[40] and GIFT[47], but the efficacy and particularly the cost-effectiveness of IUI[44–46] make IUI an optimal first-line treatment.

Pharmacologically induced ejaculation

In 1946, Guttmann was the first to use intrathecal injection of neostigmine to induce an ejaculate in men with SCI[23]. Since that time several investigators have used intrathecal neostigmine[22,31,48–51], as well as subcutaneous physostigmine[52–55], to induce ejaculation in SCI men. Neostigmine cannot transverse the blood brain barrier, necessitating intrathecal delivery. Neostigmine usually induces repeated spontaneous ejaculations approximately 2–3 h after injection[49]. Using subcutaneous physostigmine, additional penile stimulation by masturbation or vibration is necessary to induce ejaculation[52,53,55]. The exact mechanism by which these cholinesterase inhibitors induce ejaculation is unknown, but it is clear that activation of autonomic reflexes (including undesirable reflexes) at the spinal cord level is occurring. Direct stimulation of the ejaculatory spinal cord reflex center by neostigmine is probably responsible for ejaculation[20]. Subcutaneous physostigmine induces less severe autonomic changes and probably induces a partial stimulation of the ejaculatory center, lowering the threshold of inducing a reflex ejaculation with vibration, etc.[55].

Review of the literature suggests a 50% success rate in inducing ejaculation following injection of cholinesterase inhibitors in 377 SCI men[13]. A total of 21 pregnancies have been reported by these techniques coupled with artificial insemination or by coitus[13].

Unfortunately, unwanted autonomic effects are also seen with these drugs. In the case of intrathecal neostigmine, these symptoms mimic classic autonomic dysreflexia in SCI men and may include flushing, sweating, piloerection and potentially dangerous elevations of blood pressure. Indeed, Guttmann reported the death of a C6 quadriplegic from a cerebral hemorrhage induced by neostigmine[49]. The intrathecal use of neostigmine to retrieve sperm from SCI men is not recommended by the authors because it is difficult to administer, requires an intensive care unit monitoring for dysreflexia and poses substantial risk to the patient[31]. Safer alternatives are readily available.

Subcutaneous physostigmine causes parasympathetic side-effects such as nausea, vomiting, abdominal cramps and diarrhea[52]. To counteract these side-effects a peripherally acting anticholinergic should be injected prior to the subcutaneous injection of physostigmine[52,54,55]. Chapelle *et al.*[53] reported domestic use of subcutaneous physostigmine without special precautions. Clearly, the substantial blood pressure swings seen with intrathecal neostigmine are not encountered with subcutaneous physostigmine. However, the peripheral parasympathetic side-effects can be substantial, and with alternative procedures available as noted below the authors do not currently recommend subcutaneous physostigmine for ejaculation induction.

Penile vibratory stimulation

Vibratory stimulation of the penis to induce reflex ejaculation was first described by Sobrero *et al.*[56] in a group of non-SCI men. Success in men without spinal cord injury has been limited since that initial report and current thought would suggest that

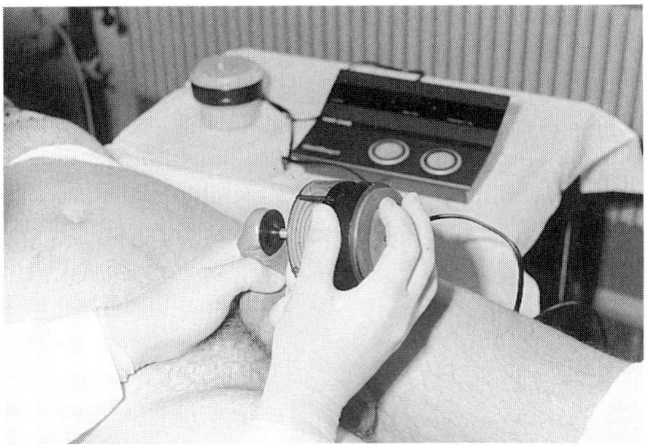

Figure 1 Application of penile vibratory stimulation. Vibrator: Modified FERTI-CARE® *clinic* version (1994) developed to meet the required frequency of 100 Hz and an amplitude of 2.5 mm[30]

vibratory stimulation is effective only in SCI men. It is largely due to Brindley[27,28] that the use of vibratory stimulation in SCI men has become widespread.

It appears that during vibratory stimulation, a normal ejaculatory reflex is induced by genital stimulation of the penis and effected via normal outflow from the thoracolumbar spinal cord. Successful ejaculation by penile vibratory stimulation in SCI men, therefore, requires an intact ejaculatory reflex arc which allows transmission of afferent stimuli to the cord, communication between the sacral and thoracolumbar regions (T11–S4) and sympathetic outflow as mentioned earlier. These neurological segments, even when isolated from the brain, will respond to vibratory stimulation of the penis in a reflex manner[57].

Vibratory stimulation should be performed with the patient in a supine or sitting position. The center of the vibrator knob is applied to the frenulum of the penis (Figure 1). The knob of the vibrator should be held in the same position until antegrade ejaculation occurs or for a maximum of 3–4 min followed by a pause of 1–2 min (one cycle). This cycle can be repeated up to six times depending on the penile skin integrity. Bruising, bleeding or superficial ulceration of the skin may occur, requiring cessation of the procedure. The time necessary to induce vibratory ejaculation in SCI men ranges from 10s–20 min[27,30,57,58].

During the vibrator stimulation procedure, characteristic reflexes may be seen. These include abdominal contractions, leg spasms, piloerection, penile erection and scrotal wall contraction. Just prior to ejaculation, rhythmic contractions of the periurethral muscles are detectable. If the procedure is stopped just as those contractions begin, multiple antegrade ejaculations may be obtained (occasionally >four within several minutes) increasing the total semen volume obtained.

Other than skin abrasions, as mentioned above, the only complication encountered commonly with vibratory stimulation is autonomic dysreflexia. In susceptible patients (complete lesions at or above T_6), sublingual nifedipine 10–20 mg is administered 10–15 minutes prior to the procedure, with nearly uniform effectiveness in controlling the blood pressure. Blood pressure monitoring during the procedure is essential in such individuals. Stopping the stimulation promptly as periurethral muscle rhythmic contractions begin also helps to limit the dysreflexia. In the event that blood pressure rises to unacceptable levels, the procedure is immediately aborted, with prompt return to baseline levels in nearly all cases. The prophylaxis regimen is then reevaluated prior to continuing.

The ejaculation rates reported after vibratory stimulation in SCI men range from 19% to 91% (Table 3)[22,27,28,55,57–63]. Several different vibrators and settings have been used and it is not possible to extract the optimum vibration variables (frequency and amplitude) from the literature.

One of the authors (JS) recently demonstrated in 25 SCI men that a vibrator output of 100 Hz and a peak-to-peak amplitude of 2.5 mm produced significantly higher ejaculation rates than a peak-to-peak amplitude of 1 mm (96% versus 32%)[30]. This indicates that an adequate peak-to-peak amplitude is essential to exceed the 'ejaculatory threshold' in the majority of SCI men. Furthermore, an ejaculation rate of 83% obtained in a subsequent prospective study of 41 SCI men verified that a frequency of 100 Hz and a peak-to-peak amplitude of 2.5 mm seems to approach the ideal vibration parameters.

During the above study[30], determinations revealed that the manufacturers' specifications regarding the peak-to-peak amplitudes were inaccurate. The considerable differences in the previously reported ejaculation rates (Table 1) may be explained by unrecognized differences between the indicated vibration variables and the actual vibra-

Table 3 Vibration variables and ejaculation rates as reported in the literature

References	*n*	*Ejaculation rates* (%)	*Vibration variables*	
			Frequency (Hz)	*Amplitude* (mm)
Whelan (1972)[59] (cited)	63	19*	?	?
Piera (1973)[22§]	101	27*	?	?
Brindley (1981)[27]	21	57†	70–100	1.6–2.4
Brindley (1984)[28¶]	93	53†	80	2.5
Francois *et al.* (1983)[60]	140	49*	?	?
Sarkarati *et al.* (1987)[61]	33	24†	80	1.6–2.4
Szasz *et al.* (1989)[57]	22	50*	120	1.0–3.0
Szasz *et al.* (1989)[57]	35	34†	?	?
Beretta *et al.* (1989)[58]	102	71†	100	?
Beilby *et al.* (1989)[62]	37	51*	?	2.0–4.0
Siösteen *et al.* (1990)[63]	32	91†	80–100	1.5–2.5
Rawicki and Hill (1991)[55]	9	44‡	80	?
Range		19–91	70–120	1.0–4.0

*No distinction between antegrade and/or retrograde ejaculations; †includes both antegrade and retrograde ejaculations; ‡only antegrade ejaculation reported; §ejaculation obtained by masturbation or penile vibratory stimulation; ¶the 21 patients from Ref. 18 are included

tor outputs. To induce ejaculation in the majority of SCI men by penile vibratory stimulation, the vibrator must produce the required output accurately.

Some predictors of ejaculatory success or failure by vibratory stimulation in SCI men can be found in the literature. Projectile, antegrade ejaculation does not commonly occur in SCI men with cord lesions below T10[28,30,57], whereas retrograde and dribbling ejaculations have been observed in SCI men with lumbar or sacral cord lesions, respectively[30,58,61]. There is a trend toward a higher number of antegrade ejaculations among the patients with cervical lesions[30]. No relation between completeness of cord lesion, patient age or years since lesion and the ejaculation response has been described[28,30,57].

The presence of both the hip flexion and bulbocavernosus reflexes is the best prognostic indicator of vibratory ejaculation success in SCI men[28,30,57]. Absence of the hip flexion and bulbocavernosus reflexes indicates damage between T11–L2 (efferent outflow of the reflex) and S2–S4 (afferent stimulation for the reflex), respectively. However, even when none of the reflexes are clinically present, ejaculation can occasionally be obtained in SCI men[30]. Despite these guidelines for prognosis there are no absolute predictors of vibratory ejaculation success or failure.

Penile vibratory stimulation is an easy, non-invasive procedure, and most SCI men with ejaculatory dysfunction should be considered candidates for vibratory stimulation prior to proceeding to more invasive procedures, such as electroejaculation. Although guidelines are not clear for taking this procedure out of the clinic setting and 'back to the bedroom', vibrator stimulation of ejaculation may be performed by the SCI patients and/or partners at home with subsequent vaginal insemination of the raw specimen. Brindley reported seven pregnancies initiated with vibrator stimulation and insemination at home[28]. Pregnancy rates in the literature are generally higher, however, when IUI is used. Also, patients at risk for autonomic dysreflexia are not candidates for initiating vibratory stimulation at home.

In a review of papers concerning vibrator stimulation of 619 SCI men, a total number of 102 pregnancies and delivery of 49 live-born children were found[13]. Pregnancies have been conceived by vaginal insemination at home or by artificial insemination using intracervical insemination and IUI. Calculation of the pregnancy rate and live birth rate is not possible due to lack of information regarding the exact number of SCI men attempting procreation, final results of ongoing pregnancies, etc.

Electroejaculation

Human electroejaculation (EEJ) was reported by Learmonth in 1931 who caused seminal emission by stimulation of presacral nerves[64]. The first rectal probe EEJ was in 1948 by Horne, Munro, and Paull who used an insulated metal urethral sound which was inserted into the rectum[65]. Of eighteen spinal cord patients attempted, semen was obtained in all, but only half of these specimens contained motile sperm. The first pregnancy by rectal probe EEJ was reported by Thomas in 1975 in a T12 paraplegic man[66]. Carol Bennett at the University of Michigan reported the first US pregnancy by electroejaculation and intrauterine insemination in 1987[67].

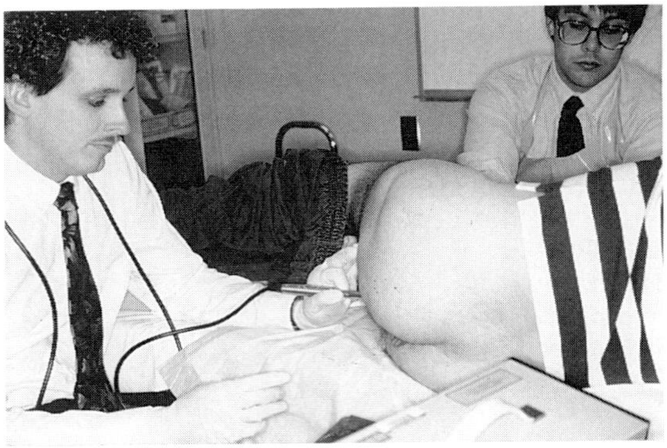

Figure 2 Electroejaculation procedure. The probe is inserted with the patient in the lateral decubitus position with electrodes facing anteriorly. The lateral decubitus position allows access to the rectum for the probe and allows the assistant to maintain easy control of the urethral meatus over the specimen container

Technique of electroejaculation

Patients are given 1.5 g sodium bicarbonate 12 h and 2 h prior to the procedure to alkalinize the urine as in patients with retrograde ejaculation. This is because with EEJ, as opposed to vibratory stimulation, a substantial portion of the semen is emitted into the bladder. In men with spinal cord injury or severe multiple sclerosis who are insensate below the level of their disease, the EEJ is performed in the clinic setting without an anesthetic. In men who are sensory intact (e.g. idiopathic anejaculation and RPLND patients) and in some spinal cord injured men with incomplete lesions, electroejaculation is too painful to be performed without a proper anesthetic. Such men are administered a spinal, epidural or general anesthetic for the procedure.

Spinal cord-injured men with lesions above T4 may experience significant autonomic dysreflexia during the procedure (see above). In general, the EEJ procedure will most likely create the most profound dysreflexia these patients have experienced. It is nearly always more substantial than that induced by vibratory stimulation. A high spinal cord-injured man with *any* history of autonomic dysreflexia is treated with prophylactic nifedipine prior to EEJ. An average sublingual dose of 20 mg is administered 15 min prior to the initiation of stimulation. A group of high lesion SCI men treated with EEJ, both with and without nifedipine, showed substantial decreases in peak systolic and diastolic blood pressures, increases in the number of stimulations possible, increased peak voltage delivery and eradication of the need to abort procedures due to elevated blood pressures when prophylaxis was given[29].

The bladder is catheterized with a plastic catheter, utilizing minimal amounts of non-toxic lubricant. Lubricants with bacteriostatic activity have been shown to be toxic to sperm[68] and are avoided. The bladder is drained absolutely dry with gentle suprapubic pressure with care taken to avoid trauma which might contaminate the specimen with red blood cells. A 'sperm-friendly' medium is instilled into the bladder.

The patient is turned on his side and rigid sigmoidoscopy performed to 15 cm to assure that no pre-existing rectal lesions are present. An appropriate size rectal probe is inserted (usually 1.25 diameter) and electricity is delivered in a progressively increasing wavelike pattern with 1–2 volt increments until antegrade ejaculation is noted by the assistant. The voltage is further increased to 50% greater than this threshold level to assure complete emptying of the seminal fluid.

During the electroejaculation process, the assistant directs the ejaculate into a specimen container and informs the operator when ejaculation begins and when it is complete, so the operator may tailor the procedure accordingly. Since there is no reflex projectile ejaculation there may be substantial amounts in the urethra at the termination of stimulation, which needs to be milked out at the end of the procedure.

A second assistant determines the blood pressure approximately every 30–60 s in the high spinal cord injured man. Despite nifedipine prophylaxis, significant hypertension may still be seen. In nearly all cases of EEJ-induced autonomic dysreflexia, the blood pressure will return to baseline promptly by stopping the electrical stimulation and removing the rectal probe.

After ejaculation is complete, the probe is withdrawn and repeat sigmoidoscopy with rectal insufflation performed to assure that no rectal injury has occurred. The patient is then turned supine again and the bladder catheterized to empty its retrograde ejaculate. The bladder is atraumatically rinsed with the medium to complete the collection.

Following the EEJ procedure, spinal cord patients are allowed to leave the clinic immediately. In a high spinal cord man who has received nifedipine, resumption of the sitting position in the wheelchair is achieved in stages to prevent postural hypotension. If postural hypotension is present, returning to the supine position for 10–15 minutes is usually adequate to allow the nifedipine effect to disappear. In men who have received an anesthetic for the EEJ procedure, standard recovery room protocols are followed.

Results of electroejaculation

At the University of Michigan, we have treated 232 men with rectal probe EEJ. Of these, the vast majority were spinal cord-injured (178). We have treated 34 men in whom an RPLND was the etiology of the anejaculation. The remainder of the patients have a variety of etiologies.

In our experience, seminal emission is achieved in virtually all patients undergoing EEJ. A high rate of inducing seminal emission has also been noted by other investigators. Three recent studies noted seminal emission rates of 81–100%[69–71]. The high emission rates are seen because the EEJ procedure does not depend upon an intact ejaculatory reflex arc to be successful. Electroejaculation probably induces seminal emission by direct stimulation of the short adrenergic neurons at the ejaculatory organs. In spinal cord-injured men with lower lesions, who lack hip flexion and bulbocavernosus reflexes (i.e. poor candidates for vibrator stimulation), EEJ can still induce seminal emission. We believe that vibratory stimulation should be tried first in SCI men for reasons mentioned above, but if ejaculation is not obtained by that method, EEJ still has an excellent chance of producing a specimen and should be offered subsequently. Similarly, in non-SCI men lacking the peripheral efferent limb of the ejaculatory reflex pathway, such as diabetic neuropaths and or after RPLND, vibrator stimulation is not an option, but EEJ successfully induces emission in all these patients.

Although the induction of seminal emission is nearly 100% in our hands, this does not mean that the ejaculate contains adequate numbers of motile sperm. In men with spinal cord injury, only 72% were deemed to have ejaculates adequate for attempts at pregnancy with artificial insemination or other ART procedures[72]. Retroperitoneal lymph node dissection patients had a rate of 87%[73]. Potential reasons for poor semen quality from EEJ is discussed further later in this chapter.

In our program, of 162 couples attempting to achieve pregnancy, 51 couples (31%) have succeeded with a total of 65 pregnancies. Intrauterine insemination (IUI) or higher technology procedures are used in conjunction with the EEJ, as we achieved no pregnancies from vaginal insemination early in the program. The cycle fecundity for intrauterine insemination is 5–10% per cycle, and with one cycle of IVF/GIFT is between 30% and 43%, depending on the etiology of the anejaculation.

We can calculate a theoretical pregnancy rate for our largest patient population, the spinal cord-injured men. In our SCI population, there has been a 72% chance of having suitable numbers of sperm on EEJ, an IUI pregnancy rate of 36% per couple and an IVF/GIFT success rate of 43% per cycle. Figure 3 shows the potential pregnancy rate for a new SCI man/partner entering our program, who are willing to go through IUI and one cycle of IVF/GIFT. Figure 4 shows the potential pregnancy rate for an SCI man determined to have adequate numbers of sperm from the initial EEJ.

It is of note that, in patients presenting for initial pregnancy attempts, the pregnancy rate per couple was 31%. On 25 occasions, couples who had a previous pregnancy returned for additional attempts. Of those 25 returning couples, 14 became pregnant for a 'secondary' fertility rate with electro-

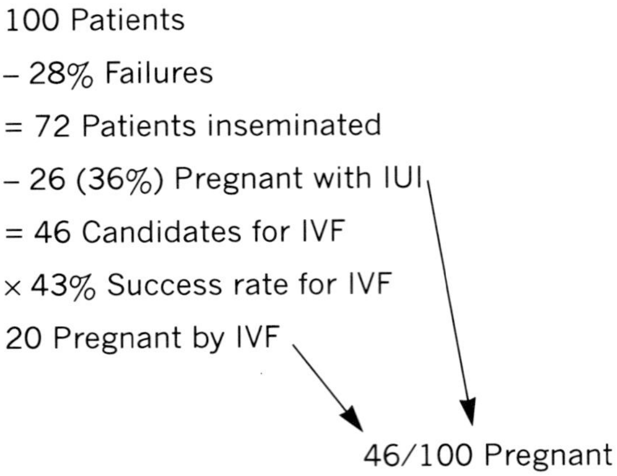

Figure 3 Chance of a spinal cord injured man achieving a pregnancy through electroejaculation and ART procedures. Data drawn from men presenting for initial attempts at electroejaculation and includes EEJ failures. 'IVF' implies *in vitro* fertilization and/or gamete intrafallopian transfer (GIFT)

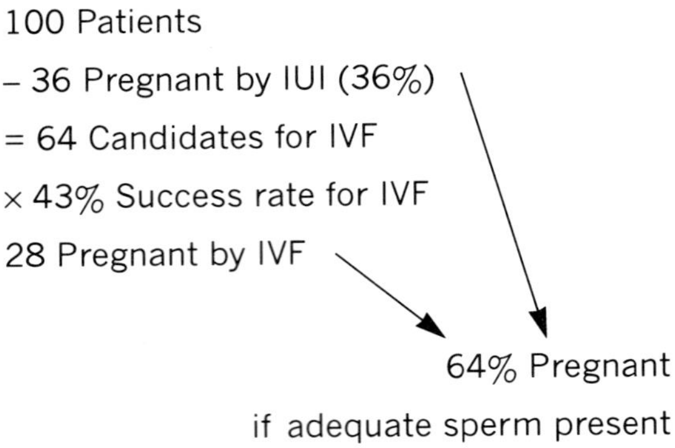

Figure 4 Chance of a spinal cord injured man achieving pregnancy through electroejaculation during initial attempt of electroejaculation. 'IVF' includes IVF-ET and GIFT procedures

ejaculation of 56%. In other words, men who have succeeded in initiating an EEJ pregnancy have a higher success rate of initiating subsequent pregnancies. A search for prognostic indicators by diagnosis, clinical situation and even semen analysis parameters, comparing successes with failures has not been fruitful in identifying men with a high chance of initiating pregnancy. These data suggest that some anejaculatory men, due to unidentified factors, have the capability of initiating a pregnancy where others will do poorly.

Our spontaneous abortion rate is slightly high at 25%, but one must note that we take great care in diagnosing pregnancy carefully. This high rate, however, does raise the possibility that either the clinical situation leading to the anejaculation, or possibly direct effects of the electroejaculation procedure are responsible for early pregnancy loss. There have been no congenital anomalies reported in any of these babies born from our program.

Pregnancy reports in the literature are sparse and usually limited to case reports. The American Fertility Society Electroejaculation Registry surveyed EEJ centers in the United States and Canada in 1993. Thirty-three centers participated in the survey, with a total of 1380 men treated. Spinal cord-injured men numbered 1081, or 78% of the population. In 604 couples interested in initiating pregnancy, 216 pregnancies were achieved[74]. Although the limited survey vehicle prevented accurate factoring of multiple pregnancies in the same couples and pregnancy outcome data, these numbers suggest that the pregnancy rate across the United States and Canada approaches 35%.

Surgical treatment of ejaculatory dysfunction

Successful retrieval of sperm from implanted sperm reservoirs in SCI men has been described[75], but alloplastic spermatoceles in SCI men have problems similar to those seen in other clinical situations. Direct aspiration of sperm from the vas deferens has been reported in only seven SCI men resulting in four pregnancies after intrauterine insemination (one case) or *in vitro* fertilization[76–79]. Belker has suggested that in selected SCI men, particularly those with chronic prostatic infection, sperm aspiration from the vas deferens may give a cleaner specimen than that obtained by other means. He has noted one such patient who had multiple failures from EEJ and artificial insemination, probably due to seminal infection. The patient had a leukocyte-free specimen on vas aspiration and initiated a pregnancy on the first attempt at vas aspiration/IUI (Belker, 1993, personal communication). This concept needs to be explored further.

Brindley has described a method to induce repeated ejaculation in SCI men by direct stimulation of the hypogastric nerve using an implanted nerve stimulator[80]. Although this is interesting, the surgery to implant such a device is a major undertaking, and the authors feel the alternatives mentioned above are preferred.

Although these surgical techniques may deserve further study, especially vas aspiration in SCI men with chronically infected semen, we feel that surgical extraction of sperm for the treatment of anejaculation is not necessary in most cases. The numbers of times surgical extraction may be performed will probably be limited by scarring. Since vibrator stimulation and EEJ can provide a reliable method of ejaculation induction without surgery and can most likely be repeated indefinitely, these methods are preferable.

THE PROBLEM OF SPERM QUALITY FROM EJACULATION INDUCTION PROCEDURES

Despite numerous methods of extracting sperm from the anejaculatory male, several common themes are seen. Pregnancy rates remain low from artificial insemination, and sperm quality is usually very poor.

One of us (DO) characterized the typical functional impairments of sperm obtained by electroejaculation[81]. In 32 anejaculatory men treated with electroejaculation, a battery of laboratory tests was performed (Table 4). The following discussion concerns the quality of the sperm obtained in that study.

Table 5 shows the average semen analysis parameters from the specimens obtained by EEJ in the study. Total sperm numbers are very high with an average *total* sperm count (antegrade and retrograde) of 2.7 *billion* sperm. Sperm motilities were very low at 10.9% in the antegrade and 6.2% in the retrograde fractions. Of note is the close approximation between the motility and the viability. The high correlation between motility and viability indicates that non-motile sperm from EEJ is non-viable, rather than just exhibiting poor motility characteristics.

Results with the bovine cervical mucus penetration tests were variable with an average mucus penetration of 19.4 mm in 30 min versus 33.0 by five comparative donor samples. Only 24% EEJ samples had normal scores of >30 mm. The average 20-h retained motility was 47% of original motility compared to 82% in the controls. Classical (not the optimized assay) hamster egg penetration assay scores were significantly lower in the electroejaculates than in donor sperm (14% penetration versus 40% penetration).

Table 4 Sperm functional testing performed on electroejaculates from 32 anejaculatory men. Reproduced from Hirsch *et al.* (1992)[82] with permission of Excerpta Medica Inc.

Analysis of the raw specimen
routine semen analysis
viability stain
bovine cervical mucus penetration test
Tests on processed semen
motility longevity
direct immunobead test
hamster penetration assay

Table 5 Average raw semen parameters in 32 anejaculatory men treated with electroejaculation. Reproduced from Hirsch *et al.* (1992)[82] with permission of Excerpta Medica Inc.

	Antegrade	*Retrograde*
pH	7.2	6.9
Volume	2.7 mL	45.5 mL
Concentration	149.3 million	65.7 million
Total sperm count	448.1 million	2308 million
Motility	10.9%	6.2%
Viability	10.4%	5.3%
Abnormal morphology	57.4%	53.8%

Although some have suggested that sperm autoimmunity may be a cause of poor sperm function[82], we did not find this to be the case. Thirty-two semen samples tested for antisperm antibodies by the direct immunobead test, and only one test was positive.

In summary, our study suggested that sperm EEJ specimens obtained from anejaculatory men exhibit low motility/viability, poor motility longevity, moderately impaired mucus penetration and decreased fertilizing capability[81].

Buch and Zorn[83] reported similar deficiencies in a cohort of patients undergoing EEJ. There was a good total sperm count, but low motility (22%), and only a minority of the patients (25%) had a normal sperm penetration assay. Also, a favorable post-thaw motility (>33% retrieval of pre-thaw motility) was seen in only 31% of patients who underwent cryopreservation testing.

Papers describing quality of sperm obtained by

vibratory stimulation[27,84] and other methods of sperm retrieval[75] show similar deficiencies. It appears clear that deficiencies in semen quality are typical in men with anejaculation, irrespective of the method used to obtain sperm.

Reasons for poor sperm quality in anejaculation

Linsenmeyer and Perkash[85] suggested seven factors that may contribute to the poor sperm quality in SCI men: recurrent urinary tract infections; type of bladder management; stasis of prostatic fluid; testicular hyperthermia; abnormal testicular histology; changes in the hypothalamic–pituitary–testicular axis; sperm antibodies; and long-term use of various medications. The relative importance of these factors is not known, but the potential damage to fertility related to some can be discussed.

Changes in testicular histology have been noted in SCI men. Hirsch *et al.*[86] demonstrated a significantly lower mean spermatid count and higher Sertoli cell count per seminiferous tubule, together with a higher Sertoli cell:spermatid ratio when compared to normal fertile controls. In other studies, abnormal as well as normal testicular histology has been found[87–89]. Despite these observations, no explanations or reasons for testicular changes have been elucidated. Neurogenic factors may possibly play a role.

Stagnation of sperm in the genital ducts in anejaculatory SCI men may cause accumulation of senescent sperm which are then ejaculated, giving rise to poor specimens. If this is true, repeated ejaculations should result in a progressive improvement in sperm quality. However, one may find studies which show improvement and other studies showing no improvement after repeated ejaculations in SCI men[58,61,63,90–92]. Whether stagnation occurs and can be remedied remains controversial.

Genitourinary infections are extremely common in SCI men. In one series of SCI men undergoing EEJ, urinary infection was seen in 41% and seminal fluid infection in 56%[93]. Recurrent infections may lead to epididymitis and epididymo-orchitis which can impair the fertility by leading to obstruction of the epididymal ducts or atrophy of the testicles. However, many SCI men with extremely poor quality ejaculates can give no history of testicular infection.

The quality of electroejaculates in SCI men performing intermittent catheterization or who have undergone sphincterotomy as methods for emptying the bladder is superior when compared to those who achieve bladder drainage with an indwelling Foley catheter or high pressure reflex voiding[72]. This may be due to inflammation of the ejaculatory ducts from a urethral catheter or high pressure voiding causing reflux of urine into the ducts. This type of reflex has been demonstrated on video urodynamics in SCI men with poor results from EEJ[72].

Elevated scrotal temperatures are known to decrease spermatogenesis[94] and this is a concern in men who are confined to a wheelchair for much of the day. In SCI men, both elevated and unchanged scrotal temperatures compared to non-injured controls have been described[95–96], but no significant correlation to poor sperm quality has been reported.

Many of the potential reasons for poor sperm quality in spinal cord patients are not applicable to other conditions. Men who have undergone RPLND have no neurological problems other than absence of emission. Their bladders function normally, they are not prone to urinary or seminal infection, yet they exhibit similar deficiencies in sperm quality[73].

Experimentally, Chang has shown by denervation of the inferior mesenteric plexus only in rats that significant epididymal changes occur. These include stagnation of sperm flow through the epididymis and change in computer determined motility characteristics. In a recent summary at the 1994 meeting of the American Society of Andrology, Chang suggested that epididymal dysfunction may result from denervation of the testis at the inferior mesenteric plexus level[97]. These experimental studies may mimic closely the clinical situation seen in patients after RPLND.

USE OF ASSISTED REPRODUCTIVE TECHNOLOGY PROCEDURES WITH EJACULATION INDUCTION

Home insemination by the patient or partner is a viable option under certain circumstances. Necessary factors include a good quality ejaculate and ability of the patient or partner to obtain the specimen at home. Potential candidates include SCI men without dysreflexia who respond to vibrator stimulation. Some men with premature and idiopathic anejaculation may also be candidates as mentioned earlier in this chapter. In SCI men, we believe that cycle fecundity will be lower with home insemination when compared to accurately timed IUI due to the poor sperm quality and impaired cervical mucus transport. Also, prolonged contact with leukocytes and bacteria in these non-washed specimens of SCI men may further impair sperm motility. Nevertheless, if ejaculation of an excellent and clean specimen can be obtained and successful vaginal insemination carried out, the costs to the patients are minimal.

Sperm processing is advisable in most patients following ejaculation induction. If IUI is being performed the seminal plasma needs to be removed prior to insemination, but other factors are also important. As mentioned earlier, the incidence of culture-proven seminal infection is 56% in spinal cord injured men undergoing EEJ[93]. Separation techniques, while isolating the motile fraction, also serve to remove bacteria, leukocytes and red blood cells from the specimen. Therefore, sperm processing adds to the safety of the procedure in preventing uterine infection.

Intrauterine insemination (IUI) is our recommended initial procedure in couples attempting to achieve pregnancy. Because of the poor penetration of bovine cervical mucus demonstrated in EEJ sperm in the laboratory, we feel that circumventing the cervical mucus is optimal.

For those couples failing intrauterine insemination, *in vitro* fertilization and adjunctive procedures (IVF/GIFT/ZIFT) should be strongly considered. Because of the poor sperm survival decreased sperm transport, and also decreased fertilizing capacity, putting the sperm in close proximity of the oocytes has the potential to have a significant impact on the pregnancy rates. Certainly our low cycle fecundity with intrauterine insemination and substantial rate with GIFT would support this notion. Since fertilizing capacity in these sperm seems to be lower than normal, the ZIFT procedure may afford an extra advantage by transferring only those eggs which fertilize. On the other hand, we have had three occasions where partners became pregnant with the GIFT procedure where there was no fertilization demonstrated *in vitro*. ZIFT would have failed in these couples.

The role of micromanipulation in an ejaculatory dysfunction treatment program remains to be determined. Pregnancies have been obtained by micromanipulation[98] and ICSI (Siösteen, 1994, personal communication) utilizing sperm obtained by ejaculation induction. Couples who fail to demonstrate fertilization during IVF should be excellent candidates for ICSI. In men whose vibrator-induced or EEJ specimens demonstrate very severe oligoasthenospermia, ICSI has the potential to improve fertility substantially.

References

1. Dubin, L. and Amelar, R. D. (1971). Etiologic factors in 1,294 consecutive cases of male infertility. *Fertil. Steril.*, **22**, 469–74
2. Thomas, A. J. (1983). Ejaculatory dysfunction. *Fertil. Steril.*, **39**, 445–54
3. Prins, G. and Zaneveld, L. (1980). Radiographic study of fluid transport in the rabbit vas deferens during sexual rest and after sexual activity. *J. Reprod. Fertil.*, **58**, 311–19
4. Masters, W. H. and Johnson, V. E. (1970). *Human Sexual Inadequacy*. (Boston: Little, Brown)
5. Kaplan, H. S. (1989). *PE – How to Overcome Premature Ejaculation*, pp. 43–60. (New York: Brunner/Mazel)
6. Stewart, D. E. and Ohl, D. A. (1989). Idiopathic anejaculation treated by electroejaculation. *Int. J. Psych. Med.*, **19**, 263–8
7. Brooks, M. E., Berezin, M. and Braf, Z. (1980). Treatment of retrograde ejaculation with imipramine. *Urology*, **15**, 353–5
8. Eppel, S. M. and Berzin, M. (1984). Pregnancy following treatment of retrograde ejaculation with clomipramine hydrochloride. A report of 3 cases. *S. Afr. Med. J.*, **66**, 889–91
9. Stewart, B. H. and Bergant, J. A. (1974). Correction of retrograde ejaculation by sympathomimetic medication: preliminary report. *Fertil. Steril.*, **25**, 1073–4
10. Abrahams, J. I., Solish, G. I., Boorjian, P. and Waterhouse, R. K. (1975). The surgical correction of retrograde ejaculation. *J. Urol.*, **114**, 888–90
11. Middleton, R. G. and Urry, R. L. (1986). The Young–Dees operation for the correction of retrograde ejaculation. *J. Urol.*, **136**, 1208–9

12. Biering-Sørensen, F. and Sønksen, J. (1992). Penile erection in men with spinal cord or cauda equina lesions. *Semin. Neurol.*, **12**, 98–105
13. Sønksen, J. and Biering-Sørensen, F. (1992). Fertility in men with spinal cord or cauda equina lesions. *Semin. Neurol.*, **12**, 106–14
14. Griffith, E. R., Tomko, M. A. and Timms, R. J. (1973). Sexual function in spinal cord-injured patients: a review. *Arch. Phys. Med. Rehab.*, **54**, 539–43
15. Comarr, A. E. (1970). Sexual function among patients with spinal cord injury. *Urol. Int.*, **25**, 134–68
16. Gott, L. J. (1981). Anatomy and physiology of male sexual response and fertility as related to spinal cord injury. In Sha'ked, A. (ed.) *Human Sexuality and Rehabilitation Medicine. Sexual Functioning Following Spinal Cord Injury*, pp. 67–73. (Baltimore, London: Williams & Wilkins)
17. Munro, D., Horne, H. W. and Paull, D. P. (1948). The effect of injury to the spinal cord and cauda equina on the sexual potency of men. *N. Engl. J. Med.*, **239**, 903–11
18. Talbot, H. (1955). The sexual function in paraplegia. *J. Urol.*, **73**, 91–100
19. Zeitlin, A. B., Cottrell, T. L. and Lloyd, F. A. (1957). Sexology of the paraplegic male. *Fertil Steril.*, **8**, 337–44
20. Bors, E. and Comarr, A. E. (1960). Neurological disturbances of sexual function with special reference to 529 patients with spinal cord injury. *Urol. Surv.*, **10**, 191–222
21. Jackson, R. W. (1972). Sexual rehabilitation after cord injury. *Paraplegia*, **10**, 50–5
22. Piera, J. B. (1973). The establishment of a prognosis for genito-sexual function in the paraplegic and tetraplegic male. *Paraplegia*, **10**, 271–8
23. Guttmann, L. (1976). The sexual problem. In Guttmann, L. (ed.) *Spinal Cord Injuries. Comprehensive Management and Research*, pp. 474–505. (Oxford: Blackwell Scientific Publications)
24. Comarr, A. E. (1985). Sexuality and fertility among spinal cord and/or cauda equina injuries. *J. Am. Paraplegia Soc.*, **8**, 67–75
25. Taylor, T. K. and Coolican, M. J. (1988). Injuries of the conus medullaris. *Paraplegia*, **26**, 393–400
26. Frankel, H. L. and Mathias, C. J. (1980). Severe hypertension patients with high spinal cord lesions undergoing electroejaculation – management with prostaglandin E_2. *Paraplegia*, **18**, 293–9
27. Brindley, G. S. (1981). Reflex ejaculation under vibratory stimulation in paraplegic men. *Paraplegia*, **19**, 299–302
28. Brindley, G. S. (1984). The fertility of men with spinal injuries. *Paraplegia*, **22**, 337–48
29. Steinberger, R. E., Ohl, D. A., Bennett, C. J., McCabe, M. and Wang, S. C. (1990). Nifedipine pretreatment for autonomic dysreflexia during electroejaculation. *Urology*, **36**, 228–31
30. Sønksen, J., Biering-Sørensen, F. and Kristensen, J. K. (1994). Ejaculation induced by penile vibratory stimulation in men with spinal cord lesion. The importance of the vibratory amplitude. *Paraplegia*, **32**, 651–60
31. Rossier, A. B., Ziegler, W. H., Duchosal, P. W. and Meylan, J. (1971). Sexual function and dysreflexia. *Paraplegia*, **9**, 51–63
32. Winfield, H. and Lange, P. (1987). Modern concepts about fertility after treatment for nonseminomatous testicular cancer. *A.U.A. Update Ser.*, **6**, 1–7
33. Donohue, J. P. (1977). Retroperitoneal lymphadenectomy: the anterior approach including bilateral suprarenal–hilar dissection. *Urol. Clin. North Am.*, **4**, 509–21
34. Donohue, J. P. and Rowland, R. G. (1981). Complications of retroperitoneal lymph node dissection. *J. Urol.*, **125**, 338–40
35. Donohue, J. P., Foster, R. S., Rowland, R. G., Bihrle, R., Jones, J. and Geier, G. (1990). Nerve-sparing retroperitoneal lymphadenectomy with preservation of ejaculation. *J. Urol.*, **144**, 287–91
36. Kedia, K., Markland, C. and Fraley, E. (1975). Sexual function following high retroperitoneal lymphadenectomy. *J. Urol.*, **114**, 237–9
37. Ross, M. A. (1993). Neuropathies associated with diabetes. *Med. Clin. North Am.*, **77**, 111–24
38. Kaiser, F. E. and Korenman, S. G. (1988). Impotence in diabetic men. *Am. J. Med.*, **85**, 147–52
39. Ellenberg, M. and Weber, H. (1966). Retrograde ejaculation in diabetic neuropathy. *Ann. Intern. Med.*, **65**, 1237–46
40. Volpe, A., Artini, P. G., Coukos, G., Uccelli, E., Marchini, E. and Genazzani, A. R. (1992). Sperm retrieval for direct intraperitoneal insemination in a diabetic with retrograde ejaculation. A case report. *J. Reprod. Med.*, **37**, 219–20
41. Valleroy, M. L. and Kraft, G. H. (1984). Sexual dysfunction in multiple sclerosis. *Arch. Phys. Med. Rehab.*, **65**, 125–8
42. Ohl, D., Grainger, R., Bennett, C., Randolph, J., Seager, S. and McCabe, M. (1989). Successful use of electroejaculation in two multiple sclerosis patients including a report of a pregnancy ultilizing intrauterine insemination. *Neurol. Urodynam.*, **8**, 195–8
43. Suominen, J. J., Kilkku, P. P., Taina, E. J. and Puntala, P. V. (1991). Successful treatment of infertility due to retrograde ejaculation by instillation of serum-containing medium into the bladder. A case report. *Int. J. Androl.*, **14**, 87–90
44. Shangold, G. A., Cantor, B. and Schreiber, J. R. (1990). Treatment of infertility due to retrograde ejaculation: a simple, cost-effective method. *Fertil. Steril.*, **54**, 175–7
45. Urry, R. L., Middleton, R. G. and McGavin, S. (1986). A simple and effective technique for increasing pregnancy rates in couples with retrograde ejaculation. *Fertil. Steril.*, **46**, 1124–7
46. van der Linden, P. J., Nan, P. M., te Velde, E. R. and

van Kooy, R. J. (1992). Retrograde ejaculation: successful treatment with artificial insemination. *Obstet. Gynecol.*, **79**, 126–8
47. Vernon, M., Wilson, E., Muse, K., Estes, S. and Curry, T. (1988). Successful pregnancies from men with retrograde ejaculation with the use of washed sperm and gamete intrafallopian tube transfer (GIFT). *Fertil. Steril.*, **50**, 822–4
48. Spira, R. (1956). Artificial insemination after intrathecal injection of neostigmine in a paraplegic. *Lancet*, **1**, 670–1
49. Guttman, L. and Walsh, J. J. (1971). Prostigmine assessment test of fertility in spinal man. *Paraplegia*, **9**, 39–51
50. Chapelle, P. A., Jondet, M., Durand, J. and Grossiord, A. (1976). Pregnancy of the wife of a complete paraplegic by homologous insemination after an intrathecal injection of neostigmine. *Paraplegia*, **14**, 173–7
51. Otani, T., Kondo, A. and Takita, T. (1986). A paraplegic fathering a child after an intrathecal injection of neostigmine: case report. *Paraplegia*, **24**, 32–7
52. Chapelle, P. A., Blanquart, F., Puech, A. J. and Held, J. P. (1983). Treatment of anejaculation in the total paraplegic by subcutaneous injection of physostigmine. *Paraplegia*, **21**, 30–6
53. Chapelle, P. A., Roby, B. A., Yakovleff, A. and Bussel, B. (1988). Neurological correlations of ejaculation and testicular size in men with a complete spinal cord section. *J. Neurol. Neurosurg. Psych.*, **51**, 197–202
54. Blockmans, D. and Steeno, O. (1988). Physostigmine as a treatment for anejaculation with paraplegic men. *Andrologia*, **20**, 311–13
55. Rawicki, H. B. and Hill, S. (1991). Semen retrieval in spinal cord injured men. *Paraplegia*, **29**, 443–6
56. Sobrero, A. J., Stearns, H. E. and Blair, J. H. (1965). Technique for the induction of ejaculation in humans. *Fertil. Steril.*, **16**, 765–7
57. Szasz, G. and Carpenter, C. (1989). Clinical observations in vibratory stimulation of the penis of men with spinal cord injury. *Arch. Sex. Behav.*, **18**, 461–74
58. Beretta, G., Chelo, E. and Zanollo, A. (1989). Reproductive aspects in spinal cord injured males. *Paraplegia*, **27**, 113–18
59. Tarabulcy, E. (1972). Sexual function in the normal and in paraplegia. *Paraplegia*, **10**, 201–8
60. Francois, N., Jouannet, P. and Maury, M. (1983). Genitosexual function of paraplegics. *J. Urol. (Paris)*, **89**, 159–64
61. Sarkarati, M., Rossier, A. B. and Fam, B. A. (1987). Experience in vibratory and electro-ejaculation techniques in spinal cord injury patients: a preliminary report. *J. Urol.*, **138**, 59–62
62. Beilby, J. A. and Keogh, E. J. (1989). Spinal cord injuries and anejaculation. *Paraplegia*, **27**, 152
63. Siösteen, A., Forssman, L., Steen, Y., Sullivan, L. and Wickstrom, I. (1990). Quality of semen after repeated ejaculation treatment in spinal cord injury men. *Paraplegia*, **28**, 96–104
64. Learmouth, J. R. (1931). A contribution to the neurophysiology of the urinary bladder in man. *Brain*, **54**, 147–76
65. Horne, H. W., Paull, D. P. and Munro, D. (1948). Fertility studies in the human male with traumatic injuries of the spinal cord and cauda equina. *N. Engl. J. Med.*, **239**, 337–48
66. Thomas, R. J., McLeish, G. and McDonald, I. A. (1975). Electroejaculation of the paraplegic male followed by pregnancy. *Med. J. Austr.*, **2**, 789–9
67. Bennett, C. J., Ayers, J. W. T., Randolph, J. F. J., Seager, S. W., McCabe, M., Moinipanah, R. and McGuire, E. J. (1987). Electroejaculation of paraplegic males followed by pregnancies. *Fertil. Steril.*, **48**, 1070–2
68. Linsenmayer, T., Wilmot, C. and Anderson, R. U. (1989). The effects of the electroejaculation procedure on sperm motility. *Paraplegia*, **27**, 465–9
69. Perkash, I., Martin, D. E., Warner, H. and Speck, V. (1990). Electroejaculation in spinal cord injury patients: simplified new equipment and technique. *J. Urol.*, **143**, 305–7
70. Lucas, M. G., Hargreave, T. B., Edmond, P., Creasey, G. H., McParland, M. and Seager, S. W. (1991). Sperm retrieval by electro-ejaculation. Preliminary experience in patients with secondary anejaculation. *Br. J. Urol.*, **67**, 191–4
71. Wang, Y. H., Chiang, H. S., Wu, C. H. and Lien, I. N. (1992). Electroejaculation in spinal cord injured males. *J. Formos. Med. Assoc.*, **91**, 413–8
72. Ohl, D. A., Bennett, C. J., McCabe, M., Menge, A. C. and McGuire, E. J. (1989). Predictors of success in electroejaculation of spinal cord injured men. *J. Urol.*, **142**, 1483–6
73. Ohl, D. A., Denil, J., Bennett, C. J., Randolph, J. F., Menge, A. C. and McCabe, M. (1991). Electroejaculation following retroperitoneal lymphadenectomy. *J. Urol.*, **145**, 980–3
74. Ohl, D. A. (1993). AFS Electroejaculation Registry. *Presented at the 1993 Annual Meeting of the American Fertility Society*, Montreal, Quebec, Canada, 14 October
75. Brindley, G. S., Scott, G. I. and Hendry, W. F. (1986). Vas cannulation with implanted sperm reservoirs for obstructive azoospermia or ejaculatory failure. *Br. J. Urol.*, **58**, 721–3
76. Berger, R. E., Muller, C. H., Smith, D., Forster, M., Moore, D., McIntosh, R. and Stewart, B. (1986). Operative recovery of vasal sperm from anejaculatory men: Preliminary report. *J. Urol.*, **135**, 948–50
77. Bustillo, M. and Rajfer, J. (1986). Pregnancy following insemination with sperm aspirated directly from vas deferens. *Fertil. Steril.*, **46**, 144–6
78. Macourt, D., Engel, S., Jones, R. F. and Zaki, M. (1991). Pregnancy by Gamete Intrafallopian Transfer (GIFT) with sperm aspirated from the vaso–epididymal junction of SCI men: Case report. *Paraplegia*, **29**, 550–3

79. Hovatta, O. and von Smitten, K. (1993). Sperm aspiration from vas deferens and *in-vitro* fertilization in cases of non-treatable anejaculation. *Hum. Reprod.*, **8**, 1689–91
80. Brindley, G. S., Sauerwein, D. and Hendry, W. F. (1989). Hypogastric plexus stimulators for obtaining semen from paraplegic men. *Br. J. Urol.*, **64**, 72–7
81. Denil, J., Ohl, D. A., Menge, A. C., Keller, L. M. and McCabe, M. (1992). Functional characteristics of sperm obtained by electroejaculation. *J. Urol.*, **147**, 69–72
82. Hirsch, I. H., Sedor, J., Callahan, H. J. and Staas, W. E. (1992). Antisperm antibodies in seminal plasma of spinal cord-injured men. *Urology*, **39**, 243–7
83. Buch, J. P. and Zorn, B. H. (1993). Evaluation and treatment of infertilility in spinal cord injured men through rectal probe electroejaculation. *J. Urol.*, **149**, 1350–4
84. Sønksen, J. O., Drewes, A. M., Biering, S. F. and Giwercman, A. J. (1991). [Vibration-induced reflex ejaculation in patients with spinal cord injuries]. *Ugeskr. Laeger*, **153**, 2888–90
85. Linsenmeyer, T. A. and Perkash, I. (1991). Infertility in men with spinal cord injury. *Arch. Phys. Med. Rehab.*, **72**, 747–54
86. Hirsch, I. H., McCue, P., Allen, J., Lee, J. and Staas, W. E. (1991). Quantitative testicular biopsy in spinal cord injured men: comparison to fertile controls. *J. Urol.*, **146**, 337–41
87. Stemmerman, G. N., Weiss, L., Averbach, O. and Friedman, M. (1950). A study of the germinal epithelium in male paraplegics. *Am. J. Clin. Pathol.*, **20**, 24–34
88. Bors, E., Engle, E. T., Rosenquist, R. C. and Holliger, V. H. (1950). Fertility in paraplegic males: a preliminary report of endocrine studies. *J. Clin. Endocrinol.*, **10**, 381–98
89. Perkash, I., Martin, D. E., Warner, H., Blank, M. S. and Collins, D. C. (1985). Reproductive biology of paraplegics: results of semen collection, testicular biopsy and serum hormone evaluation. *J. Urol.*, **134**, 284–8
90. Brindley, G. S. (1983). Physiology of erection and management of paraplegic infertility. In Hargreave, T. B. (ed.) *Male Infertility*, pp. 261–79. (Berlin: Springer-Verlag)
91. Halstead, L. S., VerVoort, S. and Seager, S. W. (1987). Rectal probe electrostimulation in the treatment of anejaculatory spinal cord injured men. *Paraplegia*, **25**, 120–9
92. Engh, E., Clausen, O. P. F., Purvis, K. and Stien, R. (1993). Sperm quality assessed by flow cytometry and accessory sex gland function in spinal cord injured men after repeated vibration-induced ejaculation. *Paraplegia*, **31**, 3–12
93. Ohl, D. A., Denil, J., Fitzgerald, S. K., McCabe, M., McGuire, E. J., Menge, A. C. and Randolph, J. F. (1992). Fertility of spinal cord injured males: effect of genitourinary infection and bladder management on results of electroejaculation. *J. Am. Paraplegia Soc.*, **15**, 53–9
94. Amelar, R. D. and Dubin, L. (1977). Other factors affecting male infertility. In Amelar, R. D., L. Dubin and P. C. Walsh (eds.) *Male Infertility*, pp. 69–102. (Philadelphia: W. B. Sauders)
95. Morales, P. A. and Hardin, J. (1958). Scrotal and testicular temperature studies in paraplegics. *J. Urol.*, **79**, 972–5
96. Brindley, G. S. (1982). Deep scrotal temperature and the effect on it of clothing, air temperature, activity, posture and paraplegia. *Br. J. Urol.*, **54**, 49–55
97. Chang, T. S. K. (1994). *Presentation to the American Society of Andrology*, Post-Graduate Course, Springfield, IL
98. Toledo, A. A., Tucker, M. J., Bennett, J. K., Green, B. G., Kort, H. I., Wiker, S. R. and Wright, G. (1992). Electroejaculation in combination with *in vitro* fertilization and gamete micromanipulation for treatment of anejaculatory male infertility. *Am. J. Obstet. Gynecol.*, **167**, 322–5

Therapeutic prospects in the treatment of the male factor 35

S. Oehninger

INTRODUCTION

Contemporary methods of assisted reproduction have undoubtedly enhanced the opportunities for conception in couples suffering from male infertility. However, the causes of male infertility are multiple, and current therapies (including assisted reproductive techniques) do not usually address an etiological or pathophysiological origin. With the exception of surgically correctable entities of the male genital tract and some ejaculatory disorders, the male factor is still treated either empirically (i.e. controversial and unproven medical therapies) or through the use of assisted reproductive techniques. Despite an explosive growth in reproductive biology research, the reality is that there has been virtually no advance in the clinical practice of male infertility except for assisted reproductive modalities. These have enhanced the clinical pregnancy rates significantly and consequently are increasingly being requested by patients desiring children.

Although efficient in some cases, assisted reproductive techniques do not directly address the underlying problem and depend upon 'getting the gametes closer together' to try to enhance the chances of fertilization. Different sperm separation methods are used to retrieve the morphologically and functionally superior sperm from the ejaculate, and these 'elite' spermatozoa are directed into the uterus (intrauterine insemination) or the Fallopian tubes (transcervical tubal insemination). In the most advanced and successful forms, sperm and oocytes are placed together either inside the Fallopian tubes (gamete intrafallopian transfer (GIFT)) or in a culture dish (*in vitro* fertilization (IVF)), followed by transfer of embryos to the uterine cavity or tubes (zygote intrafallopian transfer (ZIFT)). IVF is considered the most efficient method to treat the male factor and provides the opportunity to directly corroborate whether the crucial step of fertilization is accomplished.

IVF may circumvent different types of male factor abnormalities including some ejaculatory disorders (sometimes in combination with pharmacological interventions or electroejaculation), some congenital anomalies (combined with sperm microaspiration from the epididymis in cases of congenital absence of the vas deferens), immunological problems and idiopathic infertility (oligozoospermia, asthenozoospermia or teratozoospermia, alone or in combination)[1].

Unfortunately, over 40% of male infertility cases are still considered 'idiopathic'. On many occasions, one or more sperm features may be found to be abnormal but the lack of understanding of the subjacent pathology clearly limits the options to approach these entities in a more rational way. In this article, it is my intention to present (a) my views on the problem of 'idiopathic' male infertility, focusing on current diagnostic tools and the impact of assisted reproduction, and (b) my perception of future therapeutic prospects.

Assisted reproductive techniques, and IVF in particular, have provided a unique arena to diagnose more subtle gamete defects. It is this diagnostic aspect that I will discuss first since, in my opinion, it has led to a better understanding of sperm (dys)functions related to the process of fertilization. Only the understanding and unraveling of the facts of male reproductive physiology and how they are affected by disease, will enable us to design specific and pathophysiologically directed therapies.

CURRENT DIAGNOSIS AND MANAGEMENT OF THE MALE FACTOR

The semen analysis

The cornerstone of the andrological evaluation in all cases is a thorough history and physical evaluation followed by repeated semen analyses. Despite the significant advances, many laboratories and physicians in reproductive health care have not used or understood methodologies available for work-up of the infertile couple. The standard semen analysis still remains, in many occasions, a poorly performed test[2]. This is unfortunate because there is an important role for the *in vitro* evaluation of sperm quality in the andrology laboratory.

The ideal *in vitro* evaluation of sperm quality should simultaneously quantify attributes representing different features required for fertility[3]. Still, the relative contribution of these features for prediction of fertilization and/or pregnancy is not completely understood. In my opinion, the laboratory evaluation of sperm quality/quantity should be approached using a sequential, multistep analysis[4,5]. The initial step (or entry-level tier) consists of the so-called basic semen evaluation. This includes determination of seminal volume, pH, viscosity, presence of agglutination and sperm concentration, motility and morphology. The microscopic assessment of sperm quality can be done either using a phase-contrast microscope or utilizing a computerized system (CASA). For morphology evaluation, the strict criteria method is gaining acceptance as the most valuable technique due to its high predictive power for fertilization and pregnancy outcome in assisted reproduction[6]. A bacteriological evaluation and an immunological investigation should be performed early on to direct specific therapies.

The second step (or second-level tier) includes a more advanced assessment of sperm motion parameters using CASA, including the determination of hyperactivated motility. In addition, examination of the acrosome reaction (spontaneous and agonist-induced) and some biochemical features should be performed provided that they demonstrate a high predictive value for fertilization or pregnancy outcome. Some of these might include determination of acrosin, ATP and creatine kinase content, generation of reactive oxygen species and changes in intracellular calcium concentration in response to specific agonists. Ideally, the secondary screen would test individual sperm by flow cytometric analysis[3].

The tertiary step, probably conducted in only some selected samples, includes an evaluation of those sperm functions directly related to fertilization, i.e. sperm–zona pellucida binding and penetration, sperm–oocyte penetration, nuclear decondensation and assessment of chromatic–DNA normality[4,5].

Failure of fertilization: a sequential approach to manage the difficult patient

Severe disorders of fertilization (including failed and delayed fertilization) occur in up to 10% of IVF cycles[7,8]. Whereas these abnormalities may initially point to inadequately timed oocyte insemination or inappropriate *in vitro* culture conditions, when repetitive, they are associated with severe gamete defects that act as significant contributors[5]. Whatever the underlying causes, such factors combine to have a negative impact on the overall IVF results. Additionally, subtle gamete defects may also be responsible for failure of natural reproduction. We have used the results of predictive fertilization bioassays (hemizona assay, or HZA and hamster oocyte–sperm penetration assay, or SPA), IVF treatment, fertile donor cross-match testing using either sperm or oocytes at the time of IVF and oocyte micromanipulation for assisted fertilization, to establish a pathophysiological diagnosis in cases of recurrent failed fertilization *in vitro* (Figure 1). Disorders of sperm function manifested at the level of zona binding, zona penetration, oolemma fusion and oocyte disorders (abnormal sperm head decondensation), were identified and considered to represent the specific gamete defects that led to repetitive abnormal sperm–oocyte interaction in these patients[5,9].

These findings indicate that the sequential application of andrology tests, combined with information derived from IVF, may permit identification of specific sperm–oocyte dysfunctions. The order of progression may be important because those sperm defects that prevent tight binding of sperm to the

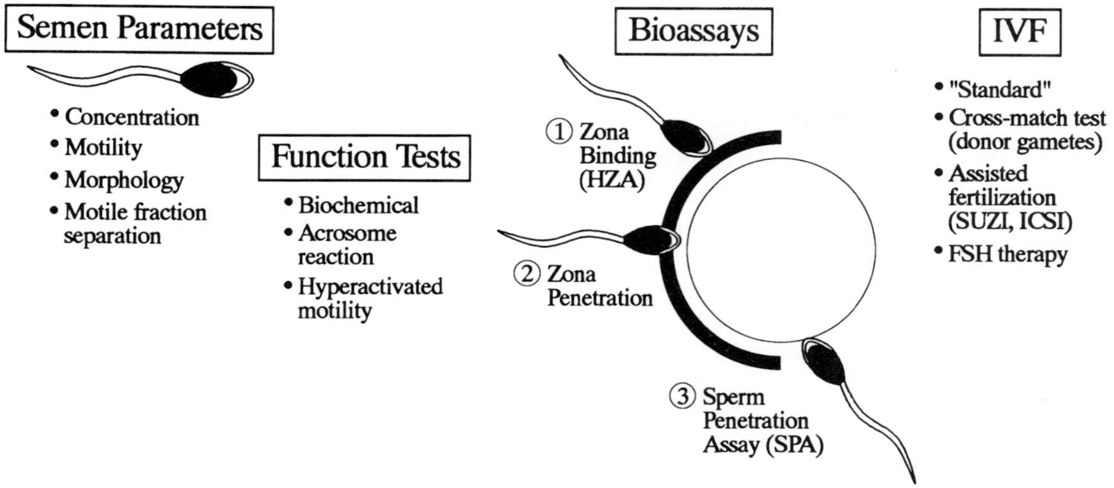

Figure 1 Diagnostic scheme to establish a stepwise progressive diagnosis in cases of recurrent failed IVF

zona pellucida or prevent its penetration will negate subsequent functional tests. Accordingly, the HZA should be performed first among the tertiary assays. Men whose specimens demonstrate adequate tight binding and penetration under HZA conditions can be examined next for oolemma fusion, sperm head decondensation and pronuclear formation capacities in sequence.

When repetitive failure of fertilization occurs and sperm defects are suspected or identified, we currently give those couples the option of systemic follicle stimulating hormone (FSH) therapy to the infertile man[10,11], or assisted fertilization techniques[12]. Although successful both in terms of fertilization and pregnancy we still consider the use of FSH therapy as experimental, and we have emphasized the need for a randomized, prospectively designed, placebo-controlled study to support the use of this therapy in severe male factor cases with failed fertilization.

Different oocyte micromanipulation techniques for assisted fertilization currently being used include partial zona dissection (PZD)[13], subzonal sperm insemination (SUZI)[14] and intracytoplasmic sperm injection (ICSI)[15]. The use of these techniques followed a multiplicity of animal studies showing the possibility of fertilization and normality of offspring[12]. Low efficiency and a limited number of delivered pregnancies were initially presented in the literature, in particular with the PZD and SUZI techniques. The improvement in methodology and sperm preparation techniques has translated into better pregnancy rates, in particular when treating couples with SUZI[15]. Recently, excellent results have been reported when using ICSI[16,17], a technique initially developed in Norfolk[18]. If these outstanding results are replicated by other centers when treating patients with recurrent failed fertilization, it may be demonstrated that ICSI is the modality of choice when assisted fertilization is needed. Clearly, these techniques have a high degree of complexity and require expensive equipment and highly qualified and skilled personnel to obtain consistent results.

RECENT PROGRESS IN MALE REPRODUCTIVE BIOLOGY AND ITS IMPACT ON THERAPEUTIC STRATEGIES

Recently, major advances have occurred in the area of molecular and cellular endocrinology of the testis, including new knowledge on gonadotropin receptors, signal transduction and regulation of spermatogenesis. In addition, facts relevant to epididymal function and some post-testicular events are beginning to be unraveled. Still, spermatogenesis cannot be readily altered for therapeutic benefit. Classical endocrinology, paracrinology, techniques of cell biology and a molecular biology approach have all contributed to the acquisition of new information.

Gonadotropins and androgens and their receptors

Many and varied hormonal treatments have been used on the presumption that gonadotropins should stimulate spermatogenesis resulting in an increased sperm number and/or function. However, pituitary and urinary gonadotropins (in particular luteinizing hormone (LH) and combinations of FSH-LH), anti-estrogens, and the rebound rise of gonadotropins after suppression with testosterone have no dramatic effect[19]. Similarly, low dose androgen and human chorionic gonadotropin (hCG) therapy may be more detrimental than beneficial. There may be a real basis for a pathophysiological-directed hormonal therapy in cases of isolated FSH deficiency and slow pulsatile LH secretion. Nevertheless, clinical trials have produced unconvincing results[20–22].

Because defects leading to sperm fertilization failure could be hypothetically due to a deficiency in the interaction of the developing sperm cell and the Sertoli cell within the seminiferous tubule, the systemic effect of FSH therapy in the context of the IVF setting has been examined[10,11]. Preliminary evidence indicates that some patients with failed fertilization may benefit from this treatment. Animal evidence (non-human primate) suggested important actions of FSH early during spermatogenesis[23] and clinical results have provided evidence for altered binding activity of serum FSH in some male infertility patients[24]. Development of a 'highly purified' FSH, a recombinant FSH and FSH analogs (agonists) will be useful for the elucidation of the physiological role of FSH and may also contribute as pharmacological interventions[25]. To this end, a theoretical conformational model of FSH has been constructed which allowed the prediction of conformational receptor binding sites. Based on these predictions, peptides could be synthesized with FSH agonistic or antagonistic effects thereby aiding in both pro-fertility and contraceptive research[25,26].

Our understanding of the molecular regulation of the gonadotropin receptors will be enhanced by the reported sequencing of the mouse LH and FSH receptor gene promoters[27], and by the understanding of the mechanisms of down-regulation of the Sertoli cell–FSH receptor[25]. The importance of oligosaccharide moieties in the gonadotropin molecule for determining biological activity has been clarified. The sugar residues, although not essential, are important for maximum gonadotropin bioactivity, probably by stabilizing the tertiary structure of the hormone[25].

Androgen receptor defects are present in some men with severe spermatogenic disorders and extensive molecular work on the androgen receptor has shown that gene mutations may lead to complete or partial androgen resistance[28]. A new open field of possible interrelationships between hormonal steroids and cerebral neurotransmitters is evolving. Depending on the phase of life, the metabolism of androgens in the brain may be crucial for 'organization' of the brain towards a male pattern, whereas at later stages 5α-reduction of androgens may be important for feedback regulation of LH secretion and, therefore, spermatogenesis control[25].

Spermatogenesis

Disorders of spermatogenesis are probably the etiologic cause in a majority of cases with 'idiopathic' male infertility. The basis of hypospermatogenesis associated with poor sperm numbers, abnormal motility and increased frequency of abnormally shaped spermatozoa is, however, still unknown. It is puzzling that despite recent major advances on basic testicular physiology there is very little understanding of the more serious causes of male infertility.

In men with 'idiopathic' infertility there is no apparent hormonal deficiency. FSH concentrations are often normal or even high. Testicular biopsy often reveals maturation arrest or quantitatively insufficient spermatogenesis. The pulsatility of GnRH may sometimes be deficient, and although serum FSH may be returned to normal levels by pulsatile GnRH therapy no improvements in semen are demonstrable[29]. Isoforms of gonadotropins with different glycosylation patterns could account for altered gonadotropin bioactivity[30]. Alternatively, defects at the FSH or androgen receptor level could be implicated either at the ligand–receptor interaction or at the post-receptor level. Errors in transcription, translation or post-translational modifications of peptides could lead to alterations in the internal milieu that are detrimental for spermatogenesis[29].

However, what paracrine factors are relevant for spermatogenesis, and can they be useful in the design of new therapies[31]? Only the final products of spermatogenesis – the spermatozoa – are readily amenable to collection and study, whereas the events of the preceding 10 weeks when these sperm were being 'manufactured' are hidden away within the testis. Ideally, what is required is a 'battery of bio-markers' (probably proteins originated in the seminiferous tubule and interstitium), detectable in semen and/or blood, which can provide a reliable and quantitative guide to specific steps of spermatogenesis[32]. Monitoring of such markers in fertile and infertile men might enable identification of the germane biochemical steps in spermatogenesis and which defects occur frequently. These could then be targeted for development of corrective therapy.

At present, however, spermatogenesis cannot be monitored by measuring Seroli/germ cell-secreted proteins (i.e. inhibin or transferrin) in semen or blood[32]. Paracrine regulation of testicular function is an interesting concept, but the nature of testicular architecture and the multiple interactions occurring at a cellular level makes the design of studies and interpretation of data generated difficult. Immunohistochemistry, mRNA expression and *in situ* hybridization suggest synthesis of a peptide but the final demonstration of specific effects of the factors isolated from testicular tissue and subsequent bioactive characterization is essential[29].

The efficiency of spermatogenesis in the human is low compared to most species. In addition to significant day to day variation in sperm output, a high frequency of abnormally shaped spermatozoa is usually observed even in the ejaculate of fertile men. Germ cell degeneration has been shown to play a pivotal role in the efficiency of spermatogenesis but its determining mechanisms and approaches for prevention remain unclear. Recently, it was shown that missing generations of germ cells along the length of human seminiferous tubules, coupled with a paucity in the number of cells within each generation, contribute to this low efficiency of spermatogenesis[33]. Missing germ cells within generations and lack of developmental synchronization may be major factors causing irregular stages of the spermatogenic cycle in humans.

The immune privilege of the testis, the blood–testis barrier and the testicular microcirculation also appear to be of utmost significance for normal spermatogenesis to ensue[34–36]. These areas of testicular physiology need a more thorough exploration since they may play a role in some forms of subfertility.

Genetics

Genetic abnormalities as a cause for male infertility become increasingly important for our understanding of 'idiopathic' infertility. The most common chromosomal abnormalities are sex chromosome aneuploidy and autosomal translocations[25]. Azoospermia and oligozoospermia occur in patients bearing deletions in the long arm of the Y chromosome[25]. Molecular biology has allowed identification of the probable sex determining gene and sequencing of the Y chromosome[37]. The analysis of terminal deletions in the Y chromosome of sterile men with a normal phenotype but azoospermia led to the assumption of a male fertility gene complex called azoospermia factor. In some of these cases, testicular biopsies reveal either arrest of spermatogenesis at the spermatogonia or early spermatocyte stage or complete absence of germ cells (Sertoli cell-only syndrome)[25].

The identification of genes expressed in a spermatogenic cell type-specific manner (i.e. proto-oncogenes) is also a valuable approach to understand the control of male germ cell differentiation. The interaction of cyclins with a serine/threonine protein kinase might be involved in the reorganization of chromatin in the sperm nucleus[25]. Consequently, such proteins might exert significant effects on processes such as spermatogenic differentiation, sperm function and fertilization.

The potential relationship between male infertility and genetic abnormalities is exemplified in other recent findings. In mice, fertility requires X–Y pairing and a Y-chromosomal 'spermiogenesis' gene mapping to the long arm[38]. The short arm of the mouse Y carries information needed for spermatogonial differentiation and the long arm includes information essential for the normal development of the sperm head (a meiotic block overcome by providing a meiotic pairing partner does not restore fertility due to abnormal sperm head anomalies).

Also in mice, transgenic animals were generated with a human epidermal growth factor (EGF) receptor cDNA[39]. EGF receptor RNA was detected in primary spermatocytes, whereas the synthesis of receptor protein was restricted to elongated spermatids. About half of the homozygous males were sterile because of sperm paralysis associated with an aberrant axonemal structure (missing of outer doublet microtubules in the midpiece), changes resembling those observed in some infertile men. These experiments showed that a sperm motility gene could be inactivated by insertion of an EGF receptor transgene leading to male infertility.

Mutations leading to sperm paralysis and male sterility have also been described in the human, the best characterized entity being the immotile-cilia syndrome[40]. Many ultrastructural defects associated with immotile spermatozoa have been described[41]. Identification of a gene whose function is restricted to spermatogenesis should greatly aid in the molecular disentangling of these processes.

The detection of microdeletions by a novel screening program (combining different hybridization techniques) should be useful in the diagnostic analysis of 'idiopathic' infertility[25]. Furthermore, defects of protamines have been observed in infertile and fertile men with a high incidence of abnormally large sperm heads in their ejaculates[42]. The authors observed a decreased proportion of P2 in relation to P1 and a decreased P2 affinity to DNA in infertile men. Therefore, potential mutations in the human P2 gene could be a cause of infertility in some patients with teratozoospermia.

Epididymal function

In recent years, the epididymis has moved from an organ of relative obscurity to almost being centerstage in a discussion on whether this human organ is truly necessary[43]. This has followed interpretation of data obtained from surgical epididymal bypass and IVF combined with sperm microsurgical aspiration from the epididymis[44]. The bulk of the evidence underscores the importance of the epididymis as an elaborate organ with androgen and temperature-dependent functions concerned with sperm maturation and storage.

The interaction of spermatozoa with epididymal secretions seems to be necessary for acquisition of functions essential for fertilization. It has been claimed that a remedy for some types of infertility might be the incubation of spermatozoa with (bioengineered?) epididymal secretions, under appropriate conditions, before insemination, IVF or other therapies[43]. Clearly, human sperm microaspirated from the epididymis (in cases of congenital absence of the vas deferens, post-inflammatory obstruction or post-vasectomy) can fertilize oocytes under *in vitro* conditions. Nevertheless, the rate of fertilization in these cases is suboptimal (∽30%), but viable pregnancies have been established following the transfer of embryos to the uterus or the Fallopian tubes[44,45]. The *in vitro* fertilizing capacity of epididymal sperm can be enhanced by improved sperm separation techniques (i.e. miniPercoll) and the use of sperm stimulants (i.e. pentoxifylline and 2-deoxyadenosine)[46]. Moreover, oocyte micromanipulation modalities are currently being used to assist fertilization with good success in preliminary reports.

The non-human primate model (cynomolgus monkey) offers the possibility to evaluate the functional and morphological features of spermatozoa microaspirated from different regions of the epididymis without the ethical constraints present in human research. We have demonstrated changes in motility patterns and acrosome reaction capacity associated with morphological differences as sperm travel through the organ[47]. This system may provide valuable information about sperm maturation– capacitation–acquisition of fertilizing capacity and is presently being examined in our laboratories.

The discovery of the association of cystic fibrosis gene mutations with bilateral congenital absence of the vas deferens makes it mandatory for these infertile couples to undergo genetic counseling[48]. One cause of azoospermia in surviving cystic fibrosis patients may be obstruction of epididymal ducts due to congestion with mucoproteins due to a mutant regulatory protein in human epididymal tissue. Less severe forms of the disease may be responsible for infertility in some men[25].

Surgical therapy

The surgical treatment of male infertility consists largely of two types of operations: (1) varicocele repair; and (2) treatment of obstructive azoospermia. Therefore, two of the known leading causes of male infertility can be directly attacked by a surgical approach that can be successful in many cases[4].

Varicocelectomy remains a controversial issue[45]. Many andrologists still question the role of varicocele and the efficacy of varicocelectomy as a treatment of male infertility. Currently, there is little doubt that varicocele is associated with a substantial risk of deteriorating testicular function with time[45]. Although the pathogenesis of altered spermatogenesis is unclear, it appears to be related to an elevated testicular temperature and altered testicular hemodynamics. It is likely that prophylactic varicocelectomy in young men with significant varicocele will reduce the incidence of future infertility[45]. In more mature men, however, the real impact of varicocelectomy still needs to be established, although men with moderate to large varicoceles typically will be offered surgical corrective therapy almost unanimously.

Technical advances have radically altered the prognosis for the treatment of obstructive azoospermia[45,49,50]. Microsurgical repair of vasal obstruction is routinely associated with patency rates >90% and pregnancy rates averaging 50%[45,49]. However, repair of epididymal obstruction remains problematic. It is clear that the more epididymis sperm are exposed to, the greater the fertilizing capacity of sperm. It has recently been shown that the best predictor of microsurgical vasoepididymostomy is the presence of sperm in the epididymal fluid at surgery[49].

Even in experienced hands, vasoepididymostomy frequently fails[45]. In these cases and in men with unreconstructible acquired or congenital lesions, microsurgically aspirated epididymal sperm can be used in conjunction with IVF to salvage pregnancy[44]. This option requires a team approach including optimal surgical technique in the male, good female response to ovarian hyperstimulation to be able to recover multiple fertilizable eggs, and state-of-the-art gamete and embryo culture techniques[45]. Nevertheless, and due to extremely poor sperm motility (and immaturity?), many of these cases are subject to oocyte micromanipulation to assist fertilization.

In vitro fertilization (IVF)

IVF has become not only a successful therapy for many male factor cases but also the ultimate test for sperm fertilizing capacity. Typically, mature (preovulatory) oocytes are inseminated with a high insemination concentration (5×10^5–1×10^6 motile sperm/mL/oocyte) whenever possible[51]. Patients with teratozoospermia and asthenozoospermia, and with at least 0.7×10^6 motile sperm recovered after swim-up or Percoll separation, yield very acceptable rates of fertilization (∽70%, compared with >90% in the non-male factor population)[52]. Because usually the female counterpart shows a favorable response to ovarian hyperstimulation, several embryos are generally available for transfer and even for cryopreservation to be transferred in future cycles.

In addition, other strategies are presently being used to try to enhance fertilization. Some programs have reported good results when using sperm function stimulants (pentoxifylline, 2-deoxyadenosine and maybe progesterone), and different sperm separation methods (Percoll, miniPercoll, swim-up, etc.)[53–57]. In this way, many male factors will have a reasonable chance to achieve a viable pregnancy through 'standard' IVF without the need for assisted fertilization. An increased insemination concentration can sometimes be obtained by inseminating oocytes in microdroplets under oil or using the technique of multiple oocytes per dish.

When severe oligozoospermia is present and the total sperm motile fraction recoverable is $<0.7\times10^6$, oocyte micromanipulation for assisted fertilization is offered to the couple. Patients with this type of severe oligo-asthenozoospermia carry a poor prognosis for fertilization in 'standard' IVF[52]. In addition, patients with severe teratozoospermia (<4% normal morphology by strict criteria), although still able to achieve fertilization, show a significantly decreased implantation rate, thereby composing a poor prognosis group for pregnancy[1,6,52].

Within this context, sperm morphology evaluation is considered critical. Morphology can be used as a biomarker of sperm dysfunctions under *in vitro* conditions[1,9,58–60]. These dysfunctions are multiple and may be all present simultaneously in the same ejaculate or not. They include: dyskinetic abnormalities (including abnormal hyperactivated motility), a deficient spontaneous and exogenously induced acrosome reaction, abnormal sperm–zona pellucida binding, a poor capacity to penetrate zona-free oocytes, and maybe defective nuclear decondensation ability and chromatin-DNA content[58–60].

Ejaculates that contain a high proportion of abnormal spermatozoa depict multiple defects at the cellular level, including an abnormal basal and stimulated intracellular calcium concentration[61], an abnormal creatine kinase content[62,63] and an enhanced capacity to generate reactive oxygen species[64]. Consequently, these spermatozoa show direct signs of deficient membrane-dependent events, as well as cytoplasmic biochemical alterations (possibly an expression of immaturity or deficiencies occurring in late spermatogenesis stages).

The HZA offers the arena in which pre-fertilization (capacitation) and fertilization events can be examined under the appropriate biological conditions, i.e. the zona pellucida[65–70]. We have shown that morphologically superior sperm (sperm with a lower creatine kinase content indicative of maturity) have a significantly higher capacity to bind to the zona pellucida[63]. Therefore, sperm–zona pellucida binding capacity assessed by the HZA reflects multiple aspects of sperm function, which explains its high predictive power for IVF outcome[5,9,58–60,71].

FUTURE DEVELOPMENTS WITH POTENTIAL THERAPEUTIC IMPLICATIONS: AREAS OF EXPECTED ADVANCE

It is expected that some of the previously discussed areas will show major advances that will enable the design of new and improved therapeutic strategies. The impact of these new therapeutic options will be significant only if they are based on and directed by newly gained pathophysiological knowledge. In my view, some of the areas of expected advancement with therapeutic implications are as shown in Table 1.

Table 1 Areas of expected advancement with therapeutical implications for the treatment of male infertility

- Endocrine
- Testis: cellular and molecular
- Testis and epididymis: paracrine and molecular
  - monitoring spermatogenesis
  - monitoring spermiogenesis
  - monitoring sperm maturation/capacitation
- Sperm and oocyte: biochemical and molecular
- Sperm transport in the female tract: dynamics and regulation

Endocrine

A therapeutic option for male factor cases of true 'endocrine' origin, suitable for systemic hormonal therapy, can possibly consist of 'purified' FSH preparations and new FSH analogs[25].

Testis: molecular and genetic

Unraveling of the genetic loci and mechanisms involved in the control of spermatogenesis is mandatory. Specific defects of the Y chromosome (and maybe others) will probably be found to be associated with severe disorders of sperm development[19]. Transgenic mouse technology has allowed the identification of genes or loci that affect the mature germ cells in two different ways[72]. First, overexpression of foreign genes in the testis can impair spermatogenesis. Secondly, the insertion of foreign DNA will occasionally disrupt an active genomic locus, causing a mutation. Some of the insertional mutants have resulted in male infertility due to a deficiency of germ cells or abnormal spermatogenesis. Identification of these disorders should lead to potential gene therapy.

Germ-line therapy is almost certainly a decade or more in the future in terms of practical clinical application[73]. Primary tasks are ways to increase the transfection rate and to provide for site-specific gene insertion. Once these problems are resolved, the adverse effects of defective genes whose expression is normally recessive could be overcome by providing a copy of the normal gene.

The problem of defective genes that are dominantly expressed is more difficult. Techniques to excise the mutant gene, prevent its expression or negate the activity of the mutant mRNA or protein would be required to prevent the manifestation of the disease. Antisense mRNA to cover the transcription initiation site on the DNA or to complex with the sense DNA are possible strategies[73].

Preimplantation genetic diagnosis is now becoming a reality in the clinical arena[73]. Several pregnancies have already been reported after IVF followed by embryo biopsy and transfer in cases of X-linked disease[73,74]. The identification and chromosomal location of genetic defects associated with male infertility may allow the application of polymerase chain reaction technology coupled with assisted reproduction in the foreseeable future. Needless to say, the ethical ramifications of such an approach become enormous and need to be addressed in conjunction[75].

Testis and epididymis: cellular and paracrine

Identification of defects that occur at a cellular level within the testis and the epididymis is surely a formidable task. This should be approached at three levels[32].

Monitoring of spermatogenesis

This focuses our attempts on measuring the levels of spermatogenesis products biosynthesized at specific times during the cycle. In this regard, experimental animal models and new methods to measure such products are needed. Success in germline cyst *in vitro* development in insects and amphibians stresses the territorial requirement of a spermatogenic cell lineage for survival[76]. Spermatogenic and somatic cell lineages may be genetically transformed to sustain a built-in differentiation program that can be monitored upon co-culture. The immortalization of mouse spermatogenic and somatic cells, and the establishment of testicular epithelial cell lines are efforts towards this goal[76].

Monitoring of spermiogenesis

Spermiogenesis is a process that, if abnormal, can lead to defects of sperm release from the seminiferous tubule and disturbances of cytoplasmic elimination late in spermatogenesis[32]. Sperm release is a highly vulnerable process, interrupted frequently by a variety of agents and conditions. Sperm may not be released at all or they may be abnormal in some way, such as having not eliminated all of their cytoplasm[72]. The Sertoli cell is a pivotal actor as a 'gatekeeper' for sperm release, and if abnormal or damaged this process would be impaired. Depletion or altered activity of pituitary and testicular hormones which act through the Sertoli cell probably cause massive failure of sperm release. Chemotherapeutic agents and other gonadotoxins may also have this deleterious effect[77].

Monitoring of sperm maturation and capacitation regulatory events

As a result of abnormal spermiogenesis (and maybe even to earlier disturbances of spermatogenesis) abnormal sperm cells appear in the ejaculate showing signs indicative of defective cytoplasmic elimination and retention of cytoplasm[77]. Those spermatozoa are found in the low density fraction of Percoll gradients and show abnormally high levels of cytoplasmic markers such as creatine kinase, superoxide dismutase, glucose-6-phosphate dehydrogenase and lactate dehydrogenease C_4[64,77,78]. Reactive oxygen species generation is associated with the low density fraction of sperm isolated via Percoll gradients, and may induce membrane lipid peroxidation[79–82]. The correlation between creatine kinase content, high reactive oxygen species generation and abnormal sperm morphology seems to be supportive of this abnormal pathophysiological mechanism[63,64]. In addition, the membrane alterations are responsible for the decreased ability of those spermatozoa to bind to and penetrate the homologous zona pellucida, and to respond inadequately to signals that trigger changes in intracellular calcium levels, the acrosome reaction and hyperactivated motility[51,83].

The knowledge of functional and morphological immaturity should help in the design of preventive and corrective therapies when dealing with ejaculated sperm. These include but are not limited to improved culture conditions, use of membrane protective agents, i.e. antioxidants and others, and better biochemical means of sperm separation.

Spermatozoa and oocyte interaction: cellular and molecular

Specific recognition events between the sperm and oocyte (and its investments) are necessary for fertilization to ensue. At the level of the zona pellucida, ZP3 is considered to have a dual role both as the primary binding site for sperm and for triggering the 'physiological' acrosome reaction[84–86]. Another zona protein, ZP2, is responsible for secondary binding allowing for zona penetration to follow[84,87]. Once in the perivitelline space, the acrosome reacted spermatozoon binds to the oolemma presumably through specific binding sites located in the post-acrosomal area. This description follows a well characterized sequence of events known in several animal species, but poorly understood in the human. HZA results used in conjunction with IVF have provided evidence that sperm–zona pellucida binding is a critical step, and that many cases with failed or very poor fertilization are due to a defective sperm–zona pellucida interaction[9,60,83]. Although other sperm defects may be present simultaneously, the unraveling of the structure and dysfunction of the sperm receptors responsible for zona pellucida and oolemma binding is crucial.

The sperm plasma membrane contains multiple domains possibly related to different functions. For example, non-genomic progesterone receptors have been characterized and may be of significance for regulation of certain functions and triggering of specific responses[88,89]. Mannose-binding sites have also been described and related to fertilization success/failure[90]. We have studied the involvement of saccharide moieties extensively (simple, conjugated and complex sugars) on sperm–zona pellucida interaction[91–94]. For example, fucoidan (a polymer of 1-sulfated fucose) is a potent inhibitor of this interaction. The demonstration of a novel structure of this complex carbohydrate may help us elucidate some of the biochemical aspects of specific gamete recognition events[95].

Multiple putative sperm ligands (or receptors) possibly involved in fertilization have been described recently[96]. In my opinion, the molecular cloning and characterization of a human recombinant ZP3 may provide the best tool for evaluation and characterization of recognition events[97–99]. This recombinant protein must be adequately glycosylated in order to express the biologic effects of 'natural' ZP3. A similar approach will possibly follow by which the cloning of ZP2 may direct the identification of a secondary sperm receptor. In this fashion, important questions about the physiology of human reproduction will be answered. Presence and quantification of these ligands by simple tests may allow for a specific diagnosis followed by a therapy directed to circumvent the particular defect.

Sperm maturation events can be approached in a similar manner. Gene products from the human epididymis that are specifically expressed in this tissue seem to be species specific, i.e. are poorly conserved. Recently, a novel human cDNA encoding a glycopeptide specifically expressed within the human epididymis has been cloned and sequenced[100]. A subclone containing the coding region of the mature peptide was used to generate a recombinant protein in a bacterial system, and the neoprotein used to generate polyclonal antisera. Immunohistochemistry and immunofluorescence showed that the peptide is present both in the epididymal surface and on the sperm surface (subacrosomal equatorial distribution on the head). These and other proteins can be tested in the HZA and analog systems for bioactivity and may lead to the identification of molecules significantly involved in sperm maturation and capacitation.

If a single defect is identified, a specific therapy may evolve. If multiple steps are deficient, then a more complex therapeutic approach could be required. Rather surprisingly, ICSI seems to bypass many types of sperm disorders as communicated in preliminary reports by some groups. It is a rather empirical approach to solve a pathological fertilization dysfunction (associated or not with sperm immaturity and capacitation deficiencies) with a surgical (microsurgical) procedure. Nevertheless, in the absence of more rational therapies, and if the technique is proven to be efficacious in cases with failed fertilization, it should be offered to couples. Current evidence seems to indicate that the normality of delivered babies after ICSI is not compromised[17]. However, caution has to be taken and a continuing evaluation of this aspect is mandatory. ICSI could then be used for assisting fertilization in the severely oligozoospermic patient and also in the patient with severe asthenozoospermia and may be even total sperm immotility. Perhaps ICSI will be the treatment of choice for those cases where microsurgical aspiration of epididymal sperm is performed.

I agree with others in advocating a very conservative approach to the use of assisted fertilization techniques, not because they are ineffective but because in many instances they can be superfluous and hence not cost-effective[101]. Assisted fertilization should only be used when prior total or significant fertilization failure has occurred or when the number of recovered sperm is limited. The use of ICSI to rescue those cycles where heavy conventional insemination has failed needs to be confirmed[101].

Spermatozoa in the female reproductive tract: dynamics and regulation

Sperm transport through the female genital tract is very poorly understood. Studies of sperm migration and storage combined with assessment of the 'physiologic' inductors of capacitation should also constitute a priority in reproductive medicine. In this regard, three different lines of investigation have been suggested: (1) development of new techniques to recover sperm successfully from different regions of the tract; (2) an *in vitro* approach to examine the modulation of reproductive tract fluids on sperm function; and (3) an *in vitro* tissue/cell culture system to investigate the interaction between the specific epithelium and sperm[102].

The available animal data suggest a highly synchronized movement of sperm through the female tract. Very little is known about physiological regulators of capacitation and sperm motility *in vivo*. It has recently been shown that ADP-ribosylation of Rho proteins inhibits sperm motility[103]. *Rho* proteins are low molecular mass GTP-binding proteins. Heterotrimeric regulatory G proteins play a major role in transducing signals across plasma membranes and have been recently found in tail spermatozoa[104,105]. These findings indicate that *Rho* proteins which reportedly regulate the microfilament system are basically involved in sperm motility. The identification of physiological regulators of sperm motility and their mechanism(s) of action will enable us to elaborate therapies that could be utilized to optimize sperm function during their journey through the female genital tract.

CONCLUDING REMARKS

Although considerable progress has been made toward understanding the physiology of the male gamete and its interaction with the oocyte, still much information remains to be discovered to develop more efficient therapeutic opportunities. As the intimate cellular and molecular events of male reproductive biology become apparent, the pathophysiology of human male infertility will be unraveled. The development and standardization of relevant clinical diagnostic tests should follow these advances. Only then will specific and more rational (pathophysiological-directed) therapeutic interventions prove efficacy.

References

1. Acosta, A. A., Oehninger, S., Morshedi, M., Swanson, R. J., Scott, R. and Irianni, F. (1989). Assisted reproduction and treatment of the male factor. *Obstet. Gynecol. Surv.*, **44**, 1–18
2. Urry, R. L. (1992). Advances in diagnosing and treating sperm problems and advanced reproductive techniques. In Smith, J. A. Jr. (ed.) *High Tech Urology: Technology Innovations and their Clinical Applications*, pp. 251–70. (Philadelphia: W. B. Saunders)
3. Amman, R. P. and Hammersted, T. (1993). *In vitro* evaluation of sperm quality: an opinion. *J. Androl.*, **14**, 397–406
4. Oehninger, S., Stecker, T. F. and Acosta, A. (1992). Male infertility: the impact of assisted reproductive technologies. *Curr. Opin. Obstet. Gynecol.*, **4**, 185–96
5. Oehninger, S., Acosta, A. A., Veeck, L., Brzyski, R. G., Kruger, T. F., Muasher, S. J. and Hodgen, G. D. (1991). Recurrent failure of *in vitro* fertilization: role of the hemizona assay (HZA) in the sequential diagnosis of specific sperm/oocyte defects. *Am. J. Obstet. Gynecol.*, **164**, 1210–5
6. Kruger, T. F., Acosta, A., Simmons, K. F., Swanson, R. J., Matta, J. F. and Oehninger, S. (1988). Predictive value of abnormal sperm morphology in *in vitro* fertilization. *Fertil. Steril.*, **49**, 112–17
7. Oehninger, S., Acosta, A. A., Kruger, T. F., Veeck, L. L., Flood, J. and Jones, H. W., Jr. (1990). Failure of fertilization in *in vitro* fertilization: the 'occult' male factor. *J.* In Vitro *Fertil. Embryo Transf.*, **5**, 181–7. Reprinted in Mishell, D. R., Paulsen, C. A. and Lobo, R. A. (eds.) *Year Book of Infertility*, p. 221. (Chicago: Year Book Medical Publishers, 1990)

8. Oehninger, S., Acosta, A. A., Veeck, L. L. and Muasher, S. J. (1989). Delayed fertilization during *in vitro* fertilization/embryo transfer cycles: analysis of causes and impact on overall results. *Fertil. Steril.*, **52**, 990–7
9. Oehninger, S., Hodgen, G. (1991). How to evaluate sperm for assisted reproduction. In DeCherney, A. (ed.) *Assisted Reproduction Reviews*, pp. 15–27. (Baltimore: Williams and Wilkins)
10. Acosta, A., Oehninger, S. and Ertunc, H. (1991). Possible role of pure FSH in the treatment of severe male-factor infertility by assisted reproduction. A preliminary report. *Fertil. Steril.*, **5**, 1150–6
11. Acosta, A. A., Khalifa, E. and Oehninger, S. (1992). Pure human follicle stimulating hormone has a role in the treatment of severe male factor infertility by assisted reproduction: Norfolk's total experience. *Hum. Reprod.*, **7**, 1067–72
12. Iritani, A. (1991). Micromanipulation of gametes for *in vitro* assisted fertilization. *Mol. Reprod. Dev.*, **28**, 199–207
13. Cohen, J., Alikani, M., Malter, H., Adler, A., Talansky, B. and Rosenwaks, Z. (1991). Partial zona dissection or subzonal sperm insertion: microsurgical fertilization alternatives based on evaluation of sperm and embryo morphology. *Fertil. Steril.*, **56**, 696–706
14. Ng, S. C., Bongso, A., Ratnam, S., Sathananthan, H., Chen, C. L. and Wong, P. C. (1988). Pregnancy after transfer of multiple sperm under the zona. *Lancet* **ii**, 790
15. Fishel, S., Dowell, K., Timson, J., Green, S., Hall, J. and Klentzeris, L. (1993). Micro-activated fertilization with human gametes. *Hum. Reprod.*, **8**, 1780–4
16. Palermo, A., Joris, H., Devroey, P. and Van Steirteghem, A. (1992). Pregnancies after intracytoplasmic injection of single spermatozoon into an oocyte. *Lancet*, **34**, 17–18
17. Van Steirteghem, A., Liu, J., Nagy, Z., Joris, H., Tournaye, H., Liebaers, I. and Devroey, P. (1993). Use of assisted fertilization. *Hum. Reprod.*, **8**, 1784–5
18. Lanzendorf, S. F., Maloney, M. K., Veeck, L. L., Slusser, J., Hodgen, G. D. and Rosenwaks, Z. (1988). A preclinical evaluation of pronuclear formation by microinjection of human spermatozoa into human oocytes. *Fertil. Steril.*, **49**, 835–42
19. Baker, W. H. G. (1993). Treatment of male infertility: what does the future hold? *Int. J. Androl.* **16**, 343–8
20. Maroulis, G. B., Parlow, A. and Marshall, I. (1977). Isolated follicle-stimulated hormone deficiency in man. *Fertil. Steril.*, **28**, 818–22
21. Gross, K., Matsumoto, A., Southworth, M. and Bremner, W. (1985). Evidence for decreased luteinizing hormone-releasing hormone pulse frequency in men with selective elevations of follicle-stimulating hormone. *J. Clin. Endocrinol. Metab.*, **60**, 197–202
22. Crottaz, B., Senn, A., Reymond, M., Rey, F., Germond, M. and Gomez, F. (1992). FSH bioactivity in idiopathic normogonadotropic oligoasthenozoospermia: double-blind trial with gonadotropin-releasing hormone. *Fertil. Steril.*, **57**, 1034–43
23. Van Alphen, M., Van de Kant, H. and DeRooig, D. (1988). Follicle-stimulating hormone stimulates spermatogenesis in the adult monkey. *Endocrinology*, **123**, 1449–55
24. Buch, J. P., Lipshulz, L. and Smith, R. (1991). Evidence for altered receptor-binding of serum follicle-stimulating hormone in male infertility. *Fertil. Steril.*, **55**, 358–62
25. Nieschlag, E., Rohre, H., Weinbauch, G., Gudemann, T., Simoni, M., Spiteri-Grech, J. and Cooper, T. (1992). Report of the Seventh European Workshop on Molecular and Cellular Endocrinology of the Testis. *Mol. Cell Endocrinol.*, **87**, R25–R42
26. Hage-van Noort, M., Puijk, W. C., Plasman, H. H., Kuperus, D., Schapper, W. M., Beekman, N. J., Grotegoed, J. A. and Meloen, R. H. (1992). Synthetic peptides based upon a three-dimensional model for the receptor recognition site of follicle-stimulating hormone exhibit antagonistic or agonistic activity at low concentrations. *Proc. Natl Acad. Sci. U.S.A.*, **89**, 3922–6
27. Huhtaniemi, I. T., Eskola, V., Pakarinen, P., Matikainen, T. and Sprengel, R. (1992). The murine luteinizing hormone and follicle-stimulating hormone receptor genes: transcription initiation sites, putative promoter sequences and promoter activity. *Mol. Cell Endocrinol.*, **88**, 55–66
28. Aiman, J. and Griffin, J. E. (1982). The frequency of androgen receptor deficiency in infertile men. *J. Clin. Endocrinol. Metab.*, **54**, 727–32
29. Spiteri-Grech, J. and Nieschlag, E. (1993). Paracrine factors relevant to the regulation of spermatogenesis: a review. *J. Reprod. Fertil.*, **98**, 1–14
30. Wang, C., Dahl, K., Leung, A., Chan, S. and Hsueh, A. (1987). Serum bioactive FSH in men with idiopathic azoospermia and oligospermia. *J. Clin. Endocrinol. Metab.*, **65**, 629–34
31. Sharpe, R. M. (1990). Intratesticular control of spermatogenesis. *Clin. Endocrinol.*, **33**, 787–807
32. Sharpe, R. M. (1992). Monitoring of spermatogenesis in man: measurement of Sertoli cell or sperm cell-secreted proteins in semen or blood. *Int. J. Androl.*, **15**, 201–10
33. Johnson, L., Chaturvedi, P. and Williams, J. (1992). Missing generations of spermatocytes and spermatids in seminiferous epithelium contributes to low efficiency of spermatogenesis in humans. *Biol. Reprod.*, **47**, 1091–8
34. Dym, M. (1994). Basement membrane regulation of Sertoli cells. *Endocr. Rev.*, **15**, 102–15
35. Ploen, L. and Setchell, B. (1992). Blood–testis barriers revisited. *Int. J. Androl.*, **15**, 1–4
36. Damber, J. E. and Bergh, A. (1992). Testicular microcirculation: a forgotten essential in Andrology? *Int. J. Androl.*, **15**, 285–92

37. Sinclair, A., Berta, M., Smith, A., Palmer, M., Hawkins, J., Griffiths, B., Smith, M., Foster, J., Fischary, A., Lovell-Badge, R. and Goodfellow, P. (1990). A gene from two human sex determining regions evokes a protein with homology to a conserved DNA binding motif. *Nature*, **346**, 240–9
38. Burgoyne, P., Mahadevan, S., Sutcliffe, M. and Palmer, S. (1992). Fertility in mice requires X–Y pairing and a Y-chromosomal 'spermiogenesis' gene mapping to the long arm. *Cell*, **71**, 391–8
39. Merlino, G., Stable, C., Theppan, C., Linton, R., Mahou, K. and Willingham, M. (1991). Inactivation of a sperm motility gene by insertion of an epidermal growth factor receptor transgene whose product is overexpressed and compartmentalized during spermatogenesis. *Genes Dev.*, **5**, 1395–406
40. Eliasson, R., Mossbey, B., Camner, P. and Atzelius, B. (1977). The immotile–cilia syndrome. A congenital ciliary abnormality as an etiologic factor in chronic airway infections and male sterility. *N. Engl J. Med.*, **297**, 1–6
41. Zamboni, L. (1987). The ultrastructural pathology of the spermatozoa as a cause of infertility: the role of electron microscopy in the evaluation of semen quality. *Fertil. Steril.*, **48**, 711–34
42. Belokopytova, I., Kostyleva, E., Tomilin, A. and Noroblev, V. (1993). Human male infertility may be due to a decrease of the protamine P2 content in human sperm chromatin. *Mol. Reprod. Dev.*, **34**, 53–7
43. Cooper, T. G. (1993). The human epididymis: is it necessary? *Int. J. Androl.*, **16**, 245–50
44. Silber, S. J., Ord, T., Balmaceda, J., Patrizio, P. and Asch, R. H. (1990). Congenital absence of the vas deferens. The fertilizing capacity of human epididymal sperm. *N. Engl. J. Med.*, **323**, 1788–92
45. Goldstein, M. (1993). Surgical therapy of male infertility. *J. Urol.*, **149**, 1374–6
46. Ord, T., Marello, E., Patrizio, P., Balmaceda, J., Silber, S. and Asch, R. (1992). The role of the laboratory in the handling of epididymal sperm for assisted reproductive technologies. *Fertil. Steril.*, **57**, 1103–6
47. Mahony, M., Oehninger, S., Doncel, G., Morshedi, M., Acosta, A. and Hodgen, G. D. (1993). Functional and morphological features of spermatozoa microaspirated from the epididymal region of cynomolgus monkeys (*Macaca fascicularis*). *Biol. Reprod.*, **48**, 613–20
48. Angulano, A., Oates, R., Amos, J., Dean, M., Gerrard, B., Stewart, C., Maher, T., White, M. and Milunsky, A. (1992). Congenital bilateral absence of the vas deferens, a primary genital form of cystic fibrosis. *J. Am. Med. Assoc.*, **267**, 1794–7
49. Neiderberger, C. and Ross, L. (1993). Microsurgical epididymovasostomy: predictors of success. *J. Urol.*, **149**, 1364–7
50. Sharlip, I. D. (1993). What is the best pregnancy rate that may be expected from vasectomy reversal? *J. Urol.*, **149**, 1469–71
51. Oehninger, S., Acosta, A. A., Morshedi, M., Veeck, L., Swanson, R. J., Simmons, K. and Rosenwaks, Z. (1988). Corrective measures and pregnancy outcome in *in vitro* fertilization in patients with severe sperm morphology abnormalities. *Fertil. Steril.*, **50**, 283–7. Reprinted in Mishell, D. R., Paulsen, C. A. and Lobo, R. A. (eds.) *Year Book of Infertility*, 1990, p. 222. (Chicago: Year Book Medical Publishers)
52. Grow, D. R., Oehninger, S., Seltman, H. J., Toner, J. P., Swanson, R. J., Kruger, T. F. and Muasher, S. J. (1994). Sperm morphology as diagnosed by strict criteria: probing the impact of teratozoospermia on fertilization rate and pregnancy outcome in a large IVF population. *Fertil. Steril.*, **62**, 559–69
53. Quinn, P. (1993). Sperm processing in assisted reproductive technology: male factor. *Semin. Reprod. Endocrinol.*, **11**, 49–55
54. Cummins, J. M. and Yovich, J. M. (1993). Sperm motility enhancement *in vitro*. *Semin. Reprod. Endocrinol.*, **11**, 56–71
55. Oehninger, S., Acosta, R., Morshedi, M., Philput, C., Swanson, R. J. and Acosta, A. A. (1990). Relationship between morphology and motion characteristics of human spermatozoa in semen and in the swim-up sperm fraction. *J. Androl.*, **11**, 446–52
56. Sueldo, C. E., Oehninger, S., Subias, E., Mahony, M., Alexander, N. J., Burkman, L. J. and Acosta, A. A. (1993). Effect of progesterone on human pellucida sperm binding and oocyte penetrating capacity. *Fertil. Steril.*, **60**, 137–40
57. Ord, T., Patrizio, P., Balmaceda, J. P. and Asch, R. H. (1993). Can severe male factor infertility be treated without micromanipulation? *Fertil. Steril.*, **60**, 110–15
58. Oehninger, S., Toner, J. P., Muasher, S. J., Coddington, C. C., Acosta, A. A. and Hodgen, G. D. (1992). Prediction of fertilization *in vitro* with human gametes: Is there a litmus test? *Am. J. Obstet. Gynecol.*, **167**, 1760–7
59. Oehninger, S. and Alexander, N. J. (1991). Male infertility: current opinion. *Obstet. Gynecol.*, **3**, 182–90
60. Oehninger, S. (1992). Diagnostic significance of sperm–zona interaction. In Smith, K. and Hodden, L. (eds.) *Reproductive Medicine Review*, pp. 57–81. (London: Edward Arnold)
61. Oehninger, S., Blackmore, P., Morshedi, M., Sueldo, C., Acosta, A. and Alexander, N. (1994). Defective calcium influx and acrosome reaction (spontaneous and progesterone-induced) in spermatozoa of infertile men with severe teratozoospermia. *Fertil. Steril.*, **61**, 349–54
62. Huszar, G. and Vigue, L. (1990). Spermatogenesis-related change in the synthesis of the creative–kinase B-type and M-type isoforms in human spermatozoa. *Mol. Reprod. Dev.*, **25**, 258–67
63. Huszar, G., Vigue, L. and Oehninger, S. (1994). Creatine kinase immunocytochemistry of human sperm–hemizona complexes: selective binding of

sperm with mature creatine kinase-staining pattern. *Fertil. Steril.*, **61**, 136–42
64. Huszar, G. and Vigue, L. (1994). Correlation between the rate of lipid peroxidation and cellular maturity as measured by creatine kinase activity in human spermatozoa. *J. Androl.*, **15**, 71–7
65. Burkman, L. J., Coddington, C. C., Franken, D. R., Kruger, T., Rosenwaks, Z. and Hodgen, G. D. (1988). The hemizona assay: development of a diagnostic test for the binding of human spermatozoa to the human zona pellucida to predict fertilization potential. *Fertil. Steril.*, **49**, 688–93
66. Franken, D. R., Burkman, L. J., Oehninger, S. C., Coddington, C. C., Veeck, L. L., Kruger, T. F., Rosenwaks, Z. and Hodgen, G. D. (1989). Hemizona assay using salt-stored human oocytes: evaluation of zona pellucida capacity for binding human spermatozoa. *Gamete Res.*, **22**, 15–26
67. Franken, D. R., Oosthuizen, T., Cooper, S., Kruger, T., Burkman, L. J., Coddington, C. C. and Hodgen, G. D. (1991). Electron microscopic evidence on the acrosomal status of bound sperm and their penetration into human hemizonae pellucida after storage in a buffered salt solution. *Andrologia*, **23**, 205–8
68. Coddington, C. C., Fulgham, D. C., Alexander, N. J., Johnson, D., Herr, J. C. and Hodgen, G. D. (1990). Sperm bound to the zona pellucida in hemizona assay demonstrate acrosome reaction when stained with T-6 antibody. *Fertil. Steril.*, **54**, 504–8
69. Oehninger, S., Mahony, M., Swanson, J. R. and Hodgen, G. D. (1993). The specificity of human spermatozoa/zona pellucida interaction under hemizona assay conditions. *Mol. Reprod. Dev.*, **35**, 59–61
70. Menkveld, R., Franken, D., Kruger, T., Oehninger, S. and Hodgen, G. (1991). Sperm selection capacity of the human zona pellucida. *Mol. Reprod. Dev.*, **30**, 346–52
71. Oehninger, S., Coddington, C. C., Scott, R., Franken, D., Acosta, A. A. and Hodgen, G. D. (1989). Hemizona assay: assessment of sperm dysfunction and prediction of *in vitro* fertilization outcome. *Fertil. Steril.*, **51**, 665–70
72. Pellas, T., Ramachandran, B., Duncan, M., Pau, S., Marone, M. and Chada, K. (1991). Germ cell deficient (GCD), an insertional mutation manifested as infertility in transgenic mice. *Proc. Natl Acad. Sci.*, **88**, 8787–91
73. Toner, J. P. and Hodgen, G. D. (1994). Future developments in reproductive biology. In Behrman, S. J., Patton Jr, G. W. and Holtz, A. (eds.) *Progress in Infertility*, 4th edn, pp. 1–36. (Boston: Little Brown and Company)
74. Handyside, A., Kontoglanni, E., Handy, K. and Winston, R. (1990). Pregnancies from biopsied preimplantation embryos sexed by Y-specific DNA amplification. *Nature*, **334**, 768
75. Robertson, J. (1992). Ethical and legal issues in preimplantation genetic swelling. *Fertil. Steril.*, **57**, 1–11
76. Kierszenbaum, A. (1994). Mammalian spermatogenesis *in vivo* and *in vitro*: a partnership of spermatogenic and somatic cell lineage. *Endocr. Rev.*, **15**, 116–34
77. Russell, L. D. (1991). The perils of sperm release: 'let my children go'. *Int. J. Androl.*, **14**, 307–11
78. Huszar, G., Vigue, L. and Corrales, M. (1990). Sperm creatine kinase activity in fertile and infertile oligospermic men. *J. Androl.*, **11**, 40–5
79. Aitken, R. J. and Clarkson, J. S. (1987). Cellular basis of defective sperm function and its association with the genesis of reactive oxygen species by human spermatozoa. *J. Reprod. Fertil.*, **81**, 459–69
80. Aitken, R. J. and Clarkson, J. S. (1988). Significance of reactive oxygen species and antioxidants in defining the efficacy of sperm preparation techniques. *J. Androl.*, **9**, 367–76
81. Aitken, R. J., Clarkson, J. S., Hargreave, T. B., Irvine, D. S. and Wu, F. C. (1989). Analysis of the relationship between defective sperm function and the generation of reactive oxygen species in cases of oligozoospermia. *J. Androl.*, **10**, 214–20
82. Aitken, R. J., Irvine, D. S. and Wu, F. C. (1991). Prospective analysis of sperm–oocyte fusion and reactive oxygen species generation as criteria for the diagnosis of infertility. *Am. J. Obstet. Gynecol.*, **164**, 542–51
83. Oehninger, S., Franken, D., Alexander, N. and Hodgen, G. (1992). Hemizona assay and its impact on the identification and treatment of human sperm dysfunction. *Andrologia*, **24**, 307–21
84. Wassarman, P. (1990). Profile of a mammalian sperm receptor. *Development*, **108**, 1–17
85. Saling, P. M. (1991). How the egg regulates sperm function during gamete interaction: facts and fantasies. *Biol. Reprod.*, **44**, 246–51
86. Jones, R. (1990). Identification and functions of mammalian sperm-egg recognition molecules during fertilization. *J. Reprod. Fertil.*, **42**, 89–105
87. Wassarman, P. M. (1990). Regulation of mammalian fertilization by zona pellucida glycoproteins. *J. Reprod. Fertil.*, **42**, 79–87
88. Tesarik, J., Menodoza, C., Moos, J. and Carreras, A. (1992). Selective expression of a progesterone receptor on the human sperm surface. *Fertil. Steril.*, **58**, 784–92
89. Tesarik, J. and Menodoza, C. (1992). Defective function of a nongenomic progesterone receptor as a sole sperm anomaly in infertile patients. *Fertil. Steril.*, **58**, 93–7
90. Benoff, S., Hurley, I., Cooper, G., Mandel, F., Hershlag, A., Schall, G. and Rosenfeld, D. (1993). Fertilization potential *in vitro* is correlated with head-specific mannose–ligand receptor expression, acrosome status and membrane cholesterol content. *Hum. Reprod.*, **8**, 2155–67
91. Oehninger, S., Acosta, A. A. and Hodgen, G. D. (1990). Antagonistic and agonistic properties of saccharide moieties in the hemizona assay. *Fertil. Steril.*, **53**, 143–9

92. Oehninger, S., Clark, G., Acosta, A. A. and Hodgen, G. D. (1991). Nature of the inhibitory effect of complex saccharide moieties on the tight binding of human spermatozoa to the human zona pellucida. *Fertil. Steril.*, **55**, 165–9
93. Oehninger, S., Clark, G., Fulgham, D., Mahony, M., Blackmore, P., Acosta, A. and Hodgen, G. D. (1992). Effect of fucoidin on human sperm-zona pellucida interactions. *J. Androl.*, **13**, 519–25
94. Mahony, M., Oehninger, S., Clark, G. F., Acosta, A. and Hodgen, G. D. (1991). Fucoidin inhibits the pellucida-induced acrosome reaction in human spermatozoa. *Contraception*, **44**, 657–65
95. Patankar, M. S., Oehninger, S., Barnett, T., Williams, R. L. and Clark, G. F. (1993). A revised structure for fuciodan may explain some of its biological activities. *J. Biol. Chem.*, **268**, 21770–6
96. Saling, P. (1989). Mammalian sperm interaction with extracellular matrices of the egg. *Oxf. Rev. Reprod. Biol.*, **11**, 339–88
97. Chamberlin, M. E. and Dean, J. (1990). Human homolog of the mouse sperm receptor. *Proc. Natl Acad. Sci. U.S.A.*, **87**, 6014–18
98. Ringuette, M. J., Chamberlin, M. E., Baur, A. W., Sobieski, D. A. and Dean, J. (1988). Molecular analysis of cDNA coding for ZP3, a sperm binding protein of the mouse zona pellucida. *Dev. Biol.*, **127**, 287–95
99. Dean, J. (1992). Biology of mammalian fertilization: role of the zona pellucida. *J. Clin. Invest.*, **89**, 1055–9
100. Osterhoff, C., Kirschoff, C., Krull, N. and Ivell, N. (1994). Molecular cloning and characterization of a novel human sperm antigen (HE2) specifically expressed in the proximal epididymis. *Biol. Reprod.*, **50**, 516–25
101. Tucker, M., Wiker, S. and Massey, J. (1993). Rational approach to assisted fertilization. *Hum. Reprod.*, **8**, 1778–85
102. Barratt, A. and Cooke, I. D. (1991). Sperm transport in the human female reproductive tract: a dynamic interaction. *Int. J. Androl.*, **14**, 394–411
103. Hinsch, K. D., Habermann, B., Hinsch, E., Pfisterer, S., Schill, W. B. and Aktories, K. (1993). ADP-ribosylatin of Rho proteins inhibits sperm motility. *FEBS Lett.*, **334**, 132–6
104. Hinsch, K. D., Hinsch, E., Aumuller, O., Tychowiecka, I., Schultz, G. and Schill, W. B. (1992). Immunological identification of G-protein α- and β-subunits in tail membranes of bovine spermatozoa. *Biol. Reprod.*, **47**, 337–46
105. Kopf, G. S. (1990). Zona pellucida-mediated signal transduction in mammalian spermatozoa. *J. Reprod. Fertil.*, **42**, 33–49

Section 4

Appendix — laboratory techniques

STAINING METHODS

Modified Papanicolaou staining procedure

Preparation of specimens

Morphology: an evenly spread thin smear, air dried and fixed in 1 : 1 ethanol : ether for 30 min and air dried.

Cytology: 1 drop of egg albumen + 1 drop of semen mixed, evenly smeared and fixed in ether : ethanol (50 : 50) for at least 30 min.

Staining procedure

(1) Dip 10 times in 80% ethyl alcohol.
(2) Dip 10 times in 70% ethyl alcohol.
(3) Dip 10 times in 50% ethyl alcohol.
(4) Dip 10 times in distilled water.
(5) Place in Mayer's hematoxylin for 5 min.
(6) Rinse in running water for 3 min.
(7) Dip twice in 0.5% hydrocholoric acid.
(8) Rinse in running water for 5 min.
(9) Place in Scott's water (20 g $MgSO_4 \times 7H_2O$, 2 g $NaHCO_3$ for 1 min.
(10) Rinse in running water for 1–5 min.
(11) Dip 10 times in 50% ethyl alcohol.
(12) Dip 10 times in 70% ethyl alcohol.
(13) Dip 10 times in 80% ethyl alcohol.
(14) Dip 10 times in 95% ethyl alcohol.
(15) Place in orange G6 for 5 min.
(16) Dip five times in 95% ethyl alcohol.
(17) Dip five times in 95% ethyl alcohol.
(18) Place in EA 50 or EA 65 stain for 5 min.
(19) Dip five times in 95% ethyl alcohol.
(20) Dip five times in 95% ethyl alcohol.
(21) Dip five times in 95% ethyl alcohol.
(22) Dip five times in absolute 1-propanol.
(23) Dip five times in 1-propanol and xylol (1 : 1).
(24) Dip 10 times in xylol.
(25) Dip 10 times in xylol.
(26) Place in xylol for 10 min.
(27) Mount immediately with DPX (BDH Ltd, UK).

Propanol can be replaced in steps 22 and 23 with ethyl alcohol

Diff-Quik staining

Diff-Quik stain is a commercially available blood cell staining kit, consisting of a fixative and two stains.

Procedure

A thin smear is prepared and air dried.

(1) Fix smears for 15 s in Diff-Quik fixative.

(2) Stain slides for 10 s in solution 1.

(3) Stain slides for 5 s in solution 2.

Between steps 1, 2 and 3 the excess solution must be drained from the slides by blotting slide edges on bibulous paper.

After step 3 the slides are washed with deionized water applied from the edges of slides to remove excessive stain.

The slides can be used mounted or unmounted.

Spermac staining

Stain is obtainable from Stain Enterprises (Wellington, RSA).

Preparation of smears

(1) Fresh semen must be diluted 1 : 1 with aqueous solution of 3% (w/v) sodium citrate (BDH 30128).

(2) Thin smears are made and air dried.

(3) Smears are fixed immediately by immersion in the fixative for 15 min minimum.

(4) Fixed air dried slides can be stored for long periods of time.

Staining procedure

(1) Before staining, wash slides by dipping gently six to seven times into tap water. Drain excess water by blotting on absorbent paper.

(2) Stain for 1 min in stain A and wash as above.

(3) Stain for 45 s to 1 min in stain B and wash as above.

(4) Stain for 1 min in stain C and wash as above.

Slides can be mounted if desired; however, stains fade over time when mounted.

Shorr staining

Reagents

(1) Ammoniacal ethanol: 95 mL of a 70% ethanol solution plus 5 mL of ammonia.

(2) Shorr stain: Merck 9275.

(3) Harris hematoxylin solution: Merck 9253.

Procedure

A thin smear is prepared and allowed to air dry.

(1) The slide is placed in 70% or 80% ethanol for 1 min.
(2) Rinse in running water 2–3 min.
(3) Place in hematoxylin for 2 min.
(4) Rinse in running water for 3 min.
(5) Dip 10 times in a 5% ammoniacal ethanol bath.
(6) Rinse in running water for 3 min.
(7) Dip 10 times in a 70% ethanol bath.
(8) Dip 10 times in a 95% ethanol bath.
(9) Place in Shorr's stain for 1 min.
(10) Dip 10 times in a 96% ethanol bath.
(11) Dip 10 times in an absolute ethanol bath.
(12) Dip 10 times in an absolute ethanol bath.
(13) Dip 10 times in xylol.
(14) Place in xylol.
(15) Mount with DPX (BDH).

SUPRAVITAL STAINING TECHNIQUES

Eosin alone (WHO)[1]

Reagents

Eosin Y: 0.5 g in 100 mL of physiological saline solution.

Procedure

(1) Mix one drop (10–15 mL) of fresh semen with one drop of 0.5% eosin solution on a microscope slide and cover with a coverslip.

(2) After 1–2 min, observe the preparation (×400) under bright light or a phase contrast microscope.

(3) A minimum of 200 spermatozoa are counted differentiating the live (unstained) gametes from the dead (stained) cells.

The eosin–nigrosin method (WHO)[1]

Reagents

(1) Eosin Y: 1 g in 100 mL of distilled water;

(2) Nigrosin: 10 g in 100 mL of distilled water.

Procedure

(1) Mix one drop of semen with two drops of 1% eosin solution.

(2) After 30 s, add three drops of 10% nigrosin solution and mix again.

(3) Place one drop of the semen–eosin–nigrosin mixture on a clear glass slide and make a smear which is then air-dried.

(4) The material is examined with 100× oil magnification. Live sperm appear white and dead sperm appear pink.

THE SUPRAVITAL NUCLEAR STAINING TEST

Methodology

Cross *et al.* (1986)[2]

Reagents

(1) Culture medium (Biggers, Whitten and Whittingham's medium) supplemented with 3 μg/mL of bovine serum albumin.

(2) Supravital stain Hoechst 33258: 1 μg/mL of culture medium.

(3) Polyvinylpyrrolidone-40:2 g in 100 mL of phosphate buffered saline, pH 7.4.

(4) Ethanol 95% (v/v).

Procedure

(1) Sperm is incubated at 37°C in 5% CO_2–95% air, in a medium containing 1 μg/mL Hoechst 33258, for 10–15 min. (After about 10 min staining, a thin bound of fluorescence appears at the posterior margin of the nucleus of some motile spermatozoa. This is considered non-specific.)

(2) Spermatozoa are then washed free of unbound stain by centrifuging them through a solution of 2% polyvinylpyrrolidone-40 in phosphate buffered saline at 900 g for 5 min. The upper portion containing free Hoechst 33258 is discarded, the spermatozoa are discarded and the spermatozoa are resuspended in 95% ethanol.

(3) After at least 30 min at 4°C the spermatozoa are dried down onto a microscope slide and mounted.

(4) This dye fluoresces an intense blue when bound to DNA. It has a limited permeability through intact cell membranes and will therefore stain only dead cells.

(5) Fluorescent nuclei indicate non-viable spermatozoa, whereas unlabeled sperm represent the vital population.

THE HYPO-OSMOTIC SWELLING TEST

Methodology

Jeyendran *et al.* (1992)[3]

Reagents

(1) *Hypo-osmotic solution*: 13.51 g fructose (MW 180.16); 7.35 g sodium citrate. 2 H_2O (MW 294.11); in 1 L of distilled water.

(2) Pipette 1 mL aliquots of hypo-osmotic solution into separate test tubes. Cap and freeze at –25°C until used.

Procedure

(1) Thaw a test tube of hypo-osmotic solution by incubation at 37°C for 10 min.

(2) Add 0.1 mL of liquefied semen to the solution and mix.

(3) Incubate the mixture for at least 30–60 min at 37°C.

(4) After incubation, place a drop of the well mixed sample on a glass slide and cover with a coverslip. Observe under a phase contrast microscope 400×) for curling of the sperm tail.

(5) Count at least 100 or 200 spermatozoa per sample, calculate the percentage of swollen sperm (typical of a reaction in the hypo-osmotic solution).

(6) If desired, the treated spermatozoa may be fixed with formaldehyde (18.5%), 0.1 mL for later observation.

Since some semen samples will have spermatozoa with curled tails before exposure to the hypo-osmotic solution test, it is useful to observe the ejaculate before exposure. The percentage of spermatozoa with curled tails in the untreated sample should be subtracted from the percentage of those which reacted in the hypo-osmotic solution test.

THE LIPID PEROXIDATION TEST

Methodology

Aitken *et al.* (1993)[4]

Reagents

(1) Culture medium (Biggers, Whitten and Whittingham's medium) (BWW).

(2) Ferrous sulphate, 7 H_2O, 4 mM/L.

(3) Sodium ascorbate, pa. 20 mM/L.

(4) Sodium dodecylsulfate, 7%.

(5) Hydrochloric acid, 0.1 M.

(6) Phosphotungstic acid, 10%.

(7) Butylated hydroxytoluene pa.

(8) 2-Thiobarbituric acid, 0.67%.

Procedure

(1) The sperm suspension in BWW is pelleted by centrifugation (500***g***) for 5 min and resuspended at 10 mL.

(2) One millilitre of this suspension is incubated at 37°C for 2 h with 10 μL ferrous sulphate and 20 μL sodium ascorbate.

(3) A thiobarbituric acid assay mixture is made up fresh every day comprising: 200 μL sodium dodecylsulfate, 2 mL hydrochloric acid, 300 μL

phosphotungstic acid, 100 μL butylated hydroxytoluene and 1 mL thiobarbituric acid.

(4) Then 200 μL of incubated sperm suspension is added to 360 μL of assay mixture and placed in water bath (100°C) for 30 min.

(5) After cooling to room temperature, the malondialdehyde–thiobarbituric acid adduct is extracted by the addition of 500 μL of butanol.

(6) The samples are read on a spectrofluorometer using wavelengths of 510 nm for excitation and 553 nm for emission.

(7) The standards are generated by incubating several dilutions of 1,1,3,3-tetraethoxypropane with equal volumes of 0.2 N hydrochloric acid overnight at room temperature.

NUCLEAR CHROMATIN DECONDENSATION STUDIES

Sodium clodecylsulfate (SDS) and dithiothreitol (DTT)

(1) Sperm in semen (0.1 mL) and in insemination medium (0.5 mL) were washed with 10 mL 0.9% sodium chloride and centrifuged at 600***g*** for 10 min.

(2) The pellet was then resuspended in 0.1 mL 50 mmol/L sodium borate buffer (pH 9.0) containing 2 mmol/L DTT prepared daily.

(3) The suspension was incubated at room temperature (18–20°C) for 30 min.

(4) Then 0.1 mL of 1% (w/v) SDS in sodium borate buffer was added and the suspension mixed gently and incubated at room temperature for 2 min.

(5) The reaction was then stopped and sperm fixed by addition of 0.2 mL of 2.5% glutaraldehyde in sodium borate buffer.

(6) The fixed suspension (15 μL) was mixed with 5 μL of 0.8% Rose Bengal in 0.9% sodium chloride on a glass slide and covered with a square (22×22 mm) glass slip and examined under a phase-contrast microscope.

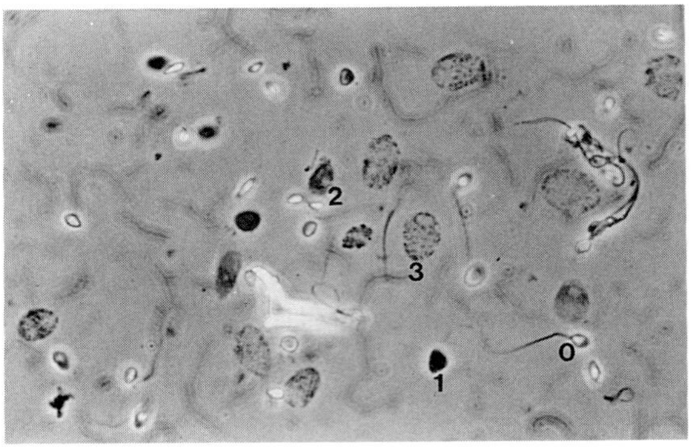

Figure 1 Different grades of nuclear swelling following treatment with DDT+SDS (see Materials and Methods) 0=non-decondensed nucleus; 1=partially decondensed nucleus; 2=markedly decondensed nucleus; 3=completely decondensed nucleus (×400 phase contrast microscope). Reproduced from Liu *et al.*[6] with permission from the Fertility Society of Australia

Sodium dodecylsulfate alone (SDS)

Sperm were washed as above, the pellet was resuspended in 0.1 mL (10%) SDS in sodium borate buffer and incubated at room temperature for 60 min, then fixed and read as above.

Sodium dodecylsulfate (SDS) and ethylenediaminetetra-acetic acid (EDTA)

Sperm were washed with 10 mL of 6 mmol/L EDTA and then prepared as for SDS alone.

For each sample, 200 sperm were classified according to similar criteria to those of Rodriguez *et al.*[5]: (Figure 1) 0 is none decondensed – normal nuclei; 1 is partially decondensed – slightly swollen nuclei with uniform purple appearance, 1.5–2 times normal sperm head size; 2 is markedly decondensed – greatly swollen nuclei with purple granular appearance, 2–4 times normal sperm head size; and 3 is grossly swollen nuclei with purple granular appearance and membrane of sperm head missing, >4 times normal sperm head size.

Acidic aniline blue (AAB)

(1) After drying, the sperm smear was fixed for 30 min in 3% glutaraldehyde in phosphate-buffered saline.

(2) The smear was stained for 15 min in 5% aqueous aniline blue (BDH Chemicals, England) in 4% acetic acid (pH 3.5).

(3) Sperm heads with immature nuclear chromatin stain dark blue with AAB and those with a mature nucleus do not stain darkly[7]. The percentage of sperm stained with aniline blue was determined by counting 200 sperm under oil immersion with 1000× magnification and bright-field illumination.

Assessment of sperm DNA normality with acridine orange (AO)

(1) After drying the sperm smear was fixed in Carnoy's solution for at least 3 h or overnight. The Carnoy's solution (three parts methanol, one part glacial acetic acid) was prepared daily.

(2) The slides were then washed in distilled water and allowed to dry for a few minutes before staining.

(3) The AO (Sigma Chemical Co., St Louis, MO) staining solution was prepared as follows: 10 mL of 1% AO in distilled water was added to a mixture of 40 mL of 0.1 M citric acid and 2.5 mL of 0.3 M $Na_2HPO_4\ 7H_2O$, pH 2.5. The AO staining solution was prepared daily. The 1% AO stock solution was stored in the dark at 4°C for 4 weeks.

(4) The sperm smear was stained for 5 min. Then the slide was gently rinsed and mounted with distilled water.

(5) The percentage of sperm with normal DNA was determined by counting 200 sperm under a fluorescence microscope (Dialux 20, Leitz, Wetzlar, Germany) with ×400 (oil lens) magnification with excitation of 450–490 nm. Sperm with normal DNA fluoresce green and those with abnormal DNA fluoresce red or yellow. It is important to score DNA normality immediately after staining.

SCREENING PROCEDURES FOR DONORS

Pre-acceptance evaluation

All semen donor applicants are required to complete an extensive medical and genetic history form of the applicant and three generations of his family members (including great-grandparents and/or first cousins). Prospective donors are told that it is their legal responsibility to inform us at the time of first interview of *all* existing medical and genetic conditions in their families. Legal consent forms for the release of rights to donor semen samples, as well as for testing for the human immunodeficiency virus and other infectious diseases are also obtained. Each application is personally interviewed and those with no major *health* and *social* risks are accepted.

Medical and genetic evaluation

Each applicant's medical and genetic history is evaluated and a complete physical examination is performed. A urine analysis with culture, as well as a complete blood count (CBC) is also performed. Jewish, French–Canadian, Mediterranean, black and Asian applicants are tested for Tay–Sachs, β-thalassemia, sickle cell and β-thalassemia and α-thalassemia, respectively. All donors should be karyotyped and evaluated for the carrier state for cystic fibrosis.

Infectious diseases evaluation

Each applicant is tested for *Chlamydia*, genital herpes, *Ureaplasma*, *Gonorrhea* and Cytomegalovirus (CMV). Those seropositive for CMV are retested for urine and semen cultures for the identification of CMV. Each applicant is also tested for hepatitis B surface antigen and total core antibody, hepatitis C antibody (second generation), syphilis, human T-cell leukemia virus-1, human immunodeficiency virus-1 and human immunodeficiency virus-2.

Evaluation of semen samples

A minimum of 2–3 samples will be evaluated with an automated semen analyzer for basic semen parameters, which also includes the evaluation of sperm morphology via the strict criteria. Samples will be checked for the presence of abnormal numbers of white blood cells, as well as for the presence of trichomonas. Only acceptable samples with acceptable parameters (>1 mL, $>60\times10^6$ concentration, >60% motility and >10% normal forms, no trichomonas, <1 million round cells) are cryopreserved and a portion of each sample is subsequently thawed for post-thaw analysis. Samples with an occasional round cell count of up to 5 million per mL are exclusively processed with Percoll and cryopreserved as 'intrauterine insemination ready'. All samples will be quarantined for a minimum of 6 months so that infectious disease evaluations can be repeated before samples are released from quarantine. Samples with poor post-thaw results will not be used for inseminations. Although samples with post-thaw motility of 25% have produced pregnancies, except on an occasional basis, samples with a motility of >40% post-thaw are mainly utilized.

Post-acceptance evaluations

Once an individual is accepted into the program, he is monitored regularly for the maintenance of his health and his blood tests are repeated several times per year before samples are released. The test for *Gonorrhea* is repeated once a week if a sample is collected in that week.

CRYOPRESERVATION OF HUMAN SEMEN

Using a programmable freezer

Freezing

(1) Allow sample to liquefy at room temperature for a maximum of 30 min.

(2) Determine basic semen parameters manually or using an automated semen analyzer (CASA).

(3) Slowly add an equal volume of Test-yolk buffer containing 12% glycerol (freezing medium, Irvine Scientific, Irvine, CA, USA) to the semen and mix gently each time a portion of the freezing medium is added. It should take about 10–15 min for this addition.

(4) Read the basic parameters of the mixture (pre-freeze analysis).

(5) Aliquot the mixture (0.5–0.8 mL/vial) into 2 mL cryo vials (Costar, Cambridge, MA, USA).

(6) Load into the automated freezer and cryopreserve as follows:

From room temperature to 5°C at 0.5°C per minute;
From 5 to 4°C at 1°C per min;
From 4 to 3°C at 2°C per min;
From 3 to 2°C at 4°C per min;
From 2 to 1°C at 8°C per min;
From 1 to 80°C at −10°C per min.

(7) Load vials on canes and plunge them into liquid nitrogen.

Thawing

Thaw vials in 37°C water bath for 5–7 min.

Manual method

Freezing

(1) Allow sample to liquefy at room temperature for a maximum of 30 min.

(2) Determine basic semen parameters manually or using an automated semen analyzer.

(3) Slowly add an equal volume of the freezing medium (see method for using a programmable freezer) to semen. Mix gently each time the medium is added. It should take approximately 10–15 min to complete the addition. Determine basic parameters of the mixture either manually or using CASA.

(4) Aliquot the mixture into cryo tubes (see method for using a programmable freezer), place tubes into a freezing tray (Taylor-Wharton, Theodore, AL, USA) and refrigerate for 45–60 min.

(5) Cryopreserve manually by placing the tray (bottom of tubes) 4 cm above liquid nitrogen for 20–30 min.

(6) Remove tubes at once, place them on a cane and plunge them into liquid nitrogen.

Thawing

Place tubes in a 37–2°C water bath for 3–5 min.

INTRAUTERINE INSEMINATION (IUI) PROCEDURES

Preparation of IUIs using Percoll

Reagents

(1) Ham's F-10, 10× concentrated (see Figure 2 for preparation method).

(2) Ham's F-10, regular strength (see Figure 3 for preparation method).

(3) Ham's F-10, regular strength with 0.2%–0.5% human serum albumin (Figure 4).

(4) One hundred per cent Percoll (isotonic Percoll, see below).

(5) Ninety-five per cent and 40% Percoll (see below).

(6) Sterile deionized distilled water.

Other materials and equipment

(1) Sterile Percoll (Catalog number P4937, Sigma).

(2) Laminar flow hood.

(3) Free-angle centrifuge.

(4) Osmometer.

(5) Carbon dioxide incubator at 37°C.

(6) Sterile tissue culture flasks, transfer pipettes, pipette tips, 15 mL conical centrifuge tubes.

Preparation of 100% Percoll

To prepare 100% Percoll (isotonic Percoll), mix nine parts of sterile well-mixed Percoll with one part Ham's F-10 10× concentrated in a laminar flow hood to maintain sterility. There is debate as to whether or not to filter sterilize the Percoll. Some centers filter sterilize after it is prepared. We recommend preparation of Percoll under the laminar flow hood so that this filtration will not be needed. Adjust the osmolality of the mixture (100% Percoll) to 280–285 mOsmol/Kg using sterile deionized distilled water. This mixture usually has an osmolality at or near 354. See Table 1 for how much of the mixture should be removed and be replaced with sterile deionized distilled water. Usually 90 mL Percoll and 10 mL Ham's F-10 10× is sufficient for 10–15 semen samples. Prepare more of 100% Percoll and store sterile for a maximum of 3 months so that 95% and 40% Percoll can be easily prepared when needed. Table 1 may be used as an easy access guide to determine the volume of medium per liter to remove and replace with water to obtain desired osmolality. The left-hand column shows unadjusted osmolality reading; the right-hand column shows volume of medium per liter to remove and replace with water in order to achieve the desired osmolality. It is important to remember that *these values are approximations*. Several attempts may be necessary to achieve the desired osmolality.

Preparation of 95% and 40% Percoll

To prepare 95% Percoll, under a laminar flow hood mix 9.5 parts (e.g. 9.5 mL) of a well-mixed 100% Percoll with 0.5 part (e.g. 0.5 mL) regular strength Ham's F-10. To prepare 40% Percoll, mix four parts (e.g. 4 mL) of a well-mixed 100% Percoll with six parts (e.g. 6 mL) regular strength Ham's F-10. See page 503 for variations in methods of Percoll preparation and separation.

Preparation of individual Percoll tubes

To prepare Percoll tubes for processing semen samples, transfer 1 mL of 95% Percoll to each 15 mL disposable polystyrene conical centrifuge tube. Using a narrow tip transfer pipette or any other narrow tip pipette, very slowly and gently overlay 1 mL of 40% Percoll on top of 95% Percoll. Gently cap the tube tightly. Several of these tubes can be prepared and labeled ahead of time for use but they must be refrigerated. We recommend that tubes prepared and refrigerated for longer than 1 month not be used. See page 503 for other methods of Percoll preparation and separation.

Cryopreservation of 'IUI ready' samples

Outline of method

(1) Allow sample to liquefy and read basic semen parameters.

Media preparation log Ham's F-10

(10X concentrated for preparation of 100% isotonic Percoll)
Date: ________________
Prepared by: ________________
Base water resistivity: ________________

It takes almost 1–2 hours to fully dissolve all components of 10× Ham's. Slight warming of the mixture to near 32–32°C may help the process

Component	*Measurement*	*Supplier: catalog no.*	*Lot no.*	*Storage place*
F-10 Nutrient Medium (Ham)	9.80 g/100 mL; one package	Gibco; 81200–040 1-800-828-6686		Refrigerator/ desicator
Lactic acid, L(+) calcium salt	0.5 mM (0.1091 g/100 mL)	Calbiochem-Behring; 4272 1-800-854-3417		Refrigerator/ desicator
Benzyl penicillin, sodium salt	0.05 g/100 mL	Sigma; P-3032 1-800-325-3010		Shelf/room temp.
Streptomycin sulfate	0.05 g/100 mL	Sigma; S1277		Refrigerator/ desicator
Sodium pyruvate	0.036 g/100 mL	Sigma; P4562		Refrigerator/ desicator
Sodium bicarbonate	2.10 g/100 mL	Sigma; S5761		Shelf/room temp.

Use Percoll (Catalog no. P4937, Sigma Co.) to prepare 100% isotonic Percoll stock. See page 52 for the preparation method.

Dispense in sterile 50 mL culture flasks and referigerate. Use within 1 month of preparation.

Dispense date: ________________
Date prepared: ________________
Ham's F-10 lot no. ________________
Expiration date: ________________
Filter type and lot number: ________________
Unadjusted osmolality: ________________
Adjusted osmolality: ________________
Unadjusted pH: ________________
Adjusted pH: ________________

Results of the mouse 2 cell embryo culture for the medium prepared
________ *Pass* (≥ 80% Mouse blastocysts and morulae combined)
________ *Retest* (< 80% Mouse blastocysts and morulae combined)
________ *Fail* (< 70% Mouse blastocysts and morulae combined)
If failed, removed from stock (refrigerator)? ________ By whom?

Figure 2 Media preparation log, Ham's F-10, 10× concentrated

Media preparation log, Ham's F-10

Date: ____________________
Prepared by: ____________________
Base water resistivity: ____________________

Component	*Measurement*	*Supplier: catalog no.*	*Lot no.*	*Storage place*
F-10 Nutrient Medium (Ham)	9.80 g/100 mL; one package	Gibco; 81200–040 1-800-828-6686-7		Refrigerator/ desicator
Lactic acid, L(+) calcium salt	0.5 mM (0.1091 g/L)	Calbiochem-Behring; 4272 1-800-854-3417		Refrigerator/ desicator
Benzyl penicillin, sodium salt	0.05 g/L	Sigma; P-3032 1-800-325-3010		Shelf/room temp.
Streptomycin sulfate	0.05 g/L	Sigma; S1277		Refrigerator/ desicator
Sodium pyruvate	0.036 g/L	Sigma; P4562		Refrigerator/ desicator
Sodium bicarbonate	2.10 g/L	Sigma; S5761		Shelf/room temp.

Dispense in sterile 50 mL culture flasks and referigerate. Incubate one flask at 37°C in 5% CO_2 and air incubator. Discard flask after 3 days of 37°C incubation.

Dispense date: ____________________
Date prepared: ____________________
Ham's F-10 lot no. ____________________
Expiration date: ____________________
Filter type and lot number: ____________________
Unadjusted osmolality: ____________________
Adjusted osmolality: ____________________
Unadjusted pH: ____________________
Adjusted pH: ____________________

Results of the mouse 2 cell embryo culture for the medium prepared

______ *Pass* (≥ 80% Mouse blastocysts and morulae combined)
______ *Retest* (< 80% Mouse blastocysts and morulae combined)
______ *Fail* (< 70% Mouse blastocysts and morulae combined)

If failed, removed from stock (refrigerator)? ________ By whom?

Figure 3 Media preparation log, Ham's F-10, regular strength

Media preparation log, Ham's F-10 and 0.5% human serum albumin

Date: ________________
Prepared by: ________________
Base water resistivity: ________________

Component	*Measurement*	*Supplier: catalog no.*	*Lot no.*	*Storage place*
F-10 Nutrient Medium (Ham)	9.80 g/100 mL; one package	Gibco; 81200–040 1-800-828-6686-7		Refrigerator/ desicator
Lactic acid, L(+) calcium salt	0.5 mM (0.1091 g/L)	Calbiochem-Behring; 4272 1-800-854-3417		Refrigerator/ desicator
Benzyl penicillin, sodium salt	0.05 g/L	Sigma; P-3032 1-800-325-3010		Shelf/room temp.
Streptomycin sulfate	0.05 g/L	Sigma; S1277		Refrigerator/ desicator
Sodium pyruvate	0.036 g/L	Sigma; P4562		Refrigerator/ desicator
Sodium bicarbonate	2.10 g/L	Sigma; S5761		Shelf/room temp.
Human serum albumin, fraction V	5 g/L = 0.5% 2 g/L = 0.2%	Irvine Scientific, 5050 1-800-437-5706		Refrigerator/ Desicator

Dispense in sterile 50 mL culture flasks labeled with the name of the medium, the date prepared, lot no., expiration date, and initials of the person who prepared the medium. Refrigerate flasks. When needed, incubate one flask at 37°C in 5% CO_2 and air incubator. Write the date incubated on the flask. Discard flask after 3 days of 37°C incubation.

Date prepared: ________________
Dispense date: ________________
Ham's F-10 lot no. ________________
Expiration date: ________________
Filter type and lot number: ________________
Unadjusted osmolality: ________________
Adjusted osmolality: ________________
Unadjusted pH: ________________
Adjusted pH: ________________

Results of the mouse 2 cell embryo culture for the medium prepared

______ *Pass* (≥ 80% Mouse blastocysts and morulae combined)
______ *Retest* (< 80% Mouse blastocysts and morulae combined)
______ *Fail* (< 70% Mouse blastocysts and morulae combined)

If failed, removed from stock (refrigerator)? ______ By whom?

Figure 4 Media preparation log, Ham's F-10 and 0.2–0.5% human serum albumin

Table 1 Osmolality correction for culture medium

Unadjusted osmolality (mOsm/kg)	*Volume of medium/L to remove and replace w/water (mL)*	*Unadjusted osmolality (mOsm/kg)*	*Volume of medium/L to remove and replace w/water (mL)*
286	3.5	306	68.6
287	7.0	307	71.7
288	10.4	308	74.7
289	13.8	309	77.7
290	17.2	310	80.6
291	20.3	311	83.6
292	24.0	312	86.5
293	27.3	313	89.5
294	30.6	314	92.4
295	33.9	315	95.2
296	37.2	316	98.1
297	40.0	317	100.9
298	43.6	318	103.8
299	46.8	319	106.6
300	50.0	320	109.4
301	53.2	321	112.1
302	56.3	322	114.9
303	59.4	323	117.6
304	62.5	324	120.4
305	65.6	325	123.1

Desired osmolality = 280–285 mOsm/kg unless a hyperosmolal medium is desired
If 2 L of medium have been made, remove twice as much as indicated above. If 100 mL of Ham's F10 10× concentrated have been made, remove 0.1 volume as indicated above
NOTE: Do not discard any medium that you remove until you have finished. It may be necessary to replace some of the medium if osmolality falls below 280 mOsm/kg. The following approximation may also be used to determine the volume of medium/L to remove and replace with water:

$$\frac{\text{(Unadjusted osmolality} - \text{desired osmolality)}}{\text{(unadjusted osmolality)}} \times \text{Volume (in mL) of medium being prepared} = \text{Volume of medium/L to remove and replace with water}$$

(2) Overlay sample on 40%/95% Percoll tubes that have come to room temperature.

(3) Balance tubes and centrifuge at 220–250***g*** for 15–20 min.

(4) Extract pellet and transfer to a sterile centrifuge tube. Add 8–10 mL of Ham's F-10 with 0.2–0.5% albumin to the recovered pellet. Centrifuge at 300–400***g*** for 7–10 min.

(5) Extract the supernate to the level determined in Table 2.

(6) Add egg yolk containing 12% glycerol (EYG) to the recovered sample at a rate of 1 mL every 10 min. Use Table 2 to determine how much EYG to add to the recovered sample.

(7) After completing the addition of EYG, read basic semen parameters of the sample. This is called a pre-freeze analysis.

(8) Dispense the sample into labeled cryo vials. Each vial should contain 0.4 mL.

(9) Refrigerate tubes for 30–45 min at 4°C.

(10) Place tray on top of 35 very high capacity tank for 45 min. The distance between the bottom of the vials and the surface of liquid nitrogen should be 5 cm.

(11) Transfer the cryo vials to cryo canes. Plunge cane into liquid nitrogen.

Detailed description of method

(1) Remove one or two 40%/95% Percoll tubes from refrigerator and allow to warm up to room temperature.

Table 2 The purpose of cryopreserving an intrauterine insemination (IUI)-ready sample is to recover an adequate number of cells in one vial to perform an IUI. Based on M. Morshedi and his colleagues' experience they have determined that approximately 40–60 million motile cells should be present per vial before freezing. This table should be used to determine the level of the medium + the pellet that should be left at the bottom of the tube, and the number of 'IUI ready' vials that can be recovered from a particular sample. Determine the number of motile cells per ejaculate by multiplying the concentration of motile by the total semen volume (i.e. the sample has a motile concentration of 100 million/mL and the semen volume is 2 mL. The number of motile cells per ejaculate equals 200 million). Use this number to determine how much medium + pellet to leave in the conical tube after washing

No. of motile cells per ejaculate ($\times 10^6$)	*Leave this volume of medium + pellet in the bottom of the tube (mL)*	*Add this volume of EYG containing 12% glycerol (mL)*	*Total freezing volume (mL)*	*Approximate no. motile cells/vial before freezing* ($\times 10^6$)	*No. of vials recovered (not including 0.4 mL post-thaw vial)*
<100	0.8	0.4	1.2	33	2
100–150	0.8	0.4	1.2	42	2
151–250	1.1	0.55	1.65	48.5	3
251–300	1.4	0.7	2.1	52.4	4
301–350	1.6	0.8	2.4	54	5
351–450	2.0	1.0	3.0	53.3	6
451–500	2.2	1.1	3.3	57.6	7
501–550	2.4	1.2	3.6	58.3	8
551–600	2.8	1.4	4.2	54.8	9
601–675	3.0	1.5	4.5	56.7	10
676–750	3.3	1.55	4.85	59.4	11
>751	3.6	1.8	5.4	>55.6	12

EYG, egg yolk containing 12% glycerol

(2) Allow sample to liquefy for a maximum of 20–30 min. Mix well and perform basic semen parameter determinations.

(3) Gently overlay a maximum of 2 mL semen on top of Percoll tube. If semen volume is >2 mL, use more tubes as needed.

(4) Centrifuge tube(s) at 220–250***g*** for 20–30 min. For good samples, 20 min is usually enough (see page 503) for different methods of handling sample for Percoll separation). Make certain tubes are *balanced well* for centrifugation so that no vibration/rattling occurs.

(5) Using a narrow tip transfer pipette, gently remove the entire pellet from the 95% Percoll fraction (bottom of tube) and transfer the pellet to another sterile 15 mL conical centrifuge tube. Make certain *not to aspirate the interface between the 40% and 95% Percoll* (remove approximately 0.8 mL of the bottom layer if the volume of the bottom layer is 1 mL). If this task is difficult, the entire seminal fluid on the top and the 40% Percoll, as well as the interface ring, can be removed first and what is left at the bottom is the sample that has to be washed for cryopreservation.

(6) Add ample amount (8–10 mL) of Ham's F-10 with 0.2–0.5% albumin to the recovered pellet, mix gently and centrifuge at 300–400***g*** for 7–10 min. Since Ham's F-10 is a carbonate/bicarbonate-based buffer, it must be incubated at 37°C in 5% carbon dioxide for at least several hours before it can be used for washing the samples. Therefore, it may be necessary to incubate one flask of the medium overnight for use the next day. When you place the Ham's F-10 in the incubator, loosen the cap slightly to establish the buffer system.

(7) Remove the tube from centrifuge immediately and extract the supernate to the level determined in Table 2.

(8) Check the basic parameters of the recovered washed and Percolled sample.

(9) Slowly, at a rate of approximately 1 mL per 10 min, add egg yolk containing 12% glycerol (EYG) to the recovered sample equal to 0.5 of

the volume of the sample (e.g. if 1 mL sample is recovered, slowly add 0.5 mL EYG to the sample). Use Table 2 as a guide for determining the volume of EYG to add to the sample.

(10) After EYG addition is complete, perform prefreeze analysis of the mixture (determination of the basic motion parameters) and aliquot it into cryo tubes. Each vial should contain 0.4 mL. Label the donor's tubes with his code and the date sample was cryopreserved. Label the patient's tubes with his name, social security, log number and the date sample was cryopreserved. Label all the tubes as '*IUI ready*' samples. Make one post-thaw vial of 4 mL.

(11) Refrigerate tubes for 30–45 min.

(12) Freeze tubes at 4 cm above liquid nitrogen (or according to your own method) for 30 min.

(13) Thaw, preferably at 40–42°C (water-bath), for 3 min or at 37°C (water bath) for 5–7 min. If 37°C incubators are used to thaw samples (not recommended), longer time is needed.

(14) The vials are now ready to be used for an intrauterine insemination.

Preparation of an IUI using Percoll separation

Outline of method

(1) Allow sample to liquefy and read basic semen parameters. If the sample is frozen, thaw it and slowly add an equal volume of Ham's F-10 to the frozen sample.

(2) Overlay sample on 40%/95% Percoll tubes that have come to room temperature.

(3) Balance tubes and centrifuge at 220–250***g*** for 15–20 min.

(4) Extract pellet and transfer to a sterile centrifuge tube. Add 4–5 mL of Ham's F-10. Mix gently. Centrifuge tube at 300–400***g*** for 5 min.

(5) Extract the supernate until near the pellet (about 0.5 mL). Add 4–5 mL of Ham's F-10. Mix gently. Centrifuge tube at 300–400***g*** for 5 min.

(6) Extract the supernate. Leave 0.4 mL or less in centrifuge tube. Sample is now ready for intrauterine inseminations.

Detailed description of the method

(1) Remove one or two 40%/95% Percoll tubes from refrigerator and allow to warm to room temperature.

(2) Allow sample to liquefy for a maximum of 20–30 min. Mix well and perform basic semen parameters determinations.

(3) Gently overlay a maximum of 2 mL semen on top of 40%/95% Percoll tube. If semen volume is more than 2 mL, use more tubes as needed.

For frozen samples, thaw vials according to recommended thawing procedures for the particular sample. In a laminar flow hood, transfer the semen into a conical centrifuge tube. Slowly add an equal volume of Ham's F-10 with 0.2–0.5% albumin to the sample at a rate of approximately 0.1 mL per min. Mix thoroughly, then gently overlay mixture on top of 40%/95% Percoll tube. No more than 2 mL should be overlaid on top of one Percoll tube.

(4) Centrifuge tube(s) at 220–250***g*** for 15–20 min. For good samples, usually 20 min is enough. Centrifuge poor quality samples for 25–30 min. If the sample is fairly good but has poor morphology, use a shorter centrifugation time (10 min). See earlier on this page for different methods of handling samples for Percoll separation. Make certain tubes are *balanced well* for centrifugation so that no vibration/rattling occurs.

(5) Using a narrow tip transfer pipette, gently remove the entire pellet from the 95% Percoll fraction (bottom of tube) and transfer the pellet to another sterile 15 mL conical centrifuge tube. Make certain *not to aspirate the interface between the 40% and 95% Percoll.* If this task is difficult, the entire seminal fluid on the top and the 40% Percoll as well as the interface ring can be removed first. Pellet remaining at the bottom must be washed before it can be used for an insemination.

(6) Add about 4–5 mL of Ham's F-10 with 0.2–0.5% albumin to the recovered pellet. Mix

gently and centrifuge at 300–400***g*** for 5 min. Since Ham's F-10 is a carbonate/bicarbonate based buffer, it must be incubated at 37°C in 5% carbon dioxide for at least several hours before it can be used for washing the samples. Therefore it may be necessary to incubate one flask of the medium overnight for use the next day. When placing the Ham's F-10 in the incubator, loosen the cap slightly to establish the buffer system.

(7) Remove the tube from the centrifuge immediately after it stops. Extract the supernate until near the pellet (leave 0.5 mL at the bottom of the tube). Sample can be washed once more following the instructions above. For *in vitro* fertilization, washing the sample a second time is strongly recommended. To obtain a more concentrated sample, you may need to remove more of the supernate (e.g. leave 0.2–0.3 mL at the bottom of tube). The recommended volume to be used for an IUI is 0.4 mL or less.

(8) Read the basic parameters of the recovered sample manually or using an automated semen analyzer.

(9) The sample is now ready to be used for an IUI. Using a micropipetete calibrated to 100 μL, transfer the sample into a properly labeled cryo vial.
  (a) *For donor IUIs*, label the cryo vial with: patient's name, date, donor code and IUI. (Figure 5 shows the format used for a donor IUI report as used by The Howard and Georgeanna Jones Institute for Reproductive Medicine). Create a donor IUI report for the sample. Using tape, place the sample in an envelope labeled with the doctor's name, patient's name and date. Place the donor IUI report in the envelope and deliver the sample to the doctor who is performing the insemination.
  (b) *For IUI using husband's samples*, label the cryo vial with: name of wife, date, husband's name, artificial insemination by husband (AIH) and IUI. Create a IUI (AIH) report for the sample. Using tape, place the sample in an envelope labeled with the doctor's name, the wife's name and the date. Place the IUI (AIH) report in the envelope and deliver the sample to the doctor who is performing the insemination.

VARIATIONS IN METHODS OF SPERM PREPARATION USING PERCOLL

Ord[157] has published several variations in methods of sperm preparation using Percoll gradient centrifugation. The following is an extraction of her work pertinent to our focus.

Several variables can influence the sperm recovery using Percoll gradients. These are:

(1) Sperm concentration in the semen;

(2) Percentage motility;

(3) Semen volume;

(4) Percentage of normal morphology;

(5) Progression;

(6) Total motile sperm in the sample; and

(7) Concentration of contaminant cells in the sample.

It is suggested that the best approach in preparing semen samples is to individualize a particular method of sperm preparation for each individual sample.

At Ord's center, there are two steps that never vary in the use of the Percoll gradient centrifugation. One is the number and density of Percoll layers used, and the other is the speed (***g***) of centrifugation. At the center, three layers of 95%, 70% and 50% Percoll are always used and the centrifugation force is always 250***g***.

However, depending on the type and quality of the semen sample being prepared, several aspects of the Percoll method is modified to accommodate for specific needs for that sample. The size of the gradient layers (e.g. 1 mL, 0.5 mL or 0.3 mL), direct layering of the samples on the Percoll gradient versus washing the sample prior to layering and the length of centrifugation time are some of these modifications (variables). One-mL Percoll layers, direct layering and a centrifugation time of 10–20 min has been suggested for samples with normal semen parameters and with normal morphology

Eastern Virginia Medical School
Cryolaboratory
The Howard and Georgeanna Jones Institute for Reproductive Medicine

601 Colley Avenue, Suite 278
Norfolk, VA 23507-1912
Office: (804) 446-5090
Laboratory: (804) 446-5029

Donor IUI report

Date:
Dr.

Please verify the following information before insemination:	
Patient's name	
Donor code	
Date sample frozen	
No. Vials processed for IUI	
Volume of processed sample sent	cc
Motility of processed sample at 37°C	%
Number of motile sperm available for IUI	$\times 10^6$

This sample is ready to be used for an Intrauterine Insemination.
Please report all pregnancies to The Jones Institute Cryo Lab.

Special instructions:

Thank you.

The Jones Institute Cryolaboratory

Figure 5 Example of Donor IUI Report as used by the Howard and Georgeanna Jones Institute for Reproductive Medicine, Norfolk, VA, USA

(>15%). For mild to moderate male factor samples, those with normal morphology of <15%, and for cryopreserved samples 0.5–mL layers and a 10–30 min centrifugation time has been suggested[157].

For cryopreserved semen samples, the following guidelines have been suggested[157]:

(1) Gradient size: 0.5 mL.

(2) Centrifugation time: 10–20 min.

(3) Centrifugation force: 250***g***.

(4) Number of Percoll layers: 3.

(5) Density of Percoll layers: 95%, 70% and 50%.

REACTIVE OXYGEN SPECIES IN DIAGNOSTIC ANDROLOGY

Measurement of generation by human sperm in suspensions using chemiluminescence

Protocol

Prepare spermatozoa by Percoll gradient centrifugation and adjust the sperm concentration to 10×10^6/mL in Biggers, Whitten and Whittingham's medium (BWW)[8].

Two hundred microliters of this sperm preparation are then carefully pipetted into a disposable luminometer container, being careful to avoid creating air bubbles.

The Berthold LB 9505 luminometer employed for these studies possesses six independent channels that are set to a temperature of 37°C.

Basal reading

0 min — Four microliters luminol (25 mM stock in dimethyl sulfoxide (DMSO) to give a final concentration of 250 μM) and 8 μL horseradish peroxidase (2 mg/mL in a phosphate buffered saline stock) are carefully added to each tube, again taking great care to avoid the formation of air bubbles. The chemiluminescent signal is then monitored for about 5 min until it has stabilized.

FMLP provocation test for leukocytes

5 min — Two microliters formyl-methionyl-leucyl-phenylalanine (FMLP; 10 mM stock in DMSO to give a final concentration of 50 μM) is then added to the reaction mixture in order to stimulate a chemiluminescent signal from any leukocytes that are present in the sperm suspension. Since FMLP receptors are not present on the surface of human spermatozoa, this signal is specific for the leukocyte population and can be calibrated with suspensions containing known numbers of polymorphonuclear leukocytes[9].

PMA response

10 min — Four microliters phorbol 12-myristrate 13-acetate (PMA; 1 mM stock in DMSO, diluted 1 : 100 to give a 10 μM working stock solution in BWW and a final concentration of 100 nM) is added to the sperm suspension after the FMLP response has subsided, which takes about 10 min. This reagent gives an indication of the contributions made by both the leukocyte and sperm subpopulations to the reactive oxygen generating capacity of the suspension.

In making these assessments, it is extremely important to realize that the capacity of a leukocyte to generate reactive oxygen species is at least 100 times higher than a spermatozoon. A very low level of leukocyte contamination can therefore have a major impact on the chemiluminescent signals generated by a given sperm suspension.

IN VITRO FERTILIZATION TECHNIQUES FOR EPIDIDYMAL SPERM

Common problems encountered with epididymal aspirations

The use of sperm surgically retrieved from different regions of the epididymis, vasa efferentia or, recently, from testicular biopsies, for *in vitro* fertilization (IVF) has posed new challenges for their handling to laboratory units.

There is no doubt that epididymal sperm has worse motility, progression and morphology than ejaculated sperm. Additionally, the total number of sperm retrieved is variable and can range from less than 1 million to more than 100 million. Further, although a great deal of attention is paid to attempting to avoid blood contamination during surgery, the epididymal aspirates are frequently contaminated with red blood cells, debris and macrophages. Therefore, in order to obtain clean samples suitable to be used for IVF, new methodologies of sperm processing and handling had to be created[10]. At the same time it was necessary to recover a final sperm sample with sufficient normal motile sperm.

This part of the appendix outlines the main methods employed in the treatment of epididymal samples.

MiniPercoll

The idea of using a reduced volume of discontinuous Percoll gradient (MiniPercoll) came after its successful application in severe male factor infertility[11].

In early work, conventional methods of semen preparation such as swim-up, wash and resuspension and sedimentation were tested, but with very poor results, and therefore they were abandoned.

During the sperm aspiration procedure each aspirate is immediately diluted with 1 mL medium (HEPES-buffered human tubal fluid [HTF], Irvine Scientific, Irvine, CA), supplemented with 0.5% human serum albumin (HSA) and an aliquot examined for the presence of motile sperm. Upon completion of sperm collection, the different aspirates are pooled together according to sperm motility and degree of blood contamination and centrifuged at 100***g*** for 10 min. Following centrifugation, the pellets are suspended in 0.3 mL of medium and layered on the MiniPercoll gradient. This consists of 0.3 mL each of 50, 70 and 95% isotonic Percoll (Parmacia, Sweden). An isotonic solution of Percoll is obtained by mixing nine parts of Percoll with one part of 10× Ham's F-10 (Gibco, I) and adding 2.1 g/L of sodium bicarbonate. To obtain the 95, 70 and 50% layers this isotonic solution is diluted with HTF and HEPES.

The discontinuous gradient is made in a 15 mL centrifuge tube by careful pipetting. The resuspended pellet of epididymal sperm is then gently layered on the 50% section. The gradients are then centrifuged at 200***g*** for 20–45 min. After centrifugation, the bottom 95% layer is recovered and washed twice with HTF to remove the Percoll. The final sperm pellet is resuspended in a culture table in 1 mL HTF + 0.5% HSA and incubated at 37% in humidified atmosphere of 5% carbon dioxide and air until the time of oocyte insemination. Table 3 illustrates the MiniPercoll steps.

The reduced volume of each Percoll layer, 0.3% versus the conventional 1.0 mL, offers several advantages:

(1) It allows better migration of sperm;

(2) It still retains the filter capacity in removing red blood cells, debris and macrophages; and

(3) It allows the recovery of high proportions of normal and motile sperm.

MiniPercoll, pentoxifylline and 2-deoxyadenosine

A recent variation in the processing of epididymal sperm has been the addition of pentoxifylline and 2-deoxyadenosine, two known sperm stimulants to miniPercoll[10]. The basic steps of this method are outlined in Table 4.

The preliminary results of Patrizio, Asch and Ord (authors of Chapter 32) were very encouraging, and the fertilization rate rose from 16% with MiniPercoll alone to 35% with MiniPercoll in conjunction with chemical stimulants. However, with more data it has become clear that:

Table 3 Steps in the use of MiniPercoll

- Epididymal sperm diluted with 1 mL HTF and pooled together
- Centrifugation at 100***g*** for 10 min
- Supernatant removed and pellet resuspended in 0.3 mL HTF
- Layering on discontinuous miniPercoll gradient (0.3 mL each of 95, 70, 50%)
- Centrifugation at 200***g*** for 20–45 min
- Ninety-five per cent layer recovered and washed twice with HTF at 100***g*** + 0.5%
- Pellet resuspended in 1 mL HTF + 0.5% HSA

HTF, HEPES – buffered human tubal fluid; HSA, human serum albumin

Table 4 Steps in the use of MiniPercoll + Pentoxifylline and 2-Deoxyadenosine

- Epididymal aspirates pooled together are incubated for 30 min with 3 mm of pentoxifylline at room temperature
- Samples centrifuged at 100***g*** for 10 min
- Supernatant removed and pellet resuspended in 0.3 mL HTF
- Layering on MiniPercoll gradient
- Centrifugation at 200***g*** for 20–45 min
- Ninety-five per cent layer recovered and incubated with 3mM of 2-deoxyadenosine for 30 min at 37°C
- Sperm washed twice and resuspended in 1 mL of culture medium

(1) There is no improvement in the number of patients who fertilize; however, those who do fertilize have more embryos available.

(2) There is no improvement in pregnancy rates.

Although we still favor the use of MiniPercoll with pentoxifylline and 2-deoxyadenosine with epididymal sperm of men, it must be remembered that, particularly with congentical absence of vas deferens (CAVD), there are cases where the fertilization rate will be very poor, even with optimizing laboratory methodologies[12].

Modification of the standard IVF method

The use of epididymal sperm for oocyte insemination also required modifications of the standard IVF methodology[13]. The modifications presented here are the same when used in dealing with extremely severe male factor samples. In brief:

(1) The oocytes are mechanically denuded of the cumulus:

(2) Use of higher numbers of sperm than the standard 100 000 motile for insemination of the oocytes. If available, or necessary, up to 1–1.5 million sperm are used;

(3) Use of 75 mm conical culture tubes for insemination of oocytes. Since sperm and oocytes aggregate at the bottom center of the culture tube, the surface area is much smaller than 35 mm Petri dishes or four-well dishes of 0.1 mL microdrops. Further, the chances for contact between gametes are maximized and, since the tube can hold 1 mL of medium, there is no risk of exhausting medium components by the large number of sperm and multiple oocytes, as might occur in a microdrop which is formed only by 0.1 mL of medium; and

(4) All the oocytes are added to the culture tube containing sperm and not vice versa, avoiding a further dilution of an already low number of sperm by separating it into multiple tubes.

Recovery of sperm from testicular biopsies

Testicular biopsies are rinsed in modified human tubal fluid (M-HTF; Irvine Scientific, Irvine, CA, USA) to remove any blood and transferred to a 60 mm Petri dish containing 1–2 mL medium.

Biopsy material is minced well with a scalpel (breaking up seminiferous tubules as much as possible). An aliquot of medium is examined for the presence of sperm. This process is continued until some free sperm, i.e. not attached to Sertoli cells, are seen. The medium is then transferred to a centrifuge tube, leaving any tissue behind, and centrifuged at 100***g*** for 10 min. The pellet is resuspended in 0.3 mL medium and layered on a miniPercoll gradient as for epididymal sperm. Sample is centrifuged for 30–45 min at 200***g***. The rest of the steps are identical to the procedure for epididymal sperm, except that the pellet is resuspended in a small volume of medium (0.1 mL) to concentrate the recovered sperm for intracytoplasmic sperm injection (ICSI).

Freezing of epididymal sperm

In the last 2 years aliquots of epididymal sperm have been frozen for future IVF attempts to avoid repetition of the surgical sperm retrieval operation.

Epididymal samples are washed and centrifuged once, concentrated to a volume of 0.3–0.6 mL and diluted 1 : 1 with freezing medium (test-yolk buffer with glycerol, Irvine Scientific, CA, USA). It is important to add the freezing medium slowly, drop by drop, over a period of 10 min. The sample is then hung over liquid nitrogen vapor overnight and plunged the next day[14].

RETRIEVAL OF RETROGRADE EJACULATE

Patient preparation

(1) 1.5 g of sodium bicarbonate 12 h and 1 h prior to procedure.

(2) Fluid restriction to limit urine production during procedure.

Sperm retrieval

Initial bladder catheterization

(1) Use plastic 14 F catheter.

(2) No preparation with betadine or other spermicidal solutions. If antibacterial is desired, may use alcohol and allow to dry prior to catheterization.

(3) Lubricant should be non-bacteriocidal/non-spermicidal (e.g. glycerine).

(4) Insert non-traumatically to avoid red blood cells in specimen.

(5) Instill 20 mL of sperm friendly medium. We use Ham's F-10, 20mM HEPES buffer, 1% human serum albumin (HSA).

Patient masturbates to orgasm

(1) Essential to have specimen cup ready in the rare case of an antegrade ejaculate!

(2) If antegrade specimen is obtained – process separately.

Retrieve retrograde sperm

(1) Catheterize again immediately after ejaculation with plastic catheter following above protocol.

(2) Drain bladder contents into specimen container.

(3) Gently irrigate with 20 mL of the buffered medium.

Post-procedure patient care

(1) Since the patient was catheterized without a sterile technique, it is prudent to prescribe antibiotics to prevent bladder or prostatic infection.

(2) Antibiotics which attain significant levels in prostatic fluid are optimal.
Suggestions: Bactrim or Septra DS, one twice daily for 5 days;
Ciprofloxacin, 250 mg twice daily for 5 days; and
Ofloxacin, 200 mg twice daily for 5 days.

Processing of specimens

(1) Prompt processing is essential to minimize contact of urine with sperm.

(2) Centrifuge at 400***g*** × 8 min.

(3) Resuspend in medium used above to about 1 ml – semen analysis.

(4) Centrifuge at 400 ***g*** for 20 min through discontinuous 40%/80% Percoll gradient; retrieve lower fraction.

(5) Centrifuge 400 ***g*** for 20 min. Resuspend in 1 mL, repeat count/motility assessment.

(6) Wash and resuspend in 250–300 μL Ham's F-10, 20 mM HEPES buffer and 5% HSA for intrauterine insemination.

PENILE VIBRATORY STIMULATION OF THE SPINAL CORD-INJURED MAN

Patient preparation

(1) Antibiotics which attain high levels in prostatic fluid (see above) are given 3 days prior to the procedure to reduce the likelihood of bacteria in the ejaculate.

(2) In individuals who may have a retrograde fraction from the procedure, sodium bicarbonate 1.5 g is taken 12 h and 1 h prior to the procedure. If the patient is known to have successful antegrade ejaculation without a retrograde fraction in several previous procedures, it is not essential to alkalinize the urine.

(3) Consider giving nifedipine prophylaxis for autonomic dysreflexia in men with a history of dysreflexia and those with complete lesions at spinal

levels at or above T6. Nifedipine dosage is 10–20 mg sublingually 10–15 min prior to the procedure.

Procedure

(1) Patients may be supine, in decubitus position or remain in the wheelchair during the procedure.

(2) Catheterization and bladder preparation as stated above (in section on retrieval of retrograde ejaculate) is optimal in men who may have a retrograde fraction during vibrator stimulation. Catheterization is optional in men who have previously demonstrated only antegrade ejaculation from the vibrator.

(3) Vibration parameters: 100 Hz frequency and 2.5 mm amplitude.

(4) Retract prepuce and place vibrator at the frenulum for 3 min stimulation periods, followed by rest periods of 1–2 min.

(5) Palpate the bulbocavernosal muscle at the penoscrotal angle during stimulation to detect the rhythmic contractions which immediately precede seminal emission. Stop stimulation at this point and collect antegrade ejaculate into specimen container. Milk the urethra to expel any intraurethral contents.

(6) Monitor blood pressure 30–60 s during stimulation to observe for autonomic dysreflexia. Abort stimulation immediately if systolic blood pressure >180 mmHg, administer nifedipine and begin again in 15 min.

(7) Repeat stimulation pattern. The procedure is terminated when no further ejaculate is obtained with stimulation, when six stimulations have been given, or when the skin condition prevents further stimulation.

(8) Catheterization of the bladder and evacuation of retrograde ejaculate in men who have a retrograde fraction is performed as discussed in the previous section.

Post-procedure care

(1) Monitor blood pressure until return to baseline.

(2) In men receiving nifedipine, resume the upright position gradually to prevent postural hypotension.

(3) Consider post-procedure antibiotic prophylaxis in men who have undergone urethral catheterization.

Processing of specimens

(1) Semen analysis of the antegrade specimen.

(2) Antegrade specimen is layered over discontinuous 40/80% Percoll gradient and centrifuged at 400***g*** for 20 min.

(3) Wash and count sperm retrieved from Percoll separation.

(4) Re-wash and suspend in 250–300 μL of Ham's + 20 mM HEPES buffer + 5% human serum albumin for intrauterine insemination.

(5) If retrograde specimen is present, process as noted in prevous section, pool with antegrade prior to final wash and resuspension.

ELECTROEJACULATION

Spinal cord-injured patient preparation

(1) Antibiotics which attain levels in prostatic fluid are given beginning 3 days prior to the procedure.

(2) The rectum is emptied the evening prior to or the morning of the procedure. Spinal cord-injured men perform their normal bowel evacuation program.

(3) Sodium bicarbonate 1.5 g is administered 12 h and 1 h prior to the procedure to alkalinize the urine.

(4) In spinal cord-injured men with a history of autonomic dysreflexia or those with complete lesions at or above T_6, give 20–30 mg of sublingual nifedipine 15 min prior to the procedure.

Non-spinal cord-injured

(1) Steps 2 and 3 for spinal cord-injured patients also apply to non-spinal cord-injured men undergoing electroejaculation.

(2) Nothing by mouth after midnight in preparation for anesthesia.

(3) Anesthesia is given for patients who are not spinal cord injured or in those spinal cord-injured men whose lesions are incomplete enough or low enough to sense pain from the electrical stimulus.

(4) General, epidural and spinal anesthesias are satisfactory for electroejaculation.

(5) Standard anesthetic protocols are used with the following additions:
  (a) General anesthesia must be very deep during stimulation, but also very short-acting due to the short duration of the procedure;
  (b) Spinal anesthesia should achieve a level above T10 or T11 and be very short in duration;
  (c) Intravenous fluids are kept to a minimum to prevent excessive urine production during the procedure.

Procedure

(1) Bladder is catheterized and medium instilled into the bladder, as detailed above (retrograde ejaculate retrieval).

(2) Perform rigid sigmoidoscopy to rule out pre-existing rectal lesions.

(3) Turn the patient in the lateral decubitus position and insert probe with electrodes facing anteriorly.

(4) Deliver electricity in a progressively increasing voltage pattern, beginning at 1–2 V and increasing 1–2 V per stimulation. Peak voltage is 50% greater than that which allows the first drop of ejaculate.

(5) Blood pressure is monitored every 30–60 s. Stop stimulation and remove the probe if systolic blood pressure is >180 mmHg. May attempt nifedipine prophylaxis and restimulation, but this is unlikely to be successful within the same day.

(6) Monitor electrode temperature continuously. Stimulation is stopped and probe removed if temperature rises >40°C.

(7) Assistant collects antegrade ejaculate into specimen container and milks urethra at the end of the procedure.

(8) If a prolonged erection is present, but no antegrade ejaculate has occurred, stop stimulation and check for retrograde ejaculate.

(9) Repeat sigmoidoscopy to check for rectal injury.

(10) Catheterize bladder and irrigate out retrograde ejaculate as detailed previously.

Post-procedure care

(1) Spinal cord-injured men are able to leave the clinic immediately after the procedure, unless they experience nifedipine-induced post-procedure hypotension.

(2) In men receiving anesthesia, follow standard recovery protocols.

(3) Consider antibiotic prophylaxis with drugs mentioned above to prevent infection from the manipulations.

Processing of specimens

(1) Follow steps outlined above for vibratory stimulation specimens.

(2) In electroejaculation, there is almost always some degree of antegrade and retrograde ejaculate, so both specimens will require processing.

(3) The specimens are pooled prior to intrauterine insemination.

References

1. World Health Organisation (1987). *Laboratory Manual for Examination of Human Semen and Semen–Cervical Mucus Interaction*. (Cambridge: Press Syndicate of the University of Cambridge)
2. Cross, N. L., Morales, P., Overstreet, J. W. and Hauson, F. W. (1986). Two simple methods for detecting acrosome-reacted human sperm. *Gamete Res.*, **15**, 213–26
3. Jeyendran, R. S., van der Ven, H. H. and Zaneveld, L. J. B. (1992). The hypo-osmotic swelling test: An update. *Arch. Androl.*, **29**, 105–16
4. Aitken, R. J., Harkiss, D. and Buckingham, D. (1993). Relationship between iron-catalyzed lipid peroxidation potential and human sperm function. *J. Reprod. Fertil.*, **98**, 257–65
5. Rodriguez, H., Ohanian, C. and Bustos-Obregon, E. (1985) Nuclear chromatin decondensation of spermatozoa *in vitro*: a method for evaluating the fertilizing ability of ovine semen. *Int. J. Androl.*, **8**, 147–58
6. Liu, D. Y., Elton, R. A., Johnston, W. I. H. and Baker, H. W. G. (1987). Spermatozoal nuclear chromatin decondensation *in vitro*: A text for sperm immaturity. Comparison with results of human *in vitro* fertilization. *Clin. Reprod. Fertil.*, **5**, 191–201
7. Dadoune, J. P., Mayaux, M. J. and Guihard-Moscato, M. L. (1988). Aniline blue staining of human spermatozoa chromatin: Evaluation of nuclear maturation. In Andre, J. J. (ed.) *The Sperm Cell*, pp. 249–52. (The Hague: Mastinus Nijhoff Publishers)
8. Biggers, J. D., Whitten, W. K. and Whittingham, D. G. (1971). The culture of mouse embryos *in vitro*. In Daniel, J. C., Jr (ed.) *Methods in Mammalian Embryology*, p. 86. (San Francisco: Freeman)
9. Krausz, C., West, K., Buckingham, D. and Aitken, R. J. (1992). Analysis of the interaction between N-formylmethionyl-leucyl-phenylalanine and human sperm suspensions: development of a technique for monitoring the contamination of human semen samples with leukocytes. *Fertil. Steril.*, **57**, 1317–25
10. Ord, T., Marello, E., Patrizio, P., Balmaceda, J. P., Silber, S. J. and Asch, R. H. (1992). The role of the laboratory in the handling of epididymal sperm for assisted reproductive technologies. *Fertil. Steril.*, **57**, 1103–6
11. Ord, T., Patrizio, P., Marello, E., Balmaceda, J. P. and Asch, R. H. (1990). MiniPercoll: A new method of semen preparation for IVF in severe male factor infertility. *Hum. Reprod.*, **5**, 987
12. Patrizio, P., Ord, T., Silber, S. J. and Asch, R. H. (1993). Cystic fibrosis mutations impair the fertilization rate of epididymal sperm from men with congenital absence of the vas deferens. *Hum. Reprod.*, **8**, 1259–63
13. Ord, T., Patrizio, P., Balmaceda, J. P. and Asch, R. H. (1993). Can severe male factor infertility be treated without micromanipulation? *Fertil. Steril.*, **60**, 110–15
14. Ord, T., Patrizio, P., Marello, E., Ord, V., Balmaceda, J. P. and Asch, R. H. (1994). Successful cryopreservation of extremely severe male factor samples allows banking to accumulate more sperm numbers for IVF. *42nd Annual Meeting Pacific Coast Fertility Meeting*, April, 1994, A4, pp. 0–8

Index